Contemporary Metabolism

Volume 1

Contemporary Metabolism

(formerly *The Year in Metabolism*)

Contemporary Metabolism

Volume 1

Edited by

Norbert Freinkel, M. D.

Kettering Professor of Medicine
Professor of Biochemistry
Director, Center for Endocrinology, Metabolism, and Nutrition
Northwestern University Medical School
Chicago, Illinois

PLENUM MEDICAL BOOK COMPANY
NEW YORK AND LONDON

ISBN-13: 978-1-4684-3449-1   e-ISBN-13: 978-1-4684-3447-7
DOI: 10.1007/978-1-4684-3447-7

© 1979 Plenum Publishing Corporation
Softcover reprint of the hardcover 1st edition 1979
227 West 17th Street, New York, N.Y. 10011

Plenum Medical Book Company is an imprint of Plenum Publishing Corporation

Contributors

Gerald D. Aurbach, M.D. • Chief, Metabolic Diseases Branch, National Institute of Arthritis, Metabolism, and Digestive Diseases, National Institutes of Health, Bethesda, Maryland 20014

Enrique Baraona, M.D. • Associate Professor of Medicine, Mount Sinai School of Medicine of the City University of New York, New York, New York 10029; Clinical Investigator, Alcoholism Research and Treatment Center, Veterans Administration Medical Center, Bronx, New York 10468

Edward M. Brown, M.D. • Senior Clinical Associate, Metabolic Diseases Branch, National Institute of Arthritis, Metabolism, and Digestive Diseases, National Institutes of Health, Bethesda, Maryland 20014

Jack W. Coburn, M.D. • Professor of Medicine, University of California at Los Angeles School of Medicine, and Chief, Nephrology Section, Medical and Research Services, Veterans Administration Wadsworth Hospital Center, Los Angeles, California 90073

Richard E. Dobbs, Ph.D. • Assistant Professor, Department of Physiology, University of Texas Southwestern Medical School, Dallas, Texas 75235; Physiologist, General Medical Research, Veterans Administration Hospital, Dallas, Texas 75216

Stefan S. Fajans, M.D. • Professor of Internal Medicine; Head, Division of Endocrinology and Metabolism; Director, Metabolism Research Unit; Director, Michigan Diabetes Research and Training Center, The University of Michigan, Ann Arbor, Michigan 48109

Irving M. Faust, Ph.D. • Assistant Professor, Department of Human Behavior and Metabolism, The Rockefeller University, New York, New York 10021

Phillip Felig, M.D. • C. N. H. Long Professor of Medicine and Vice Chairman, Department of Internal Medicine; Chief, Section of Endocrinology, Yale University School of Medicine, New Haven, Connecticut 06510

John C. Floyd, Jr., M.D. • Professor of Internal Medicine, Division of Endocrinology and Metabolism and Metabolism Research Unit; Assistant Director, Michigan Diabetes Research and Training Center, The University of Michigan, Ann Arbor, Michigan 48109

DeWitt S. Goodman, M.D. • Tilden–Weger–Bieler Professor, Department of Medicine, College of Physicians and Surgeons of Columbia University, New York, New York 10032

Jules Hirsch, M.D. • Professor and Senior Physician; Chairman, Department of Human Behavior and Metabolism, The Rockefeller University, New York, New York 10021

Patricia R. Johnson, Ph.D. • Adjunct Professor, Department of Human Behavior and Metabolism, The Rockefeller University, New York, New York 10021; Professor and Chairman, Department of Biology, Vassar College, Poughkeepsie, New York 12601

Charles R. Kleeman, M.D. • Professor of Medicine; Director of Development Office, Center for Health, Enhancement, Education, and Research, University of California at Los Angeles School of Medicine, Los Angeles, California 90073

Veikko Koivisto, M.D. • Visiting Research Fellow, Section of Endocrinology, Department of Internal Medicine, Yale University School of Medicine, New Haven, Connecticut 06510

Kiyoshi Kurokawa, M.D. • Associate Professor of Medicine, University of California at Los Angeles School of Medicine, and Assistant Chief, Nephrology Section, Medical and Research Services, Veterans Administration Wadsworth Hospital Center, Los Angeles, California 90073

Charles S. Lieber, M.D. • Professor of Medicine and Pathology, Mount Sinai School of Medicine of the City University of New York, New York, New York 10029; Director, Alcoholism Research and Treatment Center; Chief, Section and Laboratory of Liver Disease and Nutrition, Veterans Administration Medical Center, Bronx, New York 10468

Brian L. G. Morgan, Ph.D. • Staff Associate, Institute of Human Nutrition, College of Physicians and Surgeons of Columbia University, New York, New York 10032

Edwin L. Prien, Jr., M.D. • Instructor, Harvard Medical School, Boston, Massachusetts 02115; Arthritis Unit, Medical Services, Massachusetts General Hospital, Boston, Massachusetts 02114

Leon E. Rosenberg, M.D. • Professor and Chairman, Department of Human Genetics, Yale University School of Medicine, New Haven, Connecticut 06510

J. Edwin Seegmiller, M.D. • Professor, Department of Medicine, School of Medicine, The University of California San Diego, La Jolla, California 92093

Kay Tanaka, M.D. • Senior Research Scientist, Department of Human Genetics, Yale University School of Medicine, New Haven, Connecticut 06510

Roger H. Unger, M.D. • Professor, Department of Internal Medicine, University of Texas Southwestern Medical School, Dallas, Texas 75235; Staff Physician, Veterans Administration Hospital, Dallas, Texas 75216

Hibbard E. Williams, M.D. • Professor and Chairman, Department of Medicine, Cornell University Medical College, New York, New York 10021

Myron Winick, M.D. • R. R. Williams Professor of Nutrition; Professor of Pediatrics; Director, Institute of Human Nutrition, College of Physicians and Surgeons of Columbia University, New York, New York 10032

Preface

Despite a new title, *Contemporary Metabolism, Volume 1* is actually the third volume in a continuing series and succeeds *The Year in Metabolism 1975–1976* and *The Year in Metabolism 1977*. As in the earlier volumes, the same internationally recognized authorities review the noteworthy recent developments in their areas of expertise. In many instances they also address aspects that have not been considered previously.

In this volume, Dr. J. Edwin Seegmiller again updates progress in understanding disorders of purine and pyrimidine metabolism. However, particular emphasis is placed on the emerging relationships with immune mechanisms. Dr. Charles S. Lieber is joined by Dr. Enrique Baraona in a continuing review of metabolic actions of ethanol. This chapter examines effects of ethanol on protein metabolism and selected features of lipid metabolism—two areas that were not included in the earlier volumes. Dr. DeWitt S. Goodman's review of disorders of lipid and lipoprotein metabolism builds on his previous chapters, but much additional attention is directed to a critical analysis of recent advances in epidemiology and lipoprotein structures. In collaboration with Dr. Brian L. G. Morgan, Dr. Myron Winick devotes his entire chapter to a detailed review of the impact of nutrition upon brain development—an overview that has now been rendered possible by the burgeoning recent developments in this area. Dr. Hibbard E. Williams, in collaboration with Dr. Edwin L. Prien, Jr., has focused this year's chapter on renal stone diseases on calcium stones and the first double blind therapeutic trials, since these are the avenues in which the most impressive recent advances have been registered. Dr. Gerald D. Aurbach has collaborated with Dr. Edward M. Brown for the chapter on hormone receptors, cyclic nucleotides, and control of cell function. Their lucid exposition of cell biology is devoted to the new insights that have been gained via novel ligands for certain receptors, appreciation of the biosynthesis and structural properties of certain peptides, understanding of the actions of cholera toxin and calcium upon adenylate cyclase, and applications to clinical practice.

In the present volume, Dr. Stefan S. Fajans has been joined by Dr. John C. Floyd, Jr. for the third in a series of reviews of diabetes mellitus. The concept of the heterogeneity of this disorder and its complications is again underscored, and newly delineated disorders (such as those linked to receptors, antibodies to receptors, autoimmunity, etc.) as well as novel therapeutic approaches are discussed. Dr. Roger H. Unger is joined by Dr. Richard H. Dobbs in an update of glucagon metabolism. However, the regulatory roles of somatostatin and other recently described neurohumoral factors are also emphasized and a balanced recapitulation of the controversy concerning the role of glucagon in diabetes and fuel homeostasis is included. In their chapter on fuel metabolism, Drs. Phillip Felig and Veikko Koivisto present additional views regarding glucagon and somatostatin and provide a comprehensive summary of the recent clarifications concerning ketogenesis and fuel homeostasis during exercise. Dr. Jules Hirsch collaborates with Drs. Irving M. Faust and Patricia R. Johnson to address an area not considered in detail in the previous chapters on obesity. The present chapter reviews existing technology for measuring adipocyte size and number and reviews the current status of "adipocyte number" in terms of replicative mechanisms, energy economy and pathogenetic implications for obesity. Drs. Jack W. Coburn and Charles R. Kleeman are joined by Dr. Kiyoshi Kurokawa for another assessment of divalent ion metabolism; this year they have focused more narrowly on the metabolism of vitamin D and phosphorus and present a detailed analysis of the implications for pathophysiology in clinical disorders. Finally, Drs. Leon E. Rosenberg and Kay Tanaka present another major review of the metabolism of amino acids and organic acids. In the present volume their chapter is confined to an analysis of pyruvate metabolism and the specific clinical disorders that have now been linked to primary disturbances in the disposition of pyruvic acid.

The above thumbnail summary of the contents of *Contemporary Metabolism, Volume 1* clearly demonstrates the most cogent reasons for changing the name of the series. The prior title, *The Year in Metabolism,* may have been misleading and somewhat at variance with the actual product. It implied that all the new literature within a single area would be reviewed in each instance and thus each successive volume would confer "planned obsolescence" on its predecessors. In practice, this has not been the case. The authors have varied emphasis from year to year in accord with their assessment of the ongoing "action"; they have sought to achieve cumulative overview through serial presentations. And, in truth, this is the way that new knowledge in medicine evolves; everything does not "turn over" on an annual or even biennial basis. New facts emerge and concepts are revised in discontinuous fits and starts—and often the impetus arises from seemingly unrelated areas. It is the task of the discerning reviewer to identify the sprouting seedlings, and it is the challenge to his perspicacity to recognize when it is time to harvest. Serial reviews enable him to indulge in crop rotation and to plan the entire exercise in long-range dimensions.

We hope that the title "Contemporary Metabolism" conveys this philosophy more fully. It should communicate that the volumes are additive and not redundant, and that their contents should be enduring rather than ephemeral. The continuity of input by an extraordinary panel of experts, and the continuing help of Ms. Hilary Evans, Plenum Press's Senior Medical Editor, have rendered these objectives possible; the excellence of their contributions appears to have remained constant and uninfluenced by the change of title.

Norbert Freinkel, M.D.

Contents

Chapter 2
Metabolic Actions of Ethanol
Enrique Baraona and Charles S. Lieber

Chapter 3
Disorders of Lipid and Lipoprotein Metabolism
DeWitt S. Goodman

Chapter 4
Nutrition and Cellular Growth of the Brain
Myron Winick and Brian L. G. Morgan

Chapter 5
Metabolic Aspects of Renal Stone Disease
Edwin L. Prien, Jr., and Hibbard E. Williams

Chapter 6
Hormone Receptors, Cyclic Nucleotides, and Control of Cell Function
Gerald D. Aurbach and Edward M. Brown

Chapter 7
Diabetes Mellitus
Stefan S. Fajans and John C. Floyd, Jr.

Chapter 8
Glucagon and Somatostatin
Richard E. Dobbs and Roger H. Unger

Chapter 9
Recent Advances in Body Fuel Metabolism
Philip Felig and Veikko Koivisto

Chapter 10

What's New in Obesity: Current Understanding of Adipose Tissue Morphology

Jules Hirsch, Irving M. Faust, and Patricia R. Johnson

Chapter 11
Divalent Ion Metabolism
Jack W. Coburn, Kiyoshi Kurokawa, and Charles R. Kleeman

Chapter 12
Metabolism of Amino Acids and Organic Acids
Kay Tanaka and Leon E. Rosenberg

Disorders of Purine and Pyrimidine Metabolism

J. Edwin Seegmiller

1.1. Introduction

Progress during the past year in the field of aberrations of purine metabolism has extended our knowledge of the metabolic consequences of a deficiency of specific enzymes and thereby allowed formulation of better understanding of possible mechanisms involved in producing the clinical diseases. Additional patients with recently described enzyme deficiencies have been identified and have served to define more precisely the range of clinical presentations to be expected in these disorders.

One of the most impressive areas of progress has been in our understanding of the metabolic consequences of deficiency of adenosine deaminase (ADA) associated with severe combined immunodeficiency disease. This additional knowledge has led to a new unifying hypothesis

Abbreviations used in this chapter: (ADA) adenosine deaminase; (APRT) adenine phosphoribosyltransferase; (cAMP) cyclic AMP; (cGMP) cyclic GMP; (Con A) concanavallin A; (CTP) cytidine triphosphate; (dATP) deoxyadenosine triphosphate; (dCTP) deoxycytidine triphosphate; (dGTP) deoxyguanosine triphosphate; (FGAR) formyglycinamide ribonucleotide; (HPLC) high-pressure liquid chromatography; (HPRT) hypoxanthine-guanine phosphoribosyltransferase; (5-HT) 5-hydroxytryptophan; (PHA) phytohemagglutinin; (PNP) purine nucleoside phosphorylase; (PNT) purine 5'-nucleotidase; (PP-ribose-P) phosphoribosyl-1-pyrophosphate; (TTP) thymidine triphosphate; (UTP) uridine triphosphate.

J. EDWIN SEEGMILLER • Department of Medicine, School of Medicine, The University of California San Diego, La Jolla, California 92093.

(Fig. 1) for explaining the mechanisms of suppression of the immune system in deficiency of either ADA or purine nucleoside phosphorylase (PNP). It was not until excretion of large amounts of deoxynucleosides, as well as the expected ribonucleosides, was observed in children with an isolated T-cell defect associated with deficiency of the latter enzyme, PNP, that the magnitude of the turnover of deoxynucleosides in the body was appreciated. This observation focused attention on pathways for their degradation. In turn, attention was centered on a neglected role of ADA that had not previously been considered in hypotheses on the mechanism of ADA deficiency: the fact that deoxyadenosine is an even better substrate for ADA than is adenosine (Frederiksen, 1966; Agarwal *et al.*, 1975).

The possibility of deoxyadenosine rather than adenosine being the mediator of immunosuppression in adenosine deaminase deficiency is now being explored. Such a concept would readily explain a number of puzzling observations. Mills *et al.* (1976) reported the presence of substantially increased amounts of adenine in plasma and urine of an ADA-deficient child. In retrospect, one realizes that any deoxyadenosine in these fluids would have been registered as adenine in their assay by reason of degradation of this unstable nucleoside under the strongly acid conditions used for its separation and analysis. In fact, deoxyadenosine was recently found in the urine of this same ADA-deficient child (Simmonds, 1979; Goldblum *et al.*, 1979).

Further evidence of an important role for deoxyadenosine has come forth. Very large increases in the nucleotide product of deoxyadenosine, deoxyadenosine triphosphate (dATP), has also now been independently reported in erythrocytes of children with ADA deficiency by two different groups of investigators (Cohen *et al.*, 1978b; Coleman *et al.*, 1978) and increased deoxyguanosine triphosphate (dGTP) in two patients with PNP deficiency (Cohen *et al.*, 1978a). A possible theoretical basis for such an

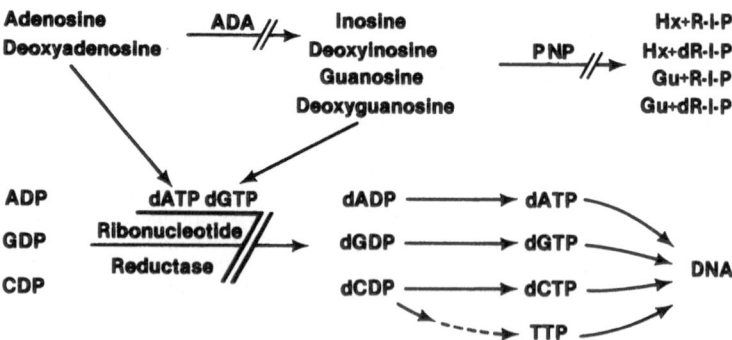

Fig. 1. Postulated mechanism of inhibition of lymphocyte proliferation in genetic deficiency of adenosine deaminase (ADA) or purine nucleoside phosphorylase (PNP).

accumulation was provided by the work of Carson *et al.* (1977b) in demonstrating that thymus had the highest activity for the kinases of deoxyadenosine and deoxyguanosine of any tissue of the body. Furthermore, they found that deoxyadenosine was a potent inhibitor of the mitogenic stimulation of peripheral blood lymphocytes and showed a 1000-fold potentiation on addition of an inhibitor of ADA. Furthermore, the inhibition could largely be prevented by addition of a pyrimidine deoxynucleoside, deoxycytidine—an observation with implications for new approaches to therapy of ADA deficiency. In addition, the deoxynucleosides deoxyinosine and deoxyguanosine were more potent inhibitors of lymphoblast growth than were the ribonucleosides inosine and guanosine. Thus, the stage has been set for a new unitary concept of the mechanism of T-cell dysfunction in these two types of immunodeficiency diseases in which deoxyguanosine accumulation might well be the proximal mediator of the isolated T-cell dysfunction in PNP deficiency, while deoxyadenosine could be a comparable inhibitor of the immune response in ADA deficiency.

Some insight is also provided into possible steps involved in inhibition of the immune response. The T cells, with their abundant deoxynucleoside kinase activity, should accumulate dGTP in PNP deficiency and dATP in ADA deficiency. As shown in Fig. 1, an imbalance of deoxynucleotide triphosphates is known to cause an inhibition of a major enzyme involved in formation of deoxynucleotides, ribonucleotide diphosphate reductase, not only in bacterial cells, but also in mammalian cells (Moore and Hurlbert, 1966; Murphree *et al.*, 1968; Tattersall *et al.*, 1975). Failure to make deoxynucleotides could then lead to a cessation of DNA synthesis and of cellular proliferation (Lowe *et al.*, 1977a). The extent to which this new hypothesis can account for the immunosuppression in these two diseases remains to be demonstrated, but it does provide a new approach toward understanding the disease and toward therapeutic intervention in the process.

Several additional families have been found with recently described enzyme defects. Two children in one family with T-cell dysfunction have been described in association with a less severe deficiency of the enzyme PNP. As might be expected, the serum urate was not as low as that of children with the severe deficiency, and they excreted not only purine nucleosides but also substantially more uric acid in the urine than did the previously described patients. As would be expected, the clinical symptoms of immunodeficiency disease were somewhat less threatening in these two children (Fox *et al.*, 1977; Osborne *et al.*, 1977; Edwards *et al.*, 1978; Gelfand *et al.*, 1978). An additional child with adenine phosphoribosyltransferase (APRT) deficiency and urinary tract obstruction from 2,8-dioxyadenine calculi was found (Barratt *et al.*, 1979; Simmonds *et al.*, 1979a), and several additional patients with deficiency of ADA were described. Eight more patients with xanthinuria were reported. In the area of pyrimidine metabolism, no new enzyme defects were found; however, seven more patients with hemolytic anemia associated with pyrimidine 5'-nucleotidase deficiency were reported (Torrance *et al.*, 1977a,b; Miwa *et al.*, 1977; Rosa *et al.*, 1977). A total of 13 patients with this disorder have now been reported. Each of them has presented with a recessively inherited congenital hemolytic anemia with basophilic stippling in the erythrocytes.

A substantial advance in biology and genetics has been made with the attempt by Dewey *et al.* (1977) to create a mouse carrying the gene for the Lesch–Nyhan syndrome. Although there is no evidence that these workers succeeded in introducing the gene into the germ cell, they did create mosaic mice with teratocarcinoma-derived mutant cells deficient in the enzyme hypoxanthine-guanine phosphoribosyltransferase (HPRT). Since these teratocarcinoma cells can be cultured *in vitro*, many other mutations could be introduced for expression in intact mice by injection of these cells into blastocysts with the intent that eventually the mutant cells would constitute the germ line of at least some of the offspring.

1.2. Purine Metabolism

At the level of basic understanding of purine nucleotide metabolism, considerable progress has been made. The newer concepts of the various factors involved in regulation of both purine synthesis *de novo* and the interconversion of purine nucleotides and the role of the "purine nucleotide cycle" in certain physiological process *in vivo* has significance for our understanding of pathological states.

1.2.1. Hypoxanthine Reutilization as a Normal Regulator of Purine Synthesis *de Novo*

The concept of an important role for hypoxanthine reutilization in regulating the rate of purine synthesis has been further consolidated (Fig. 2). Hershfield and Seegmiller (1977) found a marked increase in the rate of purine synthesis of normal human lymphoblasts when hypoxanthine is rigorously removed from the culture medium and particularly from the serum component. Indeed, under these conditions, the rate of incorporation of [^{14}C]formate into total purine compounds approached very closely that observed in cells grossly deficient in the enzyme hypoxanthine-guanine phosphoribosyltransferase. In human fibroblasts, similar results were obtained by Thompson *et al.* (1978a,b). The latter studies also clarified the curious disparate results reported earlier by Cohen *et al.* (1977), that cells cultured from a patient with PNP deficiency showed a

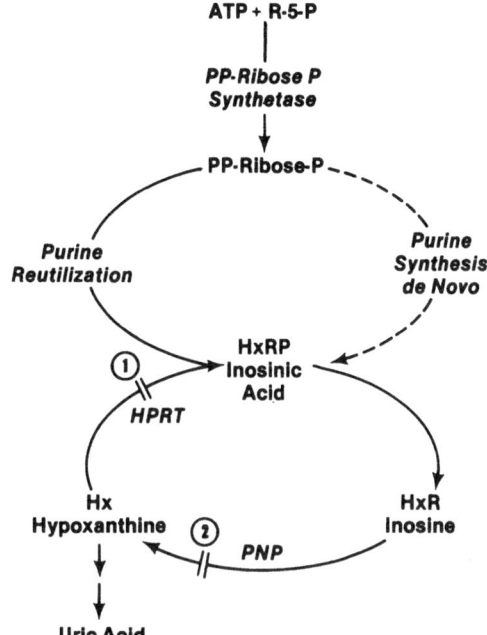

Fig. 2. Interruption of hypoxanthine reutilization cycle as a proposed mechanism of purine overproduction in ① Lesch–Nyhan syndrome [hypoxanthine-guanine phosphoribosyltransferase (HPRT) deficiency] and in ② purine nucleoside phosphorylase (PNP) deficiency.

normal rate of purine synthesis, which seemed at variance with the marked overproduction of purines shown by the affected children. Thompson *et al.* (1978a,b) found an enhanced rate of purine synthesis in PNP-deficient cells compared with normal fibroblasts only if all free purine bases and PNP enzymes were eliminated from the culture media and inosine was present. However, as might be expected, both the normal and PNP-deficient cells showed a substantial suppression of [^{14}C]formate incorporation into purine compounds in response to addition of free purines. In the absence of PNP in the media, the PNP-deficient cells were incapable of generating from inosine the hypoxanthine required for suppression of purine synthesis *de novo,* thus accounting for the purine overproduction observed in the affected children.

1.2.2. Drugs That Increase Purine Synthesis *de Novo*

Several antitumor and antiviral drugs enhance the rate of purine synthesis *de novo.* The mechanism by which the anticancer drug 2-ethylamino-1,3,4-thiadiazole causes purine overproduction in man (Seegmiller *et al.,* 1963; Krakoff, 1965) was elucidated by Nelson *et al.* (1977). The metabolic effects and antitumor activity of this drug are completely suppressed by the simultaneous addition of nicotinamide to the therapeutic regimen. These observations suggested the possibility that thiadiazole might be acting through formation of a pyrimidine nucleotide analogue (Ciotti *et al.*, 1960). This has now been proved.

Nelson *et al.* (1976) demonstrated formation of a thiadiazole-containing ribonucleotide that inhibited, very effectively, the enzyme inosinate dehydrogenase (see Fig. 3), with very little effect, presumably, on other reactions requiring pyrimidine nucleotides.

The general concept that inhibition of the conversion of inosinate to guanylate results in an excessive rate of purine synthesis was further confirmed by the work of Willis *et al.* (1978). They used another agent, ribavirin (Virazole), an antiviral and anticancer drug, which is known to inhibit, in ribonucleotide form, inosinate dehydrogenase (Streeter *et al.*, 1973). This drug was able to block the formation of guanylate in cultured human lymphoblasts and to divert large amounts of inosine into the culture medium, suggesting that any clinical use of this drug might well increase uric acid production in the human. It also provides a model system for further exploration of possible sites for metabolic blocks that could give rise to purine overproduction.

The mechanism controlling the rate of purine synthesis in Ehrlich ascites tumor cells was studied by Barankiewicz and Henderson (1977). They found an effect in the intact cell of the intracellular nucleotide concentration on activity of enzymes of purine ribonucleotide synthesis and interconversion. Blocking the conversion of inosinate to adenylate (Fig. 3) with hadacidin substantially decreased the intracellular concentrations of ATP. In a similar manner, the inhibition of inosinate conversion to guanylate with mycophenolic acid decreased the concentration within the cell of GTP, while azaserine treatment, which blocks *de novo* synthesis of purines, decreased concentrations of both ATP and GTP within the cell. Any decrease in adenine nucleotide but not of guanine nucleotide concentration substantially increased the rate of formation of phosphoribosyl-1-pyrophosphate (PP-ribose-P) by PP-ribose-P synthetase in the intact cell, with no increase in activity of PP-ribose-P synthetase and with only a minimal (7–27%), if any, increase in the first few reactions of purine synthesis. Inosinate dehydrogenase activity was increased by 43% in cells treated with azaserine. A 3-fold increase in the same enzyme was produced by treating human fibroblasts with 6-mercaptopurine (Leyva *et al.*, 1976).

A more detailed study of the metabolic effects of inhibition of growth of cultured mouse neuroblastoma cells by mycophenolic acid was presented by Cass *et al.* (1977) and of mouse lymphoma cells by Lowe *et al.* (1977b). As would be expected, this potent inhibitor of inosinate dehydrogenase reduced the intracellular concentration of GTP to 10–30% of control values, but also produced an unexpected but significant increase in the concentration of cytidine triphosphate (CTP) and uridine triphos-

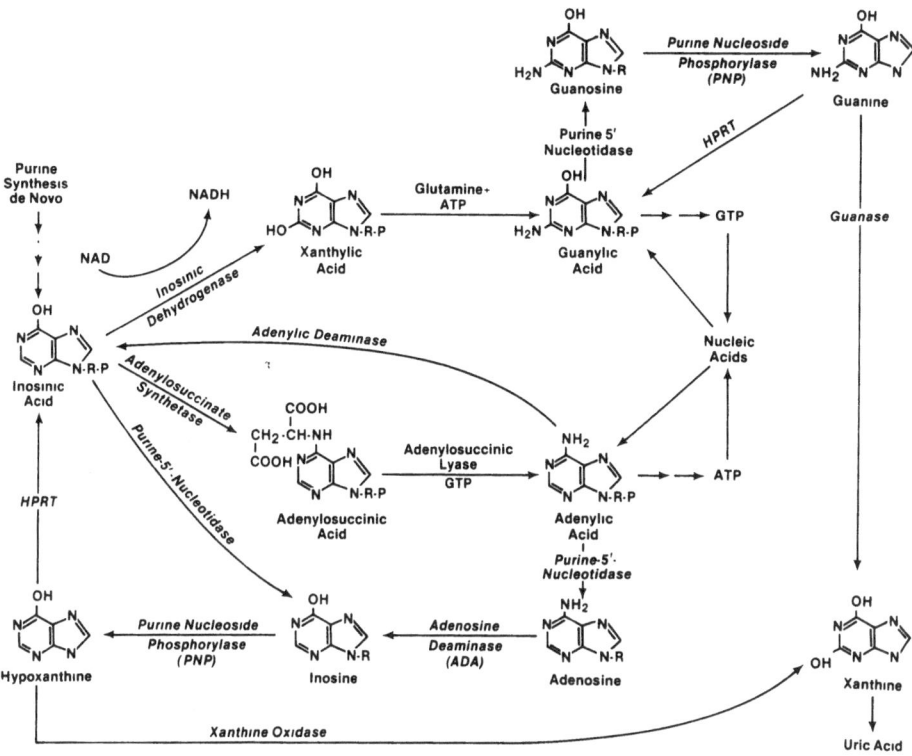

Fig. 3. Pathways of purine interconversion and catabolism.

phate (UTP). Incorporation of [³H]thymidine into DNA was suppressed to a much greater extent than was that of labeled leucine into proteins or adenosine into purine nucleotides of the cell.

1.2.3. Changes in Purine Metabolism with Cellular Proliferation

The transition of cells from a resting state, without appreciable division, to a rapidly proliferating state involves marked changes in the rate of purine metabolism. The stimulation of growth of mouse fibroblasts produced by transfer from serum-free media to complete media is accompanied by an increase in PP-ribose-P generation through an activation of preexisting enzyme rather than by an increase in amount of enzyme synthesized (Smith and Buchanan, 1977).

Additional studies in detail of the metabolism of adenosine in lymphoid cells by Harrap and Paine (1976) confirmed other reports (Snyder and Henderson, 1973; Snyder et al., 1976) of conversion of adenosine primarily to adenine nucleotides at low intracellular concentrations and a shift to deamination at high concentrations. Stimulation by mitogens produced no change in ADA activity. An unexpected finding was an increase in dATP and a marked decrease in dGTP, deoxycytidine triphosphate (dCTP), and thymidine triphosphate (TTP) concentrations in lymphocytes stimulated with phytohemagglutinin (PHA) in the presence of adenosine and the ADA inhibitor coformycin. Purine reutilization in PHA-stimulated cells was studied by Raivio and Hovi (1977, 1979).

1.2.4. Role of the Purine Nucleotide Cycle

The metabolic pathways shown in Fig. 3 provide several examples of seemingly "futile cycles" involving paths for the cyclic formation and degradation of the purine nucleotides. The significance and function of these cycles in the intact cell has been poorly understood. The "adenosine cycle" involving formation of adenosine from dephosphorylation of adenylate and its subsequent deamination was proposed by Green and Ishii (1972) as a major pathway of metabolism in mammalian cells. Brox and Henderson (1976) evaluated the quantitative importance of this pathway in intact human and mouse cells by noting the labeling of guanine nucleotides produced by addition of labeled adenine or adenosine. Less than 5% of incorporated adenine and less than 9% of incorporated adenosine was converted to guanine nucleotides, and this was reduced to only 6% by inhibition of ADA with deoxycoformycin. Evidently, deamination of adenylate is a quantitatively more important pathway than is the deamination of adenosine in the "adenosine cycle" in these cultured cells.

1.2.5. Role of the Purine Nucleotide Cycle in Transport Processes

Recent studies indicate a more important role for the purine nucleotide cycle during physiological stress of certain organs. Deamination of AMP is a major accompaniment of muscle exercise and other processes involving breakdown of ATP. The maintenance of high intracellular concentrations of nucleotides as ATP and GTP apparently protects them from degradation. Any process that lowers intracellular ATP concentration with consequent increase of cellular ADP and AMP will result in increased deamination of AMP to IMP with its accompanying generation of ammonia. Goodman and Lowenstein (1977) noted a marked increase in perfused rat skeletal muscle in concentrations of inosinate, ammonia, adenylosuccinate, and lactate in response to exercise, epinephrine, hypoxia, or cyanide at the expense of adenine nucleotides and creatine phosphate. Presumably, muscle adenylate deaminase is responsible for the ammonia generation. During recovery, the inosinate, ammonia, and lactate content are restored toward normal and a transient increase in adenylosuccinate content provides evidence of the resynthesis of adenine nucleotides. An increase in inosine and hypoxanthine content suggests a further degradation of a small portion of the nucleotides.

A similar production of ammonia and inosinate with larger amounts of inosine and hypoxanthine accompanies the loss of ATP from rat brain in response to electric shock. Adenylosuccinate can also be detected in the first minute and a half after the stimulus, thus providing evidence of operation of the same interconversion pathways *in vivo* as were previously shown *in vitro* (Schultz and Lowenstein, 1978).

Evidence of a different series of reactions leading to adenosine formation from AMP in the perfused rat heart was presented by Frick and Lowenstein (1978). Presumably, purine-5'-nucleotidase on the plasma membrane converts the adenylate to adenosine at the same time releasing the adenosine to the interior of the cell to account for the more facile uptake of labeled adenine from adenylate than from adenosine.

1.2.6. Effect of Fructose

Additional insight into the mechanism by which fructose loading leads to depletion of adenine nucleotides has come from the work of Morris *et al.* (1978). The depletion of adenine nucleotides in rat liver and renal cortex by fructose loading from the rapid and uncontrolled accumulation of fructose-1-phosphate is accompanied by a marked decrease of inorganic phosphate and is prevented by prior administration of inorganic phosphate.

During the past year, a number of reviews appeared. McKeran and Watts (1978) reviewed purine metabolism in cell physiology. Immunodeficiency disease was reviewed by Hirschhorn (1977a,b), Seegmiller (1976a, 1978a), Goldblum *et al.* (1979), and Polmar *et al.* (1979). Gout and purine metabolism was reviewed by Kelley and Wyngaarden (1978); ribonucleosides and deoxyribonucleoside metabolism, by Fox and Kelley (1978); control of purine synthesis in normal and pathological states, by Holmes *et al.* (1975, 1976), Kelley *et al.* (1975), and Wyngaarden and Holmes (1977). The mechanism of action of inhibitors of DNA synthesis was reviewed by Cozzarelli (1977). The chemistry and metabolism of adenine were reviewed by Bartlett (1977a–e) and ribonucleotide reductase by Reichard (1972).

1.3. Adenosine Deaminase Deficiency Associated with Severe Combined Immunodeficiency Disease

Substantial progress has been made in our understanding of the possible primary mediator and mechanism of the immunodeficiency produced by a gross deficiency of the enzyme ADA. This new insight has resulted largely from more detailed and reliable chemical characterization of purine metabolites excreted in the urine and of purine compounds accumulating within erythrocytes of affected patients. The recent status of our knowledge was reviewed by a number of authors (Good and Yunis, 1974; Good and Hansen, 1976; Hirschhorn, 1977a,b; Polmar, 1977; Sakura *et al.*, 1977a,b; Schwartz, R. S., 1977; Carson and Seegmiller, 1977; Seegmiller, 1976a, 1978a,b).

1.3.1. Clinical Presentation

The clinical presentation of new patients with ADA deficiency conforms, in general, to that reported in earlier cases with onset of recurrent severe infections, diarrhea, and failure to thrive, usually during the first few months or so of life, with laboratory evidence of severe impairment of T-cell function and the degrees of B-cell impairment varying from one family to another. The greater loss of T- than of B-cell function may be related to the stage of the disease. With increasing age, affected children eventually lose both T- and B-cell functions (Polmar *et al.*, 1979; Hirschhorn, 1977a,b). Infections are with fungal, protozoal, viral, and bacterial agents, reflecting the impairment of both cellular and humoral immunity. Additional cases reported by Coleman *et al.* (1978), Cohen *et al.* (1978b), Szüts *et al.* (1977), and Sakura *et al.* (1977a,b) follow the same general features. Physical examinations show very sparse or absent lymphoid tissue and often severe cutaneous infections. Laboratory tests show lymphopenia with markedly diminished response of lymphocytes to stimulation by mitogens and usually a reduction in immunoglobulin concentrations in plasma. The patients show absence of a delayed hypersensitivity response to common antigens, and their erythrocytes show less than 10% of the normal ADA activity. The tremor previously noted in one ADA-deficient patient by Polmar *et al.* (1976) has not been a notable feature of any of the additional patients reported to date.

The cartilage and boney lesions consisting of flaring of the costochondral junction is now considered by some investigators to be a relatively nonspecific response of children to other diseases as well (Rosen, 1978, personal communication). An additional child, with diminished ADA activity in erythrocytes but with 15% of normal activity in lymphocytes was detected by screening tests of the newborn in the state of New York (Hirschhorn, 1977a,b, personal communication, 1978). As in the previous patient reported by Jenkins *et al.* (1976) and Jenkins and Nurse (1976), this child showed no clinical evidence of immunodeficiency.

1.3.2. Frequency

The frequency of ADA deficiency continues to be estimated at about one third to one half of all patients with autosomal recessive type of severe combined immunodeficiency disease (Rosen, 1977, personal communication; Hirschhorn, 1977a,b). The heterozygous state in parents and siblings is detectable by the presence of reduced activity of ADA in the erythrocytes, with a 90% reliability using standard methods. The genetic polymorphism of ADA (Spencer *et al.*, 1968) is helpful in some cases in working out the genetics of inheritance. Different persons inherit different allelic forms of the enzyme, with the most prevalent enzyme pattern designated ADA-1, but rare persons exhibit another pattern, ADA-2. In addition, a null gene has been postulated to account for the inheritance in certain families. As many as 30% of the families of affected children carry a null gene for this genetic marker, if a full three generations of relatives are typed for ADA polymorphism (Hirschhorn, 1977a,b).

1.3.3. Enzyme Abnormality

The ADA activity of various organs in the normal person can be correlated roughly with the different molecular forms of the enzyme. A high-molecular-weight form of over 200,000 is found in liver, lung, kidney, and pancreas as the predominant form of the enzyme (Schrader and Stacy, 1977), and shows a lower specific activity and a diminished heat lability than does the low-molecular-weight form of 36,000, such as is found in red cells (Polmar *et al.*, 1976). The latter has a high specific activity and greater heat lability and is found predominantly in those organs with highest activity, such as thymus, spleen, and lymph node.

ADA activity is greatest in normal thymus, where it ranges from 7 to 15 times the activity found in spleen. In general, a gradual diminution in ADA activity occurs with increasing age of the subject, with differences being most marked in thymic tissue (Hirschhorn *et al.*, 1978). Tissues from a child with severe combined immunodeficiency disease, who died at 2 years of age, showed very low activities in all organs, particularly the thymus, where it was 0.2% of the activity of a group of control subjects. Spleen showed 1.1% of normal activity and lymph nodes 3.6%. The highest activity was found in the liver, where it was 30% of control values. The ADA-deficient liver showed essentially a normal pattern of distribution of residual enzyme activity between the two high-molecular-weight forms (580,000–260,000 daltons). In this patient, 62% of the activity was present as a higher-molecular-weight form, compared with 70% in the normal (Hirschhorn *et al.*, 1978).

The residual activity from the spleen of a child who died at age 2½ years with ADA deficiency and severe combined immunodeficiency disease was studied in detail by Schrader *et al.* (1978). This residual activity had a different molecular weight and different specificity for substrates and inhibitors, and did not cross-react with antibodies against highly purified ADA (Schrader *et al.*, 1976). They found small amounts of the same activity in normal spleen from which ADA had been removed by absorption on specific antibody. They therefore concluded that the residual activity is not due to a mutant form of ADA, but rather is due to another enzyme activity that is demonstrable in small amounts in normal spleen (Schrader *et al.*, 1978).

1.3.4. Screening Tests

Simplified screening tests have been designed for detection of ADA deficiency. These tests are performed on blood spotted onto filter paper, dried, and sent to the laboratory. Under these conditions, the ADA remains stable for at least 28 days in storage at room temperature. The procedure developed by Moore and Meuwissen (1974) is based on the generation of ammonia and the consequent change in pH and color of an indicator dye on incubation of the dried blood spot with adenosine. This procedure is now in use for screening of all newborns in the state of New York. The cost of the test is low; however, false-positive or false-negative results are obtained in around 2% of the patients tested (Ito *et al.*, 1977).

Ito *et al.* (1977) developed a screening method for both ADA deficiency and PNP deficiency, using similar dried blood spots absorbed on filter paper. The procedure is based on the formation of a blue insoluble formazan within a gel containing adenosine (or inosine for detection of PNP deficiency), xanthine oxidase, tetrazolium blue, and phenozine methylsulfate. Although the test is slightly more expensive than that developed by Moore and Meuwissen (1974), its accuracy is greater. Szüts *et al.* (1977) reported results of screening tests for ADA deficiency carried out in Europe.

1.3.5. Prenatal Diagnosis

The reduced enzyme activity and isoenzyme patterns present in erythrocytes are also present in fibroblasts of affected families and in amniotic cells. This fact has made possible the monitoring of at least five pregnancies at risk for ADA deficiency as ascertained by the previous birth of an affected child. In two cases, heterozygotes were identified prenatally and confirmed at birth by measurement of ADA activity in both amniotic fluid and cultured cells (Snyder, Scott, and Seegmiller, 1978, unpublished observation). One affected child was identified prenatally and two unaffected children were identified who were normal at birth, as predicted (Polmar *et al.*, 1976; Hirschhorn, 1977a,b).

1.3.6. Genetic Heterogeneity

Detailed studies of human hereditary diseases in recent years have led us to expect genetic heterogeneity in all disorders. Such genetic heterogeneity is well exemplified in ADA deficiency at both the clinical and fundamental biochemical levels. At the clinical level, all patients show impaired T-cell function, but different families vary in the degree to which ADA deficiency impairs B-cell function and in the frequency of clinical infections in affected patients. At an enzyme level, a considerable range of variation in the ADA activity was found in the different families reported (Hirschhorn, 1977a,b; Goldblum *et al.*, 1979). The amount of residual activity demonstrable in cultured fibroblasts may well be lower if cells are grown in media in which ADA contributed from fetal calf serum is inactivated or excluded (Carson and Seegmiller, 1976; Hirschhorn, *et al.*, 1976). Cultured fibroblasts also show differences in the amount of immunoreactive protein to antibody directed against ADA (Carson *et al.*, 1977a). In other cases, the residual activity showed differences from normal in thermal lability of the ADA (Coleman *et al.*, 1978). This observation might well be explained by the observations of Pollara *et al.* (1977) of a different enzyme accounting for the residual enzyme activity (see Section 1.3.3). The activity in lymphocytes is not always the same as in red cells, and this difference can account for some curious inconsistencies in clinical severity of disease. Activities of ADA in peripheral lymphocytes at 10 and 15% of normal were observed in children who had very low activities in red cells with no evidence of immunodeficiency disease (Jenkins and Nurse, 1976; Jenkins *et al.*, 1976; Hirschhorn, 1977a,b, 1978, personal communication).

1.3.7. Metabolic Studies

Additional reports of an increased intracellular concentration of adenine nucleotide in ADA deficiency have appeared, but more precise identification of some of these as deoxyribonucleotides has shifted the emphasis in concepts of pathogenesis. A high intracellular concentration of ATP in erythrocytes (Mills *et al.*, 1976) and lymphocytes was reported in ADA-deficient children (Polmar *et al.*, 1976). Schmalstieg *et al.* (1977) used high-pressure liquid chromatography (HPLC) to obtain evidence of a 4- to 8-fold increase in concentration of the purine nucleotides ADP, GTP, and ATP in the mononuclear leukocytes from a 12-month-old child with ADA deficiency, as compared with normal leukocytes analyzed simultaneously. GDP, UTP, and CTP were also increased, but to a lesser degree. The mitogenic response of the child's lymphocytes to concanavallin A (Con A) was increased 5-fold by addition of exogenous ADA, but in contrast to the patient of Polmar *et al.* (1975), added ADA had no significant effect on the proliferative response of the child's lymphocytes when stimulated with PHA. Likewise, addition of uridine, imidazole, or dibutyryl cyclic GMP (cGMP) failed to stimulate the response to PHA. The 2:1 ATP/ADP ratio in the patient's lymphocytes was abnormally low and was compared with a ratio of 5:1 in control lymphocytes, suggesting a defect in energy production by the cells, although the alternative possibility that it could result from a partial hydrolysis of ATP during preparation and shipping of the sample was not considered.

The identification of the adenine nucleotide that accumulates as ATP is now in doubt. Subsequent studies of the same patient (Simmonds *et al.*, 1978, 1979b; Kuttesch *et al.*, 1978) showed no evidence of abnormal amounts of adenine excreted in the urine, but did show a greater than 6000-fold increase in concentration of deoxyadenosine in the urine of the same affected child. They failed to find any abnormal increase in deoxyadenosine in erythrocytes, plasma, or lymphocytes of the affected child, but did consistently find substantial increases in free adenine. The possibility that the free adenine may have arisen during the sample preparation from hydrolysis of deoxyadenosine was not considered immediately, but was raised in later descriptions (Goldblum *et al.*, 1979).

Further evidence suggesting a pathogenetic role for deoxynucleosides was presented in the subsequent report by Cohen *et al.* (1978b) of a greater than 100-fold elevation in concentration of dATP in the erythrocytes of an ADA-deficient child who was immunodeficient, but not in the erythrocytes of an immunocompetent ADA-deficient patient. The increased erythrocyte dATP in two other ADA-deficient, immunodeficient patients decreased after transfusion of normal erythrocytes. The identity of the accumulated adenine nucleotide as 2'-dATP was confirmed by its cochromatography with known 2'-dATP on HPLC in a system that separates dATP from ATP. The material isolated from the erythrocytes by HPLC showed a UV absorption spectrum indistinguishable from that of dATP and was degraded to adenine after 30 min boiling with 1 M perchloric acid. After treatment with sodium periodate, a reagent that attacks ribose but not deoxyribose, the unknown material and a known sample of dATP still chromatographed at the same location in an HPLC system, while known ATP, after similar treatment, was eluted in the void volume of the column in the same position as adenine and adenosine. In an independent assay of dATP using the DNA polymerase reaction, the dATP of normal erythrocytes was 8 nmol/ml packed cells, while the same assay procedures gave 1100 nmol/ml packed cells of the ADA-deficient child. In another child who showed a comparable degree (around 1%) of ADA deficiency in erythrocytes, but no immunodeficiency, no significant accumulation of dATP was found in the erythrocytes by HPLC. This child, however, was like the !Kung child reported by Jenkins *et al.* (1976) and did show 15% of normal activity in the lymphocytes (Hirschhorn, 1978, personal communication).

The plasma and urine samples from the enzyme-deficient patients contained less than 2 μM deoxyadenosine, but in three of the four patients, adenosine or adenine or both were detectable, both of which disappeared after transfusion with normal erythrocytes.

The validity of the major observations was confirmed in an independent report of the presence of very high concentrations of dATP in erythrocytes of another ADA-deficient child (Coleman *et al.*, 1978). The child's lymphocytes showed 4.4%, and granulocytes 2.3%, of normal ADA activity. The residual activity in erythrocytes showed a substantially greater lability to heat than did that of either normal controls or the parents, with loss after heating for 1 hr at 50°C of 58% of residual ADA activity compared with an 8% loss in erythrocytes of parents or of normal subjects. The K_m and V_{max} values of the residual enzyme in the child's cells were both normal, and the mutant enzyme showed no difference from normal in electrophoretic migration. HPLC revealed the presence of over 1500 times the normal amount of dATP and over 260 times the normal amount of dADP in the child's erythrocytes. The identity of dATP was confirmed by the identification of the products formed with yeast pyrophosphatase, with alkaline phosphatase, and by its reaction with DNA polymerase, as well as by gas chromatography of the trimethylsilyl derivatives and by mass spectrometry.

1.3.8. Model Systems of Adenosine Deaminase Deficiency

A variety of inhibitors of ADA have been used to create models of the genetic disease in cells cultured *in vitro* and in experimental animals *in vivo*. The ADA inhibitor erythro-9-(2-hydroxy-3-nonyl) adenine (EHNA) was described by Schaeffer and Schwender (1974) and has a K_i of 1.6 × 10^{-9} (Agarwal *et al.*, 1977). Coformycin and deoxycoformycin show a K_i of 1 × 10^{-11} M and 2.5 × 10^{-12} (Agarwal *et al.*, 1977). These inhibitors have provided useful models for detailed biochemical study in the situation in which ADA-deficient cells or permanent cell lines are not available.

Numerous investigators have used the aforementioned inhibitors to create biochemical models of ADA deficiency in a variety of biological systems. Harrap and Paine (1976) studied cultured mouse leukemia cells and human lymphocytes, Snyder *et al.* (1978) studied human lymphoblasts, and numerous investigators studied mitogen-stimulated human lymphocytes (Fox *et al.*, 1975; Carson and Seegmiller, 1976; Harrap and Paine, 1976; Snyder *et al.*, 1976; Raivio and Hovi, 1979). Henderson *et al.* (1977) examined the specificity of the various ADA inhibitors using intact Ehrlich ascites tumor cells and cultured mouse lymphoma cells *in vitro*. Studies in intact cells showed an increasing inhibition of other enzymes of purine interconversion by EHNA at concentrations greater than 10 μM. EHNA thus proved to be the least specific inhibitor (Burridge *et al.*, 1977).

Deoxycoformycin administered to mice for up to 96 hr, at a dose producing over 95% inhibition of ADA activity in both thymus and spleen, failed to alter the proliferative responsiveness of thymus cells to stimulation by Con A *in vitro* or by mixed culture of splenic cells (Burridge *et al.*, 1977).

Gudas *et al.* (1979), using a cultured wild-type and mutant mouse T-lymphoma cells, and McBurney and Whitmore (1975), using Chinese hamster cell lines, showed that mutants lacking adenosine transport and those lacking adenosine kinase activity were resistant to the cytotoxic effects of adenosine at up to 15 μM for lymphoma lines and up to 370 μM for hamster cells, while lines lacking HPRT or APRT were fully sensitive to the killing action of adenosine. Adenosine administered at low concentrations requires phosphorylation to deplete the cells of pyrimidine nucleotides and PP-ribose-P and to promote the accumulation of orotate.

This report is at variance with the findings of Hershfield *et al.* (1977), who found a full sensitivity to adenosine toxicity in a mutant human lymphoblast line deficient in adenosine kinase, suggesting that in the human cell line, phosphorylation was not required for adenosine toxicity. A possible mechanism of such toxicity was suggested by Kredich and Martin (1977), who showed the accumulation of S-adenosylhomocysteine in cultured mouse T-lymphoma cells treated with sufficient adenosine to produce an inhibition of cell replication. This observation opens a whole new line for consideration of the mechanism of adenosine toxicity not previously considered. Presumably, DNA methylation would be inhibited *in vivo* by the high concentration of S-adenosylhomocysteine.

1.3.9. Treatment

Treatment of ADA deficiency, as with other severe combined immunodeficiency disease, is best achieved by finding a histocompatible donor for a bone marrow (Good and Yunis, 1974; Good and Hansen, 1976; Parkman, 1977; Ackeret *et al.*, 1976), fetal liver (Keightley *et al.*, 1975), or thymus epithelial transplant (Hong *et al.*, 1976) to create a chimera in which normal cells replace the defective mutant cells of the immune system.

The more specific approach to therapy first described by Polmar *et al.* (1976) consisting of transfusion of irradiated frozen erythrocytes as a source of ADA, has not been uniformly successful. Of the eight patients treated so far, four have shown some favorable response, both in their clinical improvement and in their specific tests of immune response (Polmar *et al.*, 1979). The original patient of Polmar showed a full return of immune function with the exception of a somewhat lower than normal lymphocyte count, and an inability to show a cutaneous delayed hypersensitivity. The plasma concentration of thymic hormone also increased substantially following the red cell transfusion (Polmar *et al.*, 1979).

The reason for the failure of red-cell infusion to produce a response in a portion of the patients is not entirely clear. Since the immunodeficiency appears to be acquired after birth and becomes more profound with time, presumably at some point the immunodeficiency may become irreversible due to the loss of stem cells or damage of the thymus cells. It may be that only patients with less severe enzyme deficiencies can respond to enzyme replacement (Polmar *et al.*, 1979). Schmalstieg *et al.* (1978) described in detail the poor response to transfused erythrocytes, over a 17-month period, of a 10-month-old child with profound deficiency of red cell ADA with around 1% of normal activity, and severe combined immunodeficiency disease. The irradiated erythrocytes produced a decrease in "ATP" of both lymphocytes and erythrocytes noted around 7 days after each transfusion and reduced substantially the excretion in the urine of deoxyadenosine and "adenine." The blood lymphocyte count rose and a limited increase in the response of the lymphocytes to PHA followed the transfusions. Although the serum immunoglobulin concentration increased, no specific antibody formation was elicited. Skin tests of delayed hypersensitivity remained negative. Wolf *et al.* (1976) also obtained a therapeutic response to erythrocyte transfusions and to thymosin.

The possibility of developing pharmacological agents to correct immunodeficiency disease of ADA deficiency is within reason. The increase in response to PHA produced by treatment of cells *in vitro* with lithium chloride (Polmar *et al.*, 1979) suggests this possibility, as does the use of cytidine to prevent the deoxyadenosine toxicity to PHA-stimulated human lymphocytes noted by Carson *et al.* (1977b).

1.4. Purine Nucleoside Phosphorylase Deficiency

The identification of two brothers with immunodeficiency disease associated with PNP deficiency brings the total such patients observed to date to seven in four families (Giblett *et al.*, 1975; Cohen *et al.*, 1976; Griscelli *et al.*, 1976; Hamet *et al.*, 1977; Stoop *et al.*, 1977; Fox *et al.*, 1977). The new family showed a milder form of T-cell dysfunction and excretion of large amounts of purine nucleoside in the urine, but unlike patients reported previously, the uric acid content of serum and urine was in the low normal range and the patients excreted no increased amount of orotic acid. Such differences are explainable by the incomplete deficiency in PNP and resultant less severe block in purine nucleoside degradation

(Fox *et al.*, 1977; Edwards *et al.*, 1978; Biggar *et al.*, 1978; Gelfand *et al.*, 1978). A summary of this disorder is included in several recent reviews (Hirschhorn, 1977b; Seegmiller, 1978a).

1.4.1. Clinical Presentation

The previous five patients reported with PNP deficiency (Giblett *et al.*, 1975; Hamet *et al.*, 1977; Stoop *et al.*, 1977) presented with immuno-deficiency disease of somewhat later onset than that seen in ADA deficiency. Severe anemia was a problem in one patient (Giblett *et al.*, 1975), and all previously described patients showed an enhanced suceptibility to viral diseases, particularly vaccinia, which had produced a severe infection in three patients, leading to the death of two (Hamet *et al.*, 1977; Martin, 1978, personal communication). Spastic tetraparesis is present in the patient of Stoop *et al.* (1977).

The patients all showed a marked impairment of delayed hypersensitivity and evidence of impaired T-cell function, but no evidence of B-cell dysfunction. The severe deficiency of PNP resulted in virtually no uric acid production, with serum urate values less than 1 mg/dl and urinary acid creatinine ratio of around 0.27. Yet these patients were producing and excreting an excessive amount of total purines quite comparable to that of children with the Lesch–Nyhan syndrome, but with inosine, guanosine, and the corresponding deoxyribosides in place of the excessive amounts of uric acid seen in the latter disease.

The newly described brothers showed a later onset of clinical symptoms and less severe impairment of T-cell function, in keeping with the less severe deficiency of the enzyme present in their cells (Gelfand *et al.*, 1978; Biggar *et al.*, 1978). The younger brother, age 9, had shown a normal early development with full immunization with live attenuated viruses of polio, rubella, and vaccinia carried out without incident. His growth and development were essentially normal. His first difficulties began at age 6 years, when he developed a severe bout of chicken pox. Subsequently, recurrent bacterial infections of both the upper and lower respiratory tracts and otitis media appeared. At age 8, he developed recurrent episodes of pain and swelling of the hands and feet. On physical examination, he was in the 25th percentile of weight and the 10th–20th percentile for height. His teeth showed extensive caries, and his skin showed scarring from varicella. A purulent nasal discharge was present, and the right tympanic membrane was scarred. Tonsils were present, and lymphoid tissue was palpable throughout his body. X rays showed thickened bronchial wall, and an opaque paranasal sinus and right mastoid. His granulocytes showed normal ability to kill bacteria and to respond to chemotaxis, and his complement activity was normal.

The older brother, age 10½, had onset of problems of infections at a much earlier age. Recurrent ear, sinus, and pulmonary infections began during the first months of life. He too was fully immunized without incident by 1½ years of age. At the age of 4 years, he had an episode of uncomplicated chicken pox, following which he had recurrent hospitalization for pulmonary infections and progressive pulmonary insufficiency. On physical examination, he was less than the 3rd percentile for height, and at the 10th percentile for weight, and showed a chronic purulent nasal discharge, chronic otitis media, and pulmonary rales, bilaterally, with emphysema. Bilateral chorioretinitis was present. His granulocytes and complement activity were also normal.

Studies of cell-mediated immunity revealed an absence of delayed cutaneous reactivity to a number of antigens, including dinitrochlorobenzene, and significantly reduced lymphocyte proliferative response to nonspecific mitogens, specific antigens, and allogeneic cells. The number of T cells in the peripheral blood was substantially reduced, with E-rosetting of only 20 and 31% of total lymphocytes. Serum immunoglobulin concentration and percentages of the various immunoglobulin types and C3 receptor-bearing cells were normal, and lymphocytes showed a normal ability to respond with antibody formation to specific antigens *in vivo*. *In vitro* induction of specific IgM antibody showed the presence of T-helper and T-regulator cells. Bone marrow precursor T cells formed mature T cells on treatment with thymosin, or by medium conditioned by growth of human thymic epithelium, suggesting a normal ability of these children to generate T cells and an intact thymic epithelial cell function. All attempts at reconstituting the response of lymphocytes from these children to mitogens *in vitro* were unsuccessful. These included an addition of purified PNP (Gelfand *et al.*, 1978).

1.4.2. Enzyme Abnormalities

PNP of normal human erythrocytes was purified to homogeneity by Zannis *et al.* (1978) in two steps with a yield of 56%. The native enzyme is a trimer with a molecular weight of 93,800 and subunit molecular weight of 29,700. Posttranscriptional modifications presumably account for the four different forms revealed on two-dimensional electrophoresis of the denatured enzyme.

Sandman *et al.* (1977) reported additional biochemical and immunological studies of the original patient described by Giblett *et al.* (1975). The patient's erythrocytes, lymphocytes, and cultured fibroblasts and a lymphoblast line showed normal activity of ADA, but no detectable PNP. However, the investigators failed to denote the lower limit of enzyme that could have been detected by the method they were using. PNP activity in cell lysates of the patient's mother and father was 26 and 40% of normal in erythrocytes, 48 and 40% of normal in lymphocytes, and 50 and 54% in cultured fibroblasts. No inhibitor was found in the patient's erythrocyte lysates on mixing with lysates of normal individuals. A full activity of ADA was found in the same cells of all family members. The PNP activity was also undetectable in a permanent lymphoid line established from peripheral blood lymphocytes by addition of Epstein–Barr virus (EBV). Similar studies in lymphocytes from a patient with another type of immunodeficiency showed that infection with a virus did not destroy PNP activity. On incubation of the EBV-infected lymphocytes with sheep erythrocytes, no T-cell rosettes were detected, in keeping with other studies demonstrating the B-cell characteristics of the permanent lymphoblast lines established with this virus. Incubation of the cells with polyacrylamide beads coated with anti-heavy-chain antibody yielded 65–85% B cells.

The absence of PNP in fibroblasts of affected persons suggests that amniotic fluid cells could be utilized for the prenatal diagnosis of this type of immunodeficiency, as has been reported with many other inborn errors of metabolsim (Epstein and Golbus, 1978).

PNP was grossly deficient in erythrocytes, granulocytes, and fibroblasts cultured *in vitro* from the two affected brothers in the newly discovered family (Fox *et al.*, 1977; Osborne *et al.*, 1977; Edwards *et al.*, 1978). The children each showed values in their erythrocytes 0.46% of normal, while the mother showed a value 59% of normal and the father 50% of normal. They all showed values for ADA, APRT, HPRT, and PP-ribose-P synthetase within the normal range in erythrocyte hemolysates. Fibroblasts cultured from one affected child showed values to 0.13% of normal for PNP, while granulocytes from the two children isolated from the buffy coat showed PNP activity 1.3–3.0% of normal. The erythrocyte values for ADA were elevated in both affected children.

The affinity of the enzyme in both brothers for the substrate inosine was diminished to about 10% of values found for the normal enzyme. It also showed a different migration on electrophoresis and a greater thermal lability in the presence of inosine than did normal enzyme, suggesting that this is a structural gene mutation (Fox *et al.*, 1977).

The genetic basis for the PNP deficiency in three affected patients was studied in detail by Osborne *et al.* (1977) by determining the amount of immunological reacting protein and electrophoretic migration of residual enzyme activity in erythrocyte lysates of the patients and their parents. The two brothers mentioned above showed 0.5% of normal residual enzyme activity and half the normal amount of immunological reacting protein. Each parent showed evidence of heterozygosity for a different mutation in PNP. Only one mutation accounted for the heterozygosity in the consanguineous parents of the first affected child described, who showed no detectable PNP activity and no immunological reacting protein.

1.4.3. Purine Metabolites in Urine

Unlike the previous reported patients (Cohen *et al.*, 1976; Stoop *et al.*, 1977), these patients both excreted substantial amounts of uric acid, 200 and 187 mg/24 hr, respectively. The method used for assay for inosine and guanosine also included deoxyinosine and deoxyguanosine. The total "inosine" was 4.23 mmol/24 hr in both cases, and guanosine was 0.61 and 0.65 mmol/24 hr. The calcúlated urate equivalents were 1.9 and 2.1/mg creatinine, respectively, which is substantially higher than the upper range of normal of 1.2 for children of this age (Kaufman *et al.*, 1968). The urate clearance was 5.3 and 5.0 ml/min and was within the normal range.

1.4.4. Metabolic Studies

As might be expected, the plasma concentrations of nucleosides were elevated in PNP-deficient patients. Inosine concentration was 115 μM in plasma of the patient first identified (Cohen *et al.*, 1977), and was 67 and 70 μM in the two brothers (Osborne *et al.*, 1977). The plasma inosine content of the patients of Stoop *et al.* (1977) ranged from 14 to 99 μM. Unlike that in the patient reported by Cohen *et al.* (1976), the intracellular concentration of PP-ribose-P in the erythrocytes of the two brothers was not increased. An increase in erythrocyte dGTP greater than 10-fold above normal was reported in two patients with PNP deficiency (Cohen *et al.*, 1978a).

The reduced affinity for inosine of the mutant enzyme in affected children suggested the possibility of increasing its effective activity *in vivo* by increasing the load of nucleosides presented to the enzyme by an increased rate of purine nucleotide catabolism. This activity could be increased in lysates substantially by increasing the substrate concentration. The rapid intravenous infusion of fructose increases the rate of uric acid synthesis presumably by accelerating the catabolism of hepatic adenine nucleotides to their purine nucleoside intermediates and end products (Raivio *et al.*, 1975) (see Section 1.2.6). In control subjects, it caused a prompt 25% increase in serum urate and a 40% rise in urinary uric acid content.

In contrast, the PNP-deficient subjects showed no sustained elevation over their baseline value in either serum urate or urinary uric acid or oxypurine excretion in response to fructose infusion. However, their baseline inosine excretion, which was 100 times greater than normal to start, was increased another 6-fold in the first hour after fructose infusion. Urinary guanosine, which was not detectable in normal urine, was increased from a baseline value of 1.5 to 3.9 μmol/mg creatinine within 60 min, which represented a 4- to 8-fold greater than normal increase of purine excretion accompanied by an elevation of erythrocyte PP-ribose-P concentration (Fig. 2).

The unaltered serum urate and urinary uric acid and oxypurine values indicated that the activity of the deficient enzyme, even though it has a reduced affinity for substrate (a K_m mutation), could not be augmented *in vivo* by increasing the availability of the substrates inosine and guanosine (Fox *et al.*, 1977; Edwards *et al.*, 1978). The erythrocyte inorganic phosphate concentration in normal subjects was diminished by 40–50% within the first 15 min of infusion, accompanied by a 20% decrease in erythrocyte content of PP-ribose-P and a 40–60% fall in erythrocyte ribose-5-phosphate concentrations at 1 hr. In the PNP-deficient patients, fructose infusion produced a 10–40% increase in erythrocyte inorganic phosphate concentration, a striking elevation in PP-ribose-P content, and essentially no change from baseline values of ribose-5-phosphate concentration. Serum glucose and phosphate concentrations were not substantially altered in any of the subjects during the 150 min following fructose infusion (Edwards *et al.*, 1978).

Studies of the purine catabolism in intact erythrocytes showed a conversion of 38–47% of the inosine to hypoxanthine by a 10-min incubation with normal erythrocytes in the absence of exogenous inorganic phosphate, while it was increased to 68–69% with addition of 6.25 mM inorganic phosphate. In contrast, the PNP-deficient erythrocytes showed a maximum conversion of 5% of the inosine to hypoxanthine, regardless of the amount of inorganic phosphate in the medium. Both the normal and PNP-deficient erythrocytes converted the same amount of adenosine to adenine nucleotides.

In an effort to study the effects of the aberration of nucleoside metabolism on purine interconversions in intact cells, measurement was made of the release of carbon dioxide from [7-^{14}C]orotate in intact erythrocytes from normal and PNP-deficient subjects. Erythrocytes from the PNP-deficient patients converted 45% more orotic acid to carbon dioxide over a 30-min period than did the normal and showed less suppression of PP-ribose-P synthesis by added nucleosides than did normal erythrocytes. Presumably, this is related to their inability to degrade inosine to hypoxanthine (Edwards *et al.*, 1978).

Fibroblasts cultured from an affected child compared with normal fibroblasts incorporated only 2% as much [^{14}C]inosine and 4% as much [^{3}H]guanosine into acid-precipitable nucleotides (Burke *et al.*, 1977).

1.4.5. Treatment

Attempts to treat PNP-deficient patients by enzyme replacement, as with ADA deficiency (Polmar *et al.,* 1976), have so far been ineffective. Infusion of irradiated erythrocytes produced no positive effect on lymphocyte function of one PNP-deficient patient, given at 30-day intervals over a 3-month period. At 24 days following an infusion of fresh, irradiated packed red cells, a low activity of PNP was detectable in the plasma, but none was detected in the lymphocytes. At 24 hr following the third infusion of irradiated packed red cells, a low PNP activity was detected in both erythrocytes and plasma and was within the normal range in erythrocytes. T-cell rosettes increased by 20%, but the total lymphocyte count and response of peripheral blood lymphocytes to PHA and allogeneic cells remained depressed, and immunological function remained unaltered (Sandman *et al.,* 1977).

1.4.6. Purine Nucleoside Phosphorylase Distribution in Human Tissues

PNP distribution in human tissues was reported by Carson *et al.* (1977b). It appears to be essentially uniformly distributed throughout all the tissues analyzed, with no increased activity in thymus tissue. Nevertheless, Borgers *et al.* (1977) described a histochemical method for detection of PNP in circulating human lymphocytes. They reported a correlation between the number of PNP-positive cells and the number of E-rosette-forming cells in the same blood samples of healthy and diseased people, and proposed that it might be a useful marker for T cells in man. They also reported additional evidence for the presence of PNP activity in T cells and not in B cells from experiments in which PNP activity and surface membrane immunoglobulins are simultaneously demonstrated on the same preparations. These results showed that the bulk of lymphocytes that are reactive for PNP do not reveal surface membrane immunoglobulins and that most Ig-bearing cells are unreactive for PNP. An ultramicrochemical method for determination of PNP suitable for assay of single cells was described by Uitendaal *et al.* (1978).

1.5. Biochemical Basis of the Immunodeficiency in Adenosine Deaminase and Purine Nucleoside Phosphorylase Deficiency

The precise biochemical mechanism relating the primary enzyme defects in nucleoside metabolism to the immunodeficiency disease is still not well understood; however, considerable progress has been made in our understanding of this relationship, particularly during the past year. The first hypothesis relating PNP and ADA deficiency to a common mechanism was that the substantial accumulation of inosine that occurs in the plasma of PNP-deficient children (see Section 1.4.4) acts as an end-product inhibitor of ADA, and thus a primary and secondary ADA deficiency would be responsible for both immune defects (Cohen *et al.*, 1976; Ullman *et al.*, 1976; Seegmiller *et al.*, 1977a,b). Osborne *et al.* (1978) provided evidence against this concept from a kinetic analysis of ADA. No measurable product inhibition, by up to 2mM inosine, was observed on ADA purified from human red cells and assayed by conversion of [^{14}C]adenosine to inosine.

1.5.1. Ribonucleoside Accumulation

Accumulation of adenosine as a mediator of ADA deficiency has been a working hypothesis for the mechanism of immunosuppression. Schmalstieg *et al.* (1978) and Mills *et al.* (1976) reported plasma concentration of adenosine of 1–2 μM. This concentration approaches the range required to exhibit the cytotoxic action on lymphocytes in the presence of an inhibitor of ADA (Wolberg *et al.*, 1975). The 10-fold accumulation of ATP in the lymphocytes (Polmar *et al.*, 1976; Schmalstieg *et al.*, 1977) and lesser accumulations in the erythrocytes (Mills *et al.*, 1976) were taken as indirect evidence of the validity of this concept (Meuwissen *et al.*, 1975; Seegmiller, 1976a, 1978a,b; Polmar *et al.*, 1977). The failure to detect any appreciable accumulation of adenosine in serum or urine argued against this concept, but was attributed to the alternate pathway for adenosine utilization via adenosine kinase, which has a higher affinity for the substrate, and constitutes a major pathway in most physiological conditions (Snyder *et al.*, 1976; Benke and Dittmar, 1976; Perret and Dean, 1977). The most convincing evidence against a role for adenosine as a mediator of immunodeficiency was provided by Polmar *et al.* (1977) PHA-stimulated lymphocytes from an ADA-deficient child in remission from erythrocyte transfusions showed no difference from normal lymphocytes in their sensitivity to inhibition by adenosine.

1.5.2. Pyrimidine Starvation

A direct consequence of adenosine toxicity, in a variety of cultured lymphoid cells, is a lowering of the intracellular concentration of pyrimidine nucleotides associated with very low concentrations of PP-ribose-P (Green and Chan, 1973; Snyder *et al.*, 1977, 1978). Although uridine corrects a part of the adenosine toxicity in cells cultured *in vitro*, it has not been effective therapy in the few patients in whom it has been tried, nor has it countered the decrease in cytotoxic response of lymphocytes produced by adenosine and ADA inhibitors (Parkman *et al.*, 1975; Wolberg *et al.*, 1975; Polmar *et al.*, 1976; Goldblum *et al.*, 1979). Furthermore, PP-ribose-P-dependent reactions occur at normal rates in ADA-deficient lymphocytes (Raivio *et al.*, 1977). Most decisive, however, is the finding of an increase, rather than a decrease, of pyrimidine nucleotides in lymphocytes of an ADA-deficient patient (Schmalsteig *et al.*, 1977).

1.5.3. Possible Role of Cyclic AMP

A possible role for cyclic AMP (cAMP) as a mediator of immuno-suppression has been a recurring hypothesis. Ullman *et al.* (1976) provided strong arguments against cAMP being involved in adenosine toxicity. A mutant mouse lymphoma line that was deficient in cAMP receptors was nevertheless equally sensitive to adenosine toxicity as the parental strain. More convincing evidence of the possible role for cAMP was presented by Schmalstieg *et al.* (1977), who reported, without presenting specific data, a 2- to 3-fold increase in the concentration of cAMP in ADA-deficient lymphocytes. This concentration was decreased some 21% by incubation with exogenous ADA added to the lymphocyte suspension, whereas no change was observed when the same amount of ADA was added to normal cells. The addition of dibutyryl cGMP failed to stimulate the response of this child's lymphocytes to PHA.

Studies by Polmar *et al.* (1979) on lymphocytes from a patient in remission from red cell transfusion (see Section 1.3.9) provided additional indirect evidence for a role of increased cAMP concentrations in suppressing the ability of lymphocytes to respond to the mitogen PHA, as measured by [^{3}H]thymidine incorporation. No direct assessments were made of the intracellular concentration of cAMP, but deductions were possible from the response of the cells to a variety of agents known to influence cAMP concentrations. Either theophylline, which elevates cAMP by inhibiting its metabolism by a phosphodiesterase, or a specific inhibitor of the same enzyme depressed [^{3}H]thymidine incorporation of ADA-deficient lymphocytes to a significantly greater extent than it did that of normal lymphocytes at the same concentration. Norepinephrine, which stimulates adenylate cyclase activity and cAMP synthesis, also inhibited the response. Other potent inducers of cAMP synthesis, the prostaglandins E_1 and E_2, produced an exquisitely sensitive inhibition of the response, while prostaglandin E_{2d}, which does not enhance cAMP synthesis, showed no such effect. Further indirect pharmacological evidence was provided by the use of the inhibitor of cAMP synthesis lithium chloride, which markedly enhanced [^{3}H]thymidine incorporation of ADA-deficient lymphocytes at concentrations that either inhibited or had no effect on normal lymphocytes. The possibility that this effect was mediated by activation of the lymphocyte adenosine receptors was proposed by A. L. Schwartz *et al.* (1979). Turpin *et al.* (1977) confirmed in fat cells *in situ* the earlier work of Fain and Wieser (1975) in demonstrating a role for adenosine in modulating hormone-stimulated lipolysis in isolated rate epididymal fat cells.

1.5.4. Deoxyribonucleoside Accumulation

The surprisingly large amounts of deoxyribonucleosides excreted along with ribonucleosides in the urine of PNP-deficient patients (Cohen *et al.*, 1976; Stoop *et al.*, 1977) focused attention on the importance of the deoxynucleoside degradation pathway (Snyder and Henderson, 1973). Deoxyadenosine has a higher affinity than adenosine for ADA and was identified in the urine of an ADA-deficient child instead of the expected adenosine (Simmonds *et al.*, 1978; Goldblum *et al.*, 1979). Carson *et al.* (1977b) provided additional reasons for considering deoxyadenosine as a potential mediator by showing that thymus carries the highest activity of deoxynucleoside kinase of any human tissue. They also demonstrated the greater toxicity of deoxyadenosine as compared with adenosine in the proliferative response of cultured human cells. In addition, deoxyguanosine and deoxyinosine showed comparable toxicity, and both showed greater toxicity than the corresponding ribonucleosides. The subsequent identification of increased quantities of dATP in erythrocytes of ADA-deficient children (Cohen *et al.*, 1978b; Coleman *et al.*, 1978) and the decrease in dATP following therapeutic infusion of irradiated erythrocytes provided the next link. Even in the absence of ADA inhibitors (Tattersall *et al.*, 1975), deoxyadenosine was a more potent inhibitor of the mitogen response of human lymphocytes than was adenosine, and was greatly potentiated by ADA inhibitors (Harrap and Paine, 1976). The latter workers also noted a curious increase in dATP content of these cells in the presence of adenosine and deoxycoformycin. Transport of deoxyadenosine into murine leukemia cells was studied by Kessel (1978).

At present, no one doubts that the increased "ATP" reported in lymphocytes of ADA-deficient children is largely dATP, since the analytical systems were not specific. Donofrio *et al.* (1978) have demonstrated the presence of increased dATP in lymphocytes from children with ADA deficiency, and an increased dGTP was reported in erythrocytes of PNP-deficient children (Cohen *et al.*, 1978a). Likewise, an increase in dATP was shown by Bluestein *et al.* (1979) in mitogen-stimulated normal human lymphocytes in the presence of deoxycoformycin.

The mechanism by which an accumulation of dATP in the case of ADA deficiency or dGTP in the case of PNP deficiency could lead to immunosuppression is suggested by the marked effect of accumulation of these substances on the activity of ribonucleoside diphosphate reductase (Fig. 1), an enzyme required for formation of deoxyribonucleotides of both purines and pyrimidines (Moore and Hurlbert, 1966; Murphree *et al.*, 1968; Krygier and Momparler, 1971; Reichard, 1972). If an inadequate supply of these other deoxynucleotides were indeed the cause of failure of these cells to proliferate, we would expect them to grow after being provided with another source for deoxynucleotides. Deoxyadenosine expanded the dATP pool and reduced formation of all other deoxynucleotides, while deoxyguanosine expanded the dGTP pool and reduced rather specifically the concentration of dCTP in human lymphocytes during mitogenic stimulation (Tattersall *et al.*, 1975).

1.5.5. Implications for Therapy

If an inhibition of ribonucleotide reductase by accumulated dATP in patients with ADA deficiency and accumulated dGTP in patients with PNP deficiency is indeed a valid mechanism for the immunosuppression in these disorders, we might expect a correction of the toxic action of these substances by providing deoxyribonucleotides from an external source. Carson *et al.* (1977b) demonstrated a 70% correction of the toxic effects of deoxyadenosine in PHA-stimulated, ADA-inhibited human lymphocytes by deoxycytidine addition. Bluestein *et al.* (1979) were able to correct fully the toxic suppression by combinations of deoxyguanosine and deoxypyrimidine nucleosides. The enhancement of PHA response of lymphocytes from an ADA-deficient patient by addition of lithium chloride (Polmar *et al.*, 1979) provides an additional concept for further investigation. These findings in the human cells, cultured *in vitro,* point the direction for more definitive studies of new therapeutic agents of possible value for patients with these inherited types of immunodeficiency.

1.6. Purine 5'-Nucleotidase Deficiency in Hypogammaglobulinemia

The previous report of the low activity of purine 5'-nucleotidase (PNT) in peripheral blood mononuclear cells from patients with nonfamilial adult onset (variable) primary hypogammaglobulinemia (Johnson, S. M., *et al.,* 1977) was extended in additional studies from the same laboratory (Webster *et al.,* 1978).

1.6.1. Clinical Categories with Low Purine 5'-Nucleotidase

The later report expands substantially the number of patients studied (Webster *et al.*, 1978). However, only 8 of 21 patients with adult onset of agammaglobulinemia showed values for PNT in mononuclear cells below the normal range compared with 9 of 11 patients in the earlier report of S. M. Johnson *et al.* (1977). Additional diseases in which very low PNT activity was found included 1 patient with the Wiskott–Aldrich syndrome, 1 patient with an immunodeficiency state associated with red blood cell aplasia, 3 patients with isolated IgA deficiency, and 1 of 2 patients with congenital dwarfism and immune deficiency.

Of the 7 patients in the latter four categories, 5 showed values for PNT less than 10% of the mean value for the normal, and 6 were below the lower limits found in the normal. Although 5 patients with sex-linked recessive agammaglobulinemia showed values somewhat lower than a mean value for the normal, they were not outside the normal range. In 3 of these patients, ADA activity was over twice the mean normal value in lymphocytes, but not in erythrocytes.

In addition, these investigators explored the possibility that adult-onset types of agammaglobulinemia could represent variants of ADA or PNP deficiency. No such variants were found to account for adult onset of agammaglobulinemia. A variety of other enzyme activities were measured and found to be in the normal range. These included HPRT, APRT, PP-ribose-P synthetase, and PP-ribose-P amidotransferase activity. The PP-ribose-P contents of the cells were all in the normal range. In 2 of 6 patients with adult onset of hypogammaglobulinemia, values for PP-ribose-P synthetase activity of erythrocytes was around twice the mean normal value and clearly above the normal range. PNT is also markedly diminished or undetectable in most patients with chronic lymphocytic leukemia (Quagliata *et al.*, 1974; Lopes *et al.*, 1973; Marique and Hildebrand, 1973). The decreased enzyme level has remained for more than 24 months of observation. Lymphocytes from 103 other patients with a wide variety of clinical disorders were examined and a marked decrease in PNT found as a transient event only in the early phase of infectious mononucleosis and in 2 patients with acute lymphocytic leukemia (Quagliata *et al.*, 1974).

1.6.2. Enzyme Characteristics

Webster *et al.* (1978) took special precautions to show the specificity of the PNT activity that is diminished in lymphocytes from the patients described above. The PNT activity was uninfluenced by various concentrations of inhibitors of alkaline and acid phosphatase, including cysteine,

β-glycerophosphate, and sodium potassium tartrate. None of these agents produced any significant inhibition. In contrast, the more specific 5'-nucleotidase inhibitor TTP produced 84% inhibition, while ATP produced 94% inhibition. The mononuclear cells had no nonspecific phosphatase activity detectable using p-nitrophenylphosphate as substrate.

Additional studies of the series of possible substrates showed the ready conversion of 5'-AMP, 5'-IMP, 5'-GMP, and 5'-UMP to the corresponding nucleosides by mononuclear cells of both normal subjects and at substantially lower rates by hypogammaglobulinemia patients. Both PHA and Con A inhibited the 5'-nucleotidase activity of the mononuclear cells either after preincubation with the cells or when added to the assay mixture. The Con A inhibition was reversed by adding α-methyl-D-mannoside, but this had no effect on the inhibition caused by PHA, and α-methyl-D-mannoside had virtually no effect when it was added to the assay alone.

1.7. Adenine Phosphoribosyltransferase Deficiency

A total of four patients in three families have now been described with APRT deficiency since the original description by Cartier *et al.* in 1974 and a more detailed report by Debray *et al.* (1976). A more comprehensive description of the clinical features of the two brothers described in the second known family (Simmonds *et al.*, 1976b, 1977; Van Acker *et al.*, 1977a) appeared in the past year (Van Acker *et al.*, 1977b). In addition, a new case, not previously reported, was described (Barratt *et al.*, 1979; Simmonds *et al.*, 1979a). In each family, evidence was found for a recessive mode of inheritance. Clinical features indicate that this is a benign disorder except for the propensity to form calculi in the urinary tract, composed of the sparingly soluble substance 2,8-dihydroxyadenine. Such calculi have now been identified in three of the four known patients with this metabolic disorder.

1.7.1. Clinical Presentation

The major clinical symptoms of patients with APRT deficiency are attributed to the excretion in the urine of a very sparingly soluble product of adenine metabolism, 2,8-dihydroxyadenine. The second known patient with this disorder, a 2-year-old boy, had gravel, crystals, and small calculi in his urine from birth, and after 9 months of age frequently developed episodes of abdominal colic, dysuria, and pain in the uretha (Van Acker *et al.*, 1977a,b). Clinical examination showed no abnormal findings other than a marked hyperlaxity of the joints and muscular hypertonia when he was first seen at age 20 months. The patient was unable to walk without aid, which may have been the result of a low-protein diet prescribed for control of stone formation. Urine analysis reported "uric acid" crystals in the urine. He was treated with *allopurinol*, 200 mg/day, and bicarbonate with little change in stone formation. On reinvestigation at 31 months of age, he weighed 14 kg and the hypotonia had diminished appreciably; he was now able to walk normally. All routine laboratory examinations were normal. The urinary sediment contained numerous round crystals, which, on routine analysis, were again reported as "pure uric acid." An older brother was found to have the same biochemical features, but had never developed clinical symptoms from stone or gravel formation (see Section 1.7.3).

The one additional patient described by Barratt *et al.* (1979) and Simmonds *et al.* (1979a,b) was a third child of consanguineous Arab parents. Birth was normal and she appeared perfectly well until 1 year of age, when she began to suffer repeated attacks of abdominal pain with fever, which were diagnosed as repeated urinary tract infections. At 21 months of age, she was referred to London for investigation of lithiasis, and an intravenous pyelogram showed a nonfunctioning left kidney and a radiolucent calculus in the pelvis of the right kidney. Physical examination was unremarkable, and neurological examination was entirely normal; however, urine culture showed a growth of *Klebsiella aerogenes* with numerous leukocytes, red cells, and debris. Surgeons removed a calculus obstructing the left lower ureter and another calculus from the pelvis of the right kidney. These calculi were friable, greyish in color, and on routine thermogravimetric analysis (Rose, G. A., and Woodfine, 1976) were reported as "uric acid."

1.7.2. Composition of Calculi

More detailed examination, with more sophisticated methods, was required to identify the true composition of the stones. An acid extract of the stones showed the characteristic UV absorption spectrum of 2,8-dihydroxyadenine at pH 2 and 10. Further identification was obtained by high-voltage electrophoresis and chromatography, as previously described by Simmonds *et al.* (1976b). These same methods had been used earlier to identify the presence of 2,8-dihydroxyadenine in the urinary sediment and gravel of the second patient identified with APRT deficiency (Van Acker *et al.*, 1977a,b).

1.7.3. Purine Metabolites in the Urine and Plasma

The more detailed examination of purine metabolites excreted in the urine in the members of the second known family (Van Acker *et al.*,

1977a,b), led to the identification of the same metabolic abnormality in the 7-year-old brother of the propositus, who had no clinical symptoms whatever. Both siblings excreted increased amounts of adenine in the urine, amounting to 13.8 mg/24 hr for the propositus and 27 mg/24 hr for the unaffected brother. These values are more than 10–20 times the amount of adenine excreted by a normal adult. They also both excreted lesser amounts of 8-hydroxyadenine, 2.4 and 1.0 mg/24 hr, and substantial amounts of 2,8-dihydroxyadenine, 23.6 and 42.0 mg/24 hr. The amount of uric acid excreted, 120 and 291 mg/24 hr for the propositus and the unaffected brother, respectively, was within normal range. The plasma uric acid was 3.3 mg/dl in both brothers.

The same analytical methods were applied to the urine of the propositus in the third family (Barratt *et al.*, 1979; Simmonds *et al.*, 1979a,b). The molar proportions of the various purine compounds in the urine were: uric acid, 59.5%; xanthine, 2.6%; hypoxanthine, 3.0%; adenine, 11%; 8-hydroxyadenine, 5.2%; 2,8-dihydroxyadenine, 18.6%.

The total uric acid excretion was within the normal range for the child and was in the upper range of normal for one of her parents. Her serum urate was 4, while that of her parents was 5.0 and 3.0 mg/dl. Plasma uric acid concentration was also in the normal range in the two brothers. Adenine was present in detectable amounts only in the urine of the homozygote.

1.7.4. Adenine Phosphoribosyltransferase Activity in Erythrocytes

The activity of APRT in lysed erythrocytes in the family reported by Van Acker *et al.* (1977a,b) was less than 1% of the normal in the patient and his asymptomatic brother and was 53% of normal in the father and 47% of normal in the mother. In the patient described by Barratt *et al.* (1979) and Simmonds *et al.* (1979a), the value was 2.2% of normal in the propositus and 24 and 34% of normal in the parents. One older sibling also showed a value of 27%, well within the heterozygote range. These values are quite in agreement with previous studies (Kelley *et al.*, 1968), in which around one fourth of the normal activity was found in the carrier state for this disorder. At that time, it was postulated that the enzyme might well be a dimer and that only dimers containing both normal subunits would be enzymatically active to account for the relatively low values found in the heterozygotes.

1.7.5. Treatment

In the patient reported by Van Acker *et al.* (1977a,b), allopurinol at 10 mg/kg per 24 hr was effective in substantially reducing the excretion in the urine of 2,8-dihydroxyadenine to values around one third of those observed in the control period. Simultaneously, the excretion of free adenine more than doubled. The total amount of adenine and its metabolites could be substantially lowered by placing the patient on a diet low in purines. Under these conditions, with allopurinol, the 2,8-dihydroxyadenine virtually disappeared from the urine. This combination of allopurinol and a low-purine diet has maintained the patient free of stones. The simultaneous administration of alkali may have contributed to the failure of an earlier unsuccessful treatment with allopurinol, since the solubility of 2,8-dihydroxyadenine is decreased at alkaline pH (Simmonds *et al.*, 1979a).

In the patient of Barratt *et al.* (1979), a dose of 10 mg allopurinol/kg per 24 hr was ineffective in preventing formation of additional concretions in the urinary tract. The dose was therefore raised to 20 mg/kg per 24 hr, which did appear to be effective. The dose was subsequently reduced to 15 mg/kg per 24 hr for maintenance therapy, with cessation of the crystalluria.

1.7.6. Metabolic Significance

Unlike the consequences of gross deficiency of the analogous enzyme, HPRT (see Section 1.8), deficiency of APRT apparently had no effect on the rate of purine synthesis *de novo* either *in vitro* in lymphoblast lines selected for APRT deficiency, after mutagenesis (Spector *et al.*, 1978), or in the patients *in vivo*, as shown by the normal uric acid production. This observation in the homozygote provides further confirmation that the heterozygote state is also without significant metabolic effects. Its past association with certain members of families with gout is entirely fortuitous and reflects the population in which the screening test was conducted. Studies by Dean and Perrett (1976) show no difference in heterozygotic and normal erythrocytes in their ability to metabolize adenine at the low concentrations of adenine normally found in the serum, thus providing a biochemical basis for the observation that heterozygotes are essentially normal, since they can metabolize the available adenine adequately.

1.7.7. Frequency

A spectrophotometric determination of APRT activity in erythrocytes that is suitable for screening was presented by L. A. Johnson *et al.* (1977a), who found a frequency of 3 heterozygotes in 700 normal blood donors, an incidence of 1 in 233, not significantly different from that previously observed in patients with gout. The calculated frequency of the disease should therefore be 1 homozygote per 217,000 births, a frequency comparable to many other rare inborn errors of metabolism.

The discovery of an additional case of APRT deficiency reported from the same laboratory over such a short period of time also indicates that this metabolic defect may indeed be more common than has previously been suspected, and that the routine test for uric acid in urinary concretions may be quite inadequate and responsible for our failure to identify the patients homozygotic for APRT deficiency. An additional clinical observation that could be of help to the urologist in identifying this condition is the observation that uric acid stones are hard and tend to be yellow, while 2,8-dihydroxyadenine stones are friable and gray-blue on being crushed. Any child with urinary calculi that give a positive test for uric acid should also have the calculus examined more closely by UV absorption spectrum at pH 2 for the possible presence of 2,8-dihydroxyadenine.

1.8. Hypoxanthine-Guanine Phosphoribosyltransferase Deficiency

The present state of our knowledge of the relationship of the clinical presentation to the metabolic aberrations associated with HPRT deficiency and the mechanism responsible for the various clinical features of the disease was reviewed recently by Seegmiller (1976a,b), Fox (1976), Galton *et al.* (1977), Kelley and Wyngaarden (1978), McKeran and Watts (1978), Becker (1979), and Astakhova and Usova (1977), and was presented at several recent symposia (*Ciba Foundation Symposium No. 48*, 1977; Müller *et al.*, 1977a,b).

1.8.1. Genetic Heterogeneity

The genetic heterogeneity of the disease is apparent at both clinical and basic levels of consideration. The clinical presentation of severe neurological involvement with choreoathetosis, spasticity, mental retardation, compulsive self-mutilation, and marked overproduction of uric acid still constitutes the classic Lesch–Nyhan syndrome; however, the mental retardation generally seems to be rather minimal in most cases. Recently, sporadic phenocopies have been found without HPRT deficiency (Nyhan, 1978, personal communication). The compulsive self-mutilation is also quite variable from time to time, and in age of onset, and reflects in part the severity of the basic HPRT deficiency. The possibility of modifier genes that may affect the expression of the neurological features of the disease must also be considered (Edelstein *et al.*, 1978).

Additional evidence has been presented for the genetic heterogeneity in the mutation occurring at the HPRT locus. A very pertinent indication of this heterogeneity is the amount of enzymatically inactive protein present that reacts with antibody produced against highly purified HPRT.

Upchurch *et al.* (1975) reported a normal amount of immunologically cross-reactive material in 1 of 14 patients and no detectable cross-reacting protein in the remaining 13, raising the possibility of a defect in synthesis or an enhanced degradation of the mutant enzyme protein. Bakay *et al.* (1977b) found no immunologically cross-reactive material in two patients who had 2.5 and 4.6% of normal HPRT activity in their erythrocytes, while hemolysates from a patient with 50% of normal activity did contain substantial amounts of cross-reactive protein. Evidently, in some cases, the mutant gene is able to produce an enzymatically inefficient product that does not react with antibody against the normal enzyme. In a sensitive radioimmunoassay capable of detecting and quantitating as little as 20 ng HPRT, Ghangas and Milman (1975) found no detectable immunologically cross-reacting protein in HPRT-deficient hemolysates in 15 of 16 patients with the Lesch–Nyhan syndrome. Only 1 patient's hemolysates showed a normal amount of such material.

Fox and Lacroix (1977) found a different pattern of isozymes in hemolysates from four patients with partial HPRT deficiency, as compared with the normal. The patients' patterns were also different from each other. These observations suggest that electrophoretic variation is a common occurrence in this mutation and support the existence of structural gene mutations with genetic heterogeneity in this disorder.

Willers *et al.* (1977) showed the expected correlations among degree of HPRT deficiency, [^{14}C]hypoxanthine uptake, and resistance to growth inhibition by 8-azaguanine of fibroblast strains from patients with severe and with partial HPRT deficiency. They also confirmed the greater heat lability of HPRT from patients compared with that of normal subjects.

1.8.2. Enzyme Characteristics

A subunit molecular weight of 34,500 was reported for HPRT enzyme purified from human erythrocytes by Arnold and Kelley (1971), while that from mouse was 27,000 (Hughes *et al.*, 1975) and from hamster 25,000 (Olsen and Milman, 1974a). This disparity was resolved when Olsen and Milman (1974b) showed a resolution of the single band obtained from human erythrocytes by Arnold and Kelley (1971) by separation on sodium dodecyl sulfate–polyacrylamide gels with the HPRT activity being associated with a minor component of subunit molecular weight 26,000. The native enzyme purified by Olsen and Milman (1977) 13,000-fold from human erythrocytes had a molecular weight of 81,000–83,000, as determined by sedimentation equilibrium centrifugation. Again, a subunit molecular weight of 26,000 was found, suggesting that the native enzyme is a trimer. The amino acid composition was determined and three peaks of enzyme activity were found on isoelectric focusing at positions corresponding to pHs of 5.6, 5.7, and 5.9. The enzyme immunoprecipitated from HeLa or human lymphoblast extracts after two-dimensional polyacrylamide gel electrophoresis displayed only a single spot located at the same position as the most basic of the erythrocyte isoenzymes focusing at pH 5.9, while that from erythrocyte lysates showed two major spots (Ghangas and Milman, 1977). These differences suggest that the isoenzyme of red cells results from posttranscriptional modification of the primary gene product. The possibility of deamidation of the HPRT enzyme with aging of erythrocytes was proposed. The HPRT in hemolysate from a Lesch–Nyhan patient migrated to an even more basic position, indicating a mutation of the structural gene.

New insight into the nature of the genetic events that accompany the development of HPRT deficiency in human cells and in their revertants was obtained by Milman et al. (1976) from studies using two-dimensional polyacrylamide gel electrophoresis (O'Farrell, 1975). From HeLa cells, he selected 24 HPRT-deficient mutant clones by using thioguanine as a selective agent after mutagenizing with ethyl methanesulfonate or N-methyl-N'-nitro-N-nitrosoguanadine for 24 hr. After the cells were labeled with [^{35}S]methionine, a two-dimensional polyacrylamide gel electrophoresis was performed and the protein location identified by radioautography or by staining for protein. The untreated HeLa cells, and the crude or purified red cell HPRT, showed a protein spot on the gel that coincided in position, indicating the same molecular weight of 26,000, and the same charge with an isoelectric focusing position of pH 6. As might be expected, it was the only protein spot missing from 24 HeLa mutants lacking HPRT activity. One additional mutant with less than 0.10% HPRT enzyme activity showed the full amount of antigenic HPRT protein and migrated to a different position on the two-dimensional gels. The protein disappeared on passing the extract through Sepharose-conjugated antibody to HPRT, indicating that it is an altered form of HPRT that may be a missense mutant (Milman et al., 1976).

Detailed study of HPRT revertants provided new insight into the basic genetic events responsible (Milman et al., 1976). Five independently isolated revertants of the single mutant clone mentioned above showed spots corresponding to that of the wild-type HeLa HPRT as well as that of the mutant clone extract. The appearance of the two spots suggests that the revertants may synthesize HPRT from two separate genes, one producing the wild-type protein and the other producing the mutant protein. The revertants also differed from the wild-type HeLa in producing a high frequency of spontaneously arising HPRT-deficient clones, which retained the mutant enzyme, while no spontaneous HPRT mutants occurred from wild-type. Presumably, the HPRT protein must have been synthesized from a newly activated and previously silent wild-type gene. A similar type of activation was reported by Bakay *et al.* (1973) and by Croce *et al.* (1973) in hybrid cells. A similar finding by Kahan and DeMars (1975) was attributed to a derepression of the inactive X chromosome in human female cells hybridized with mouse cells. In more detailed studies, Milman *et al.* (1977) found evidence for the presence of the aforementioned mutant protein, as compared with the wild-type.

1.8.3. Enzyme Assays

L. A. Johnson *et al.* (1977b) reported a simplified spectrophotometric assay based on a measurement of residual hypoxanthine remaining after reaction with the red cell lysate, in which both the lysate protein and the inosine monophosphate produced in the reaction are removed by precipitation with lanthanum phosphate. Giacomello and Salerno (1977) described a continuous spectrophotometric analytical system in which oxidation of NADH is measured in a coupled series of reactions generating pyruvate. They propose its use for screening red cell lysates for HPRT deficiency. Singh *et al.* (1976) reported a micromethod for determining HPRT activity in amniotic cells cultured directly on microtest plates, which are then used as reaction vessels for measuring the activity of 500–10,000 cells. Radioactive reaction products are then separated by thin-layer chromatography and should allow prenatal diagnosis of Lesch–Nyhan syndrome to be made within 7–10 days of the time of amniocentesis. Hösli *et al.* (1977) described the use of an ultramicromethod in which cells are cultured on plastic sheets and, after lyophilization, leaflets containing 5 cells are cut away and incubated with substrate in a volume of 0.3 μl. The diagnosis of an affected male fetus was thus made by examining 50 cells and confirmed on cells grown from the fetus aborted at 20 weeks with prostaglandin. The radioautographic method (Fujimoto *et al.*, 1968) was applied directly to amniotic cells cultured on cover slips to provide a more rapid and definitive identification not only of hemizogotes but also of heterozygotes from the presence of normal and mutant cells (Halley and Heukels-Dully, 1977).

The range of mutational events impairing the HPRT enzyme function is obviously large and influences the clinical presentation. Sweetman *et al.* (1977b) described a diminished affinity of HPRT enzyme for purine substrates in a patient with gout. This raises the possibility of additional such K_m mutations being missed in gouty patients because of the conventional routine use of saturating concentrations for measurement of enzyme activity.

One new observation by Willers *et al.* (1977) was an increase of up to 3-fold in HPRT activity after lyophilization and extraction of the sediment of lysed fibroblasts from patients with the Lesch–Nyhan syndrome and the variants. No such activation was observed in fibroblasts from healthy controls. This observation suggested a possible association of HPRT with the cell membranes with a rearrangement of the active site of the enzyme during its release from the membrane after lyophilization. An analogous activation of the deficient enzyme, on being mixed with normal enzymes, on electrophoresis in gels had been reported earlier by Bakay and Nyhan (1972).

Rozen et al. (1977) described, as part of a general diagnostic method using fibroblasts, a method of identifying HPRT deficiency in affected fibroblasts. The ratio of incorporation of [^{14}C]hypoxanthine/[^{3}H]thymidine into trichloracetic-acid-insoluble material was between 0 and 4% of the ratio obtained in normal fibroblasts.

Detailed studies allowed the identification of families in which a new mutation has occurred (McKeran et al., 1975; Francke et al., 1976; Bakay et al., 1977a). A substantially lower frequency of new mutations in mothers of affected children was found than would be expected on theoretical grounds, with some suggestion that the mutation may have come from the germ line of a maternal grandfather of affected children (Francke et al., 1976). Morton and Lalouel (1977) raised some objections to possible ascertainment bias in the identification of the families involved and pointed out the need to use segregation analysis for such studies. These objections were met in a response by Francke et al. (1977).

Mizuno et al. (1976) reported the autopsy of a patient with Lesch–Nyhan syndrome, which again, as with previously reported autopsies, showed no specific pathological features except delayed physical development. New observations were the presence of calculi, presumed from their staining properties to be xanthine scattered in the kidneys, brain, thymus, and thyroid glands; yet no symptoms of calculi of the urinary tract had been observed during life. Another curious aberration noted was the finding of a normal activity of HPRT in the liver but grossly deficient activities in all other tissues. The renal calculi were identified as 65–75% xanthine with traces of phosphate by analysis with column chromatography. Strauss et al. (1978) used DEAE–dextran as an effective helper agent for allowing entry of purified HPRT enzyme into deficient cells to achieve between 3 and 4% of the normal cellular enzyme activity in cultured Chinese hamster cells.

1.8.4. Genetic Transformation

Chromosomes were used to provide the HPRT locus to HPRT-deficient Chinese hamster fibroblasts (McBride and Ozer, 1973), and the same type of transfer of genetic information with chromosomes was achieved using the HPRT-deficient mouse cell (Degnen *et al.*, 1976). Mukherjee *et al.* (1978) were able to increase the frequency of genetic transformation by isolated chromosomes as much as 10-fold by enclosing the chromosome in phospholipid vesicles.

An instability of the chromosomes in an HPRT-deficient line of Chinese hamster cells was described by Nebola and Spurna (1977), with a higher frequency of deletions and rearrangements of some heterochromatic segments of the X chromosomes than in the parental strain.

1.8.5. Neurological Disorders

The precise way by which a gross deficiency of HPRT enzyme leads to the severe neurological and behavior abnormalities in this disease continues to be a provocative and challenging area for investigation. In contrast to the elevated activities of dopamine-β-hydroxylase activity in the plasma of 3 Lesch–Nyhan patients noted by Rockson *et al.* (1974), Lake and Ziegler (1977) found low activities of dopamine-β-hydroxylase averaging 51% of normal activity in plasma of 14 Lesch–Nyhan patients. Despite an elevated pulse rate, the children with Lesch–Nyhan syndrome showed normal concentrations of norepinephrine in plasma, no elevation in concentrations immediately after venipuncture, and a diminished increment compared with controls on assuming a sitting position. The explanation proposed for these observations is the relative disuse from infancy of the sympathetic nervous system in Lesch–Nyhan patients because of the lack of demand for noradrenergic responsiveness to standing posture, thus resulting in a diminished need for synthesis of norepinephrine and its synthetic enzymes.

Another approach to investigation of the central nervous system abnormalities in this disease was suggested by Mizuno and Yugari (1974, 1975), who reported cessation of self-mutilation on administration of 5-hydroxytryptophan (5-HT) to children with the Lesch–Nyhan syndrome. Workers in England (Frith *et al.*, 1976) and the United States (Ciaranello *et al.*, 1976) were unable to confirm this observation. Nyhan (1976, 1977) and Sweetman *et al.* (1977a) investigated the metabolic and behavioral effects of administration of 5-HT with and without carbidopa (MK-486), an inhibitor of the decarboxylase responsible for removing 5-HT from the peripheral circulation. By preventing peripheral metabolism, carbidopa promotes prolonged higher concentrations of 5-HT in the serum and the central nervous system. They also measured the end product of 5-HT metabolism, the excretion of 5-hydroxyindoleacetic acid (HIAA) in the urine. While Mizuno and Yugari (1975) reported excretion of normal amounts of HIAA in the urine of their four patients, Sweetman *et al.* (1977a) found a mean value for HIAA excretion in nine patients with

Lesch–Nyhan syndrome to be 8.6 μg/kg creatinine, which was significantly greater than the mean value of 5.1 found for five normal males of similar age. The administration of 5-HT resulted in a large increase in excretion of HIAA, which was approximately proportional to the amount of 5-HT administered. The simultaneous administration of carbidopa greatly reduced excretion of HIAA, indicating that peripheral decarboxylation and oxidation of 5-HT was the major source of urinary HIAA.

The effect of this combined therapy with two drugs on the behavior of patients with the Lesch–Nyhan syndrome was variable. Some patients showed no response, while most responded. However, despite increased dosage, all developed tolerance to 5-HT within a 3-month period. An unusual and unexpected finding was a 4-fold increase in glycine excretion of children receiving carbidopa, with no consistent changes in other amino acids. Three of five patients showed an increase in plasma glycine concentrations on treatment with carbidopa; however, the values did not exceed the normal range found in plasma. These results suggest the possibility that carbidopa may inhibit glycine metabolism, as well as the aromatic amino acid decarboxylase. The investigative use of 5-HT was reviewed by Zarcone and Guilleminault (1977).

HPRT-deficient neuroblastoma cells in culture and HPRT-deficient mouse glioma cells showed an increased intracellular concentration of glycine, a putative neurotransmitter (Skaper and Seegmiller, 1976b, 1977).

Another metabolic abnormality that has been found so far only in cultured cells deficient in HPRT enzyme is a decrease in monoamine oxidase activity. This decrease was observed in cultured human fibroblasts (Breakefield *et al.*, 1976; Roth *et al.*, 1976; Edelstein *et al.*, 1978), as well as in a mouse neuroblastome line cultured *in vitro*, in which the mutation for HPRT deficiency had been selected (Breakefield *et al.*, 1976), and in rat glioma cell lines in which the HPRT mutation had been selected (Skaper and Seegmiller, 1976a). The amount of enzyme activity varied with the stage of growth and species (Hawkins and Breakefield, 1978). Of special interest was the observation of an enhanced supernormal activity of monoamine oxidase in fibroblasts from the patient of Catel and Schmidt (1959) and reported later by Manzke (1976), who showed no evidence of self-mutilation, although he was severely incapacitated with cerebral palsy (Edelstein *et al.*, 1978).

Children with the Lesch–Nyhan syndrome are incapable of learning from aversive stimuli (Anderson *et al.*, 1977). A similar behavior abnormality in the Brattelboro rat carrying a genetic deficiency in vasopressin can be corrected by administering vasopressin. This learning deficit in children with the Lesch–Nyhan syndrome is overcome in part if the children are given an intranasal solution of a long-lasting vasopressin analogue (Anderson *et al.,* 1979). The drug, however, was ineffective in preventing the self-mutilating behavior of Lesch–Nyhan children. Jochmus *et al.* (1977) reported some success in modifying the self-destructive behavior of affected children by establishing an alternative behavior. Arima (1976) reported on the involuntary movement.

The presence of a similar pattern of self-mutilation among patients with Gilles de la Tourette syndrome with their compulsive tics and abusive foul language prompted investigation of HPRT activity in patients with this disorder. Van Woert *et al.* (1977) found no difference in the activity of either enzyme in fresh hemolysates from 18 normal subjects and 17 patients with Gilles de la Tourette syndrome; however, on isoelectric focusing, these investigators reported multiple peaks of enzyme activity that were not found in erythrocyte lysates of normal subjects. They postulated the presence of a "factor" that would alter the isoelectric point of HPRT in erythrocytes. 5-HT and carbidopa greatly reduced the self-mutilation and tics in some of the affected patients, leading these workers to conclude, without convincing evidence, that HPRT enzyme may be less stable than normal in these affected children. G. G. Johnson *et al.* (1977) examined by isoelectric focusing the HPRT in red cell lysates of six unrelated male patients with the Gilles de la Tourette syndrome. All six showed normal total HPRT activity, and this enzyme was separable into multiple isoenzyme forms by electrophoresis and electrofocusing that were indistinguishable from HPRT enzyme patterns of normal individuals.

1.8.6. Attempts to Produce a Hypoxanthine-Guanine-Phosphoribosyltransferase-Deficient Mouse

A major deterrent to detailed investigation of the mechanism by which HPRT deficiency produces the neurological symptoms in the human is the inaccessibility of the central nervous system. A novel approach toward obtaining an experimental model of this disease was made by Dewey *et al.* (1977). These investigators made use of the observation that teratocarcinoma cell lines of mice cultured *in vitro* can be inserted into the blastocyst of another genetic strain of mouse, which then allows the previously malignant cells to participate successfully in normal embryogenesis, and tumor-free viable mosaic mice are obtained (Mintz and Illmensee, 1975). Implantation of an HPRT-deficient line of teratocarcinoma cells selected *in vitro* raised the possibility of obtaining chimeric mice that are mosaic for HPRT deficiency. This has now been obtained by Dewey *et al.* (1977). Retention of the severe HPRT deficiency in the differentiated state was documented in extracts of mosaic tissue by a depressed specific activity of the enzyme and also by the presence of unlabeled clones in autoradiographs of explanted cells incubated with [³H]hypoxanthine. In some mosaic mice, certain tissue showed the mutant strain cell. The low frequency of HPRT-deficient cells found in blood suggests the presence of a particularly strong selection against the HPRT mutation in the developing hematopoietic system of the mosaic mice, which is in agreement with the absence of HPRT-deficient cells in the hematopoietic system of human heterozygotes who are also mosaics for the severe deficiency (Nyhan *et al.*, 1970).

The obtaining of a line of mice carrying the HPRT-deficient gene for generating the Lesch–Nyhan syndrome would be dependent on the mutant cell line's being incorporated into the germ cell line of the mosaic. Such an incorporation into the germ cell was observed in early studies by Mintz and Illmensee (1975). The remarkable implications of this development are discussed by Heath (1978).

1.8.7. Mechanism of Excessive Purine Synthesis

The mechanism by which a deficiency of HPRT leads to an excessive rate of purine production has been further clarified. The central role of an increased intracellular concentration of PP-ribose-P in determining the activity of the presumed rate-limiting reaction of the enzyme PP-ribose-P amidotransferase and its additional controlling role as a rate-limiting substrate for this enzyme (Seegmiller, 1976a) continues to dominate the prevailing views (Becker, 1979; Fox and Kelley, 1978; Fox, 1976; Kelley and Wyngaarden, 1978; Wyngaarden, 1976).

New insight into more details of the mechanism of purine overproduction has come from the work of Hershfield and Seegmiller (1977) and Thompson *et al.* (1978a,b). Normal lymphoblasts deprived of hypoxanthine are capable of increasing their rate of purine synthesis to produce large amounts of purines quite comparable to the amount produced by HPRT-deficient cells from children with the Lesch–Nyhan syndrome. Deprivation of hypoxanthine also increases intracellular concentration of PP-ribose-P so that the underlying mechanism may still center on the key role of this metabolite. It also serves to accentuate the importance of hypoxanthine reutilization from peripheral blood as a normal factor suppressing the rate of purine synthesis *de novo*. A very high turnover rate of hypoxanthine has been demonstrated in the human in previous studies (Engelman *et al.*, 1964; Sorensen, 1970).

The availability of hypoxanthine as a determinant of the rate of purine synthesis provides a unifying concept for the bases of purine overproduction in two well-defined enzyme defects of childhood. The virtual absence of HPRT makes children with the Lesch–Nyhan syndrome unable to reutilize hypoxanthine, while children with immunodefi-

ciency disease from PNP deficiency (see Section 1.4 and Fig. 2) are unable
to generate hypoxanthine from inosine (Cohen *et al.*, 1976; Thompson *et
al.*, 1978a,b). Earlier reports of an enhanced rate of PP-ribose-P synthesis
through an increased activity of the enzyme PP-ribose-P synthetase in cells
from children with the Lesch–Nyhan syndrome (Graf *et al.*, 1975; Martin,
D. W., and Maler, 1976; Reem, 1975) are not in agreement with the
earlier work of Rosenbloom *et al.* (1968) or Becker *et al.* (1973), nor were
they supported by more recent work by Reem (1977) or by Benke and
Dittmar (1977). The latter workers showed a curious stimulation of PP-
ribose-P synthetase activity by the addition of aminopterin to HPRT-
deficient cells. This stimulation can best be explained by the block in
purine synthesis *de novo* produced by aminopterin, since the same effect
was observed by blocking purine synthesis *de novo* with azaserine (Barankiewicz and Henderson, 1977) (Section 1.2.2). Whether or not a similar
stimulation in PP-ribose-P synthetase activity is produced by the orotate
used in the assay of Graf *et al.* (1975) remains to be determined.

1.8.8. Other Metabolic Correlations

A low serum folate concentration of HPRT-deficient patients
prompted Giliberti *et al.* (1977) to investigate indices of folate metabolism
in such a patient. Loading tests with glycine resulted in a substantially
smaller increase in plasma concentration of serine than was seen in the
three normal control subjects. Excretion of formiminoglutamic acid in the
24-hr urine was around twice the normal value and was increased over 6-
fold by a load of histidine, while the value in the normal urine was
increased only 5-fold. The urinary excretion of aminoimidazole carboxamide in the 24-hr urine was 3- to 6-fold greater than that of control
subjects, but was not significantly altered by loads of methionine, serine,
glycine, or histidine.

Lowy and Williams (1977) demonstrated a 10- to 35-fold increase in
[^{14}C]formate labeling of inosinic acid on addition of aminoimidazole
carboxamide to both normal and HPRT-deficient cells. Presumably, this
substance is phosphorylated by APRT and then acts as a receptor for
formyl groups, and provides a potential way to circumvent the HPRT
deficiency in purine reutilization.

1.9. Increased Phosphoribosyl-1-Pyrophosphate Synthetase Activity

An increased activity of PP-ribose-P synthetase is another cause of
increased intracellular PP-ribose-P concentration and purine overproduc-

tion in some patients with gouty arthritis. This separate mutation provides additional confirmation of the important role of PP-ribose-P concentration in the regulation of purine synthesis *de novo*. Again, genetic heterogeneity is found in the types of mutations giving rise to the increase in PP-ribose-P synthetase. In one family (Sperling *et al.*, 1978a), the mutation affects the regulatory site on the enzyme and produces a decreased ability to respond to normal concentrations of feedback inhibitors. In others, it produces an alteration at the catalytic site that in one family increases the affinity of the enzyme for ribose-5-phosphate, while in still other families it results in a high specific activity of the enzyme with normal kinetics (Becker, 1976, 1977; Becker *et al.*, 1977).

1.9.1. Enzyme Characteristics

The enzyme PP-ribose-P synthetase was purified to homogeneity and the effects of substrate activators and inhibitors on the quaternary structure of the enzyme were assessed by Becker *et al.* (1977) and L. J. Meyer and Becker (1977). It is composed of single polypeptide subunits of molecular weight 33,200 that undergo a reversible self-association to a number of polymeric states under the influence of enzyme concentration and various ligands. Aggregated forms containing 2, 4, 8, 16, and 32 subunits have been identified. Association to the 16 and 32 subunits results from incubation of the enzyme with magnesium ion, inorganic phosphate, magnesium ATP, or purine nucleotide inhibitors of activity as well as reaction products. Increased enzyme concentration also favors more extensive subunit self-association. The largest aggregated forms of the enzyme composed of 16 and 32 subunits are fully active, while the monomeric and smaller aggregated forms containing 2, 4, and 8 subunits show a minimal or no enzyme activity, leading to the conclusion that the activity of PP-ribose-P synthetase in cells resides in the largest aggregates. The inhibitory effects of the purine nucleotides ADP and GDP appear to result from a direct inactivation of the larger enzyme aggregates rather than from interference with the aggregation process itself. On the other hand, the inhibitor 2,3-diphosphoglycerate may well be exerting its effect through a disassociation of the enzyme into smaller inactive forms, although this possibility remains to be proved.

1.9.2. Inheritance

The pedigree of two families carrying increased PP-ribose-P synthetase has been compatible with either autosomal or X-linked transmission. More definitive evidence of X-linkage would be provided by the demonstration of both normal and mutant cell types in fibroblasts cultured from a heterozygote female resulting from the random inactivation of one of the two X chromosomes. Zoref *et al.* (1975, 1977a,b) presented evidence suggestive of both normal and mutant cell populations in fibroblasts cultured from the mother of two affected patients. The evidence was based largely on the greater resistance of the mutant cells to a lethal decrease in purine synthesis produced by methylmercaptopurine ribonucleoside.

More direct evidence of two such cell populations was presented by Yen *et al.* (1978), who cloned out fibroblast sublines from the daughter of an affected patient. Some clones showed the normal activity found in her mother's cells; others showed the increased activity characteristic of her father's cells. Her erythrocyte lysates showed activities of PP-ribose-P synthetase quite comparable to that of her father and her affected paternal uncle. Two bands of enzyme activity corresponding to the normal and mutant PP-ribose-P synthetase were found in fibroblast lysates from the daughter after electrophoresis on cellulose acetate strips. In contrast, only mutant enzyme was detectable in fibroblast lysates derived from the father or from the daughter's cloned fibroblasts carrying high activity, and only the normal enzyme pattern was found on electrophoresis of her clones carrying the normal enzyme activity. These studies provide convincing evidence for assigning the structural gene for human PP-ribose-P synthetase to the X chromosome. The failure to find evidence of normal enzyme in erythrocytes or lymphocyte lysates from the daughter suggests either nonrandom X-chromosomal inactivation in precursors of these cells or selection against hematopoietic cells bearing the normal enzyme, after the random X-chromosomal inactivation that occurs early in zygote development.

1.9.3. Biochemical Studies

Evidence was found for the participation of PP-ribose-P as a determinant of the rate of purine synthesis *de novo* in normal epitheliallike liver cells maintained in long-term culture (Bashkin and Sperling, 1978). Factors known to increase PP-ribose-P synthesis such as incubation with a high inorganic phosphate concentration resulted in acceleration of purine synthesis. At the physiological concentrations of inorganic phosphate, the concentration of ribose-5-phosphate was not limiting for PP-ribose-P synthetase. Similar results were found from studies of rat liver *in vivo* by Lalanne and Henderson (1975).

Blinov *et al.* (1976) reported a decrease of PP-ribose-P synthetase associated with a low intracellular concentration of PP-ribose-P in erythrocytes of patients with microspherocytic and hypoplastic anemia. A spectrophotometric assay for PP-ribose-P synthetase was described by Ferrari *et al.* (1978).

1.10. Xanthinuria

More general interest in disorders of purine metabolism character-ized by hypouricemia has resulted in an increasing number of patients with hypouricemia associated with xanthinuria being detected (Kelley, 1975b) (see also Section 1.5). This diagnosis is now of importance in that it identifies persons who have around a 30% chance of developing concre-tions of the urinary tract composed of xanthine. It should not be a deterrent to pregnancy (Chalmers, 1977).

1.10.1. Conditions Associated with Hypouricemia

The determination of the urinary excretion of uric acid and oxypu-rines must be made to distinguish xanthinuria from hypouricemia result-ing from an enhanced rate of excretion of uric acid either induced by drugs such as chlorprothixene ingestion in excess (Weinshilboum *et al.*, 1975) or from genetic abnormalities in tubular reabsorption of urate (Simkin *et al.*, 1974). Hypouricemia is also found in patients with PNP deficiency (see Section 1.4).

1.10.2. Clinical Presentation

In 22 of the 35 patients with xanthinuria reported to date, the disease has been asymptomatic, while 13 patients developed symptoms of uroli-thiasis. Frayha *et al.* (1977) reported 3 new patients with hereditary xanthinuria and reviewed the 27 previously known cases. In 2 siblings, the disease was asymptomatic and detected by the discovery of hypouricemia while the familial hyperlipidemia was being evaluated. In a second family, xanthinuria was discovered in a 66-year-old man who gave a history of having passed a urinary calculus in 1973 that was not analyzed, with no recurrences since that time.

Yokoyama *et al.* (1977) reported an additional patient from Japan, a 9-year-old boy, whose parents were first cousins, who presented with a 1-year history of recurrent colic, right flank pain with nausea and vomiting, and acute urinary retention. Physical examination showed, in addition to a distended bladder, a palpable small bean-size hard mass along the urethra at the penoscrotal junction, which was also detected by peripheral calcifi-cation on X ray. The mass was readily replaced into the bladder and then removed by cystotomy. It consisted of a hard brown stone measuring 11 × 9 × 16 mm and weighing 0.2 g. It showed lamellar structure, was brown to chocolate in color and was composed of 93.8% xanthine. Serum urate was 1.2–1.4 mg/dl. The identification of xanthine in the calculus was made by mass spectrometry, UV spectrophotometric measurements, and atomic absorption analysis.

The urine contained over 60 times as much oxypurine as uric acid and 20 times the normal amount. The ratio of hypoxanthine to xanthine was 1:4.6. These investigators report having found 52 cases of xanthine stone in the literature, 14 of which were reported in Japan, with xanthine calculi appearing at ages ranging from infancy to over 70 years of age.

Other clinical symptoms have included muscle pain, cramps, and myopathy in 3 and arthritis in 3, presumably secondary to the demonstrated accumulation of xanthine crystals in the tissues (Seegmiller, 1978a). The renal clearance of xanthine was 6 times greater than that of hypoxanthine.

Auscher *et al.* (1977a,b) reported briefly a family with 4 siblings afflicted with xanthinuria, 2 of whom had developed xanthine lithiasis and a 5th with gouty arthritis and uric acid kidney stones.

Sperling *et al.* (1978b) reported a gouty patient with partial deficiency of HPRT who passed xanthine stones in the urine while taking 300 mg allopurinol/day. On this dose of allopurinol, his 24-hr urinary uric acid decreased from pretreatment values of 1450 mg/24 hr to 600 mg/24 hr, but as would be expected with an HPRT-deficient patient, total purine synthesis was not decreased substantially. The deficit in uric acid excretion appeared as oxypurines (hypoxanthine plus xanthine), which increased to an excretion of 600 mg/24 hr. This is the first report of xanthine stones in a gouty patient treated with allopurinol, although several reports of xanthine stones in Lesch–Nyhan patients treated with allopurinol have appeared (Seegmiller, 1976b).

1.11. Gouty Arthritis

The many varied facets of gouty arthritis were included in recent reviews (Wyngaarden and Kelley, 1976, 1978; Kelley, 1977a,b; Honig *et al.*, 1977; Seegmiller, 1976a, 1978a; Rodnan, 1977; Becker, 1979), in an international symposium of purine metabolism (Müller *et al.*, 1977a,b), and at an international workshop (Scott and Hiisi-Brummer, 1975).

1.11.1. Hyperuricemia

The recognition that hyperuricemic body fluids are supersaturated with response to monosodium urate is not often emphasized (Watts,

1977). The hyperuricemia required for the precipitation of urate crystals in tissues and the development of gouty arthritis is generated by both environmental and genetic factors. The long-suspected possibility that the correlation of obesity with gout might be a result of a more discerning palate and greater ability of such patients to enjoy their food and drink was raised by Kahn (1976) (Editorial, 1976). No change in their appreciation of gustatory or olfactory sensations was brought about by lowering their serum urate concentration.

The magnitude of the environmental contribution is demonstrated by the marked increase in hyperuricemia and gout noted with the development of more affluent societies. Such an increase occurred in Japan concurrent with the adoption of a more Western style of dietary habits since World War II (Nishioka *et al.*, 1974, 1975). The incidence of hyperuricemia and gout is also increasing less dramatically in Western Europe. Increases in serum urate since World War II have been noted in populations in Germany and Britain (Scott *et al.*, 1977) and in Finland (Isomäki and Von Essen, 1977). Among blacks in South Africa, no gout was found, but the serum urate increased with increasing sophistication of lifestyle as shown in comparative values from rural villages to urban centers (Beighton *et al.*, 1977). In Copenhagen, de Muckadell and Gyntelberg (1976) showed an increased frequency of gout. They found a surprising reversal in the perception of the disease generally held in that gout was more prevalent among the lower social class males, than in those of the upper classes. A detailed study of the Maoris by B. S. Rose (1975) also implicates a Western diet and lifestyle as being the major cause of the very high frequency of gout among the Maoris.

Current examples of environmental factors causing hyperuricemia have been presented. A recent case of saturnine gout, porphyrinuria, and lead nephropathy described by Orfanos and Künzig (1975) occurred in a printer after prolonged professional exposure to lead. Infusion of calcium EDTA produced a significantly higher excretion of lead in his 24-hr urine than in the 24-hr urine of a control subject. Much more common causes of hyperuricemia are the diuretics used in treatment of hypertension and cardiac failure (Healey, 1977). In studies of a recent series of 300 men, Helgeland *et al.* (1978) found a correlation among increases in serum triglycerides, in serum urate concentrations, and in body weight with thiazide treatment. Ethambutol used in treatment of tuberculosis is also known to cause a hyperuricemia, and Self *et al.* (1977) described the development of acute gouty arthritis in such a patient. Niemi (1977) described the unusual problems of a woman receiving the diuretic furosemide, which is also known to increase serum urate concentrations. She developed a panniculitis of the anterior aspects of her legs associated with a subcutaneous fat necrosis as the only cutaneous signs of gout. She gave no history of articular symptoms and none was present, but urate crystals surrounded by granulomata were found on biopsy of the affected subcutaneous area.

1.11.2. Diagnosis

The diagnosis of gouty arthritis continues to be based largely on clinical features of the disease. In 85–95% of patients with gout, urate crystals can be identified in the synovial fluid by inspection under cross-polarizing filters under the microscope. However, examples are known in which initial arthrocentesis failed to show the presence of urate crystals only to have them demonstrated on a subsequent tap 5–24 hr later (Schumacher *et al.*, 1975). Microcrystals of monosodium urate were found within the phagocytic cells of a synovial biopsy upon examination with electron microscopy, even though no crystals were detected with ordinary light microscopy.

The American Rheumatism Association has presented diagnostic criteria for gout (Wallace *et al.*, 1977). Sales (1977) also provided a number of guidelines to avoid common diagnostic pitfalls in the diagnosis of gouty arthritis.

Simkin (1977) presented a provocative theory to account for several puzzling clinical features of gout in which the urate would be concentrated within the joint to create more supersaturated conditions during the resolution of traumatic or other effusions as a result of the rate of egress of urate from the effusion being about half that of water.

The value of xeroradiography in defining more precisely bony erosions in an extreme case of gouty arthritis was reported by Mödder and Künzig (1976), although X rays are of value only to a limited extent generally and then in rather far advanced cases of gout. Resnick (1977) presented a detailed and helpful review of the radiographic manifestations of gouty arthritis.

Needle biopsy with detailed examination of the fluid under cross-polarizing filters and of the tissue specimen by both light and electron microscopy was of value in showing the early changes of synovial membrane in both gout and chondrocalcinosis (Lenz *et al.*, 1976). Rosenthal (1977) reported on the value of a simple commercial system "urotest" available for demonstrating the presence of birefringent crystals in tissues or synovial effusions, using polarizing filters.

A most unusual report in this day and age records consecutive stages of progression in joint destruction over the years 1962–1975 in 250 patients with gout followed at the Institute of Rheumatology in Warsaw, Poland (Kawenoki-Minc *et al.*, 1975, 1977). It is difficult to understand how such a failure in therapy could occur in light of our present knowledge. No mention of the cause is made in the text, and the authors concluded that sodium urate deposits in articular tissues determine the progression of arthropathy. A phalangeal metastasis from bronchogenic carcinoma was described by Vaezy and Budson (1978) in a patient who presented with symptoms suggestive of gouty arthritis.

1.11.3. Disorders Associated with Gout

Eckes (1975) reported the simultaneous occurrence of cirrhosis, sarcoidosis, and gout in three additional patients. He raised the possibility that a common genetic factor may underlie the cirrhosis and gout and that the sarcoidosis is pathogenetically unrelated. Against such an association was the finding of hyperuricemia in only 7 of 52 men and 3 of 63 women with cirrhosis. These findings suggest that hyperuricemia is not a common characteristic of sarcoid arthritis (Lambert and Wright, 1977). Three patients with a rather unusual complication of gout, the development of a carpal tunnel syndrome, were reported by Pledger *et al.* (1976), Künzer (1975), and Wolfensberger (1976), and were treated by surgical decompression.

Hyperuricemia and gout found in a patient with Down's syndrome were attributed to a low renal clearance of uric acid (Nishida *et al.,* 1976). Subsequently, no difference in serum urate or PP-ribose-P concentration was found in blood samples collected from 20 institutionized patients with Down's syndrome in Japan, as compared with 16 mentally retarded subjects matched for age and sex at the same institution (Nishida *et al.,* 1977).

1.11.4. The Kidney and Gout

The role of the kidney in generation of hyperuricemia and conversely the role of hyperuricemia in the development of gouty nephropathy or kidney stones were reviewed by Holmes and Kelley (1975), Emmerson and Row (1975), Emmerson (1976), Gonick (1977), Klinenberg (1977), Fleisch *et al.* (1976), Bluestone *et al.* (1977), and Simmonds (1979). The latter author describes a subgroup of young gouty female patients who show distinctive dominantly inherited familial renal lesions and are unable to concentrate urine and show no hypertension.

Urate crystals are common in the urine of neonates, and colic associated with urinary uric acid crystals is occasionally seen in the newborn nursery. Urate crystals are also frequently seen at autopsy in the renal pyramids of newborn infants, regardless of the cause of death. Yet urate nephropathy as the cause of renal insufficiency in the newborn infant has been reported only rarely (Raivio, 1976). Such an entity was invoked to account for renal failure in three infants presenting with oliguria, a marked hyperuricemia, and renal enlargement seen on intravenous pyelography or [^{131}I]hippuran renography with very slow visualization of the renal outline and absence of appearance of contrast material in the bladder. The pyelography also appeared to be therapeutic, presumably by reason of the osmotic diuresis produced by the contrast material (Ahmadian and Lewy, 1977).

Another pediatric problem that has emerged is the increased uric acid excretion that results from administration of high doses of purine-rich pancreatic extract to patients with cystic fibrosis. Nousia-Arvanitakis *et al.* (1977) were able to achieve a therapeutic effect with lower doses of pancreatic extract that did not lead to complications from hyperuricosuria.

The relatively frequent finding of an association between hyperuricemia and development of calcium-containing stones of the urinary tract has been noted for many years (Coe, 1977). J. L. Meyer *et al.* (1976) provided some evidence that seed crystals of anhydrous uric acid can induce epitaxial crystal growth of calcium oxalate monohydrate from its metastable supersaturated solution. Despite the close similarities between the crystal lattices of some faces of the two crystal types, the induction period required for such heterogenous nucleation by the seed material was about half the time required for spontaneous precipitation in the absence of such agents. This fact has created some doubt as to whether crystals of uric acid have an influence on the formation of calcium oxalate lithiasis in the short period of time that it resides within the renal collecting system. Pak *et al.* (1977) provided evidence that supersaturation of sodium urate occurs in urine at urate concentrations above 300 mg/liter and pH above 6.0. These results suggest that a nidus of sodium urate could potentially form in the urine of such patients and serve as seed crystals for the subsequent precipitation of calcium-containing stones. This would account for the fact that such stones, rather than uric acid, are formed in some patients with a normal calcium and excessive uric acid excretion in the urine, and would also explain the beneficial effects of allopurinol treatment noted by Coe (1977) (see Section 1.11.8).

Simmonds *et al.* (1976a) presented evidence that the pig kidney eliminates uric acid by filtration and secretion only. Logan *et al.* (1976) propose use of the woolly monkey as a primate model for investigation of enzyme replacement strategies in gout, since it lacks uricase.

1.11.5. Association of Hyperuricemia and Vascular Disease

Hyperuricemia has long been recognized as a risk factor in vascular disease; however, in recent years, most investigators have relegated it to the concurrent hyperlipidemia that accompanies hyperuricemia, and have not regarded it as an independent risk factor.

A reconsideration of this association is appropriate in view of the report of a multicenter combined study showing a 46% reduction in mortality from recurrent myocardial infarction produced by treatment with sulfinpyrazone, a uricosuric drug (Sherry et al., 1978). Among 733 patients with a recent myocardial infarction treated with sulfinpyrazone (800 mg/day), the death rate was 5.1% as compared with 9.5% among 742 placebo-treated patients. Of particular significance was the fact that the frequency of recurrent myocardial infarctions was not altered, but rather the survival from the attacks was substantially increased, by sulfinpyrazone therapy. The authors attribute this to the specific effect of sulfinpyrazone in reducing the adhesiveness of platelets. It also suggests the possibility that sulfinpyrazone treatment might alter the outcome in other patients with their first acute myocardial infarction.

In view of these remarkable results, a more detailed survey is presented of involvement of the cardiovascular system in patients with gout. Most rheumatologists are impressed with the increased frequency with which they see calcification of the major vessels in patients with gouty arthritis.

Ginsberg et al. (1977b) described an interaction between crystals of monosodium urate and platelets that proceeds in two phases: (1) a secretory phase involving the rapid, active release of serotonin, ATP, and ADP with little loss of lactic dehydrogenase or β-glucuronidase, followed by (2) a lytic phase involving the slower loss of all platelet constituents. Both phases are inhibited by iodoacetate or dinitrophenol, suggesting an energy requirement for the process. An electron photomicrograph showed lysis of washed platelets that appeared to contain crystals. The possibility that a similar type of interaction might be occurring at a variety of sites of urate crystal deposition, leading to release of platelet constituents as a component stage in the pathogenesis of gouty inflammation or atherosclerosis, was suggested.

A substantial increase in platelet count and aggregation induced by either ADP or thrombin in platelet-rich plasma from rats made hyperuricemic with a diet rich in nucleic acids and including oxonate was reported by Winocour et al. (1976, 1977). Of particular note, however, was the fact that the serum urate of these treated animals (3.5 mg/dl) was substantially lower than the saturation level required in the human for formation of monosodium urate crystals; therefore, the effect may well be mediated by the urate molecule rather than by crystals. May and Robert (1975) reported on the frequency with which attacks of gout and attacks of angina or acute myocardial ischemic episodes are correlated in patients with gout, and interpret it as evidence of the "gouty heart," presumably because of the presence of deposits of urates within the heart. Newland

(1975) provided a hypothetical mechanism by which this could occur in which hyperuricemia leads to an increased aggregation of platelets as an initial event in thrombosis and thus increases the incidence of thrombosis and arterial disease in hyperuricemic persons. He proposed that the hypouricemic action of some oral anticoagulants may be a part of their effectiveness in treatment of thromboses and occlusive arterial disease. A recurrent phlebitis responding to colchicine was described in a hyperuricemic nongouty patient (Pasero, 1977). Additional references from the older literature pertinent for consideration of the association of cardiovascular disease and hyperuricemia include the following: a report of a patient with primary gout with myocardial involvement by Pund *et al.* (1960), a decreased platelet survival time in patients with gout (Mustard *et al.*, 1963), specific vascular changes in gout by Traut *et al.* (1954), a tophus in the mitral valve in gout by Bunim and McEwen (1940), and reference to the gouty heart by Hench and Darnell (1933).

1.11.6. Association of Hyperuricemia with Avascular Necrosis of the Femoral Head

The association of hyperuricemia with avascular necrosis of the head of the femur was studied by Mielants *et al.* (1975) in 35 patients with this disorder. Patients with avascular necrosis showed a significant increase in the concentration of triglycerides, cholesterol pre-β lipoprotein, and uric acid in the serum. Although the serum urate was higher in the 3 patients with gout in this series, no significant difference was observed between the lipid and lipoprotein concentrations in the gouty patients as compared with the nongouty patients in this series. They found no statistical difference between the lipid, lipoprotein, and uric acid levels in patients with avascular necrosis receiving corticosteroids or using alcohol as compared with those not taking these drugs, and proposed that the initiating event may well lie in the lipid disturbance. A larger series of patients was reviewed by Lequesne *et al.* (1975). They found 14 cases of avascular necrosis of the femoral head among 651 patients with gout over a 10-year period. Among these gouty patients, there was a clear preponderance in males and a slight tendency to be bilateral and occurrence at a slightly earlier age than in the nongouty. The gout always preceded the necrosis by an average of 7½ years. Only one patient gave an obvious history of a painful crisis in the hip that could be attributed to acute gout. Affected patients tended to have increased triglycerides and hypercholesterolemia, and the mechanism proposed is a formation of microparticulate fatty emboli that may obstruct, among others, the terminal arteries of the femoral head.

1.11.7. Acute Attack of Gout

Malawista (1977) reviewed details of gouty inflammation in which a greater role is proposed for urate crystal deposition in the periarticular tissues than in the intraarticular space. Ginsberg *et al.* (1977a) reported the absorption of lysomal enzymes to monosodium urate crystals following the crystal-induced dissolution of peripheral blood leukocytes. The possible role of protein absorption to monosodium urate, calcium pyrophosphate dihydrate, and silica crystals in the pathogenesis of the induced inflammation was discussed by Kozin and McCarty (1976).

1.11.8. Treatment

The treatment of gout was reviewed by Seegmiller (1974), Scott (1977), and Kelley (1975a,c, 1976). The drug benzbromarone has been in use for several years in Europe as maintenance therapy for controlling the serum urate of patients with gouty arthritis (Heel *et al.*, 1977). The mechanism of its action is shown to be a uricosuria with a 4-fold increase in clearance of urate with respect to creatinine over control values achieved within 2–4 hr of drug administration with a drop in the mean serum uric acid of 6 patients from control values of 7.8 to 4.3 within 24 hr. The uricosuric action was completely blocked by pyrazinamide and partially inhibited by acetyl salicylic acid or sulfinpyrazone. No elevation of urinary oxypurines was observed following benzbromarone ingestion (Sinclair and Fox, 1975). Similar results were obtained by Sorensen and Levinson (1976). Bröll *et al.* (1975) maintained 34 gouty patients on benzbromarone, including 2 women and 32 men, between the age of 32 and 66 years, for over 6 months with reduction of the mean serum urate from 7 to less than 4 mg/dl by the 4th week of treatment. A total of 32 patients showed a positive therapeutic effect. This was achieved in 16 patients with 100 mg daily, in 8 patients with 150 mg daily, and in 10 patients with 200 mg daily. It was well tolerated. In only 2 patients was the medication discontinued because of diarrhea.

Ascorbic acid has been identified in the past as a natural substance that may be responsible for development of nonurate chromogens in the serum when urate determinations are performed by the colormetric methods (Seegmiller, 1974). Another effect of ascorbic acid was described by Stein *et al.* (1976). A dose of 4 g produced a substantial uricosuria with over a 100% increase in fractional clearance of uric acid. In 3 subjects who ingested 8 g ascorbic acid for 3–7 days, the serum urate decreased by 1.2–3.1 mg/dl as a result of a sustained uricosuria. With the tendency of ascorbic acid to produce a very acid urine, it could also conceivably contribute to development of calculi of the urinary tract. Conger and Falk

(1977) concluded from studies of rats treated with diuretics and the uricase inhibitor oxonic acid that a high renal tubular fluid flow, whether induced by solute or water diuresis, is a primary mechanism of protection against acute uric acid blockade of the renal tubules. In their study, alkalinization of the urine played a relatively minor preventive role.

The effectiveness of several newer antirheumatic drugs in controlling acute attacks of gout has been evaluated. Fenoprofen calcium administered for a duration not exceeding 8 days was a very effective drug in 27 patients with 36 joints affected with acute gouty arthritis (Wanasukapunt et al., 1976). Ibuprofen was very effective in treatment of a stubborn case of polyarticular gout (Franck and Brown, 1976). Sturge et al. (1977) found naproxen to be as effective as phenylbutazone in terminating acute attacks of gout of 41 patients in a multicenter trial in Britain.

Briney et al. (1975) presented evidence of arrest of renal deterioration and in some instances actual improvement of renal function after adequate control of uric acid production and serum urate concentrations have been achieved with allopurinol administration. Even though the allopurinol is a very effective therapeutic agent, it may cause many serious side effects. These include arteritis, toxic epidermal necrolysis, interstitial nephritis, agranulocytosis, and granulomatous hepatitis, as well as the less serious gastrointestinal intolerance, skin eruptions, and hematologic abnormalities. In some patients, symptoms have suggested a malignant disease. Calin (1978) described a patient who gave a history of 3-month weight loss, anorexia, weakness, nonspecific abdominal pain, and an abnormal increase in carcinoembryonic antigen suggesting a malignancy. He had been receiving diuretic therapy for fluid retention and allopurinol medication for his hyperuricemia and suspected gout. A scheduled laparotomy was canceled when he developed a vasculitis associated with an elevation of serum creatinine. By stopping all therapy, the patient made a dramatic medical recovery, with complete restoration of weight and health. Appelboom and Famaey (1977) found the same therapeutic effects in 30 patients with gout, whether allopurinol was administered in 3 doses of 100 mg each through the day or as a single tablet of 300 mg taken each morning. Such a result would be expected from the long half-life of the oxidation product, oxipurinol, in the body.

The effectiveness of allopurinol in preventing calcium oxalate stone formation (see Section 1.11.4) was further evaluated in a group of patients by Coe (1977). In agreement with his earlier report, treatment with thiazide or allopurinol, or both, over a period of 625 patient years, reduced the frequency of new stone formation from an expected value of 220 to 22. A group of 34 patients without discernible metabolic disturbances and treated only with increased fluid intake and dietary advice formed 29 new stones, compared with a predicted 33. A similar group of

30 patients treated with thiazide and allopurinol formed 6 stones, compared with a predicted 32. Coe concluded that the combination of thiazide and allopurinol is an effective way to prevent recurrent calcium oxalate stone formation.

With the frequent association of hyperuricemia and gout in patients receiving thiazide diuretics, a new diuretic, antihypertensive drug related in structure to ethacrynic acid, which also has uricosuric action, holds promise of simplifying therapy of some patients (Reese and Steele, 1976). This drug, ticrynafen, was used in a double-blind study to treat 20 hypertensive patients on a 6-week regime of either ticrynafen or hydrochlorothiazide. Of particular interest was the striking decrease of serum urate to less than half the pretreatment level in patients receiving ticrynafen. Both groups showed a similar reduction in blood pressure, in body weight, and in serum potassium. This drug was well tolerated (Nemati *et al.*, 1977). Similar results were reported by Lemieux *et al.* (1977) with the additional observation of the development of a metabolic alkalosis and a hypocalciuria. Ticrynafen is also capable of inhibiting urate secretion by the renal tubule of the dalmatian dog.

Colchicine still holds a venerable position as a specific drug for treatment of acute gout; however, the precise mechanism of action of colchicine is still not well understood. It interferes with microtubule formation within the cell. The filamentous arrangement of proteins of high molecular weight localized along the intracellular microtubules was disrupted by colchicine treatment of cultured 3T3 cells (Sherline and Schiavone, 1977). An antagonistic effect of adenosine and colchicine on cell shape was noted in hamster lung fibroblasts or SV 40-transformed 3T3 cells. This effect was apparently not mediated by changes in intracellular cAMP concentrations (Yin and Berlin, 1975). The induction of amyloid in the mouse by casein injection can be successfully blocked by the administration of colchicine (Shirahama and Cohen, 1974). Cortese *et al.* (1977) used podophyllotoxin, another substance that arrests mitoses, as a probe for the colchicine-binding site on tubulin.

1.11.9. Metabolic Factors That Contribute to Hyperuricemia

By measurement of the 24-hr excretion of uric acid on a diet virtually free of purines (Seegmiller, 1974, 1976a,b; Watts, 1977), an inherent metabolic and genetically determined overproduction of uric acid as a major cause of hyperuricemia can be readily detected provided the patient has good renal function. Around 10–15% of gouty patients show evidence of excretion of uric acid in excess of 600 mg/day, according to a panel of clinicians (Watts, 1977). The percentage of patients with purine overproduction is increased in patients with onset of gout at an early age.

In 26 patients with juvenile gout, ages 15–34, Babucke and Mertz (1976) found that half of them excreted more than 600 mg uric acid/24 hr on a purine-free diet, with a mean value of 828 ± 128, and the reminder showed a mean value of 432 ± 133 mg/24 hr. Of these patients, 7 showed a uric acid/creatinine ratio greater than 0.5 with a mean value of 0.67, ranging from 0.5 to 1.45. These patients also showed a higher serum urate of 10 compared with the 19 hypoexcretors who showed a serum urate of 9.

Chanard et al. (1977) proposed another method for evaluating the rate of purine synthesis de novo in which the incorporation of [^{14}C]formate into formyglycinamide ribonucleotide (FGAR) in circulating blood lymphocytes in vitro after treatment of the cells with azaserine was used. Among 27 patients with gout not taking allopurinol, FGAR synthesis was normal in 5 and increased in all the others. FGAR synthesis was decreased in all patients with renal failure, whatever the therapy. However, FGAR synthesis remained increased in patients with primary gout complicated with renal insufficiency.

A novel theory for a function for xanthine and uric acid as regulators of plasma hypoxanthine concentration by acting as inhibitors of xanthine oxidase was proposed by Smythe (1977). The oxidation of hypoxanthine by xanthine oxidase is competitively inhibited by xanthine at physiologic concentrations. The fact that this is also a substrate and is itself converted to uric acid in place of hypoxanthine was not elaborated on. They proposed that urate was an inhibitor of xanthine oxidase as well. With its $K_{i_{urate}}$ equivalent to 27 mg/dl, the inhibition expected at the concentration of urate usually encountered would be minimal. However, Bergman (1978, personal communication) maintains that uric acid is not an inhibitor of xanthine oxidase.

Alterations of carbohydrate metabolism are known to influence the rate of formation of uric acid. Forster and Hoos (1977) reported consistent production of hyperuricemia and increased purine synthesis in man and in oxonate-treated rats by rapid infusion of fructose, sorbitol, or xylitol. Allopurinol pretreatment prevents the rise in serum urate in man induced by xylitol. A complication of the clinical use of xylitol has been development of calcium oxalate deposits in the renal tubules found at autopsy. These findings led Hauschild et al. (1976) to investigate the organic acids excreted in the urine after xylitol infusion. An increase in glycolic and tetronic acids occurred after xylitol infusion, but not with glucose infusion. However, there was no evidence of any increase in oxalate excretion in any of the patients studied.

The absence of glucose-6-phosphatase in patients with Type 1 glycogen storage disease (Von Gierke's disease) is associated with a marked hyperuricemia and overproduction of uric acid. Benke and Gold (1978) reported a substantial decrease in [^{14}C]glycine incorporation into urinary uric acid with a lowered intracellular concentration of PP-ribose-P of erythrocytes on the addition of continuous nocturnal oral feedings by vivonex infusion. It also enhanced the renal excretion of uric acid, as would be expected from the accompanying decrease in serum lactate. They concluded that such management could very well reduce the risk of developing gouty arthritis. Roe and Kogut (1977) showed a decrease in serum urate and in blood inorganic phosphate as a result of fructose infusion in five patients with Type 1 glycogen storage disease. No change in uric acid excretion in the urine was produced; however, glucagon injection increased uric acid excretion and serum urate concentrations with a lowering of blood inorganic phosphate. They proposed an enhanced purine nucleotide catabolism, a lowered intracellular phosphate, and a resulting increase in purine synthesis as the cause of the hyperuricemia and excessive purine synthesis of these children.

The known enzyme defects associated with purine overproduction in gouty patients were reviewed by several authors (Becker, 1976; Seegmiller, 1976a,b, 1978a; Kelley, 1977b; Wyngaarden and Kelley, 1978). Models of additional enzyme defects that could cause purine overproduction have come from studies of drugs that increase the rate of purine synthesis *in vivo,* by interfering with the interconversions of purine nucleotides (see Section 1.2.2). The genetically determined deficiency of these enzymes has not yet been identified, but might well account for some of the patients with gout and purine overproduction.

1.12. Decreased Adenylate Deaminase Activity

Kar and Pearson (1973) reported diminished activity of adenylate deaminase in muscle biopsies of eight patients with Duchenne muscular dystrophy, an X-linked disease. Values obtained in two obligate heterozygotes were slightly below the range found in biopsies of six control subjects. The low values were associated with decreased creatine kinase, noncollagen protein, and severely affected muscles in only one patient with Duchenne dystrophy, but were found in three patients with myotonic dystrophy, one patient with inflammatory myopathy, and three patients with miscellaneous myopathies. Properties of the enzyme purified 20,000-fold to homogeneity from red cells were described by Yun and Suelter (1978).

1.13. Abnormalities of Pyrimidine Metabolism

Earlier studies by Geiger and Yamasaki (1956) provided some evidence in support of cytidine and uridine being important metabolites generated by the liver for use by the brain. T. F. J. Martin and Tashjian (1978) have now provided evidence that thyrotropin-releasing hormone increases uridine phosphorylation, but not its uptake by rat pituitary cells cultured *in vitro*. They therefore infer that this hormone must be a modulator of uridine kinase activity of these cells.

A new agent of possible value for study of pyrimidine metabolism was described by Swyryd *et al.* (1974). This compound, N-(phosphonacetyl)-L-aspartate, is an analogue of the activated complex in the reaction catalyzed by aspartate transcarbamylase and is a potent and specific inhibitor of the enzyme with a K_i of 1×10^{-9} M. Resistance to the drug is accompanied by a large increase in the aspartate transcarbamylase activity in the mutant cells.

1.13.1. Ammonia and Pyrimidine Nucleotide Synthesis

Although ammonia is not the physiological substrate for the first enzyme of pyrimidine synthesis, cytoplasmic carbamylphosphate synthetase, it is a substrate for the mitochondrial enzyme carrying out the synthesis of this substance. The excretion of orotic acid in the urine of patients with a variety of metabolic disorders, leading to an accumulation of ammonia, is presumed to act by stimulating carbamylphosphate synthesis within the mitochondria. At the high concentrations generated, carbamylphosphate then leaks into the cytoplasm where it is a rate-limiting substrate for pyrimidine nucleotide synthesis. Further evidence of such a pathway was provided by Colombo *et al.* (1977) from studies of enzymes of ammonia detoxication after a portacaval shunt in the rat. This operation produced a 2-fold increase in plasma ammonia and a 2- to 4-fold increase in excretion of orotic acid in the urine, accompanied by a 10- to 30-fold increase in activity of carbamylphosphate synthetase, a 2½-fold increase in aspartate transcarbamylase, and a 2- to 3-fold increase in ornithine carbamyltransferase within 30 days after the portacaval shunt.

1.13.2. Pyrimidine 5′-Nucleotidase Deficiency

It seems likely that deficiency of PNT, first described by Valentine *et al.* (1974), will prove to be a fairly common cause of nonspherocytic hemolytic anemia. The normal enzyme was purified to 250,000-fold from human erythrocytes (Torrance *et al.*, 1977c). It shows a molecular weight of 28,000 by gel filtration, with a K_m of purified enzyme of 10 μM, compared with 40 μM when measured in hemolysates. Inorganic phosphate was a competitive inhibitor of the enzyme, and its presence in hemolysate may be responsible for increasing the K_m of the enzyme under these conditions. Torrance *et al.* (1977b) described a simple and rapid radiometric assay for the enzyme that is based on the binding of unreacted [^{14}C]cytidine monophosphate to the barium sulfate precipitate used in the deproteinizing process.

Several additional new patients were reported, including two cases by Torrance et al. (1977b), three cases in a Japanese family (Miwa et al., 1977), and one from South Africa (Torrance et al., 1977a). Rosa et al. (1977) reported a new case in a large family from Guadalupe in the West Indies. In each case, the patient presented with a chronic hereditary hemolytic anemia with marked basophilic stippling associated with a high glutathione content of the cell. The enzyme activity of the deficient red cells ranged from 4 to 14% of normal, and in each family reported, an intermediate activity of the enzyme in erythrocytes of both parents was found, indicative of a recessive mode of inheritance. The presence of an alteration in the electrophoretic pattern, a difference in heat stability as affected by pH, and a difference in K_m from that of the enzyme from normal subjects is evidence of a structural gene mutation.

Paglia et al. (1977) extended their earlier studies to evaluate the metabolic significance of an inhibition of PNT they noted in patients with lead poisoning. They found a general correlation between the blood lead concentration and the degree of inhibition of PNT, with values 13–28% of the mean activity in normal control erythrocytes. Even greater degrees of inhibition of the enzyme activities were found when compared with normal blood specimens of comparably increased reticulocytes in young cells. Most of the patients had a mild or moderate anemia, and moderate basophilic stippling, evident in Wright-stained peripheral smears. The greatest accumulation of pyrimidine-containing nucleotides occurred in the two patients with the highest blood lead concentration.

1.13.3. Orotic Aciduria

No additional cases of primary hereditary orotic aciduria due to deficiency of orotate decaboxylase and orotate phosphoribosyltransferase have been reported, but the condition was reviewed by Kelley and Smith (1978). The appearance of a secondary orotic aciduria in other metabolic disturbances continues to be taken as an indicator of deranged pyrimidine nucleotide metabolism. Cohen et al. (1977) described a modest orotic aciduria consisting of a greater than 6- to 8-fold increase in urinary orotic acid excretion in two children with hereditary immunodeficiency disease, associated with PNP deficiency. Since adenosine toxicity in cultured cells creates an excretion of orotic acid associated with a very low intracellular concentration of PP-ribose-P, Snyder et al. (1977, 1978) proposed that the presence of orotic aciduria in these children reflects a lowered intra-cellular PP-ribose-P in at least some cells of the body. Potassium oxonate treatment of mice produced a 10- to 30-fold increase in the urinary excretion of orotic acid (Mangoff and Milner, 1978).

1.14. Abnormalities of DNA Repair (Xeroderma Pigmentosum)

The clinical symptoms of this disease, consisting of sunlight-induced pigmentation abnormalities and numerous malignancies on areas of the skin exposed to sunlight, are produced by a rare autosomal recessive defect in enzymes involved in the excision and repair of DNA damaged by UV irradiation. Progressive mental retardation, degeneration of the nervous system with motor incoordination, and other neurological abnormalities are seen in some patients. The clinical and biochemical features were reviewed by Robbins et al. (1974) and Cleaver (1978). Cell fusions of fibroblasts cultured from certain pairs of patients result in a mutual repair of the defect, demonstrating the heterogeneity of the genetic lesion. The number of complementation groups so identified that are indicative of separate mutations that can cause defective DNA repair was increased from four (Kraemer et al., 1975a) to five (Kraemer et al., 1975b).

The defect is present in the peripheral lymphocytes, and permanent lymphoid lines have been established from affected patients (Andrews et al., 1974). Patients with the most severe neurological abnormalities had the least effective DNA repair (Andrews et al., 1976a; Cheng et al., 1976). Fibroblasts from affected patients show a greater reduction in ability to form colonies after UV irradiation than do normal strains, (Robbins et al., 1976). A similar type of inability has been noted in fibroblasts from patients with Cockayne's syndrome; however, these two disorders are clinically quite different, and the basis for the phenomena is not yet understood (Andrews et al., 1976b; Yoder et al., 1976). Heterokaryons, formed from fusing fibroblasts from affected patients belonging to different complementation groups, are as capable of restoring biological activity to UV-damaged adenovirus 2 as are normal cells, although the unfused cells show a diminished ability (Day et al., 1975). The abnormality in DNA repair evidently increases the cytotoxicity and mutagenicity of polycyclic hydrocarbon compounds in vitro (Maher et al., 1977).

1.15. Purine and Pyrimidine Compounds as Inhibitors of Viral and Cellular Proliferation

Constraints of space prevent any detailed discussion; however, a fairly detailed listing and description of antineoplastic and immunosuppressive drugs was presented by Sartorelli and Johns (1975).

1.15.1. Effective Clinical Treatment of Herpes Encephalitis with Adenine Arabinoside

The clinical effectiveness of adenine arabinoside in treatment of Type 1 herpes simplex encephalitis was evaluated by Whitley *et al.* (1977). In 28 patients in whom the diagnosis was proved by virus isolation from a brain biopsy, treatment reduced mortality from 70 to 28%. Furthermore, 50% of the survivors had only moderately debilitating or no neurological sequelae, and none of the treated patients showed any evidence of acute toxicity from the drug.

1.15.2. New Antiviral Agents

Elion *et al.* (1977) described a new type of antiviral drug that is a derivative of guanosine—acycloguanosine. It is phosphorylated by a virus specific kinase to the di- and triphosphates. The latter compounds inhibit viral DNA polymerase 10–30 times more effectively than cellular DNA polymerase and are effective in controlling herpes encephalitis in mice *in vivo*. Zamecnik and Stephenson (1978) reported another approach to antiviral therapy in which a tridecamer sequence of deoxynucleotides complementary to the reiterated terminal sequences of Rous sarcoma virus was used to inhibit production of this virus in virus-infected cultures of chick embryo fibroblasts. The same sequence was also an efficient inhibitor of translation of proteins specified by viral RNA (Stephenson and Zamecnik, 1978).

ACKNOWLEDGMENTS

This work was supported in part by grants AM-13622 and GM-17702 from the United States Public Health Service, and grants from the Kroc Foundation.

References

Ackeret, C., Plüss, H. J., and Hitzig, W. H., 1976, Hereditary severe combined immunodeficiency and adenosine deaminase deficiency, *Pediatr. Res.* **10**:67–70.

Agarwal, R. P., Sagar, S. M., and Parks, R. E., Jr., 1975, Adenosine deaminase from human erythrocytes: Purification and effects of adenosine analogs, *Biochem. Pharmacol.* **24**:693–701.

Agarwal, R. P., Spector, T., and Parks, R. E., Jr., 1977, Tight binding inhibitors—IV. Inhibition of adenosine deaminase by various inhibitors, *Biochem. Pharmacol.* **26**:359–367.

Ahmadian, Y., and Lewy, P. R., 1977, Possible urate nephropathy of the newborn infant as a cause of transient renal insufficiency, *J. Pediatr.* **91**:96–100.

Anderson, L., Dancis, J., Alpert, M., and Herrmann, L., 1977, Punishment learning and self-mutilation in Lesch–Nyhan disease, *Nature (London)* **265**:461–463.

Anderson, L. T., David, R., Bonnet, K., and Dancis, J., 1979, Passive avoidance learning in Lesch–Nyhan disease: Effect of a varopressin analogue, *Life Sci.* (in press).

Andrews, A. D., Robbins, J. H., Kraemer, K. H., and Buell, D. N., 1974, Brief communication: Xeroderma pigmentosum long-term lymphoid lines with increased ultraviolet sensitivity, *J. Natl. Cancer Inst.* **53**:691–693.

Andrews, A. D., Barrett, S. F., and Robbins, J. H., 1976a, Relation of D.N.A. repair processes to pathological aging of the nervous system in xeroderma pigmentosum, *Lancet* **1**:1318–1320.

Andrews, A. D., Yoder, F. W., Barrett, S. F., Petinga, R. A., and Robbins, J. H., 1976b, Cockayne's syndrome fibroblasts have decreased colony-forming ability but normal rates of unscheduled DNA synthesis after ultraviolet irradiation, *Clin. Res.* **24**:624A (abstract).

Appelboom, P., and Famaey, J. P., 1977, Allopurinol et hyperuricimie goutteuse: A propos de 30 cas traites par une dose quotidienne unique, *Bruxelles-Med.* **57**:133–137.

Arima, M., 1976, Involuntary movement in Lesch–Nyhan syndrome, *Brain Nerv.* **28**:1170–1173.

Arnold, W. J., and Kelley, W. N., 1971, Human hypoxanthine-guanine phosphoribosyltransferase, *J. Biol. Chem.* **246**:7398–7404.

Astakhova, L. N., and Usova, I., 1977, Pathogenesis, clinical picture, diagnosis and treatment of Lesch–Nyhan syndrome, *Pediatriya* **3**:86–89.

Auscher, C., deGery, A., Pasquier, C., and Delbarre, F., 1977a, Xanthinuria, lithiasis and gout in the same family, *Adv. Exp. Med. Biol.* **76A**:405–411.

Auscher, C., Pasquier, C., de Gery, A., Weissenbach, R. and Delbarre, F., 1977b, Xanthinuria: Study of a large kindred with familial urolithiasis and gout, *Biomed. Express (Paris)* **27**:57–59.

Babucke, G., and Mertz, D. P., 1976, The hypoexcretors and hyperproducers of uric acid among juvenile gout patients, *Med. Welt* **27**:558–562.

Bakay, B., and Nyhan, W. L., 1972, Activation of variants of hypoxanthine-guanine phosphoribosyltransferase by the normal enzyme, *Proc. Natl. Acad. Sci. U.S.A.* **69**:2523–2527.

Bakay, B., Croce, C. M., Koprowski, H., and Nyhan, W. L., 1973, Restoration of hypoxanthine phosphoribosyl transferase activity in mouse IR cells after infusion with chick-embryo fibroblasts, *Proc. Natl. Acad. Sci. U.S.A.* **70**:1998–2002.

Bakay, B., Francke, U., Nyhan, W. L., and Seegmiller, J. E., 1977a, Experience with detection of heterozygous carriers and prenatal diagnosis of Lesch–Nyhan disease, *Adv. Exp. Med. Biol.* **76A**:351–358.

Bakay, B., Graf, M., Carey, S., and Nyhan, W. L., 1977b, Study of immunoreactive material in patients with deficient HPRT activity, *Adv. Exp. Med. Biol.* **76A**:361–369.

Barankiewicz, J., and Henderson, J. F., 1977, Effect of lowered intracellular ATP and GTP concentrations on purine ribonucleotide synthesis and interconversion, *Can. J. Biochem.* **55**:257–262.

Barratt, T. M., Simmonds, H. A., Cameron, J. S., Potter, C. F., Rose, G. A., Arkell, D. G., and Williams, D. I., 1979, Complete deficiency of adenosine phosphoribosyltransferase: A third case presenting as renal stones in a young child, *Arch. Dis. Child.* (in press).

Bartlett, G. R., 1977a, Adenine: Chemistry, analytical methods, sources, purity, and specifications, *Transfusion* **17**:333–338.

Bartlett, G. R., 1977b, Biology of free and combined adenine: Distribution and metabolism, *Transfusion* **17**:339–350.

Bartlett, G. R., 1977c, Metabolism by the rabbit of intravenously administered adenine, *Transfusion* **17**:351–357.

Bartlett, G. R., 1977d, Formation of oxyadenine metabolites in the rabbit after intravenous administration of adenine, *Transfusion* **17**:358–366.

Bartlett, G. R., 1977e, Metabolism by man of intravenously administered adenine, *Transfusion* **17**:367–373.

Bashkin, P., and Sperling, O., 1978, Some regulatory properties of purine biosynthesis *de novo* in long-term cultures of epithelial-like rat liver cells, *Biochim. Biophys. Acta* **538**:505–511.

Becker, M. A., 1976, Patterns of phosphoribosylpyrophosphate and ribose-5-phosphate concentration and generation in fibroblasts from patients with gout and purine overproduction, *J. Clin. Invest.* **57**:308–318.

Becker, M. A., 1977, Fibroblast phosphoribosylpyrophosphate and ribose-5-phosphate concentration and generation in gout with purine overproduction, *Adv. Exp. Med. Biol.* **76A**:270–279.

Becker, M. A., 1979, Abnormalities of PRPP metabolism leading to an overproduction of uric acid, in: *Handbook of Experimental Pharmacology* (I. M. Weiner and W. N. Kelley, eds.) (in press).

Becker, M. A., Meyer, L. J., and Seegmiller, J. E., 1973, Gout with purine overproduction due to increased phosphoribosylpyrophosphate synthetase activity, *Am. J. Med.* **55**:232–242.

Becker, M. A., Meyer, L. J., Huisman, W. H., Lazar, C., and Adams, W. B., 1977, Human erythrocyte phosphoribosylpyrophosphate synthetase: Subunit analysis and states of subunit association, *J. Biol. Chem.* **252**:3911–3918.

Beighton, P., Solomon, L., Soskolne, C. L., and Sweet, M. B. E., 1977, Rheumatic disorders in the South African Negro. Part IV: Gout and hyperuricaemia, *S. Afr. Med. J.* **51**:969–972.

Benke, P. J., and Dittmar, D., 1976, Purine dysfunction in cells from patients with adenosine deaminase activity, *Pediatr. Res.* **10**:642–646.

Benke, P. J., and Dittmar, D., 1977, Phosphoribosylpyrophosphate synthesis in cultured human cells, *Science* **198**:1171–1173.

Benke, P. J., and Gold, S., 1978, Purine metabolism in therapy of Von Gierke's disease, *Pediatr. Res.* **12**:204–206.

Biggar, W. D., Giblett, E. R., Ozere, R. L., and Grover, B. D., 1978, A new form of nucleoside phosphorylase deficiency in two brothers with defective T-cell function, *J. Pediatr.* **92**:354–357.

Blinov, M. N., Kamyshentsev, M. V., Luganova, I. S., Filanovskaia, L. I., and Filippova, V. N., 1976, Phosphoribosylpyrophosphate and its metabolic enzymes in the erythrocytes in certain forms of anemia, *Vopr. Med. Khim.* **22**:456–462.

Bluestein, H. G., Carson, D., Willis, R. C., Thompson, L. F., Matsumoto, S., and Seegmiller, J. E., 1979, Accumulation of deoxyribonucleotide as a possible mediator of immunosuppression in hereditary deficiency of adenosine deaminase and purine nucleoside phosphorylase, *J. Assoc. Am. Phys.* (in press).

Bluestone, R., Waisman, J., and Klinenberg, J. R., 1977, The gouty kidney, *Semin. Arthritis Rheum.* **7**:97–113.

Borgers, M., Vergaegen, H., DeBrabander, M., Thoné, F., Van Reempts, J., and Geuens, G., 1977, Purine nucleoside phosphorylase, a possible histochemical marker for T-cells in man, *J. Immunol. Methods* **16**:101–110.

Breakefield, X. O., Castiglione, C. M., and Edelstein, S. B., 1976, Monoamine oxidase activity decreased in cells lacking hypoxanthine phosphoribosyltransferase activity, *Science* **192**:1018–1020.

Briney, W. G., Ogden, D., Bartholomew, B., and Smyth, C. J., 1975, The influence of allopurinol on renal function in gout, *Arthritis Rheum.* **18**:877–881.

Bröll, H., Sochor, H., Tausch, G., and Eberl, R., 1975, Long-term therapy with benzbromarone in uric arthritis, *Wien. Med. Wochenschr.* **125**:546–548.

Brox, L. W., and Henderson, J. F., 1976, The "adenosine cycle" is not a significant route of purine metabolism in mammalian cells, *Can. J. Biochem.* **54**:200–202.

Bunim, J. J., and McEwen, C., 1940, Tophus of the mitral valve in gout, *Arch. Pathol.* **29**:700–704.

Burke, W. C., Chen, S.-H., Scott, C. R., and Ammann, A. J., Jr., 1977, Incorporation of purine nucleosides in cultured fibroblasts from a patient with purine nucleoside phosphorylase deficiency and associated T-cell immunodeficiency, *J. Cell. Physiol.* **92**:109–113.

Burridge, P. W., Paetkau, V., and Henderson, J. F., 1977, Studies of the relationship between adenosine deaminase and immune function, *J. Immunol.* **119**:675–678.

Calin, A., 1978, Allopurinol toxicity masquerading as malignancy, *J. Am. Med. Assoc.* **239**:497.

Carson, D. A., and Seegmiller, J. E., 1976, Effect of adenosine deaminase inhibition upon human lymphocyte blastogenesis, *J. Clin. Invest.* **57**:274–282.

Carson, D. A., and Seegmiller, J. E., 1977, Relationship of adenosine deaminase and nucleoside phosphorylase deficiency to immunodeficiency, *Arthritis Rheum.* **20**(Suppl.):S235–S240.

Carson, D. A., Goldblum, R., Keightly, R., and Seegmiller, J. E., 1977a, Immunoreactive adenosine deaminase (ADA) in cultured fibroblasts from patients with combined immunodeficiency disease, *Adv. Exp. Med. Biol.* **76A**:463–470.

Carson, D. A., Kaye, J., and Seegmiller, J. E., 1977b, Lymphospecific toxicity in adenosine deaminase deficiency and purine nucleoside phosphorylase deficiency: Possible role of nucleoside kinase(s), *Proc. Natl. Acad. Sci. U.S.A.* **74**:5677–5681.

Cartier, M. P., Hamet, M., and Hamburger, J., 1974, A new metabolic disease:

The complete deficit of adenine phosphoribosyltransferase and lithiasis of 2,8-dihydroxyadeine, *C. R. Acad. Sci. Paris* **279**:883–886.

Cass, C. E., Lowe, J. K., Manchak, J. M., and Henderson, J. F., 1977, Biological effects of inhibition of guanine nucleotide synthesis by mycophenolic acid in cultured neuroblastoma cells, *Cancer Res.* **37**:3314–3320.

Catel, V. W., and Schmidt, J., 1959, Über familiare gichtische Diathese in Verdendung mit zerebralen und renalen Symptomen bei eimem Kleinkind, *Dtsch. Med. Wochenschr.* **84**:2145–2147.

Chalmers, R. A., 1977, Xanthinuria and pregnancy, *Lancet* **2**:301.

Chanard, J., Kamoun, P., Pleau, J.-M., Brami, M., Brunois, J.-P., and Funck-Brentano, J.-L., 1977, Mesure de la biosynthèse *de novo* des bases puriques dans les hyperuricémies, *Nouv. Presse Med.* **6**:2579–2582.

Cheng, W. S., Andrews, A. D., Whang-Peng, J., and Robbins, J. H., 1976, Lymphocyte cell lines for study of spontaneous and UV-light-induced sister chromatid exchanges in xeroderma pigmentosum, *Clin. Res.* **24**:624A (abstract).

Ciaranello, R. D., Anders, T. F., Barchas, J. D., Berger, P. A., and Cann, H. M., 1976, The use of 5-hydroxytryptophan in a child with Lesch–Nyhan syndrome, *Child Psychiatry Hum. Dev.* **7**:127–133.

Ciba Foundation Symposium No. 48, 1977, *Purine and Pyrimidine Metabolism*, Elsevier/Excerpta Medica, North-Holland, Amsterdam.

Ciotti, M. M., Humphreys, S. R., Venditti, J. M., Kaplan, N. O., and Goldin, A., 1960, The antileukemic action of two thiadiazole derivatives, *Cancer Res.* **20**:1195–1201.

Cleaver, J. E., 1978, Xeroderma pigmentosum, in: *The Metabolic Basis of Inherited Disease* (J. B. Stanbury, J. B. Wyngaarden, and D. S. Frederickson, eds.), pp. 1072–1095, McGraw-Hill, San Francisco.

Coe, F. L., 1977, Treated and untreated recurrent calcium nephrolithiasis in patients with idiopathic hypercalciuria, hyperuricosuria, or no metabolic disorder, *Ann. Intern. Med.* **87**:404–410.

Cohen, A., Doyle, D., Martin, D. W., Jr., and Ammann, A. J., 1976, Abnormal purine metabolism and purine overproduction in a patient deficient in purine nucleoside phosphorylase, *N. Engl. J. Med.* **295**:1449–1454.

Cohen, A., Staal, G. E. J., Ammann, A. J., and Martin, D. W., Jr., 1977, Orotic aciduria in two unrelated patients with inherited deficiencies of purine nucleoside phosphorylase, *J. Clin. Invest.* **60**:491–494.

Cohen, A., Gudas, L. J., Ammann, A. J., Staal, G. E. J., and Martin, D. W., Jr., 1978a, Deoxyguanosine triphosphate as a possible toxic metabolite in the immunodeficiency associated with purine nucleoside phosphorylase deficiency, *J. Clin. Invest.* **61**:1405–1409.

Cohen, A., Hirschhorn, R., Horowitz, S. D., Rubinstein, A., Polmar, S. H., Hong, R., and Martin, D. W., Jr., 1978b, Deoxyadenosine triphosphate as a potentially toxic metabolite in adenosine deaminase deficiency, *Proc. Natl. Acad. Sci. U.S.A.* **75**:472–476.

Coleman, M. S., Donofrio, J., Hutton, J. J., Hahn, L., Daoud, A., Lampkin, B., and Dyminski, J., 1978, Identification and quantitation of adenine deoxynucleotides in erythrocytes of a patient with adenosine deaminase deficiency and severe combined immunodeficiency, *J. Biol. Chem.* **253**:1619–1626.

Colombo, J. P., Berüter, J., Bachman, C., and Peheim, E., 1977, Enzymes of ammonia detoxification after portacaval shunt in the rat, *Enzyme* **22**:391–398.

Conger, J. D., and Falk, S. A., 1977, Intrarenal dynamics in the pathogenesis and prevention of acute nephropathy, *J. Clin. Invest.* **59**:786–793.

Cortese, F., Bhattacharyya, B., and Wolff, J., 1977, Podophyllotoxin as a probe for the cholchicine binding site of tubulin, *J. Biol. Chem.* **252**:1134–1140.

Cozzarelli, N. R., 1977, The mechanism of action of inhibitors of DNA synthesis, *Annu. Rev. Biochem.* **46**:641–668.

Croce, C. M., Bakay, B., Nyhan, W. L., and Koprowski, H., 1973, Reexpression of the rat hypoxanthine phosphoribosyltransferase gene in rat–human hybrids, *Proc. Natl. Acad. Sci. U.S.A.* **70**:2590–2594.

Day, R. S., Kraemer, K. H., and Robbins, J. H., 1975, Complementing xeroderma pigmentosum fibroblasts restore biological activity to UV-damaged DNA, *Mutat. Res.* **28**:251–255.

Dean, B. M., and Perrett, D., 1976, Studies on adenine and adenosine metabolism by intact human erythrocytes using high performance liquid chromatography, *Biochim. Biophys. Acta* **437**:1–21.

Debray, H., Cartier, P., Temstet, A., and Cendron, J., 1976, Child's urinary lithiasis revealing a complete deficit in adenine phosphoribosyltransferase, *Pediatr. Res.* **10**:762–766.

Degnen, G. E., Miller, I. L., Eisenstadt, J. M., and Adelberg, E. A., 1976, Chromosome-mediated gene transfer between closely related strains of cultured mouse cells, *Proc. Natl. Acad. Sci. U.S.A.* **73**:2838–2842.

deMuckadell, O. B., and Gyntelberg, F., 1976, Occurrence of gout in Copenhagen males aged 40–59, *Int. J. Epidemiol.* **5**:153–158.

Dewey, M. J., Martin, D. W., Jr., Martin, G. R., and Mintz, B., 1977, Mosaic mice with teratocarcinoma-derived mutant cells deficient in hypoxanthine phosphoribosyltransferase, *Proc. Natl. Acad. Sci. U.S.A.* **74**:5564–5568.

Donofrio, J., Coleman, M. S., Hutton, J. J., Daoud, A., Lampkin, B., and Dyminski, J., 1978, Overproduction of adenine deoxynucleosides and deoxynucleotides in adenosine deaminase deficiency with severe combined immunodeficiency disease, *J. Clin. Invest.* **62**:884–887.

Eckes, L., 1975, The simultaneous occurrence of psoriasis, sarcoidosis and gout, *Hautarzt* **26**:357–361.

Edelstein, S. B., Castiglione, C. M., and Breakefield, X. O., 1978, Low monoamine oxidase activity in Lesch–Nyhan fibroblasts, *J. Neurochem.* **31**:1247–1255.

Editorial, 1976, Gout for gourmets, *Lancet* **2**:777.

Edwards, N. L., Gelfand, E. W., Biggar, D., and Fox, I. H., 1978, Partial deficiency of purine nucleoside phosphorylase: Studies of purine and pyrimidine metabolism, *J. Lab. Clin. Med.* **91**:736–749.

Elion, G. B., Furman, P. A., Fyfe, J. A., deMiranda, P., Beauchamp, L., and Schaeffer, H. J., 1977, Selectivity of action of an antiherpetic agent, 9-(2-hydroxyethoxymethyl) guanine, *Proc. Natl. Acad. Sci. U.S.A.* **74**:5716–5720.

Emmerson, B. T., 1976, Gout, uric acid and renal disease, *Med. J. Aust.* **1**:403–405.

Emmerson, B. T., and Row, P. G., 1975, An evaluation of the pathogenesis of the gouty kidney (editorial), *Kidney Int.* **8**:65–71.

Engelman, K., Watts, R. W. E., Klinenberg, J. R., Sjoerdsma, A., and Seegmiller, J. E., 1964, Clinical, physiological and biochemical studies of a patient with xanthinuria and pheochromocytoma, *Am. J. Med.* **37**:839–861.

Epstein, C. J., and Golbus, M. S., 1978, The prenatal diagnosis of genetic disorders, *Annu. Rev. Med.* **29**:117–128.

Fain, J. N., and Wieser, P. B., 1975, Effects of adenosine deaminase on cyclic adenosine monophosphate accumulation, lipolysis and glucose metabolism of fat cells, *J. Biol. Chem.* **250**:1027–1034.

Ferrari, M., Giacomello, S., Salerno, C., and Messina, E., 1978, A spectrophotometric assay for phosphoribosylpyrophosphate synthetase, *Anal. Biochem.* **89**:355–360.

Fleisch, H., Robertson, W. G., Smith, L. H., and Vahlensieck, W. (eds.), 1976, *Urolithiasis Research*, Plenum Press, New York, 582 pp.

Forster, H., and Hoos, I., 1977, Carbohydrates induced increase in uric acid synthesis: Studies in human volunteers and in laboratory rats, *Adv. Exp. Med. Biol.* **76A**:519–528.

Fox, I. H., 1976, Inborn errors of purine and pyrimidine metabolism, *Clin. Perinatol.* **3**:133–140.

Fox, I. H., and Kelley, W. N., 1978, The role of adenosine and 2′-deoxyadenosine in mammalian cells, *Annu. Rev. Biochem.* **47**:655–686.

Fox, I. H., and Lacroix, S., 1977, Electrophoretic variation in the partial deficiency of hypoxanthine-guanine phosphoribosyltransferase, *J. Lab. Clin. Med.* **90**:25–29.

Fox, I. H., Keystone, E. C., Gladman, D. D., Moore, M., and Cane, D., 1975, Inhibition of mitogen mediated lymphocyte blastogenesis by adenosine, *Immunol. Commun.* **4**:419–427.

Fox, I. H., Andres, C. M., Gelfand, E. W., and Biggar, D., 1977, Purine nucleoside phosphorylase deficiency: Altered kinetic properties of a mutant enzyme, *Science* **197**:1084–1086.

Franck, W. A., and Brown, M. M., 1976, Ibuprofen in acute polyarticular gout, *Arthritis Rheum.* **19**:269.

Francke, U., Felsenstein, J., Gartler, S. M., Migeon, B. R., Dancis, J., Seegmiller, J. E., Bakay, B. (F)., and Nyhan, W. L., 1976, The occurrence of new mutants in the X-linked recessive Lesch–Nyhan disease, *Am. J. Hum. Genet.* **28**:123–137.

Francke, U., Felsenstein, J., Gartler, S. M., Nyhan, W. L., and Seegmiller, J. E., 1977, Answer to criticism of Morton and Lalouel, *Am. J. Hum. Genet.* **29**:307–311.

Frayha, R. A., Salti, I. S., Arnaout, A., Khatchadurian, A., and Uthman, S. M., 1977, Hereditary xanthinuria: Report on three patients and short review of the literature, *Nephron* **19**:328–332.

Frederiksen, S., 1966, Specificity of adenosine deaminase toward adenosine and 2′-deoxyadenosine analogues, *Arch. Biochem. Biophys.* **113**:383–388.

Frick, G. P., and Lowenstein, J. M., 1978, Vectorial production of adenosine by 5′-nucleotidase in the perfused rat heart, *J. Biol. Chem.* **253**:1240–1244.

Frith, C. D., Johnstone, E. C., Joseph, M. H., Powell, R. J., and Watts, R. W. E., 1976, Double-blind clinical trial of 5-hydroxytryptophan in a case of Lesch–Nyhan syndrome, *J. Neurol. Neurosurg. Psychiatry* **39**:656–662.

Fujimoto, W. Y., Seegmiller, J. E., Uhlendorf, B. W., and Jacobson, C. B., 1968, Biochemical diagnosis of an X-linked disease *in utero, Lancet* **2**:511–512.

Galton, D. J., Betteridge, D. J., Taylor, K. G., Holdsworth, G., and Stocks, J., 1977, Defects of enzyme regulation in metabolic disease, *Clin. Sci. Mol. Med.* **53**:197–203.

Geiger, A., and Yamasaki, S., 1956, Cytidine and uridine requirement of the brain, *J. Neurochem.* **1**:93–100.

Gelfand, E. W., Dosch, H.-M., Biggar, W. D., and Fox, I. H., 1978, Partial purine nucleoside phosphorylase deficiency: Studies of lymphocyte function, *J. Clin. Invest.* **61**:1071–1080.

Ghangas, G. S., and Milman, G., 1975, Radioimmune determination of hypoxanthine phosphoribosyltransferase crossreacting material in erythrocytes of Lesch–Nyhan patients, *Proc. Natl. Acad. Sci. U.S.A.* **72**:4147–4150.

Ghangas, G. S., and Milman, G., 1977, Hypoxanthine phosphoribosyltransferase: Two dimensional gels from normal and Lesch–Nyhan hemolysates, *Science* **196**:1119–1120.

Giacomello, A., and Salerno, C., 1977, A continuous spectrophotometric assay for hypoxanthine-guanine phosphoribosyltransferase, *Anal. Biochem.* **79**:263–267.

Giblett, E. R., Ammann, A. J., Wara, D. W., Sandman, R., and Diamond, L. K., 1975, Nucleoside-phosphorylase deficiency in a child with severely defective T-cell immunity and normal B-cell immunity, *Lancet* **1**:1010–1013.

Giliberti, P., Pignero, A., and Tancredi, F., 1977, Metabolism dell'acido folico nella sindrome di Lesch–Nyhan, *Minerva Pediatr.* **29**:697–702.

Ginsberg, M. H., Kozin, F., Chow, D., May, J., and Skosey, J. L., 1977a, Absorption of polymorphonuclear leukocyte lysosomal enzymes to monosodium urate crystals, *Arthritis Rheum.* **20**:1538–1542.

Ginsberg, M. H., Kozin, F., O'Malley, M., and McCarty, D. J., 1977b, Release of platelet constituents by monosodium urate crystals, *J. Clin. Invest.* **60**:999–1007.

Goldblum, R. M., Schmalstieg, F. C., Nelson, J. A., and Mills, G. C., 1979, Adenosine deaminase (ADA) and other enzyme abnormalities in immune deficiency states, in: *Proceedings of the Birth Defects Conference,* Memphis, Tennessee (in press).

Gonick, H. C., 1977, Kidney in patients with abnormalities in uric acid metabolism, *Contrib. Nephrol.* **7**:79–96.

Good, R. A., and Hansen, M. A., 1976, Primary immunodeficiency diseases, *Adv. Exp. Med. Biol.* **73B**:155–178.

Good, R. A., and Yunis, E., 1974, Association of autoimmunity, immunodeficiency and aging in man, rabbits, and mice, *Fed. Proc. Fed. Am. Soc. Exp. Biol.* **33**:2040–2050.

Goodman, M. N., and Lowenstein, J. M., 1977, The purine nucleotide cycle: Studies of ammonia production by skeletal muscle *in situ* and in perfused preparations, *J. Biol. Chem.* **252**:5054–5060.

Graf, L. H., Jr., McRoberts, J. A., Harrison, T. M., and Martin, D. W., Jr., 1975, Increased PRPP synthetase activity in cultured rat hepatoma cells containing mutations in the hypoxanthine-guanine phosphoribosyltransferase gene, *J. Cell. Physiol.* **88**:331–342.

Green, H., and Chan, T. S., 1973, Pyrimidine starvation induced by adenosine in fibroblasts and lymphoid cells: Role of adenosine deaminase, *Science* **182**:836–837.

Green, H., and Ishii, K., 1972, On the existence of a guanine nucleotide trap, the role of adenosine kinase and a possible cause of excessive purine production in mammalian cells, *J. Cell Sci.* **11**:173–177.

Griscelli, C., Hamet, M., and Ballet, J.-J., 1976, Third Workshop of the International Cooperative Group for Bone Marrow Transplantation in Man, New York.

Gudas, L. J., Cohen, A., Ullman, B., and Martin, D. W., Jr., 1979, Analysis of adenosine-mediated pyrimidine starvation using cultured wild-type and mutant mouse T-lymphoma cells, *Somat. Cell Genet.* **4** (in press).

Halley, D., and Heukels-Dully, M. J., 1977, Rapid prenatal diagnosis of the Lesch–Nyhan syndrome, *J. Med. Genet.* **14**:100–102.

Hamet, M., Griscelli, C., Cartier, P., Ballay, J., and Hösli, P., 1977, A second case of inosine phosphorylase deficiency with severe T-cell abnormalities, *Adv. Exp. Med. Biol.* **76A**:477–480.

Harrap, K. R., and Paine, R. M., 1976, Adenosine metabolism in cultured lymphoid cells, in: *Advances in Enzyme Regulation,* Vol. 15 (G. Weber, ed.), pp. 169–193, Pergamon Press, New York.

Hauschild, S., Chalmers, R. A., Lawson, A. M., Schultis, K., and Watts, R. W. E., 1976, Metabolic investigations after xylitol infusion in human subjects, *Am. J. Clin. Nutr.* **29**:258–273.

Hawkins, M., Jr., and Breakefield, X. O., 1978, Monoamine oxidase A and B in cultured cells, *J. Neurochem.* **30**:1391–1398.

Healey, L. A., 1977, Management of gouty arthritis induced by thiazide, *Med. Times* **105**(66):26D–30D.

Heath, J. K., 1978, The man-made mouse, *Nature (London)* **271**:610–611.

Heel, R. C., Brogden, R. N., Speight, T. M., and Avery, G. S., 1977, Benzbromarone: A review of its pharmacological properties and therapeutic use in gout and hyperuricaemia, *Drugs* **14**:349–366.

Helgeland, A., Hjermann, I., Holme, I., and Leren, P., 1978, Serum triglycerides and serum uric acid in untreated and thiazide-treated patients with mild hypertension, *Am. J. Med.* **64**:34–38.

Hench, P. S., and Darnall, C. M., 1933, A clinic on acute, old-fashioned gout; with special reference to its inciting factors, *Med. Clin. North Am.* **16**:1371–1393.

Henderson, J. F., Brox, L., Zombor, G., Hunting, D., and Lomax, C. A., 1977, Specificity of adenosine deaminase inhibitors, *Biochem. Pharmacol.* **26**:1967–1972.

Hershfield, M. S., and Seegmiller, J. E., 1977, Regulation of *de novo* purine synthesis in human lymphoblasts: Similar rates of *de novo* synthesis during growth by normal cells and mutants deficient in hypoxanthine-guanine phosphoribosyltransferase activity, *J. Biol. Chem.* **252**:6002–6010.

Hershfield, M. S., Snyder, F., and Seegmiller, J. E., 1977, Adenine and adenosine are toxic to human lymphoblast mutants deficient in adenine phosphoribosyltransferase or adenosine kinase, *Science* **197**:1284–1286.

Hirschhorn, R., 1977a, Adenosine deaminase deficiency and immunodeficiencies, *Fed. Proc. Fed. Am. Soc. Exp. Biol.* **36**:2166–2170.

Hirschhorn, R., 1977b, Defects of purine metabolism in immunodeficiency disease, in: *Progress in Clinical Immunology*, Vol. 3 (R. S. Schwartz, ed.), pp. 67–83, Grune & Stratton, San Francisco.

Hirschhorn, R., Beratis, N., and Rosen, F. S., 1976, Characterization of residual enzyme activity in fibroblasts from patients with adenosine deaminase deficiency and combined immunodeficiency: Evidence for a mutant enzyme, *Proc. Natl. Acad. Sci. U.S.A.* **73**:213–217.

Hirschhorn, R., Martiniuk, F., and Rosen, F. S., 1978, Adenosine deaminase activity in normal tissues and tissues from a child with severe combined immunodeficiency and adenosine deaminase deficiency, *Clin. Immunol. Immunopathol.* **9**:287–292.

Holmes, E. W., Jr., and Kelley, W. N., 1975, An analysis of the bidirectional transport of uric acid by the human nephron, *Arthritis Rheum.* **18**(Suppl.):811–815.

Holmes, E. W., Jr., Wyngaarden, J. W., and Kelley, W. N., 1975, Regulation of human glutamine phosphoribosylpyrophosphate amidotransferase by interconversion of two forms of the enzyme, in: *Isozymes II: Physiological Function* (C. L. Markert, ed.), pp. 425–437, Academic Press, New York.

Holmes, E. W., Kelley, W. N., and Wyngaarden, J. B., 1976, Control of purine biosynthesis in normal and pathological states, *Bull. Rheum. Dis.* **26**:848–853.

Hong, R., Santosham, M., Shulte-Wissermann, H., Horowitz, S., Hsu, S. H., and Winkelstein, J. A., 1976, Reconstitution of B and T lymphocyte function in severe combined immunodeficiency disease after transplantation with thymic epithelium, *Lancet* **2**:1270–1272.

Honig, S., Gorevic, P., Hiffstein, S., and Weissman, G., 1977, Crystal deposition disease: Diagnosis by electron microscopy, *Am. J. Med.* **63**:161–164.

Hösli, P., de Bruyn, C. H. M. M., Oerlemans, F. J. J. M., Verjaal, M., and Nobrega, R. E., 1977, Rapid prenatal diagnosis of HG-PRT deficiency using ultramicrochemical methods, *Hum. Genet.* **37**:195–200.

Hughes, S. H., Wahl, G. M., and Capecchi, M. R., 1975, Purification and characterization of mouse hypoxanthine-guanine phosphoribosyltransferase, *J. Biol. Chem.* **250**:120–126.

Isomäki, H., and von Essen, R., 1977, Gout is on the increase in Finland, *Duodecim* **93**:1090–1098.

Ito, K., Sakura, N., Usui, T., and Uchino, H., 1977, Screening for primary immunodeficiencies associated with purine nucleoside phosphorylase deficiency or adenosine deaminase deficiency, *J. Lab. Clin. Med.* **90**:844–848.

Jenkins, T., and Nurse, G. T., 1976, Biomedical studies on the desert dwelling hunter-gatherers of Southern Africa, *Prog. Med. Genet.* **1**:211–281.

Jenkins, T., Rabson, A. R., Nurse, G. T., and Lane, A. B., 1976, Deficiency of adenosine deaminase not associated with severe combined immunodeficiency, *J. Pediatr.* **89**:732–736.

Jochmus, I., Koch, A., and Wilhelmstroop-Meyer, A., 1977, Verhaltenstherapie der Autoaggressionen beim Lesch–Nyhan-Syndrom, *Monatsschr. Kinderheilkd.* **125**:839–841.

Johnson, G. G., Pepple, J. M., Singer, H. S., and Littlefield, J. W., 1977, HGPRT in the Gilles de la Tourette syndrome, *N. Engl. J. Med.* **297**:339.

Johnson, L. A., Gordon, R. B., and Emmerson, B. T., 1977a, Adenine phosphoribosyltransferase: A simple spectrophotometric assay and the incidence of mutation in the normal population, *Biochem. Genet.* **15**:265–272.

Johnson, L. A., Gordon, R. B., and Emmerson, B. T., 1977b, Hypoxanthineguanine phosphoribosyltransferase: A simple spectrophotometric assay, *Clin. Chim. Acta* **80**:203–207.

Johnson, S. M., Asherson, G. L., Watts, R. W. E., North, M. E., Allsop, J., and Webster, A. D. B., 1977, Lymphocyte-purine 5'-nucleotidase deficiency in primary hypogammaglobulinaemia, *Lancet* **1**:168–170.

Kahan, B., and DeMars, R., 1975, Localized derepression on the human inactive X chromosome in mouse–human cell hydrids, *Proc. Natl. Acad. Sci. U.S.A.* **72**:1510–1514.

Kahn, M. F., 1976, Goutte, obésité et plaisirs de la table: Comparison entre 40 gotteux et 40 temoins, *Nouv. Presse Med.* **5**:1897–1898.

Kar, N. C., and Pearson, C. M., 1973, Muscle adenylic acid deaminase activity, *Neurology* **23**:478–482.

Kaufman, J. M., Greene, M. L., and Seegmiller, J. E., 1968, Urine uric acid to creatinine ratio: A screening test for inherited disorders of purine metabolism, *J. Pediatr.* **73**:583–592.

Kawenoki-Minc, E., Eyman, E., Leo, W., and Werynska-Przybylska, J., 1975, Wylyw roznych metod leczenia na rozwoj artropatii chorego na dne: Obserwacja 155 pacjentow, *Rheumatologia* **13**:263–270.

Kawenoki-Minc, E., Maldyk, E., and Polowiec, Z., 1977, Consecutive stages of arthropathy progression in patients with gout, *Z. Rheumatol.* **36**:106–111.

Keightley, R. G., Lawton, A. R., Cooper, M. D., and Yunis, E. J., 1975, Successful fetal liver transplantation in a child with severe combined immunodeficiency, *Lancet* **2**:850–853.

Kelley, W. N., 1975a, Effects of drugs on uric acid in man, *Annu. Rev. Pharmacol.* **15**:327–350.

Kelley, W. N., 1975b, Hypouricemia, *Arthritis Rheum.* **18**(Suppl.):731–738.

Kelley, W. N., 1975c, Pharmacologic approach to the maintenance of urate homeostasis, *Nephron* **14**:99–115.

Kelley, W. N., 1976, Current therapy of gout and hyperuricemia, *Hosp. Pract.* **11**:69–76.

Kelley, W. N., 1977a, Introduction: Symposium on gout and related disorders of purine metabolism—A quarter century of progress, *Arthritis Rheum.* **20**(Suppl.):S219–S220.

Kelley, W. N., 1977b, Inborn errors of purine metabolism, *Arthritis Rheum.* **20**(Suppl.):S221–S227.

Kelley, W. N., and Smith, L. H., Jr., 1978, Hereditary orotic aciduria, in: *The Metabolic Basis of Inherited Disease* (J. B. Stanbury, J. B. Wyngaarden, and D. S. Frederickson, eds.), pp. 1045–1071, McGraw-Hill, New York.

Kelley, W. N., and Wyngaarden, J. B., 1978, The Lesch–Nyhan Syndrome, in: *The Metabolic Basis of Inherited Disease* (J. B. Stanbury, J. B. Wyngaarden, and D. S. Frederickson, eds.), pp. 1011–1036, McGraw-Hill, New York.

Kelley, W. N., Levy, R. I., Rosenbloom, F. M., Henderson, J. F., and Seegmiller, J.

E., 1968, Adenine phosphoribosyltransferase deficiency: A previously undescribed genetic defect in man, *J. Clin. Invest.* **47**:2281–2289.

Kelley, W. N., Holmes, E. W., and Van der Weyden, M. B., 1975, Current concepts on the regulation of purine biosynthesis *de novo* in man, *Arthritis Rheum.* **18**(Suppl.):673–680.

Kessel, D., 1978, Transport of nonphosphorylated nucleoside, 5′-deoxyadenosine, by murine leukemia L1210 cells, *J. Biol. Chem.* **253**:400–403.

Klinenberg, J. R., 1977, Renal stones associated with disorders of purine metabolism, *Arthritis Rheum.* **20**(Suppl.):S228–S234.

Kozin, F., and McCarty, D. J., 1976, Protein adsorption to monosodium urate, calcium pyrophosphate dihydrate, and silica crystals: Relationship to the pathogenesis of crystal induced inflammation, *Arthritis Rheum.* **19**:433–438.

Kraemer, K. H., Coon, H. G., Petinga, R. A., Barrett, S. F., Rahe, A. E., and Robbins, J. A., 1975a, Genetic heterogeneity in xeroderma pigmentosum: Complementation groups and their relationship to DNA repair rates, *Proc. Natl. Acad. Sci. U.S.A.* **72**:59–63.

Kraemer, K. H., De Weerd-Kastelein, E. A., Robbins, J. H., Keijzer, W., Barrett, S. F., Petinga, R. A., and Bootsma, D., 1975b, Five complementation groups in xeroderma pigmentosum, *Mutat. Res.* **33**:327–340.

Krakoff, I. H., 1965, Increase in uric acid biosynthesis produced by 2-substituted thiadiazoles, *Arthritis Rheum.* **8**:836–839.

Kredich, N. M., and Martin, D. W., Jr., 1977, Role of S-adenosylhomocysteine in adenosine mediated toxicity in cultured mouse T lymphoma cells, *Cell* **12**:931–938.

Krygier, V., and Momparler, R. L., 1971, Mammalian deoxynucleoside kinases, *J. Biol. Chem.* **246**:2752–2757.

Künzer, W., 1975, A rare surgical emergency: Calcium gout complicated by acute carpal tunnel, *Arch. Fr. Pediatr.* **32**:293.

Kuttesch, J. F., Schmalstieg, F. C., and Nelson, J. A., 1978, Analysis of adenosine and other adenine compounds in patients with immunodeficiency diseases, *J. Liq. Chromatogr.* **1**:97–109.

Lake, C. R., and Ziegler, M. G., 1977, Lesch–Nyhan syndrome: Low dopamine-β-hydroxylase activity and diminished sympathetic response to stress and posture, *Science* **196**:905–906.

Lalanne, M., and Henderson, J. F., 1975, Effects of hormones and drugs on phosphoribosylpyrophosphate concentrations in mouse liver, *Can. J. Biochem.* **53**:394–399.

Lambert, J. R., and Wright, V., 1977, Serum uric acid levels in psoriatic arthritis, *Ann. Rheum. Dis.* **36**:264–267.

Lemieux, G., Gougoux, A., Vinay, P., Kiss, A., and Baverel, G., 1977, The metabolic effects of tienilic acid, a new diuretic with uricosuric properties in man and dog, *Adv. Exp. Med. Biol.* **76B**:334–341.

Lenz, W., Klein, W., and Huth, F., 1976, Needle biopsy in gout and pseudogout, *Beitr. Pathol.* **157**:161–182.

Lequesne, M., Bensasson, M., Kahn, M. F., and de Sèze, S., 1975, Hyperuricemia and femur head osteonecrosis (FHON), *Rev. Rhum. Mal. Osteoartic.* **42**:177–183.

Leyva, A., Holmes, E. W., Jr., and Kelley, W. N., 1976, Effect of 6-mercaptopurine on inosinic acid dehydrogenease in cultured human fibroblasts, *Biochem. Pharmacol.* **25**:527–532.

Logan, D. C., Wilson, D. E., Flowers, C. M., Sparks, P. J., and Tyler, F. H., 1976, Uric acid catabolism in the woolly monkey, *Metabolism* **25**:517–522.

Lopes, J., Zucker-Franklin, D., and Silber, R., 1973, Heterogeneity of 5′-nucleotidase activity in lymphocyte in chronic lymphocytic leukemia, *J. Clin. Invest.* **52**:1297–1300.

Lowe. J. K., Gowans, B., and Brox, L., 1977a, Deoxyadenosine metabolism and toxicity in cultured L5178Y cells, *Cancer Res.* **37**:3013–3017.

Lowe, J. K., Brox, L., and Henderson, J. F., 1977b, Consequences of inhibition of guanine nucleotide synthesis by mycophenolic acid and virazole, *Cancer Res.* **37**:736–743.

Lowy, B. A., and Williams, M. K., 1977, The synthesis of inosine 5′-phosphate in the hypoxanthine-guanine phosphoribosyltransferase-deficient erythrocyte by alternate biochemical pathways, *Pediatr. Res.* **11**:691–694.

Maher, V. M., McCormick, J. J., Grover, P. L., and Sims, P., 1977, Effect of DNA repair on the cytotoxicity and mutagenticity of polycyclic hydrocarbon derivatives in normal and xeroderma pigmentosum human fibroblasts, *Mutat. Res.* **43**:117–138.

Malawista, S. E., 1977, Gouty inflammation, *Arthritis Rheum.* **20**:S241–S248.

Mangoff, S. C., and Milner, J. A., 1978, Oxonate-induced hyperuricemia and orotic aciduria in mice, *Proc. Soc. Exp. Biol. Med.* **157**:110–115.

Manzke, H., 1976, Variabel Expressivat der Gerwirkung beim Lesch–Nyhan Syndrom, *Dtsch. Med. Wochenschr.* **11**:428–429.

Marique, D., and Hildebrand, J., 1973, Evidence for a 5′-nucleotidase in human leukemic leukocytes, *Clin. Chim. Acta* **45**:93–98.

Martin, D. W., Jr., and Maler, B. A., 1976, Phosphoribosylpyrophosphate synthetase is elevated in fibroblasts from patients with the Lesch–Nyhan syndrome, *Science* **193**:408–411.

Martin, T. F. J., and Tashjian, A. H., Jr., 1978, Thyrotopin-releasing hormone modulation of uridine uptake in rat pituitary cells, *J. Biol. Chem.* **253**:106–115.

May, V., and Robert, H., 1975, Coronary insufficiency in patients with gout, *Rev. Rhum. Mal. Osteoartic.* **42**:471–474.

McBride, O. W., and Ozer, H. L., 1973, Transfer of genetic information by purified metaphase chromosomes, *Proc. Natl. Acad. Sci. U.S.A.* **70**:1258–1262.

McBurney, M. W., and Whitmore, G. F., 1975, Mutants of Chinese hamster cells resistant to adenosine, *J. Cell. Physiol.* **85**:87–99.

McKeran, R. O., and Watts, R. W. E., 1978, Purine metabolism and cell physiology, in: *Recent Advances in Endocrinology and Metabolism* (J. L. H. O'Riordan, ed.), pp. 219–252, Churchill Livingstone, New York.

McKeran, R. O., Andrews, T. M., Howell, A., Gibbs, D. A., Chinn, S., and Watts, R. W. E., 1975, The diagnosis of carrier state for the Lesch–Nyhan syndrome, *Q. J. Med.* **44**:189–205.

Meuwissen, H. J., Pollara, B., Pickering, R. J., Porter, I. H., Hook, E. B., and

Kelley, S. (eds.), 1975, *Combined Immunodeficiency Disease and Adenosine Deaminase Deficiency*, Academic Press, New York, 321 pp.

Meyer, J. L., Bergert, J. H., and Smith, L. H., 1976, The epitaxially induced crystal growth of calcium oxalate by crystalline uric acid, *Invest. Urol.* **14**:115–119.

Meyer, L. J., and Becker, M. A., 1977, Human erythrocyte phosphoribosylpyrophosphate synthetase: Dependence of activity on state of subunit association, *J. Biol. Chem.* **252**:3919–3925.

Mielants, H., Veys, E. M., DeBussere, A., and Van der Jeught, J., 1975, Avascular necrosis and its relation to lipid and purine metabolism, *J. Rheumatol.* **2**:430–436.

Mills, G. C., Schmalstieg, F. C., Trimmer, K. B., Goldman, A. S., and Goldblum, R. M., 1976, Purine metabolism in adenosine deaminase deficiency, *Proc. Natl. Acad. Sci. U.S.A.* **73**:2867–2871.

Milman, G., Lee, E., Ghangas, G. S., McLaughlin, J. R., and George, M., Jr., 1976, Analysis of HeLa cell hypoxanthine phosphoribosyltransferase mutants and revertants by two-dimensional polyacrylamide gel electrophoresis: Evidence for silent gene activation, *Proc. Natl. Acad. Sci. U.S.A.* **73**:4589–4593.

Milman, G., Krauss, S. W., and Olsen, A. S., 1977, Tryptic peptide analysis of normal and mutant forms of hypoxanthine phosphoribosyltransferase from HeLa cells, *Proc. Natl. Acad. Sci. U.S.A.* **74**:926–930.

Mintz, B., and Illmensee, K., 1975, Normal genetically mosaic mice produced from malignant teratocarcinoma cells, *Proc. Natl. Acad. Sci. U.S.A.* **72**:3585–3589.

Miwa, S., Nakashima, K., Fujii, H., Matsumoto, M., and Nomura, K., 1977, Three cases of hereditary hemolytic anemia with pyrimidine 5′-nucleotidase deficiency in a Japanese family, *Hum. Genet.* **37**:361–364.

Mizuno, T.-I., and Yugari, Y., 1974, Self-mutilation in the Lesch–Nyhan syndrome, *Lancet* **1**:761.

Mizuno, T., and Yugari, Y., 1975, Prophylactic effect of L-5-hydroxytryptophan on self-mutilation in the Lesch–Nyhan syndrome, *Neuropaediatrie* **6**:13–23.

Mizuno, T., Endoh, H., Konishi, Y., Akaoka, M., and Akaoka, I., 1976, An autopsy case of the Lesch–Nyhan syndrome: Normal HGPRT activity in liver and xanthine calculi in various tissues, *Neuropaediatrie* **7**:351–355.

Mödder, U., and Künzig, M., 1976, A case of extreme gouty arthritis, shown xeroradiographically, *Roentgenblaetter* **29**:96–100.

Moore, E. C., and Hurlbert, R. B., 1966, Regulation of mammalian deoxyribonucleotide biosynthesis by nucleotides as activators and inhibitors, *J. Biol. Chem.* **241**:4802–4809.

Moore, E. C., and Meuwissen, H. J., 1974, Screening for ADA deficiency, *J. Pediatr.* **85**:802–804.

Morris, R. C., Jr., Nigon, K., and Reed, E. B., 1978, Evidence that the severity of depletion of inorganic phosphate determines the severity of the disturbance of adenine nucleotide metabolism in the liver and renal cortex of the fructose-loaded rat, *J. Clin. Invest.* **61**:209–220.

Morton, N. E., and Lalouel, J. M., 1977, Genetic epidemiology of Lesch–Nyhan disease, *Am. J. Hum. Genet.* **29**:304–307.

Mukherjee, A. B., Orloff, S., Butler, J. D., Triche, T., Lalley, P., and Schulman, J.

D., 1978, Entrapment of metaphase chromosomes into phospholipid vesicles (lipochromosomes): Carrier potential in gene transfer, *Proc. Natl. Acad. Sci. U.S.A.* **75**:1361–1365.

Müller, M. M., Kaiser, E., and Seegmiller, J. E. (eds.), 1977a, *Advances in Experimental Medicine and Biology*, Vol. 76A, *Purine Metabolism in Man II: Regulation of Pathways and Enzyme Defects*, Plenum Press, New York, 641 pp.

Müller, M. M., Kaiser, E., and Seegmiller, J. E. (eds.), 1977b, *Advances in Experimental Medicine and Biology*, Vol. 76B, *Purine Metabolism in Man II: Physiology, Pharmacology, and Clinical Aspects*, Plenum Press, New York, 373 pp.

Murphree, S., Moore, E. C., and Beall, P. T., 1968, Regulation by nucleotides of the activity of partially purified ribonucleotide reductase from rat embryos, *Cancer Res.* **28**:860–863.

Mustard, J. F., Murphy, E. A., Ogryzlo, M. A., and Smythe, H. A., 1963, Blood coagulation and platelet economy in subjects with primary gout, *Can. Med. Assoc. J.* **89**:1207–1211.

Nebola, M., and Spurna, V., 1977, Chromosomal characteristic of Chinese hamster cells and their HGPRT-deficient mutant line, *Folia Biol. (Prague)* **23**:222–224.

Nelson, J. A., Rose, L. M., and Bennett, L. L., Jr., 1976, Effects of 2-amino-1,3,4-thiadiazole on ribonucleotide pools of leukemia L1210 cells, *Cancer Res.* **36**:1375–1378.

Nelson, J. A., Rose, L. M., and Bennett, L. L., Jr., 1977, Mechanism of action of 2-amino-1,3,4-thiadiazole (NSC 4728), *Cancer Res.* **37**:182–187.

Nemati, M., Kyle, M. C., and Freis, E. D., 1977, Clinical study of ticrynafen: A new diuretic, antihypertensive, and uricosuric agent, *J. Am. Med. Assoc.* **237**:652–657.

Newland, H., 1975, Hyperuricemia in coronary, cerebral and peripheral arterial disease: An explanation, *Med. Hypotheses* **1**:152–155.

Niemi, K.-M., 1977, Panniculitis of the legs with urate crystal deposition, *Arch. Dermatol.* **113**:655–656.

Nishida, Y., Akaoka, I., Nishizawa, T., Maruki, M., Aikawa, T., Mitamura, T., Yokohari, R., and Horiuchi, Y., 1976, A case of gouty arthritis associated with Down's syndrome, *J. Ment. Defic. Res.* **20**:277–283.

Nishida, Y., Akaoka, I., Nishizawa, T., Maruki, M., and Maruki, K., 1977, Synthesis and concentration of 5-phosphoribosyl-1-pyrophosphate in erythrocytes from patients with Down's syndrome, *Ann. Rheum. Dis.* **36**:261–263.

Nishioka, K., Hirose, K., and Mikanagi, K., 1974, Clinical study of gout and hyperuricemia in Japan (1), *Ryumachi, J. Jpn. Rheum. Assoc.* **14**:95–105.

Nishioka, K., Mikanagi, K., and Hirose, K., 1975, Clinical study of gout and hyperuricemia in Japan (II), *Ryumachi, J. Jpn. Rheum. Assoc.* **15**:141–153.

Nousia-Arvanitakis, S., Stapleton, F. B., Linshaw, M. A., and Kennedy, J., 1977, Therapeutic approach to pancreatic extract-induced hyperuricosuria in cystic fibrosis, *J. Pediatr.* **90**:302–305.

Nyhan, W. L., 1976, Behavior in the Lesch–Nyhan syndrome, *J. Autism Child. Schizophr.* **6**:235–252.

Nyhan, W. L., 1977, Genetic heterogeneity at the locus for hypoxanthine-guanine phosphoribosyltransferase, in: *Ciba Found. Symp. No. 48: Purine and Pyri-*

midine Metabolism, pp. 65–82, Elsevier/Excerpta Medica, North-Holland, Amsterdam.

Nyhan, W. L., Bakay, B., Connor, J. D., Marks, J. F., and Keele, D. K., 1970, Hemizygous expression of glucose-6-phosphate dehydrogenase in erythrocytes of heterozygotes for the Lesch–Nyhan syndrome, *Proc. Natl. Acad. Sci. U.S.A.* **65**:214–218.

O'Farrell, P. H., 1975, High resolution two-dimensional electrophoresis of proteins, *J. Biol. Chem.* **250**:4007–4021.

Olsen, A. S., and Milman, G., 1974a, Chinese hamster hypoxanthine-guanine phosphoribosyltransferase: Purification, structural and catalytic properties, *J. Biol. Chem.* **249**:4030–4037.

Olsen, A. S., and Milman, G., 1974b, Subunit molecular weight of human hypoxanthine-guanine phosphoribosyltransferase, *J. Biol. Chem.* **249**:4038–4040.

Olsen, A. S., and Milman, G., 1977, Human hypoxanthine phosphoribosyltransferase: Purification and properties, *Biochemistry* **16**:2501–2505.

Orfanos, C. E., and Künzig, M., 1975, Chronic lead poisoning: Lead gout with giant tophi on the skin, nepropathy and porphyrinopathy, *Hautarzt* **26**:581–584.

Osborne, W. R. A., Chen, S.-H., Giblett, E. R., Biggar, W. D., Ammann, A. A., and Scott, C. R., 1977, Purine nucleoside phosphorylase deficiency: Evidence for molecular heterogeneity in two families with enzyme-deficient members, *J. Clin. Invest.* **60**:741–746.

Osborne, W. R. A., Chen, S.-H., and Scott, C. R., 1978, Use of the integrated steady state rate equation to investigate product inhibition of human red cell adenosine deaminase and its relevance to immune dysfunction, *J. Biol. Chem.* **253**:323–325.

Paglia, D. E., Valentine, W. N., and Fink, K., 1977, Lead poisoning: Further observations on erythrocyte pyrimidine-nucleotidase deficiency and intracellular accumulation of pyrimidine nucleotides, *J. Clin. Invest.* **60**:1362–1366.

Pak, C. Y. C., Waters, O., Arnold, L., Holt, K., Cox, C., and Barilla, D., 1977, Mechanism for calcium urolithiasis among patients with hyperuricosuria, *J. Clin. Invest.* **59**:426–431.

Parkman, R., 1977, Treatment of immunodeficiency diseases by organ transplantation, in: *Progress in Clinical Immunology*, Vol. 3 (R. S. Schwartz, ed.), pp. 85–102, Grune & Stratton, New York.

Parkman, R., Gelfand, E. W., Rosen, F. S., Sanderson, A., and Hirschhorn, R., 1975, Severe combined immunodeficiency and adenosine deaminase deficiency, *N. Engl. J. Med.* **292**:714–719.

Pasero, G., 1977, Recurrent gouty phlebitis without articular gout, *Adv. Exp. Med. Biol.* **76B**:245–248.

Perrett, D., and Dean, B., 1977, The functions of adenosine deaminase in the human erythrocyte, *Biochem. Biophys. Res. Commun.* **77**:374–378.

Pledger, S. R., Hirsch, B., and Freiberg, R. A., 1976, Bilateral carpal tunnel syndrome secondary to gouty tenosynovitis, in: *Clinical Orthopaedics and Related Research*, Vol. 118 (M. R. Urist, ed.), pp. 188–189, J. B. Lippincott, Philadelphia.

Pollara, B., Schrader, W. P., and Meuwissen, H. J., 1977, Tissue adenosine deaminase activity in an adenosine deficient–combined immunodeficiency disease patient, *Pediatr. Res.* **11**:722A(abstract).

Polmar, S. H., 1977, Lymphocyte enzyme deficiencies and the metabolic basis of immunodeficiency disease, *Clin. Haematol.* **6**:423–438.

Polmar, S. H., Wetzler, E. M., Stern, R. C., and Hirschhorn, R., 1975, Restoration of *in vitro* lymphocyte responses with exogenous adenosine deaminase in a patient with severe combined immunodeficiency, *Lancet* **2**:743–746.

Polmar, S. H., Stern, R. C., Schwartz, A. L., Wetzler, E. M., Chase, P. A., and Hirschhorn, R., 1976, Enzyme replacement therapy for adenosine deaminase deficiency and severe combined immunodeficiency, *N. Engl. J. Med.* **295**:1337–1343.

Polmar, S. H., Wetzler, E. M., and Stern, R. C., 1977, Immunopharmacologic studies of adenosine deaminase deficient lymphocytes, *Pediatr. Res.* **11**:723A (abstract).

Polmar, S. H., Wetzler, E. M., and Stern, R. C., 1979, Adenosine deaminase deficiency: Enzyme replacement therapy and investigations of the biochemical basis of immunodeficiency, in: *Inborn Errors of Immunity and Phagocytes* (E. Wamberg and E. Guttler, eds.), NTP Press, Lancaster, England (in press).

Pund, E. E., Jr., Hawley, R. L., McGee, H. J., and Blount, S. G., 1960, Gouty heart, *N. Engl. J. Med.* **263**:835–838.

Quagliata, F., Faig, D., Conlyn, M., and Silber, R., 1974, Studies on the lymphocyte 5′-nucleotidase in chronic lymphocyte leukemia, infectious mononucleosis, normal subpopulations, and phytohemagglutinin-stimulated cells, *Cancer Res.* **34**:3197–3202.

Raivio, K. O., 1976, Neonatal hyperuricemia, *J. Pediatr.* **88**:625–630.

Raivio, K. O., and Hovi, T., 1977, Adenine and adenosine metabolism in phytohemagglutinin-stimulated normal human lymphocytes, *Adv. Exp. Med. Biol.* **76A**:448–455.

Raivio, K. O., and Hovi, T., 1979, Purine reutilization in phytohemagglutinin-stimulated human T-lymphocytes, *Exp. Cell Res.* (in press).

Raivio, K. O., Becker, M. A., Meyer, L. J., Greene, M. L., Nuki, G., and Seegmiller, J. E., 1975, Stimulation of human purine synthesis *de novo* by fructose infusion, *Metabolism* **24**:861–869.

Raivio, K. O., Schwartz, A. L., Stern, R. C., and Polmar, S. H., 1977, Adenine and adenosine metabolism in lymphocytes deficient in adenosine deaminase activity, *Adv. Exp. Med. Biol.* **76A**:456–462.

Reem, G. H., 1975, Phosphoribosylpyrophosphate overproduction, a new metabolic abnormality in the Lesch–Nyhan syndrome, *Science* **190**:1098–1099.

Reem, G. H., 1977, Purine biosynthesis in mutant mamallian cells, in: *Ciba Found. Symp. No. 48: Purine and Pyrimidine Metabolism,* pp. 105–137, Elsevier/ Excerpta Medica, North-Holland, Amsterdam.

Reese, O. G., Jr., and Steele, T. H., 1976, Renal transport of urate during diuretic-induced hypouricemia, *Am. J. Med.* **60**:973–977.

Reichard, P., 1972, Control of deoxyribonucleotide synthesis *in vitro* and *in vivo,* *Adv. Enzyme Regul.* **10**:3–16.

Resnick, D., 1977, The radiographic manifestations of gouty arthritis, in: *CRC Crit. Rev. Diagnostic Imaging,* Vol. 9, pp. 265–335.

Robbins, J. H., Kraemer, K. H., Jutzner, M. A., Festoff, B. W., and Coon, H. G., 1974, Xeroderma pigmentosum: An inherited disease with sun sensitivity, multiple cutaneous neoplasms, and DNA repair, *Ann. Intern. Med.* **80**:221–248.

Robbins, J. H., Kraemer, K. H., and Andrews, A. D., 1976, Inherited DNA repair defects in *H. sapiens:* Their relation to UV-associated processes in xeroderma pigmentosum, in: *Biology of Radiation Carcinogenesis* (J. M. Yuhas, R. W. Tennant, and J. D. Regan, eds.), pp. 115–127, Raven Press, New York.

Rockson, S., Stone, R., Van der Weyden, M., and Kelley, W. N., 1974, Lesch–Nyhan syndrome: Evidence for abnormal adrenergic function, *Science* **186**:934–935.

Rodnan, G. P., 1977, Growth and development of rheumatology in the United States—A bicentennial report, *Arthritis Rheum.* **20**:1149–1168.

Roe, T. E., and Kogut, M. D., 1977, The pathogenesis of hyperuricemia in glycogen storage disease Type I, *Pediatr. Res.* **11**:664–669.

Rosa, R., Rochant, H., Dreyfus, B., Valentin, C., and Rosa, J., 1977, Electrophoretic and kinetic studies of human erythrocytes deficient in pyrimidine 5'-nucleotidase, *Hum. Genet.* **38**:209–215.

Rose, B. S., 1975, Gout in Maoris, *Semin. Arthritis Rheum.* **5**:121–145.

Rose, G. A., and Woodfine, C., 1976, The thermogravimetric analysis of renal stones in clinical practice, *Br. J. Urol.* **48**:403–412.

Rosenbloom, F. M., Henderson, J. F., Caldwell, I. C., Kelley, W. N., and Seegmiller, J. E., 1968, Biochemical bases of accelerated purine biosynthesis *de novo* in human fibroblasts lacking hypoxanthine-guanine phosphoribosyltransferase, *J. Biol. Chem.* **243**:1166–1173.

Rosenthal, M., 1977, Experiences with uricotest, a simple device for the demonstration of birefringent crystals in tissue, *Praxis* **66**:617–618.

Roth, J. A., Breakefield, X. O., and Castiglione, C. M., 1976, Monoamine oxidase and catechol-O-methyltransferase activities in cultured human skin fibroblasts, *Life Sci.* **19**:1705–1710.

Rozen, R., Buhl, S., Mohyuddin, F., Caillibot, V., and Scriber, C. R., 1977, Evaluation of metabolic pathway activity in cultured skin fibroblasts and blood leukocytes, *Clin. Chim. Acta* **77**:379–386.

Sakura, N., Usui, T., and Ito, K., 1977a, Congenital immunodeficiency syndrome with adenosine deaminase and purine nucleoside phosphorylase deficiencies (1), *Nippon Rinsho* **35**:2397–2403.

Sakura, N., Usui, T., and Ito, K., 1977b, Congenital immunodeficiency with adenosine deaminase and purine nucleoside phosphorylase deficiency (2), *Nippon Rinsho* **35**:2564–2580.

Sales, L. M., 1977, Foibles and fallacies in the diagnosis of arthritis, *South. Med. J.* **70**:1314–1316.

Sandman, R., Ammann, A. J., Grose, C., and Wara, D. W., 1977, Cellular immunodeficiency associated with nucleoside phosphorylase deficiency, *Clin. Immunol. Immunopathol.* **8**:247–253.

Sartorelli, A. C., and Johns, D. G. (eds.), 1975, *Antineoplastic and Immunosuppressive Agents* I and II (*Handbook of Experimental Pathology*, Vol. 38), Springer-Verlag, New York, Heidelberg, Berlin.

Schaeffer, H. J., and Schwender, G. F., 1974, Enzyme inhibitors 26: Bridging hydrophobic and hydrophyllic regions of adenosine deaminase with some 9-(2-hydroxy-3-alkyl) adenines, *J. Med. Chem.* **17**:6–8.

Schmalstieg, F. C., Nelson, J. A., Mills, G. C., Monahan, T. M., Goldman, A. S., and Goldblum, R. M., 1977, Increased purine nucleotides in adenosine deaminase-deficient lymphocytes, *J. Pediatr.* **91**:48–51.

Schmalstieg, F. C., Mills, G. C., Nelson, J. A., May, L. T., Goldman, A. S., and Goldblum, R. M., 1978, Limited effect of erythrocyte and plasma infusions in adenosine deaminase deficiency, *J. Pediatr.* **93**:597–604.

Schrader, W. P., and Stacy, A. R., 1977, Purification and subunit structure of adenosine deaminase from human kidney, *J. Biol. Chem.* **252**:6409–6415.

Schrader, W. P., Stacy, A. R., and Pollara, B., 1976, Purification of human erythrocyte adenosine deaminase by affinity column chromatography, *J. Biol. Chem.* **251**:4026–4032.

Schrader, W. P., Pollara, B., and Meuwissen, H. J., 1978, Characterization of the residual adenosine deaminating activity in the spleen of a patient with combined immunodeficiency disease and adenosine deaminase deficiency, *Proc. Natl. Acad. Sci. U.S.A.* **75**:446–450.

Schultz, V., and Lowenstein, J. M., 1978, The purine nucleoside cycle, *J. Biol. Chem.* **253**:1938–1943.

Schumacher, H. R., Jimenez, S. A., Gibson, T., Pascual, E., Traycoff, R., Dorwart, B. B., and Reginato, A. J., 1975, Acute gouty arthritis without urate crystals identified on initial examination of synovial fluid: Report on nine patients, *Arthritis Rheum.* **18**:603–612.

Schwartz, A. L., Stern, R. C., and Polmar, S. H., 1979, Demonstration of an adenosine receptor on human lymphocytes *in vitro* and its possible role in the adenosine deaminase deficient form of severe combined immunodeficiency disease, *Clin. Immunol. Immunopathol.* (in press).

Schwartz, R. S. (ed.), 1977, *Progress in Clinical Immunology*, Vol. 3, Grune & Stratton, New York, 208 pp.

Scott, J. T., 1977, Choice of treatment in gout, *Practitioner* **219**:469–474.

Scott, J. T., and Hiisi-Brummer, L., 1975, Etiopathogenesis of the gouty arthritis, *Scand. J. Rheumatol.* **12**(Suppl.):140–141.

Scott, J. T., Sturge, R. A., Kennedy, A. C., Hart, D. P., and Buchanan, W. W., 1977, Serum uric acid levels in England and Scotland, in: *Advances in Experimental Medicine and Biology*, Vol. 76B, *Purine Metabolism in Man II: Physiology, Pharmacology, Clinical Aspects* (M. M. Müller, E. Kaiser, and J. E. Seegmiller, eds.), pp. 214–222, Plenum Press, New York.

Seegmiller, J. E., 1974, Diseases of purine and pyrimidine metabolism, in: *Duncan's Diseases of Metabolism*, 7th ed. (P. K. Bondy and L. E. Rosenberg, eds.), pp. 655–774, W. B. Saunders, Philadelphia.

Seegmiller, J. E., 1976a, Disorders of purine and pyrimidine metabolism, in: *The Year in Metabolism 1975–1976* (N. Freinkel, ed.), pp. 213–258, Plenum Medical Book Company, New York.

Seegmiller, J. E., 1976b, Inherited deficiency of hypoxanthine-guanine phosphoribosyltransferase in X-linked uric aciduria (the Lesch–Nyhan syndrome and its variants), in: *Advances in Human Genetics*, Vol. 6 (H. Harris and K. Hirschhorn, eds.), pp. 75–163, Plenum Press, New York.

Seegmiller, J. E., 1978a, Disorders of purine and pyrimidine metabolism, in: *The*

Year in Metabolism 1977 (N. Freinkel, ed.), pp. 253–325, Plenum Medical Book Company, New York.

Seegmiller, J. E., 1978b, Progress in understanding the mechanism of immunodeficiency disease associated with defects in purine metabolism, *Monogr. Hum. Genet.* **10**:88–91.

Seegmiller, J. E., Grayzel, A. I., Liddle, L., and Wyngaarden, J. B., 1963, The effect of 2-ethylamino-1,3,4-thiadiazole on the incorporation of glycine into urinary purines and uric acid in man, *Metabolism* **12**:507–515.

Seegmiller, J. E., Watanabe, T., and Schreier, M. H., 1977a, The effect of adenosine on lymphoid cell proliferation and antibody formation, in: *Ciba Found. Symp. No. 48: Purine and Pyrimidine Metabolism*, pp. 249–266, Elsevier, Amsterdam.

Seegmiller, J. E., Watanabe, T., Schreier, M. H., and Waldmann, T. A., 1977b, Immunological aspects of purine metabolism, in: *Advances in Experimental Medicine and Biology*, Vol. 76A, *Purine Metabolism in Man II: Regulation of Pathways and Enzyme Defects* (M. M. Müller, E. Kaiser, and J. E. Seegmiller, eds.), pp. 412–433, Plenum Press, New York.

Self, T. H., Fountain, F. F., Taylor, W. J., Jr., and Sutliff, W. D., 1977, Acute gouty arthritis associated with the use of ethambutol, *Chest* **71**:561–562.

Sherline, P., and Schiavone, K., 1977, Immunofluorescence localization of proteins of high molecular weight along intracellular microtubules, *Science* **198**:1038–1040.

Sherry, S., and Committee, 1978, The Anturane Reinfarction Trial Research Group (S. H. Kanse, chairman): Sulfinpyrazone in the prevention of cardiac death after myocardial infarction, *N. Engl. J. Med.* **298**:289–295.

Shirahama, T., and Cohen, A. S., 1974, Blockage of amyloid induction by colchicine in an animal model, *J. Exp. Med.* **140**:1102–1107.

Simkin, P. A., 1977, The pathogenesis of podagra, *Ann. Intern. Med.* **86**:230–233.

Simkin, P. A., Skeith, M. D., and Healey, L. A., 1974, Suppression of uric acid secretion in a patient with renal hypouricemia, *Adv. Exp. Med. Biol.* **41B**:723–728.

Simmonds, H. A., 1979, Crystal induced nephropathy: A current view, *Eur. J. Rheum. Inflamm.* (in press).

Simmonds, H. A., Hatfield, P. J., Cameron, J. S., and Cadenhead, A., 1976a, Uric acid excretion by the pig kidney, *Am. J. Physiol.* **230**:1654–1661.

Simmonds, H. A., Van Acker, K. J., Cameron, J. S., and Snedden, W., 1976b, The identification of 2,8-dihydroxyadenine, a new component of urinary stones, *Biochem. J.* **157**:485–486.

Simmonds, H. A., Van Acker, K. J., Cameron, J. S., and McBurney, A., 1977, Purine excretion in complete adenine phosphoribosyltransferase deficiency: Effect of diet and allopurinol therapy, in: *Advances in Experimental Medicine and Biology*, Vol. 76B, *Purine Metabolism in Man II: Physiology, Pharmacology, Clinical Aspects* (M. M. Müller, E. Kaiser and J. E. Seegmiller, eds.), pp. 304–311, Plenum Press, New York.

Simmonds, H. A., Panayi, G. S., and Corrigall, V., 1978, A role for purine metabolism in the immune response: Adenosine-deaminase activity and deoxyadenosine catabolism, *Lancet* **1**:60–63.

Simmonds, H. A., Rose, G. A., Potter, C. F., Sahota, A., Barratt, T. M., Williams, D. I., Arkell, D. G., Van Acker, K. T., and Cameron, J. S., 1979a, A further case of adenine phosphoribosyltransferase deficiency presenting with supposed "uric" acid stones: Pitfalls of diagnosis, *Proc. R. Soc. Med.* (in press).

Simmonds, H. A., Sahota, A., Potter, C. F., and Cameron, J. S., 1979b, Purine metabolism and immunodeficiency: Urinary purine excretion as a diagnostic screening test in adenine deaminase and purine nucleoside phosphorylase deficiency, *Clin. Sci. Mol. Med.* (in press).

Sinclair, D. S., and Fox, I. H., 1975, The pharmacology of hypouricemic effect of benzbromarone, *J. Rheum.* **2**:437–445.

Singh, S., Willers, I., and Goedde, H. W., 1976, A rapid micromethod for prenatal diagnosis of Lesch–Nyhan syndrome, *Clin. Genet.* **10**:12–15.

Skaper, S. D., and Seegmiller, J. E., 1976a, Hypoxanthine-guanine phosphoribosyltransferase mutant glioma cells: Diminished monoamine oxidase activity, *Science* **194**:1171–1173.

Skaper, S. D., and Seegmiller, J. E., 1976b, Increased concentrations of glycine in hypoxanthine-guanine phosphoribosyltransferase-deficient mouse neuroblastoma cells, *J. Neurochem.* **26**:689–694.

Skaper, S. D., and Seegmiller, J. E., 1977, Elevated intracellular glycine associated with hypoxanthine-guanine phosphoribosyltransferase deficiency in glioma cells, *J. Neurochem.* **29**:83–86.

Smith, M. L., and Buchanan, J. M., 1977, Purine biosynthesis during transition from resting to growing fibroblasts, *Fed. Proc. Fed. Am. Soc. Exp. Biol.* **36**:798 (abstract).

Smythe, H. A., 1977, Xanthine and uric acid as xanthine oxidase inhibitors, *Arthritis Rheum.* **20**:135–136.

Snyder, F. F., and Henderson, J. F., 1973, Alternative pathways of deoxyadenosine and adenosine metabolism, *J. Biol. Chem.* **248**:5899–5904.

Snyder, F. F., Mendelsohn, J., and Seegmiller, J. E., 1976, Adenosine metabolism in phytohemagglutinin-stimulated human lymphocytes, *J. Clin. Invest.* **58**:654–666.

Snyder, F. F., Hershfield, M. S., and Seegmiller, J. E., 1977, Purine toxicity in human lymphoblasts, in: *Advances in Experimental Medicine and Biology,* Vol. 76A, *Purine Metabolism in Man II: Regulation of Pathways and Enzyme Defects* (M. M. Müller, E. Kaiser, and J. E. Seegmiller, eds.), pp. 30–39, Plenum Press, New York.

Snyder, F. F., Hershfield, M. S., and Seegmiller, J. E., 1978, Cytotoxic and metabolic effects of adenosine and adenine upon human lymphoblasts, *Cancer Res.* **38**:2357–2362.

Sorensen, L. B., 1970, Mechanism of excessive purine biosynthesis in hypoxanthine-guanine phosphoribosyltransferase deficiency, *J. Clin. Invest.* **49**:968–978.

Sorensen, L. B., and Levinson, D. J., 1976, Clinical evaluation of benzbromarone: A new uricosuric drug, *Arthritis Rheum.* **19**:183–190.

Spector, E. B., Hershfield, M. S., and Seegmiller, J. E., 1978, Purine reutilization and synthesis *de novo* in long-term human lymphocyte cell lines deficient in adenine phosphoribosyltransferase activity, *Somat. Cell. Genet.* **4**:253–264.

Spencer, N., Hopkinson, D. A., and Harris, H., 1968, Adenosine deaminase polymorphism in man, *Ann. Hum. Genet.* **32**:9–14.

Sperling, O., Boer, P., Brosh, S., Zoref, E., and deVries, A., 1978a, Overproduction disease in man due to enzyme feedback resistance mutation, *Enzyme* **23**:1–9.

Sperling, O., Brosh, S., Boer, P., Liberman, U. A., and deVries, A., 1978b, Urinary xanthine stones in an allopurinol-treated gouty patient with partial deficiency of hypoxanthine-guanine phosphoribosyltransferase, *Isr. J. Med. Sci.* **14**:288–292.

Stein, H. B., Hasan, A., and Fox, I. H., 1976, Ascorbic acid-induced uricosuria: A consequence of megavitamin therapy, *Ann. Intern. Med.* **84**:385–388.

Stephenson, M. L., and Zamecnik, P. C., 1978, Inhibition of Rous sarcoma viral RNA translation by a specific oligodeoxyribonucleotide, *Proc. Natl. Acad. Sci. U.S.A.* **75**:285–288.

Stoop, J. W., Zegers, B. J. M., Hendricks, G. F. M., Siegenbeek van Heukelom, H. L., Staal, G. E. M., deBree, P. K., Wadman, S. K., and Ballieux, R. E., 1977, Purine nucleoside phosphorylase deficiency associated with selective cellular immunodeficiency, *N. Engl. J. Med.* **296**:651–655.

Strauss, M., Theile, M., and Geissler, E., 1978, The incorporation of homologous and heterologous hypoxanthine-guanine phosphoribosyltransferase into mutant cells, *Biochim. Biophys. Acta* **538**:11–22.

Streeter, D. G., Witkowski, J. T., Khare, G. P., Sidwell, R. W., Bauer, R. J., Robins, R. K., and Simon, L. N., 1973, Mechanism of action of 1-B-D ribofuranosyl-1,2,4-triazole-3-carboxamide (virazole), a new broad spectrum antiviral agent, *Proc. Natl. Acad. Sci. U.S.A.* **70**:1174–1178.

Sturge, R. A., Scott, J. T., Hamilton, E. B. D., Liyanage, S. P., Dixon, St. J., and Engler, C., 1977, Multicentre trial of naproxen and phenylbutazone in acute gout, *Ann. Rheum. Dis.* **36**:80–82.

Sweetman, L., Borden, M., Kulovich, S., Kaufman, I., and Nyhan, W. L., 1977a, Altered excretion of 5-hydroxyindoleacetic acid and glycine in patients with the Lesch–Nyhan disease, in: *Advances in Experimental Medicine and Biology,* Vol. 76A, *Purine Metabolism in Man II: Regulation of Pathways and Enzyme Defects* (M. M. Müller, E. Kaiser, and J. E. Seegmiller, eds.), pp. 398–404, Plenum Press, New York.

Sweetman, L., Borden, M., Lesch, P., Bakay, B., and Becker, M. A., 1977b, Diminished affinity for purine substrates as a basis for gout with mild deficiency of hypoxanthine-guanine phosphoribosyltransferase, in: *Advances in Experimental Medicine and Biology,* Vol. 76A, *Purine Metabolism in Man II: Regulation of Pathways and Enzyme Defects* (M. M. Müller, E. Kaiser, and J. E. Seegmiller, eds.), pp. 319–325, Plenum Press, New York.

Swyryd, E. A., Seaver, S. S., and Stark, G. R., 1974, N-(phosphonacetyl)-L-aspartate, a potent transition state analog inhibitor of aspartate transcarbamylase, blocks proliferation of mammalian cells in culture, *J. Biol. Chem.* **249**:6945–6950.

Szüts, P., Havass, Z., and Boda, D., 1977, Adenosine deaminase defect of erythrocytes and combined immune defect: A new metabolic disease. First experiences with screening test of the disease and quantitative determination of enzyme activity, *Orv. Hetil.* **118**:2457–2460.

Tattersall, M. H. N., Ganeshaguru, K., and Hoffbrand, A. V., 1975, The effect of external deoxyribonucleosides on deoxyribonucleoside triphosphate concentrations in human lymphocytes, *Biochem. Pharmacol.* **24**:1495–1498.

Thompson, L. F., Willis, R. C., Stoop, J. W., and Seegmiller, J. E., 1978a, Purine metabolism in cultured human fibroblasts derived from patients deficient in enzymes of the purine salvage pathway, *Monogr. Hum. Genet.* **10**:100–103.

Thompson, L. F., Willis, R. C., Stoop, J. W., and Seegmiller, J. E., 1978b, Purine metabolism in cultured human fibroblasts derived from patients deficient in hypoxanthine-guanine phosphoribosyltransferase, purine nucleoside phosphorylase, or adenosine deaminase, *Proc. Natl. Acad. Sci. U.S.A.* **75**:3722–3726.

Torrance, J. D., Karabus, C. D., Shinier, M., Meltzer, M., Katz, J., and Jenkins, T., 1977a, Haemolytic anaemia due to erythrocyte pyrimidine 5'-nucleotidase deficiency, *S. Afr. Med. J.* **52**:671–673.

Torrance, J., West, C., and Beutler, E., 1977b, A simple rapid radiometric assay for pyrimidine-5'-nucleotidase, *J. Lab. Clin. Med.* **90**:563–568.

Torrance, J. D., Whittaker, D., and Beutler, E., 1977c, Purification and properties of human erythrocyte pyrimidine 5'-nucleotidase, *Proc. Natl. Acad. Sci. U.S.A.* **74**:3701–3704.

Traut, E. F., Knight, A. A., Szanto, P. B., and Passerelli, E. W., 1954, Specific vascular changes in gout, *J. Am. Med. Assoc.* **156**:591–593.

Turpin, B. P., Duckworth, W. C., and Solomon, S. S., 1977, Perfusion of isolated rat adipose cells, *J. Clin. Invest.* **60**:442–448.

Uitendaal, M. P., de Bruyn, C. H. M. M., Oei, T. L., Hösli, P., and Griscelli, C., 1978, A new ultramicrochemical assay for purine nucleoside phosphorylase, *Anal. Biochem.* **84**:147–153.

Ullman, B., Cohen, A., and Martin, D. W., Jr., 1976, Characterization of a cell culture model for the study of adenosine deaminase and purine nucleoside phosphorylase-deficient immunologic disease, *Cell* **9**:205–211.

Upchurch, K. S., Leyva, A., Arnold, W. J., Holmes, E. W., and Kelley, W. N., 1975, Hypoxanthine phosphoribosyltransferase deficiency: Association of reduced catalytic activity with reduced levels of immunologically detectable enzyme protein, *Proc. Natl. Acad. Sci. U.S.A.* **72**:4142–4146.

Vaezy, A., and Budson, D. C., 1978, Phalangeal metastases from bronchogenic carcinoma, *J. Am. Med. Assoc.* **239**:226–227.

Valentine, W. N., Fink, K., Paglia, D. E., Harris, S. R., and Adams, W. S., 1974, Hereditary hemolytic anemia with human erythrocyte pyrimidine 5'-nucleotidase deficiency, *J. Clin. Invest.* **54**:866–879.

Van Acker, K. J., Simmonds, H. A., and Cameron, J. S., 1977a, Complete deficiency of adenine phosphoribosyltransferase: Report of a family, in: *Advances in Experimental Medicine and Biology*, Vol. 76A, *Purine Metabolism in Man II: Regulation of Pathways and Enzyme Defects* (M. M. Müller, E. Kaiser, and J. E. Seegmiller, eds.), pp. 295–302, Plenum Press, New York.

Van Acker, K. J., Simmonds, H. A., Potter, C., and Cameron, J. S., 1977b,

Complete deficiency of adenine phosphoribosyltransferase: Report of a family, *N. Engl. J. Med.* **297**:127—132.

Van Woert, M. H., Yip, L. C., and Balis, M. E., 1977, Purine phosphoribosyltransferase in Gilles de la Tourette syndrome, *N. Engl. J. Med.* **296**:210–212.

Wallace, S. L., Robinson, H., Masi, A. T., Decker, J. L., McCarty, D. J., and Yü, T.-F., 1977, Preliminary criteria for the classification of the acute arthritis of primary gout, *Arthritis Rheum.* **20**:895–900.

Wanasukapunt, S., Lertratanakul, Y., and Rubinstein, H. M., 1976, Effect of fenoprofen calcium on acute gouty arthritis, *Arthritis Rheum.* **19**:933–935.

Watts, R. W. E. (chairman), 1977, Panel discussion: Hyperuricemia as a risk factor, *Adv. Exp. Med. Biol.* **76B**:342–364.

Webster, A. D. B., North, M., Allsop, J., Asherson, G. L., and Watts, R. W. E., 1978, Purine metabolism in lymphocytes from patients with primary hypogammaglobulinaemia, *Clin. Exp. Immunol.* **31**:456–463.

Weinshilboum, R. M., Goldstein, J. L., and Kelley, W. N., 1975, Prolonged hypouricemia associated with acute chloroprothixene ingestion, *Arthritis Rheum.* **18**(Suppl.):739–742.

Whitley, R. J., Soong, S.-J., Dolin, R., Galasso, G. J., Ch'ien, L. T., Alford, C. A., and Collaborative Study Group, 1977, Adenine arabinoside therapy of biopsy-proved herpes simplex encephalitis, *N. Engl. J. Med.* **297**:289–294.

Willers, I., Held, K. R., Singh, S., and Goedde, H. W., 1977, Genetic heterogeneity of hypoxanthine-phosphoribosyl transferase in human fibroblasts of 3 families, *Clin. Genet.* **11**:193–200.

Willis, R. C., Carson, D. A., and Seegmiller, J. E., 1978, Adenosine kinase initiates the major route of ribavirin activation in a cultured human cell line, *Proc. Natl. Acad. Sci. U.S.A.,* **75**:3042–3044.

Winocour, P. D., Munday, K. A., Taylor, T. G., and Turner, M. R., 1976, Platelet aggregation in rats made hyperuricaemic with nucleic acid-rich diets containing oxonate, an inhibitor of uricase, *Proc. Nutr. Soc.* **35**:54A–55A.

Winocour, P. D., Turner, M. R., Taylor, T. G., and Munday, K. A., 1977, Gout and cardiovascular disease, *Lancet* **1**:959–960.

Wolberg, G., Zimmerman, T. P., Hiemsra, K., Winston, M., and Chu, L. C., 1975, Adenosine inhibition of lymphocyte mediated cytolysis: Possible role of cyclic adenosine monophosphate, *Science* **187**:957–959.

Wolf, J., Reid, R., Anderson, J., Rebuck, J., Lightbody, J., Johnson, R., Uberti, J., and Weiss, L., 1976, Transplantation, bacterial challenges on pulmonary and alveolar macrophages. Cellular immunodeficiency associated with ADA deficiency: Treatment with thymosin and ADA enzyme replacement, *J. Reticuloendothel. Soc.* **20**:48A.

Wolfensberger, C., 1976, Ein seltener chirurgischer Notfall: Akutes Karpaltunnelsyndrom bei Kalgich, *Helv. Chir. Acta* **43**:147–150.

Wyngaarden, J. B., 1976, Regulation of purine biosynthesis and turnover, *Adv. Enzyme Regul.* **14**:25–42.

Wyngaarden, J. B., and Holmes, E. W., Jr., 1977, Molecular nature of enzyme regulation, in: *Ciba Found. Symp. No. 48: Purine and Pyrimidine Metabolism*, pp. 43–64, Elsevier/Excerpta Medica, North-Holland, Amsterdam.

Wyngaarden, J. B., and Kelley, W. N., 1976, *Gout and Hyperuricemia*, Grune & Stratton, New York, 512 pp.

Wyngaarden, J. B., and Kelley, W. N., 1978, Gout, in: *The Metabolic Basis of Inherited Disease* (J. B. Stanbury, J. B. Wyngaarden, and D. S. Frederickson, eds.), pp. 916–1010, McGraw-Hill, New York.

Yen, R. C. K., Adams, W. B., Lazar, C., and Becker, M. A., 1978, Evidence for X-linkage of human phosphoribosylpyrophosphate synthetase, *Proc. Natl. Acad. Sci. U.S.A.* **75**:482–485.

Yin, H. H., and Berlin, R. D., 1975, The relation of endogeneous adenosine cyclic 3':5'-monophosphate to the antagonistic effects of adenosine and colchicine on cell shape, *J. Cell. Physiol.* **85**:627–634.

Yoder, F. W., Brumback, R. A., Andrews, A. D., Peck, G. L., and Robbins, J. H., 1976, A comparison of some clinical manifestations of Cockayne's syndrome and xeroderma pigmentosum, *Clin. Res.* **24**:624A (abstract).

Yokoyama, M., Suzuki, T., Aso, Y., and Akaoka, I., 1977, A xanthine stone in a xanthinuric boy: A biochemical case study, *J. Urol.* **118**:651–653.

Yun, S.-L., and Suelter, C. H., 1978, Human erythrocyte 5'-AMP aminohydrolase, *J. Biol. Chem.* **253**:404–408.

Zamecnik, P. C., and Stephenson, M. L., 1978, Inhibition of Rous sarcoma virus replication and cell transformation by a specific oligodeoxynucleotide, *Proc. Natl. Acad. Sci. U.S.A.* **75**:280–284.

Zannis, V., Doyle, D., and Martin, D. W., Jr., 1978, Purification and characterization of human erythrocyte purine nucleoside phosphorylase and its subunits, *J. Biol. Chem.* **253**:504–510.

Zarcone, V., and Guilleminault, G., 1977, 5-Hydroxytryptophan as an investigative tool in neurological and psychiatric disorders, in: *Neuroregulators and Psychiatric Disorders* (E. Usdin, ed.), pp. 188–192, Oxford University Press, New York.

Zoref, E., Sperling, O., and deVries, A., 1975, Characterization of purine metabolism in cultured fibroblasts from a gouty family with feedback-resistant phosphoribosylpyrophosphate synthetase, *Isr. J. Med. Sci.* **11**:1216–1217.

Zoref, E., deVries, A., and Sperling, O., 1977a, Evidence for X-linkage of phosphoribosyl-pyrophosphate synthetase in man: Studies with cultured fibroblasts from a gouty family with mutant feedback-resistant enzyme, *Hum. Hered.* **27**:73–80.

Zoref, E., deVries, A., and Sperling, O., 1977b, Transfer of resistance to selective conditions from fibroblasts with mutant feedback-resistant phosphoribosylpyrophosphate synthetase to normal cells: A form of metabolic cooperation, in: *Advances in Experimental Medicine and Biology*, Vol. 76A, *Purine Metabolism in Man II: Regulation of Pathways and Enzyme Defects* (M. M. Müller, E. Kaiser, and J. E. Seegmiller, eds.), pp. 80–84, Plenum Press, New York.

Metabolic Actions of Ethanol

Enrique Baraona and Charles S. Lieber

2.1. Effects of Ethanol on Protein Metabolism

Two of the earliest and most conspicuous features of the hepatic damage produced by alcohol are the deposition of fat and the enlargement of the liver. This hepatomegaly was traditionally attributed to the accumulation of lipids. However, in animals fed alcohol-containing diets, lipids account for only half the increase in liver dry weight (Lieber *et al.*, 1965), and it was recently shown that the other half is almost totally accounted for by an increase in proteins (Baraona *et al.*, 1975) (Fig. 1). The increase involves mainly soluble proteins, the accumulation of which is accompanied by a proportional retention of water. The increases in lipid, protein, and water result in increased size of the hepatocytes. Since the number of hepatocytes and the hepatic content of DNA do not change after alcohol treatment, the hepatomegaly is entirely accounted for by the increased cell volume.

2.1.1. Origin of the Increased Liver Protein

It was reported more than ten years ago that in rats alcohol consumption results in proliferation of the smooth membranes of the endoplasmic reticulum (Iseri *et al.*, 1966). This finding was subsequently

ENRIQUE BARAONA and CHARLES S. LIEBER • Alcoholism Research and Treatment Center, Veterans Administration Medical Center, Bronx, New York 10468; Mount Sinai School of Medicine of the City University of New York, New York, New York 10029.

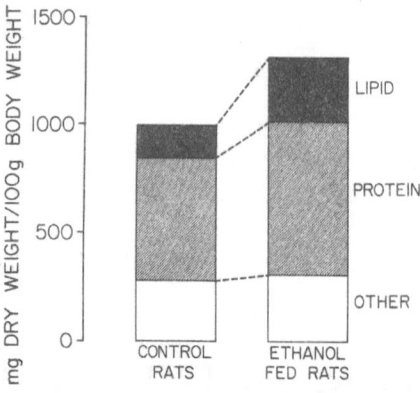

Fig. 1. Effects of ethanol feeding on hepatic lipid and protein contents. From Baraona *et al.* (1975).

confirmed (Lane and Lieber, 1966; Rubin *et al.*, 1968; Carulli *et al.*, 1971) and established on a biochemical basis by the demonstration of an increase in both phospholipids and total protein content of the smooth membranes (Ishii *et al.*, 1973). The mechanism of this microsomal alteration remains unknown. By analogy with the proliferation of this organelle induced by other drugs or foreign compounds that utilize microsomal enzymes during their metabolism, the alcohol-induced hypertrophy has been linked to the fact that alcohol can be oxidized by a microsomal ethanol-oxidizing system (MEOS) (Lieber and DeCarli, 1970a), in addition to the predominant alcohol dehydrogenase (ADH) pathway of the cytosol. The rise in microsomal protein, however, accounts for only 30% of the total protein increase. Mitochondria are also grossly altered after alcohol administration (Iseri *et al.*, 1966; Lane and Lieber, 1966; Rubin *et al.*, 1972). Swollen and giant mitochondria are commonly observed, but total mitochondrial proteins do not contribute significantly to the total increase in liver protein. More than half the total increase in liver protein is actually due to increased soluble proteins of the cytosol (Baraona *et al.*, 1975) (Fig. 2).

2.1.2. Type of Proteins That Accumulate after Chronic Alcohol Consumption

Contrasting with the lack of changes in the concentration of total hepatic proteins, the concentration of some proteins (such as albumin and transferrin) that are primarily destined for export into the plasma was found significantly increased in the liver of ethanol-fed rats, whereas the concentration of soluble constituent proteins (such as ferritin) decreased (Baraona *et al.*, 1975, 1977). The increased concentration of export proteins reflects an even greater increase in the amount per total liver, since alcohol administration produced hepatomegaly. Conversely, decreased concentration of constituent proteins after alcohol feeding may merely reflect dilution in enlarged protein and water pools. These observations pose a general problem in the interpretation of protein concentrations or enzyme activities after alcohol treatment when expressed solely per gram of liver or per gram of protein without concomitant assessment of the liver size.

It was shown, in the case of albumin, that the increase involves precursor proteins (such as proalbumin) as well as mature serum albumin (Baraona *et al.*, 1977). The current theory is that proteins destined for export are synthesized by bound ribosomes, discharged into the cysterna of the rough endoplasmic reticulum, and then transported to the smooth endoplasmic reticulum and Golgi apparatus (Peters, 1962; Glaumann, 1970; Glaumann and Ericsson, 1970; Peters *et al.*, 1971; Morgan and Peters, 1971a,b; Redman and Cherian, 1972). This theory, supported by biochemical evidence, has been disputed in the case of albumin because of electron-microscopic evidence that indicates direct discharge of albumin from bound ribosomes into the cytosol (Lin and Chang, 1975). Though immunoreactive albumin accumulates preferentially in the cytosol and transferrin in the microsomal fraction, after ethanol feeding, the concentration of these proteins increased in both compartments. Since no evidence of leakage from the microsomes was obtained, the possibility that the cytosol could serve as a storage site of retained proteins must be considered.

It must be pointed out, however, that the increases in these two export proteins (albumin and transferrin) account for only a small fraction of the total increase in soluble proteins. Thus, the major contributor to the ethanol-induced accumulation of liver protein has not been identified as yet.

2.1.3. Mechanisms of the Alcohol-Induced Accumulation of Liver Protein

Accumulation of protein in the liver could result from increased production, decreased disposition, or a combination of both mechanisms.

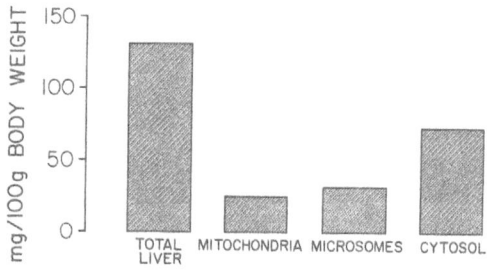

Fig. 2. Distribution among subcellular fractions of the increase in liver protein induced by ethanol feeding. From Baraona *et al.* (1975).

Reduced disposition, in turn, could be due to decreased proteolysis or
delayed secretion into the plasma.

2.1.3.1. Effects of Ethanol on Protein Synthesis

There is a consensus that acute ethanol administration inhibits the
synthesis of both constituent and export proteins of the liver. This view is
supported mainly by experimental evidence that has been obtained after
addition of ethanol to various *in vitro* preparations, such as perfused livers
(Rothschild *et al.*, 1971; Kirsch *et al.*, 1973; Chambers and Piccirillo, 1973;
Morland, 1975), liver slices (Perin *et al.*, 1974; Sorrell *et al.*, 1977a),
microsomes (Renis *et al.*, 1975), ribosomes (Kuriyama *et al.*, 1971; Perin
and Sessa, 1975), and mitochondria (Rubin *et al.*, 1970; Renis *et al.*, 1975).
In vivo, however, the acute effects of ethanol on protein synthesis have
been less consistent. No change in the synthesis of total liver protein was
found after administration of ethanol (3–6 g/kg body weight) to naïve rats
(Seakins and Robinson, 1964; Ashworth *et al.*, 1965; Moojerkea and
Chow, 1969; Morland, 1974a). In one study in which subcellular fractions
were separated, acute administration of 5 g ethanol/kg body weight
decreased [^{14}C]leucine incorporation into mitochondrial protein markedly and in microsomal protein slightly (Renis *et al.*, 1975). Decreased
hepatic production of export proteins (such as albumin and transferrin)
was demonstrated after acute administration of ethanol (3 g/kg) to the rat
in vivo (Jeejeebhoy *et al.*, 1972). Similarly, inhibition of the hepatic production of serum lipoproteins was reported after acute ethanol administration, especially when high ethanol concentrations are achieved either *in
vitro* (Schapiro *et al.*, 1964) or *in vivo* (Dajani and Kouyoumjian, 1967;
Madsen, 1969). However, no changes, or even an increase, in lipoprotein
production were observed with more moderate doses both *in vitro* (Gordon, 1972) and *in vivo* (Elko *et al.*, 1961; Seakins and Robinson, 1964;
Wooles, 1966; Hirayama and Hiroshige, 1970; Baraona *et al.*, 1973;
Abrams and Cooper, 1976). Hypo- and hyperlipemic effects of ethanol
were produced by varying the dose of alcohol administered (Estler, 1975).
It is not clear whether the decreased production of plasma proteins is due
solely to a defect in synthesis or to a concomitant impairment of secretion.
Indeed, delayed appearance in the plasma of newly labeled albumin and
fibrinogen was observed after acute administration of ethanol *in vivo*
(Jeejeebhoy *et al.*, 1972). Also, *in vitro*, it was noted recently that the
ethanol-induced inhibition in the incorporation of either leucine or glucosamine into proteins released in the media by liver slices is greater than
the effects on tissular protein (Sorrell *et al.*, 1977a). Thus, it appears
reasonable to conclude that the acute inhibitory effects of ethanol on

protein synthesis are exaggerated by the *in vitro* conditions, suggesting that these effects may be greatly compensated by regulatory mechanisms operating *in vivo*. In addition, some degree of anoxia is almost unavoidable in *in vitro* preparations, and anoxia was shown to enhance the toxic effects of ethanol on protein synthesis (Jeejeebhoy *et al.*, 1975).

The acute inhibitory effects of ethanol on protein synthesis may not pertain to the conditions prevailing in alcoholics or in animals in which metabolic adaptations have developed in response to prolonged alcohol exposure. In keeping with this possibility, the ethanol-induced inhibition of albumin synthesis observed in naïve animals was not reproduced when ethanol was administered after chronic alcohol consumption (Jeejeebhoy *et al.*, 1975). Similar discrepancies between the acute and chronic effects of ethanol on protein synthesis were reported in isolated mice ribosomes (Kuriyama *et al.*, 1971) and rat microsomes (Renis *et al.*, 1975); these organelles exhibit enhanced ability to incorporate amino acids into protein when obtained from ethanol-fed animals, whereas they have reduced ability when obtained from naïve animals given an acute dose of alcohol.

Studies of protein synthesis after chronic ethanol administration have yielded conflicting results. Decreased incorporation of labeled amino acids into liver proteins was found by Banks *et al.* (1970) in rats fed the ethanol-containing diets described by Porta *et al.* (1968), and by Morland (1974b) after several weeks of administration of a mixture of solid and liquid diets containing ethanol. Moreover, the latter investigator showed that livers isolated from alcohol-fed rats have decreased ability to incorporate amino acids into protein after stimulation with dexamethasone, and reduced activity of enzymes (tryptophan oxygenase, tyrosine aminotransferase) involved in protein metabolism (Morland, 1974b). A common feature of these studies was the inability to produce either fatty liver or hepatomegaly or significant weight gain after administration of the alcohol-containing diets, suggesting that ethanol administration may have been associated with some degree of undernutrition. Therefore, the effects of chronic alcohol administration on protein synthesis were reassessed by Baraona *et al.* (1977) using rats pair-fed the liquid diets described by DeCarli and Lieber (1967). Under these conditions, rats gained weight at a rate of 3–4 g/day, the weight gain being slightly less in the alcohol-fed rats than in the controls despite isocaloric feeding. The inefficiency of ethanol calories to promote growth and weight gain compared with that of calories from other nutrients has been previously emphasized (Pirola and Lieber, 1972). Moreover, despite a 9.4% lower body weight, ethanol-fed rats had hepatomegaly and fatty liver. Contrasting with the previous reports, the incorporation of leucine into protein was not decreased. Moreover, as previously reported in other species (Shaw and Lieber, 1976), alcohol feeding increased the concentration of leucine (and other branched-chain amino acids) in the plasma and to an even greater extent in the liver, diluting the specific activity of the tracer in the amino acid precursor pools. When the dilution of the amino acid pool was corrected and the rates of protein synthesis were calculated according to Morgan and Peters (1971a,b), protein synthesis was shown to be enhanced by chronic ethanol administration.

The changes in total liver protein represent a balance of effects on individual proteins that may differ considerably. In keeping with this interpretation, it was found in alcohol-fed rats that mitochondrial protein synthesis is decreased (Rubin et al., 1970), despite the increase in the synthesis of total liver protein.

The mechanism of these effects of ethanol on protein synthesis is unknown. Most of the studies concerning the mechanism have been carried out after acute ethanol administration and mainly in vitro. In contrast to the acute inhibition of protein synthesis produced in the liver, ethanol does not affect protein synthesis in tissues with low or no capacity to oxidize alcohol, such as spleen, pancreas, diaphragm, bone marrow (Perin and Sessa, 1975), and heart (Schreiber et al., 1972), whereas significant inhibition is produced by its metabolite, acetaldehyde. An exception to this rule is the brain, which contains very little ADH activity; nevertheless, its ability to synthesize proteins is inhibited by ethanol, both acutely and chronically (Kuriyama et al., 1971; Tewari and Noble, 1971; Renis et al., 1975). In liver, the inhibition of ADH by pyrazole or 4-methyl-pyrazole markedly decreases the rate of ethanol oxidation and prevents the ethanol-induced inhibition on the synthesis of total proteins (Perin et al., 1974; Perin and Sessa, 1975), glycoproteins (Sorrell et al., 1977a), and depending on the nutritional conditions, also that of albumin (Rothschild et al., 1977). These observations indicate that the agent responsible for these alterations is a product of ethanol oxidation, rather than ethanol itself.

Two major consequences of the oxidation of alcohol in the liver have been postulated to play a role in the inhibition of protein synthesis: the shifting of the redox state (due to the increased NADH/NAD ratio) and the generation of acetaldehyde, a product that can react directly with various amino acids or sulfydryl groups of enzymes. The effects of agents that mimic alcohol-induced redox changes (such as sorbitol) and those that tend to correct this alteration (such as pyruvate or methylene blue) on the ethanol-induced inhibition of protein synthesis have been variable depending on the protein studied. While the inhibition of leucine incorporation into protein of liver slices was shown to be reversible, reproduced by sorbitol, and prevented by agents that antagonize the redox shift produced by ethanol (Perin et al., 1974; Perin and Sessa, 1975), the inhibition of glycoprotein synthesis by liver slices was found to be irreversible (Sorrell *et al.*, 1977b), not prevented by pyruvate or methylene blue, and reproduced by acetaldehyde (Sorrell *et al.*, 1977a). On the other hand, the inhibitory effect of acetaldehyde on protein synthesis was partially prevented by addition of substrates that decrease the NADH/NAD ratio (Perin and Sessa, 1975), suggesting that part of the effects of acetaldehyde may also be mediated by its ability to shift redox state.

In addition to studies on the agent responsible for the inhibitory effects of ethanol, several investigators have addressed the question of what step of protein metabolism serves as target for this inhibitory effect. The acute inhibition of albumin production induced by ethanol is associated with disaggregation of polysomes, especially those bound to the rough endoplasmic reticulum (Rothschild *et al.*, 1971, 1974). These bound polysomes are involved in the synthesis of export proteins (Redman, 1969; Hicks *et al.*, 1969). In addition, ethanol produces detachment of the polysomes and ribosomes from the endoplasmic membrane (Jeejeebhoy *et al.*, 1972; Rothschild *et al.*, 1974). These effects are aggravated by fasting, which by itself decreases the aggregation of ribosomes into polysomes (Rothschild *et al.*, 1968). However, the administration of the polyamine spermine, which favors the ribosome–membrane attachment, restored the aggregation of membrane-bound polysomes (as well as that of free polysomes), but did not prevent the ethanol-induced inhibition of albumin synthesis, unless arginine was added (Oratz *et al.*, 1976). Morphologically, the alterations of the rough endoplasmic reticulum occurred at higher ethanol doses than those necessary to demonstrate inhibition of albumin production *in vivo* (Jeejeebhoy *et al.*, 1972). These dissociations and others between the state of polysomal aggregation and protein synthesis (Rothschild *et al.*, 1977) suggest that the polysomal alteration is not generally the rate-limiting step in the inhibitory effect of ethanol on protein synthesis, though it might become limiting under certain conditions such as fasting. Moreover, ethanol (and acetaldehyde) added *in vitro* to isolated ribosomes (Kuriyama *et al.*, 1971) or polysomes (Perin and Sessa, 1975) incubated with the pH 5 enzyme fraction inhibited protein synthesis only when concentrations higher than those likely to be found *in vivo* were used (Kuriyama *et al.*, 1971). Also, the ability of microsomal preparations to synthesize protein *in vitro* was unaffected by previous intragastric administration of 5 g ethanol/kg body weight, a dose that produced decreased amino acid incorporation into microsomal protein *in vivo* (Renis *et al.*, 1975). These observations suggest that the inhibitory effect of ethanol does not take place directly at the ribosomal level.

The acute effects of ethanol on protein synthesis and on polysome aggregation can be reversed by massive supplementation with amino acids (Rothschild *et al.*, 1971; Jeejeebhoy *et al.*, 1972; Kirsch *et al.*, 1973; Perin and Sessa, 1975). This observation suggests that the primary target for the ethanol effect may be the availability of amino acids for protein synthesis. Ethanol could interfere with the availability of amino acids for protein synthesis by inhibiting the inward transport or by favoring utilization for purposes other than protein synthesis. It was reported that ethanol (in concentrations of 200 mg/100 ml) inhibits the uptake of some amino acids, particularly alanine and α-aminoisobutyric acid, both in isolated perfused livers and *in vivo* (Chambers and Piccirillo, 1973). This alteration appears to be linked to the redox shift produced by ethanol, since sorbitol and lactate reproduced and pyruvate or fructose prevented the ethanol-induced inhibition of the hepatic uptake of α-aminoisobutyric acid, an amino acid analogue that is actively transported by mammalian tissues without being metabolized or incorporated into protein (Chambers and Piccirillo, 1973). The uptake of leucine (which uses a different carrier system) was less sensitive to the inhibitory effect and required higher concentrations of ethanol (400 mg/100 ml) (Chambers and Piccirillo, 1973). Despite the lack of effect on uptake, leucine incorporation into protein was markedly inhibited by ethanol (Chambers and Piccirillo, 1973; Perin and Sessa, 1975; Sorrell *et al.*, 1977a). It was hypothesized by Perin and Sessa (1975) that the shift of the redox potential toward a reduced state produced by the oxidation of ethanol could enhance utilization of amino acids for the provision of the oxidized members of redox-dependent reactions (e.g., pyruvate–lactate, oxaloacetate–malate), decreasing their availability for protein synthesis. An alternative possibility is direct condensation of acetaldehyde with amino acids, rendering them unsuitable for incorporation into protein (Perin and Sessa, 1975; Sorrell *et al.*, 1977a).

The acute inhibitory effect of ethanol on protein synthesis disappears after prolonged alcohol consumption, and it is actually replaced by a stimulatory effect for reasons that have not as yet been clarified. Livers from alcoholics or animals given alcohol chronically display striking paucity of rough endoplasmic reticulum when examined by electron microscopy. This is associated with marked proliferation of the smooth membranes (Iseri *et al.*, 1966; Lane and Lieber, 1966). On a biochemical basis, there is also a 15% decrease in rough microsomal protein and RNA, with a somewhat lesser decrease in phospholipids per gram of liver in ethanol-fed rats compared with controls (Ishii *et al.*, 1973). Since the liver weight and volume (and the size of the hepatocyte) increase by 20–30%, the morphological impression and the biochemical data may reflect only a lesser contribution of the rough endoplasmic reticulum to the alcoholic hepatomegaly than that of other subcellular fractions. The state of ribosomal aggregation after chronic alcohol administration is unknown. If the ability of ethanol to promote a marked shift in redox potential is indeed responsible for the acute inhibitory effects, one would expect these effects to decrease after chronic alcohol consumption in view of the evidence that the redox changes generated by the oxidation of ethanol are attenuated after prolonged alcohol intake (Domschke *et al.,* 1974). Moreover, as indicated later in this review, there is suggestive evidence for increased proteolysis in alcohol-fed animals, which could lead to greater amino acid availability than in naïve animals. Chronic alcohol consumption not only prevents the acute inhibitory effects of ethanol, but actually enhances the net rate of protein synthesis for reasons that again are not clear. Enhanced protein synthesis may contribute to the development of hepatomegaly. The stimulatory effect of alcohol consumption on synthesis affected to the same degree total liver proteins and those proteins that are primarily destined for export, such as proalbumin (Baraona *et al.,* 1977). Nevertheless, while total protein concentration remained unchanged, the concentration of export protein increased, indicating that these changes cannot be accounted for solely by an overall increase in synthesis.

2.1.3.2. Effects of Ethanol on Protein Secretion

A secretory defect was recently documented in rats fed alcohol-containing diets by the observation of delayed appearance of newly labeled albumin and transferrin in the serum with a corresponding retention of these newly labeled proteins in the liver (Baraona and Lieber, 1977; Baraona *et al.,* 1977) (Fig. 3).

As previously mentioned, delayed appearance of newly labeled albumin and fibrinogen was observed by Jeejeebhoy *et al.* (1972) after an acute dose of ethanol. Moreover, Sorrell *et al.* (1977b) reported that ethanol inhibits the incorporation of leucine or glucosamine into proteins released by liver slices more than into tissular proteins, indicating either a preferential inhibitory effect of ethanol on the synthesis of exportable protein or a secretory defect. More recent preliminary studies (Tuma and Sorrell, 1977) also favor the possibility that the acute inhibitory effects of ethanol are exerted not only on protein synthesis but also on secretion. After chronic alcohol feeding, the secretory defect results in significant accumulation of exportable protein inside the liver. The contribution of this retention to the total increase in soluble protein remains to be determined. It is likely that export proteins other than albumin and transferrin could also be retained. The degree of retention may be particularly important for those export proteins (such as lipoproteins) the production of which is greatly enhanced by ethanol feeding (Baraona and Lieber, 1970; Baraona *et al.,* 1973).

Most of the plasma proteins (with the exception of albumin) are exported from the liver in the form of glycoproteins. The incorporation of glucosamine into glycoproteins is inhibited by acute ethanol administra-

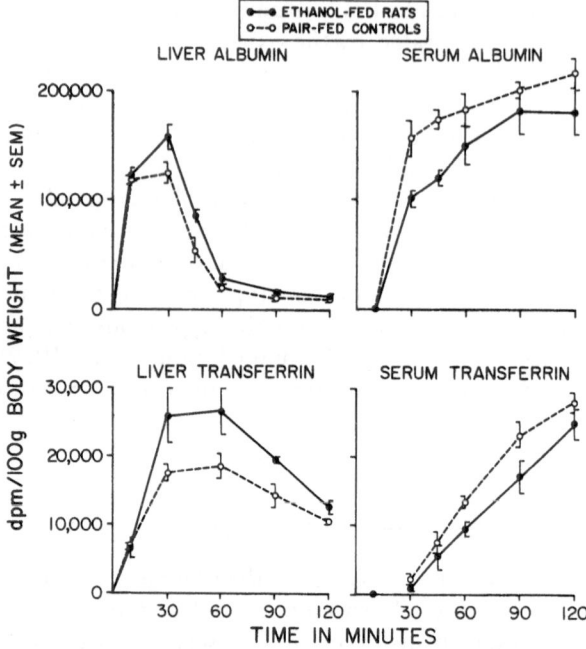

Fig. 3. Incorporation of intravenously injected [^{14}C] leucine into liver and serum albumin and transferrin at various time intervals in rats pair-fed either ethanol-containing or control diets. Labeling of liver albumin (30–45 min after injection) and of liver transferrin (30–90 min) was significantly greater in ethanol-fed rats, whereas labeling of serum albumin and transferrin (same time periods) was significantly reduced in these rats, compared with controls. From Baraona *et al.* (1977).

tion both *in vivo* (Moojerkea and Chow, 1969) and *in vitro* (Sorrell *et al.*, 1977a). This acute inhibitory effect of ethanol takes place during the formation of the precursor UDP-*N*-acetylglucosamine, which decreases after ethanol treatment (Moojerka and Chow, 1969; Sorrell *et al.*, 1977a), but it has been suggested that ethanol may also inhibit further steps in the glycosylation process, including the final attachment to the protein moiety (Sorrell *et al.*, 1977a). It appears paradoxical, however, that the activity of the glycosyl-transferases responsible for the carbohydrate binding to protein in the Golgi apparatus increases already 16 hr after an acute ethanol dose and even more after chronic ethanol feeding (Gang *et al.*, 1973). Moreover, a defect in glycosylation cannot account for the concomitant impairment in the secretion of albumin, a protein that does not require glycosylation. Therefore, attention was focused on a final secretory step affecting both glycoproteins and nonglycoproteins. Drugs (such as colchicine and Vinka alkaloids) that alter microtubules have been reported to impair secretion of macromolecules from various organs, including the liver (LeMarchand *et al.*, 1973, 1974; Stein and Stein, 1973; Stein *et al.*, 1974; Redman *et al.*, 1975). It was recently shown (Baraona *et al.*, 1977) in alcohol-fed rats that the defect in export was associated with a significant decrease in the content of polymerized tubulin, the major chemical component of microtubules. That this biochemical change was indeed due to a decrease in microtubules was recently documented morphologically (Baraona *et al.*, 1977; Matsuda *et al.*, 1978). The microtubules of ethanol-fed rats were not only decreased in number, but also differed qualitatively from normal microtubules, being generally shorter and significantly thicker (Matsuda *et al.*, 1978).

Incubation of hepatocytes with ethanol reproduced the microtubular alterations observed *in vivo*. These effects were prevented by pyrazole, indicating that they are linked to derangements generated by the oxidation of ethanol, rather than to ethanol itself. Moreover, serial additions of acetaldehyde with maintenance of concentrations similar to those reported to occur *in vivo* ($<200\ \mu$M) reproduced the effects of ethanol on both polymerized tubulin and visible microtubules (Baraona *et al.*, 1977). More recent experiments (Matsuda *et al.*, 1978) indicate that another product of ethanol metabolism, acetate, has similar inhibitory effects. Acetaldehyde (but not acetate) was also incriminated in the inhibitory effect of ethanol on the secretion of glycoproteins (Sorrell *et al.*, 1977a,b; Tuma and Sorrell, 1977). The respective roles and the mechanism of action of these metabolites have not been elucidated.

2.1.3.3. Effects of Ethanol on Protein Catabolism

It can be calculated from the data of Baraona *et al.* (1977) that the difference between the rate of synthesis of proalbumin and the rate of release of albumin into the serum should result in an accumulation of albumin far greater than that actually measured. Thus, it is likely that most of the retained proteins undergo degradation. The rate of proteolysis is generally assessed in the liver from the release of branched-chain amino acids (leucine, isoleucine, and valine), when reincorporation into protein can be suppressed or accounted for (Khairallah and Mortimore, 1976), since these amino acids are not significantly metabolized in the liver (Mortimore and Mondon, 1970). Adapting this method to isolated hepatocytes from normal rats, Morland and Bessesen (1977) found no changes in the rate of proteolysis after the addition of ethanol. However, these results may not pertain to the conditions of animals fed ethanol chronically, in which the concentration of branched-chain amino acids (such as leucine) increases in both liver and plasma, with a concentration gradient favoring release from liver to plasma (Baraona *et al.*, 1977). Also in keeping with the possibility of increased proteolysis in ethanol-fed animals are the reports of increased urinary nitrogen excretion (Klatskin, 1961; Rodrigo *et al.*, 1971).

2.1.4. Summary of the Alcohol-Induced Alterations of Hepatic Protein Metabolism and Possible Consequences

The acute inhibitory effect of alcohol on hepatic protein synthesis cannot persist for a significant length of time; otherwise, it would lead to rapid atrophy of the liver and reduced plasma protein concentrations, two complications that occur only at terminal stages of alcoholic liver disease. In fact, early stages are characterized by hepatomegaly (with increased content of liver protein) and no alteration in most plasma proteins. In fact, after chronic alcohol consumption, the synthesis of total liver protein increases.

An impairment in the secretion of exportable proteins can be demonstrated early in the course of alcoholic liver damage. This results in retention of export proteins in the liver and delayed appearance in the plasma. It is not known to what extent the retention of this type of protein contributes to the total increase in soluble protein that occurs in the liver after chronic alcohol consumption. The alteration in export does not produce significant changes in the plasma concentrations of most proteins. In this regard, the increased synthesis of precursors of exportable protein may represent a compensatory effort to maintain plasma levels even at the expense of further hepatic accumulation and probably enhanced degradation. With progression of liver damage, further deterioration of the secretory process or impaired synthesis may result in the low plasma protein levels that characterize advanced stages of alcoholic liver disease. The defect in export is associated with qualitative and quantitative alterations of microtubules, a cytoskeletal organelle required for normal export of macromolecules. The alteration of this organelle and the increased hepatic content in soluble protein (with parallel retention of water) produce swelling of the hepatocyte and disorganization of the subcellular architecture. These lesions may result in the "ballooning" of liver cells, a lesion commonly encountered in alcoholics in association with inflammation and necrosis.

2.2. Effects of Ethanol on Lipid Metabolism

2.2.1. Liver Lipids

Alcohol consumption promotes accumulation in the liver of the three main lipid classes: triglycerides, cholesterol (mainly its ester forms), and phospholipids. These alterations are considered to be due primarily to interference with the disposition of lipids reaching the liver from various sources (Fig. 4). Lipids are disposed by oxidation or by release either into the plasma or into the bile. Decreased fatty acid oxidation produced by ethanol has been demonstrated in liver slices (Lieber and Schmid, 1961; Blomstrand *et al.*, 1973), perfused livers (Lieber *et al.*, 1967), isolated hepatocytes (Ontko, 1973), and *in vivo* (Blomstrand and Kager, 1973). This effect offers the most likely explanation for the deposition in the liver of dietary fat (when available) or fatty acids derived from endogenous synthesis (in the absence of dietary fat) after chronic alcohol consumption. Fatty acid oxidation is impaired by both functional and structural changes that take place in the mitochondria (Rubin *et al.*, 1972; Cederbaum *et al.*, 1975; Matsuzaki and Lieber, 1977).

The disposition of cholesterol is also altered. The main pathway for cholesterol catabolism is bile salt formation, which decreases in ethanol-fed rats (Lefevre *et al.*, 1972). This alteration was recently attributed to decreased activity of cholesterol-7α hydroxylase (Lakshmanan and Veech, 1977).

The third major pathway for disposition of lipids from the liver is the production of serum lipoproteins, which was shown to be increased in rats fed alcohol-containing diets (Baraona and Lieber, 1970; Baraona *et al.*, 1973). This stimulation involves very-low-density (VLDL) and high-den-

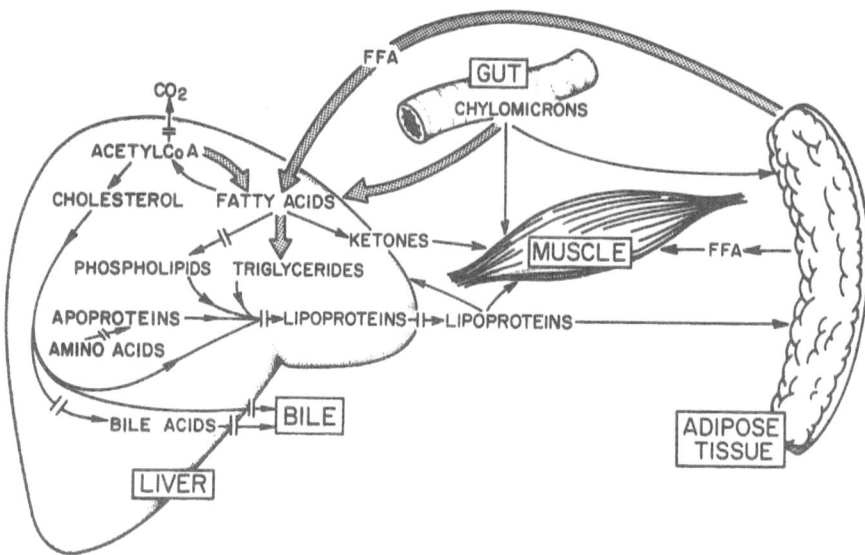

Fig. 4. Theoretical mechanisms for the development of alcoholic fatty liver. Ethanol intake could result in fatty liver either by enhancing the pathways illustrated by heavy arrows or by blocking those illustrated by broken lines. From Lieber (1979).

sity (HDL) lipoproteins, the two proteins produced by the liver, as well as low-density lipoproteins (LDL), a product of VLDL metabolism (Baraona and Lieber, 1970). At the early stage of alcoholic liver damage (fatty liver), the greatest increase occurs in VLDL. Full development of alcoholic hyperlipemia in the rat coincides with cessation of the active accumulation of fat in the liver (Lieber and DeCarli, 1970b). Nevertheless, fatty liver does not disappear on continued alcohol administration, illustrating a relative deficiency of the hyperlipemic response to rid the liver of fat. It has been postulated (Lieber et al., 1977) that this inability may be linked to the associated effects of ethanol on the secretion of exportable proteins (Baraona et al., 1977), hyperlipemia representing a balance between two opposite effects of ethanol: increased lipoprotein synthesis and delayed secretion into the plasma. Moreover, after prolonged and continuous alcohol intake, the relative deficiency in the lipoprotein response becomes an absolute one. Progressive alcoholic liver damage is associated with a decrease in the magnitude of alcoholic hyperlipemia, mainly at the expense of triglyceride-carrying lipoproteins (Marzo et al., 1970). Preliminary results in nonhuman primates fed alcohol-containing diets indicate that the decrease in hyperlipemia and serum VLDL with advancing liver disease coincides with exaggeration of the hepatic steatosis (Borowsky et al., 1976).

In the course of alcoholic liver disease, there are not only quantitative changes in the magnitude of the hyperlipemia, but also qualitative changes in serum lipoproteins. While the alcohol-induced increase in VLDL may represent a compensatory mechanism to counteract liver fat accumulation, the increase in HDL is poorly understood. The reported negative correlation between serum HDL levels and the incidence of coronary heart disease has revived the interest in the possible relationships between alcohol consumption and the development of atherosclerosis. Both the metabolic alterations of serum lipoproteins and the role of alcohol on the development of ischemic heart disease were the subject of studies to be summarized in the two following sections.

2.2.2. Alcohol-Induced Alterations in the Metabolism of Serum Lipoproteins

Accumulation of lipid in the blood occurs when its rate of entry into the blood exceeds its rate of removal. Thus, hyperlipemia can be produced either by an excessive production and release of lipoprotein into circulation or by defective removal or by a combination of both mechanisms. Positive evidence for increased serum lipoprotein production was obtained previously in ethanol-fed rats (Baraona and Lieber, 1970; Baraona et al., 1973). Increased splanchnic production of triglycerides was also observed after ethanol infusion to men submitted to hepatic vein catherization (Wolfe *et al.,* 1976). Secretion of VLDL-triglycerides increased in four of five subjects after alcohol, though this increase was insufficient to raise serum VLDL concentrations. It must be pointed out that these results were obtained after a 69-hr fast, and the blood ethanol levels achieved were very low (3–5 mM).

Contrasting with the stimulatory effect of ethanol on lipoprotein production, no changes were observed in the removal of lipids from circulation (Lieber *et al.,* 1966; Baraona and Lieber, 1970), except in a selected group of alcoholics with marked hyperlipemia in whom a persistent decrease in lipoprotein lipase activity was associated with alcohol abuse (Losowsky *et al.,* 1963). These studies were limited to the clearance of chylomicron-triglycerides. However, it has been recently recognized that the removal of chylomicrons is a two-step process whereby most of the triglycerides are removed by extrahepatic tissues by the action of lipoprotein lipase, leaving a "remnant" particle, relatively enriched in cholesterol esters, that is subsequently removed from circulation by the liver. Therefore, the effects of chronic ethanol administration on chylomicron removal were recently reassessed by Redgrave and Martin (1977). By feeding rats with a modified liquid diet containing 36% of calories as ethanol, these investigators produced hyperlipemia in the ethanol-fed rats and studied the removal of chylomicrons doubly labeled with [^{3}H]cholesterol and [^{14}C]palmitate. After infusion of these chylomicrons at a constant rate, the ethanol-fed rats developed higher levels of radioactivity in the plasma than the controls. ^{3}H-labeled cholesterol esters were removed from the plasma of normal rats less efficiently than were ^{14}C-labeled triglycerides, and in alcohol-fed rats, the clearance of cholesteryl esters was particularly delayed. The clearance of chylomicron-tiglycerides followed a similar trend, but the possibility of increased recirculation of labeled fatty acid in contaminating VLDL-triglycerides cannot be excluded. These experiments suggest that the hepatic step of chylomicron removal may be altered after chronic ethanol administration and that accumulation of chylomicron remnants could contribute cholesterol esters and triglycerides during alcoholic hyperlipemia. VLDL shares similar catabolic pathways with chylomicrons, except that a fraction of the remnant VLDL escapes complete hepatic degradation and appears as LDL, the catabolism of which occurs mainly in extrahepatic tissues. Thus, the liver removes most of the cholesterol esters and some of the triglycerides of chylomicrons and VLDL. However, the retention of cholesterol-ester-enriched remnant alone does not account for the hyperlipemia induced by alcohol in both man and animals, since the predominant increase occurs in triglycerides with a much lesser increase in cholesterol esters.

At more severe stages of alcoholic liver disease, the lipoprotein changes are indistinguishable from those occurring in liver diseases of other etiologies (Seidel *et al.*, 1970; Papadopoulos and Charles, 1970; Muller *et al.*, 1974). Sabesin *et al.* (1977) recently described such changes in patients with alcoholic hepatitis and laboratory evidence of intrahepatic cholestasis. There were striking alterations of the composition and ultra-structure of serum lipoproteins. Lipid stain after agarose electrophoresis showed disappearance of α- and pre-β lipoproteins and the presence of a single band of abnormal motility in the β area in the acute phase of the disease, with progressive normalization during recovery. VLDL (which normally migrate in a pre-β position) and HDL (which normally migrate in an α position) can be obtained by ultracentrifugation. Electron micro-graphs of negatively stained lipoprotein fractions revealed bilamellar vesicles and chains of stacked discs of variable size in the HDL and some of the LDL fractions. Their lipid composition was also markedly altered. There was a decrease in esterified cholesterol in all lipoprotein fractions, a decrease in lipids in HDL, and an increase in LDL fractions. The disap-pearance of α lipoproteins has been attributed to its decreased lipid content, whereas that of pre-β lipoproteins has been attributed to a lack of apoprotein A, which alters electrophoretic motility (Seidel *et al.*, 1972). These changes can be attributed, at least in part, to the concomitant decrease of lecithin:cholesterol acyltransferase (LCAT) activity. This activity requires an enzyme and HDL, which provide the activator and substrates for the enzyme. All the components of this system are pro-duced by the liver. Some of the lipoprotein alterations found in liver diseases resemble those found in patients with congenital deficiency of the LCAT enzyme, but it is not known whether the defective activity in patients with liver disease is due to defective enzyme, HDL components, or a combination of factors. The major role of this activity is to promote esterification of cholesterol derived from the membranes of most tissues and its transport to the liver, where it is finally excreted mainly as bile salts. Though this process occurs primarily in HDL, there is exchange of lipids with other lipoproteins. In addition, this process is associated with transfer of various apoproteins between lipoprotein fractions. Some of these apo-proteins appear to be required for the adequate removal of triglyceride-carrying lipoproteins. The LDL fraction of these patients contains a lipoprotein of very abnormal composition (lipoprotein X) associated with cholestasis (Seidel *et al.*, 1969, 1970), and also a triglyceride-rich lipopro-tein (β_2LP) that appears to be a remnant of either chylomicrons or VLDL (Muller *et al.*, 1974). The retention of the latter remnant is associated with decreased activity of hepatic triglyceride lipase in liver disease of various etiologies (Muller *et al.*, 1974; Freeman *et al.*, 1977), including alcoholism. These observations suggest that the lipoprotein abnormalities in alcoholics are multifactorial: some changes reflect alterations in production, whereas others indicate alterations in metabolism and removal.

2.2.3. Alcohol, Coronary Heart Disease, and High-Density Lipoproteins

The role of alcohol in the development of atherosclerosis and coronary heart disease (its most severe complication) has been a matter of controversy since the beginning of the century. In the last century, the opinion prevailed that alcohol could be an etiological factor in these diseases. This view was challenged by the observation of Cabot (1904), who showed that the incidence of atherosclerotic lesions in autopsies from patients with a history of alcoholism was remarkably low. A dissenting opinion was adopted by Wilens (1947), who indicated that the low incidence of atherosclerosis in chronic alcoholism could be due to the young age of the alcoholics in the necropsy material and to a relatively infrequent association between alcoholism and other conditions known to favor the development of atherosclerosis, such as hypertension, diabetes, and obesity. He noted, however, that alcoholics had a decreased tendency to develop lesions in the heart and brain in the presence of hypertension. While further studies confirmed the low incidence of coronary heart disease in alcoholics who died with cirrhosis of the liver (Hall *et al.*, 1953; Grant *et al.*, 1959; Howell and Manion, 1960), others failed to observe significant correlations (Spain and Bradess, 1957), or showed negative correlation with cirrhosis, but not with alcoholism (Hirst *et al.*, 1965).

Both Ruebner *et al.* (1961) and Parrish and Eberly (1961) interpreted the rarity of myocardial infarction in cirrhosis as a statistical fallacy, resulting from the low likelihood that two fatal diseases will occur together. Furthermore, in autopsy series, there is a heavy contribution of cases with atherosclerotic and hypertensive heart disease. As a consequence, other subgroups may exhibit an apparent "protective" effect. In autopsy series composed of victims of automobile accidents or other sudden deaths, either there was no correlation between alcoholism and atherosclerosis (Viel *et al.*, 1966) or even a positive correlation was reported (Lifsic, 1976). These series, in contrast, are heavily weighed with cases of alcoholism. Prospective clinical studies have shown either positive correlations (Tibblin *et al.*, 1975; Hrubec *et al.*, 1976) or no correlation (Paul *et al.*, 1963; Morris *et al.*, 1966; Sackett *et al.*, 1968; Myrhed, 1974). A major problem with these epidemiological studies has been the validity of the controls, since alcoholism involves a variety of psychological, sociological, and probably biochemical and genetic determinants that are difficult to match. Moreover, alcoholism is frequently associated with recognized risk factors of coronary heart disease, such as smoking. When most of these factors are considered, a negative correlation between alcohol consumption and coronary heart disease has emerged in several, but not all, recent studies (Klatsky *et al.*, 1974; Stason *et al.*, 1976). In a recent retrospective study (Barboriak *et al.*, 1977), the severity of arteriographically demonstrable coronary lesions in patients with angina pectoris or previous myocardial infarction or both was less in drinkers than in abstainers of similar age, despite a higher incidence of smoking and hypertriglyceridemia among drinkers.

A particularly significant study is that of Yano *et al.* (1977), which was done in a cohort of 7705 Japanese men living in Hawaii. The alcohol consumption recorded at the entry examination was correlated with the development of coronary heart disease; in a 6-year follow-up period, 294 subjects developed definitive manifestations of coronary heart disease. Of these, 59% were nondrinkers, whereas only 47% of the subjects without coronary heart disease were nondrinkers. A negative association between moderate alcohol consumption (11–60 ml alcohol/day) and age-adjusted incidence of coronary heart disease was found, independently of the type of alcoholic beverage consumed. By contrast, there was a trend toward higher incidence of coronary insufficiency among those subjects with the largest alcohol consumption (>40 ml alcohol/day). The incidence of coronary heart disease was highest for ex-drinkers, lowest for current drinkers, and intermediate for lifetime teetotalers. The negative association between moderate alcohol consumption and coronary heart disease became stronger if other risk factors, such as smoking, were taken into account. Since such moderate alcohol consumption has become common in modern societies, one wonders whether the apparent protection toward coronary disease is due to some other factor associated with the change in lifestyle. Only an experimental approach could provide perfectly matched controls. However, such studies have been hampered by the late development of adequate animal models of both atherosclerosis and alcoholism. The classic work of Eberhard (1936), which showed, in rabbits, protection by alcohol against the atherosclerotic lesions induced by diets, was recently confirmed (Goto *et al.*, 1974). Using different animal species, however, other investigators failed to detect any protective effect (Nichols *et al.*, 1956; Nikkila and Ollila, 1959; Gottlieb *et al.*, 1959).

The mechanism for the apparent protective effect of alcohol on the development of coronary heart disease is unknown. In view of the negative correlation between the incidence of coronary heart disease and the levels of serum HDL, it has been speculated that the effect of alcohol could be mediated by its ability to increase serum levels of this lipoprotein fraction. Indeed, high concentrations of HDL occur in alcoholics (Johansson and Laurell, 1969; Johansson and Medhus, 1974; Castelli *et al.*, 1977), and an elevation was noted in animals fed alcohol (Baraona and Lieber, 1970). The high levels of HDL might promote increased transport of cholesterol from peripheral tissues to the liver, where it is excreted (mainly as bile salts). However, at least in rats, ethanol inhibits rather than enhances bile salt production (Lefevre *et al.*, 1972). Alternatively, HDL could inhibit the uptake of LDL-cholesterol by vascular cells (Carew *et al.*, 1976; Miller, N. E., *et al.*, 1977).

2.2.4. Conclusion

Alcohol consumption promotes the accumulation of all lipid classes in the liver and increases the concentration of the two major serum lipoproteins (VLDL and HDL) as well as their metabolic products (LDL and various remnants). The rise in triglyceride-carrying VLDL is probably due to increased hepatic production, in response to an excess of hepatic fatty acids. However, this mechanism is not sufficient to prevent fatty liver development. The mechanism of the increase in plasma HDL is unknown. The negative correlation between the incidence of atherosclerosis and moderate alcohol consumption suggests that the increased serum levels of HDL after alcohol could play a key role in enhancing cholesterol removal from peripheral tissues.

ACKNOWLEDGMENTS

Original studies from the authors' laboratory referred to in this paper were supported in part by the Medical Research Service of the Veterans Administration and by USPHS grants AA 03508, AA 00224, and AM 12511.

References

Abrams, M. A., and Cooper, C., 1976, Quantitative analysis of metabolism of hepatic triglyceride in ethanol-treated rats, *Biochem. J.* **156**:33–46.

Ashworth, C. T., Johnson, C. F., and Wrightsman, F. J., 1965, Biochemical and morphologic correlations of hepatic protein synthesis in acute ethanol intoxication in rats, *Am. J. Pathol.* **46**:757–773.

Banks, W. L., Kline, E. S., and Higgins, E. S., 1970, Hepatic composition and metabolism after ethanol consumption in rats fed liquid purified diets, *J. Nutr.* **100**:581–594.

Baraona, E., and Lieber, C. S., 1970, Effects of chronic ethanol feeding on serum lipoprotein metabolism in the rat, *J. Clin. Invest.* **49**:769–778.

Baraona, E., and Lieber, C. S., 1977, Effects of ethanol on hepatic protein synthesis and secretion, in: *Currents in Alcoholism,* Vol. I (F. A. Seixas, ed.), pp. 33–46, Grune & Stratton, New York.

Baraona, E., Pirola, R. C., and Lieber, C. S., 1973, Pathogenesis of postprandial hyperlipemia in rats fed ethanol-containing diets, *J. Clin. Invest.* **52**:296–303.

Baraona, E., Leo, M. A., Borowsky, S. A., and Lieber, C. S., 1975, Alcoholic hepatomegaly: Accumulation of protein in the liver, *Science* **190**:794–795.

Baraona, E., Leo, M. A., Borowsky, S. A., and Lieber, C. S., 1977, Pathogenesis of alcohol-induced accumulation of protein in the liver, *J. Clin. Invest.* **60**:546–554.

Barboriak, J. J., Rimm, A. A., Anderson, A. J., Schmidhoffer, M., and Tristani, F. E., 1977, Coronary artery occlusion and alcohol intake, *Br. Heart J.* **39**:289–293.

Blomstrand, R., and Kager, L., 1973, The combustion of triolein-1-^{14}C and its inhibition by alcohol in man, *Life Sci.* **13**:113–123.

Blomstrand, R., Kager, L., and Lantto, O., 1973, Studies on the ethanol-induced decrease of fatty acid oxidation in rat and human liver slices, *Life Sci.* **13**:1131–1141.

Borowsky, S. A., Perlow, W., Baraona, E., and Lieber, C. S., 1976, Disappearance of alcoholic hyperlipemia as a sign of advancing liver damage, *Gastroenterology* **70**:978A–120.

Cabot, R. C., 1904, The relation of alcohol to arteriosclerosis, *J. Am. Med. Assoc.* **43**:774–775.

Carew, T. E., Hayes, S. B., Koschinsky, T., and Steinberg, D., 1976, A mechanism by which high-density lipoproteins may slow the atherogenic process, *Lancet* **1**:1315–1317.

Carulli, N., Manenti, F., Gallo, M., and Salvioli, G. F., 1971, Alcohol–drugs interaction in man: Alcohol and tolbutamide, *Eur. J. Clin. Invest.* **1**:421–424.

Castelli, W. P., Gordon, T., Hjortland, M. C., Kagan, A., Doyle, J. T., Hames, C. G., Hulley, S. B., and Zukel, W. J., 1977, Alcohol and blood lipids, *Lancet* **2**:153–155.

Cederbaum, A. I., Lieber, C. S., Beattie, D. S., and Rubin, E., 1975, Effect of chronic ethanol ingestion on fatty acid oxidation by hepatic mitochondria, *J. Biol. Chem.* **250**:5122–5129.

Chambers, J. W., and Piccirillo, V. J., 1973, Effects of ethanol on amino-acid uptake and utilization by the liver and other organs of rats, *Q. J. Stud. Alcohol* **34**:707–717.

Dajani, R. M., and Kouyoumjian, C., 1967, A probable direct role of ethanol in the pathogenesis of fat infiltration in the rat, *J. Nutr.* **91**:535–539.

DeCarli, L. M., and Lieber, C. S., 1967, Fatty liver in the rat after prolonged intake of ethanol with a nutritionally adequate new liquid diet, *J. Nutr.* **91**:331–336.

Domschke, S., Domschke, W., and Lieber, C. S., 1974, Hepatic redox state: Attenuation of the acute effects of ethanol induced by chronic ethanol consumption, *Life Sci.* **15**:1327–1334.

Eberhard, T. P., 1936, Effect of alcohol on cholesterol-induced atherosclerosis in rabbits, *Arch. Pathol.* **21**:616–627.

Elko, E. E., Wooles, W. R., and DiLuzio, N. R., 1961, Alterations and mobilization of lipids in acute ethanol-treated rats, *Am. J. Physiol.* **201**:923–926.

Estler, C.-J., 1975, Comparison of hepatic triglyceride content and hepatic lipid secretion after various doses of ethanol, *Biochem. Pharmacol.* **24**:1871–1873.

Freeman, M., Kuiken, L., Ragland, J. B., and Sabesin, S. M., 1977, Hepatic triglyceride lipase deficiency in liver disease, *Lipids* **12**:443–445.

Gang, H., Lieber, C. S., and Rubin, E., 1973, Ethanol increases glycosyl transferase activity in the hepatic Golgi apparatus, *Nature (London) New Biol.* **243**:123–125.

Glaumann, H., 1970, Studies on the synthesis and transport of albumin in microsomal subfractions from rat liver, *Biochim. Biophys. Acta* **224**:206–218.

Glaumann, H., and Ericsson, J. L. E., 1970, Evidence for the participation of the Golgi apparatus in the intracellular transport of nascent albumin in the liver cell, *J. Cell Biol.* **47**:555–567.

Gordon, E. R., 1972, Effect of an intoxicating dose of ethanol on lipid metabolism in an isolated perfused rat liver, *Biochem. Pharmacol.* **21**:2991–3004.

Goto, Y., Kikuchi, H., Abe, K., Nagahashi, Y., Ohiro, S., and Kudo, H., 1974, The effect of ethanol on the onset of experimental atherosclerosis, *Tohoku J. Exp. Med.* **114**:35–43.

Gottlieb, L. S., Broitman, S. A., Vitale, J. J., and Zamcheck, N., 1959, The influence of alcohol and dietary magnesium upon hypercholesterolemia and atherogenesis in the rat, *J. Lab. Clin. Med.* **53**:433–441.

Grant, W. C., Wasserman, F., Rodensky, P. L., and Thomson, R. V., 1959, The incidence of myocardial infarction in portal cirrhosis, *Ann. Intern. Med.* **51**:774–779.

Hall, E. M., Olsen, A. Y., and Davis, F. E., 1953, Portal cirrhosis: Clinical and pathological review of 782 cases from 16,600 necropsies, *Am. J. Pathol.* **29**:993–1027.

Hicks, S. J., Drysdale, J. W., and Munro, H. N., 1969, Preferential synthesis of ferritin and albumin by different populations of liver polysomes, *Science* **164**:584–585.

Hirayama, C., and Hiroshige, K., 1970, Effect of α-tocopherol and tocopheronolactone on ethanol induced fatty liver and triglyceridemia, *Experientia* **26**:1306–1308.

Hirst, A. E., Hadley, G. G., and Gore, I., 1965, The effect of chronic alcoholism and cirrhosis of the liver on atherosclerosis, *Am. J. Med. Sci.* **249**:143–149.

Hrubec, Z., Cederlöf, R., and Friberg, L., 1976, Background of angina pectoris: Social and environmental factors in relation to smoking, *Am. J. Epidemiol.* **103**:16–29.

Howell, W. L., and Manion, W. C., 1960, The low incidence of myocardial infarction in patients with portal cirrhosis of the liver: A review of 636 cases of cirrhosis of the liver from 17,731 autopsies, *Am. Heart J.* **60**:341–344.

Iseri, O. A., Lieber, C. S., and Gottlieb, L. S., 1966, The ultrastructure of fatty liver induced by prolonged ethanol ingestion, *Am. J. Pathol.* **48**:535–555.

Ishii, H., Joly, J.-G., and Lieber, C. S., 1973, Effect of ethanol on the amount and enzyme activities of hepatic rough and smooth microsomal membranes, *Biochim. Biophys. Acta* **291**:411–420.

Jeejeebhoy, K. N., Phillips, M. J., Bruce-Robertson, A., Ho, J., and Sodtke, U., 1972, The acute effect of ethanol on albumin, fibrinogen and transferrin synthesis in the rat, *Biochem. J.* **126**:1111–1126.

Jeejeebhoy, K. N., Bruce-Robertson, A., Ho, J., and Sodtke, U., 1975, The effect of ethanol on albumin and fibrinogen synthesis *in vivo* and in hepatocyte suspensions, in: *Alcohol and Abnormal Protein Synthesis* (M. A. Rothschild, M. Oratz, and S. S. Schreiber, eds.), pp. 373–391, Pergamon Press, New York.

Johansson, B. G., and Laurell, C. B., 1969, Disorders of serum α-lipoproteins after alcoholic intoxication, *Scand. J. Clin. Lab. Invest.* **23**:231–233.

Johansson, B. G., and Medhus, A., 1974, Increase in plasma α-lipoproteins in chronic alcoholics after acute abuse, *Acta Med. Scand.* **195**:273–277.

Khairallah, E. K., and Mortimore, G. E., 1976, Assessment of protein turnover in perfused rat liver: Evidence for amino acid compartmentation from differential labeling of free and t-RNA bound valine, *J. Biol. Chem.* **251**:1375–1384.

Kirsch, R. E., Frith, L. O., Stead, R. H., and Saunders, S. J., 1973, Effect of alcohol on albumin synthesis by the isolated perfused rat liver, *Am. J. Clin. Nutr.* **26**:1191–1194.

Klatskin, G., 1961, The effect of ethyl alcohol on nitrogen excretion in the rat, *Yale J. Biol. Med.* **34**:124–143.

Klatsky, A. L., Friedman, G. D., and Siegelaub, A. B., 1974, Alcohol consumption before myocardial infarction: Results from the Kaiser–Permanente epidemiologic study of myocardial infarction, *Ann. Intern. Med.* **81**:294–301.

Kuriyama, K., Sze, P. Y., and Rauscher, G. E., 1971, Effects of acute and chronic ethanol administration on ribosomal protein synthesis in mouse brain and liver, *Life Sci.* **10**(Part 2):181–189.

Lakshmanan, M. R., and Veech, R. L., 1977, Short- and long-term effects of ethanol administration *in vivo* on rat liver HMG-CoA reductase and cholesterol 7α-hydroxylase activities, *J. Lipid Res.* **18**:325–330.

Lane, B. P., and Lieber, C. S., 1966, Ultrastructural alterations in human hepatocytes following ingestion of ethanol with adequate diets, *Am. J. Pathol.* **49**:593–603.

Lefevre, A. F., DeCarli, L. M., and Lieber, C. S., 1972, Effect of ethanol on cholesterol and bile acid metabolism, *J. Lipid Res.* **13**:48–55.

LeMarchand, Y., Singh, A., Assimacopoulos-Jeannet, F., Orci, L., Rouiller, C., and Jeanrenaud, B., 1973, A role for the microtubular system in the release of very low density lipoproteins by perfused mouse livers, *J. Biol. Chem.* **248**:6862–6870.

LeMarchand, Y., Patzelt, C., Assimacopoulos-Jeannet, F., Loten, E. G., and Jeanrenaud, B., 1974, Evidence for a role of the microtubular system in the secretin of newly synthesized albumin and other proteins by the liver, *J. Clin. Invest.* **53**:1512–1517.

Lieber, C. S., 1979, *Medical Aspects of Alcoholism,* W. P. Saunders, Philadelphia (in press).

Lieber, C. S., and DeCarli, L. M., 1970a, Hepatic microsomal ethanol-oxidizing system: *In vitro* characteristics and adaptive properties *in vivo, J. Biol. Chem.* **245**:2505–2512.

Lieber, C. S., and DeCarli, L. M., 1970b, Quantitative relationship between amount of dietary fat and severity of alcoholic fatty liver, *Am. J. Clin. Nutr.* **23**:474–478.

Lieber, C. S., and Schmid, R., 1961, The effect of ethanol on fatty acid metabolism: Stimulation of hepatic fatty acid synthesis *in vitro*, *J. Clin. Invest.* **40**:394–399.

Lieber, C. S., Jones, D. P., and DeCarli, L. M., 1965, Effects of prolonged ethanol intake: Production of fatty liver despite adequate diets, *J. Clin. Invest.* **44**:1009–1021.

Lieber, C. S., Spritz, N., and DeCarli, L. M., 1966, Role of dietary, adipose, and endogenously synthesized fatty acids in the pathogenesis of the alcoholic fatty liver, *J. Clin. Invest.* **45**:51–62.

Lieber, C. S., Lefevre, A., Spritz, N., Feinman, L., and DeCarli, L. M., 1967, Difference in hepatic metabolism of long- and medium-chain fatty acids: The role of fatty acid chain length in the production of alcoholic fatty liver, *J. Clin. Invest.* **46**:1451–1460.

Lieber, C. S., Baraona, E., Borowsky, S. A., and Leo, M. A., 1977, Effect of ethanol on lipoprotein and protein export from the liver and its relationship to progressive alcoholic liver injury, in: *Membrane Alterations as Basis of Liver Injury* (L. Bianchi, H. Popper, and W. Reutter, eds.), pp. 327–341, MTP Press, Lancaster, England.

Lifsic, A. M., 1976, Alcohol consumption and atherosclerosis, *Bull. WHO* **53**:623–630.

Lin, C.-T., and Chang, J. P., 1975, Electron microscopy of albumin synthesis, *Science* **190**:465–467.

Losowsky, M. S., Jones, D. P., Davidson, C. S., and Lieber, C. S., 1963, Studies of alcoholic hyperlipemia and its mechanism, *Am. J. Med.* **35**:794–803.

Madsen, N. P., 1969, Reduced serum low-density lipoprotein levels after acute ethanol administration, *Biochem. Pharmacol.* **18**:261–262.

Marzo, A., Ghirardi, P., Sardini, D., Prandini, B. D., and Albertini, A., 1970, Serum lipids and total fatty acids in chronic alcoholic liver disease at different stages of cell damage, *Klin. Wochenschr.* **48**:949–950.

Matsuda, Y., Baraona, E., Salaspuro, M., and Lieber, C. S., 1978, Pathogenesis and role of microtubular alterations in alcohol induced liver injury, *Fed. Proc. Fed. Am. Soc. Exp. Biol.* **37**:402.

Matsuzaki, S., and Lieber, C. S., 1977, Increased susceptibility of hepatic mitochondria to the toxicity of acetaldehyde after chronic ethanol consumption, *Biochem. Biophys. Res. Commun.* **75**:1059–1065.

Miller, N. E., Weinstein, D. B., Carew, T. E., Koschinsky, T., and Steinberg, D., 1977, Interaction between high density and low density lipoproteins during uptake and degradation by cultured human fibroblasts, *J. Clin. Invest.* **60**:78–88.

Moojerkea, S., and Chow, A., 1969, Impairment of glycoprotein synthesis in acute ethanol intoxication in rats, *Biochim. Biophys. Acta* **184**:83–94.

Morgan, E. H., and Peters, T., Jr., 1971a, The biosynthesis of rat serum albumin. V. Effect of protein depletion and refeeding on albumin and transferrin synthesis, *J. Biol. Chem.* **246**:3500–3507.

Morgan, E. H., and Peters, T., Jr., 1971b, Intracellular aspects of transferrin synthesis and secretion in the rat, *J. Biol. Chem.* **246**:3508–3511.

Morland, J., 1975, Incorporation of labelled amino acids into liver protein after acute ethanol administration, *Biochem. Pharmacol.* **24**:439–442.

Morland, J., 1974b, Effects of chronic ethanol treatment on tryptophan oxygenase, tyrosine aminotransferase and general protein metabolism in the intact and perfused rat liver, *Biochem. Pharmacol.* **23**:21–35.

Morland, J., and Bessesen, A., 1977, Inhibition of protein synthesis by ethanol in isolated rat liver parenchymal cells, *Biochim. Biophys. Acta* **474**:312–320.

Morris, J. N., Kagan, A., Pattison, D. C., Gardner, M. J., and Raffle, P. A. B., 1966, Incidence and prediction of ischemic heart-disease in London busmen, *Lancet* **2**:553–559.

Mortimore, G. E., and Mondon, C. E., 1970, Inhibition by insulin of valine turnover in the liver: Evidence for a general control of proteolysis, *J. Biol. Chem.* **245**:2375–2383.

Muller, P., Fellin, R., Lanbrecht, J., Agostini, B., Wieland, H., Rost, W., and Speidel, D., 1974, Hypertriglyceridaemia secondary to liver disease, *Eur. J. Clin. Invest.* **4**:419–428.

Myrhed, M., 1974, Alcohol consumption in relation to factors associated with ischemic heart disease, *Acta Med. Scand. Suppl.* **567**:1–93.

Nichols, C. W., Jr., Siperstein, M. D., Gaffey, W., Lindsay, S., and Chaikoff, I. L., 1956, Does the ingestion of alcohol influence the development of arteriosclerosis in fowls?, *J. Exp. Med.* **103**:465–475.

Nikkila, E. A., and Ollila, O., 1959, Effect of alcohol ingestion on experimental chicken atherosclerosis, *Circ. Res.* **7**:588–594.

Ontko, J. A., 1973, Effects of ethanol on the metabolism of free fatty acids in isolated liver cells, *J. Lipid Res.* **14**:78–86.

Oratz, M., Rothschild, M. A., and Schreiber, S. S., 1976, Alcohol, amino acids, and albumin synthesis. II. Alcohol inhibition of albumin synthesis reversed by arginine and spermine, *Gastroenterology* **71**:123–127.

Papadopoulos, N. M., and Charles, M. A., 1970, Serum lipoprotein patterns in liver disease, *Proc. Soc. Exp. Biol. Med.* **134**:797–799.

Parrish, H. M., and Eberly, A. L., 1961, Negative association of coronary atherosclerosis with liver cirrhosis and chronic alcoholism—statistical fallacy, *J. Indiana State Med. Assoc.* **54**:341–347.

Paul, O., Lepper, M. H., Phelan, W. H., Dupertuis, G. W., Macmillan, A., McKean, H., and Park, H., 1963, A longitudinal study of coronary heart disease, *Circulation* **28**:20–31.

Perin, A., and Sessa, A., 1975, *In vitro* effects of ethanol and acetaldehyde on tissue protein synthesis, in: *The Role of Acetaldehyde in the Actions of Ethanol*, Satellite Symposium of the 6th International Congress of Pharmacology, Helsinki (K. O. Lindros and C. J. P. Eriksson, eds.), Vol. 23, pp. 105–122, The Finnish Foundation for Alcohol Studies, Helsinki.

Perin, A., Scalabrino, G., Sessa, A., and Arnaboldi, A., 1974, *In vitro* inhibition of protein synthesis in rat liver as a consequence of ethanol metabolism, *Biochim. Biophys. Acta* **366**:101–108.

Peters, T., Jr., 1962, The biosynthesis of rat serum albumin. II. Intracellular phenomena in the secretion of newly formed albumin, *J. Biol. Chem.* **237**:1186–1189.

Peters, T., Jr., Fleischer, B., and Fleischer, S., 1971, The biosynthesis of rat serum albumin. IV. Apparent passage of albumin through the Golgi apparatus during secretion, *J. Biol. Chem.* **246**:240–244.

Pirola, R. C., and Lieber, C. S., 1972, The energy cost of the metabolism of drugs, including ethanol, *Pharmacology* **7**:185–196.

Porta, E. A., Koch, O. R., Gomez-Dumm, C. L. A., and Hartroft, W. S., 1968, Effects of dietary protein on the liver of rats in experimental chronic alcoholism, *J. Nutr.* **94**:437–446.

Redgrave, T. G., and Martin, G., 1977, Effects of chronic ethanol consumption on the catabolism of chylomicron triacylglycerol and cholesteryl ester in the rat, *Atherosclerosis* **28**:69–80.

Redman, C. M., 1969, Biosynthesis of serum proteins and ferritin by free and attached ribosomes of rat liver. *J. Biol. Chem.* **244**:4308–4315.

Redman, C. M., and Cherian, M. G., 1972, The secretory pathways of rat serum glycoproteins and albumin: Localization of newly formed proteins within the endoplasmic reticulum, *J. Cell Biol.* **52**:231–245.

Redman, C. M., Banerjee, D., Howell, K., and Palade, G. E., 1975, Colchicine inhibition of plasma protein release from rat hepatocytes, *J. Cell Biol.* **66**:42–59.

Renis, M., Giovine, A., and Bertolino, A., 1975, Protein synthesis in mitochondrial and microsomal fractions from rat brain and liver after acute and chronic ethanol administration, *Life Sci.* **16**:1447–1457.

Rodrigo, C., Antezana, C., and Baraona, E., 1971, Fat and nitrogen balances in rats with alcohol-induced fatty liver, *J. Nutr.* **101**:1307–1310.

Rothschild, M. A., Oratz, M., Mongelli, J., and Schreiber, S. S., 1968, Effects of a short-term fast on albumin synthesis studied *in vivo*, in the perfused liver, and on amino acid incorporation by hepatic microsomes, *J. Clin. Invest.* **47**:2591–2599.

Rothschild, M. A., Oratz, M., Mongelli, J., and Schreiber, S. S., 1971, Alcohol-induced depression of albumin synthesis: Reversal by tryptophan, *J. Clin. Invest.* **50**:1812–1818.

Rothschild, M. A., Oratz, M., and Schreiber, S. S., 1974, Alcohol, amino acids, and albumin synthesis, *Gastroenterology* **67**:1200–1213.

Rothschild, M. A., Oratz, M., and Schreiber, S. S., 1977, The effects of ethanol and acetaldehyde on albumin synthesis, *Clin. Res.* **25**:516A.

Rubin, E., Hutterer, F., and Lieber, C. S., 1968, Ethanol increases hepatic smooth endoplasmic reticulum and drug-metabolizing enzymes, *Science* **159**:1469–1470.

Rubin, E., Beattie, D. S., and Lieber, C. S., 1970, Effects of ethanol on the biogenesis of mitochondrial membranes and associated mitochondrial functions, *Lab. Invest.* **23**:620–627.

Rubin, E., Beattie, D. S., Toth, A., and Lieber, C. S., 1972, Structural and functional effects of ethanol on hepatic mitochondria, *Fed. Proc. Fed. Am. Soc. Exp. Biol.* **31**:131–140.

Ruebner, B. H., Miyai, K., and Abbey, H., 1961, Low incidence of myocardial infarction in hepatic cirrhosis—a statistical artefact?, *Lancet* **2**:1435–1436.

Sabesin, S. M., Hawkins, H. L., Kuiken, L., and Ragland, J. B., 1977, Abnormal plasma lipoproteins and lecithin-cholesterol acyltransferase deficiency in alcoholic liver disease, *Gastroenterology* **72**:510–518.

Sackett, D. L., Epid, M. S., Gibson, R. W., Bross, I. D. J., and Pickren, J. W., 1968, Relation between aortic atherosclerosis and the use of cigarettes and alcohol; an autopsy study, *N. Engl. J. Med.* **279**:1413–1420.

Schapiro, R. H., Drummey, G. D., Shimizu, Y., and Isselbacher, K. J., 1964, Studies on the pathogenesis of ethanol-induced fatty liver. II. Effect of ethanol on palmitate-1-C^{14} metabolism by isolated perfused rat liver, *J. Clin. Invest.* **43**:1338–1347.

Schreiber, S. S., Briden, K., Oratz, M., and Rothschild, M. A., 1972, Ethanol, acetaldehyde and myocardial protein synthesis, *J. Clin. Invest.* **51**:2820–2826.

Seakins, A., and Robinson, D. S., 1964, Changes associated with the production of fatty livers by white phosphorus and by ethanol in the rat, *Biochem. J.* **92**:308–312.

Seidel, D., Alaupovic, P., and Furman, R. H., 1969, A lipoprotein characterizing obstructive jaundice. I. Method for quantitative separation and identification of lipoproteins in jaundice subjects, *J. Clin. Invest.* **48**:1211–1223.

Seidel, D., Alaupovic, P., Furman, R. H., and McConathy, W. J., 1970, A lipoprotein characterizing obstructive jaundice. II. Isolation and partial characterization of the protein moieties of low density lipoproteins, *J. Clin. Invest.* **49**:2396–2407.

Seidel, D., Greten, H., Geisen, H. P., Wengeler, H., and Wieland, H., 1972, Further aspects on the characterization of high and very low density lipoproteins in patients with liver disease, *Eur. J. Clin. Invest.* **2**:359–364.

Shaw, S., and Lieber, C. S., 1976, Characteristic plasma amino acid abnormalities in the alcoholic: Respective role of alcoholism, nutrition and liver injury, *Clin. Res.* **24**:291A.

Sorrell, M. F., Tuma, D. J., and Barak, A. J., 1977a, Evidence that acetaldehyde irreversibly impairs glycoprotein metabolism in liver slices, *Gastroenterology* **73**:1138–1141.

Sorrell, M. F., Tuma, D. J., Schafer, E. C., and Barak, A. J., 1977b, Role of acetaldehyde in the ethanol-induced impairment of glycoprotein metabolism in rat liver slices, *Gastroenterology* **73**:137–144.

Spain, D. M., and Bradess, V. A., 1957, Sudden death from coronary atherosclerosis, *Arch. Intern. Med.* **100**:228–231.

Stason, W. B., Neff, R. K., Miettinen, O. S., and Jick, H., 1976, Alcohol consumption and non-fatal myocardial infarction, *Am. J. Epidemiol.* **104**:603–608.

Stein, O., and Stein, Y., 1973, Colchicine-induced inhibition of very low density lipoprotein release by rat liver *in vivo*, *Biochim. Biophys. Acta* **306**:142–147.

Stein, O., Sanger, L., and Stein, Y., 1974, Colchicine-induced inhibition of lipoprotein and protein secretion into the serum and lack of interference with secretion of biliary phospholipids and cholesterol by rat liver *in vivo*, *J. Cell Biol.* **62**:90–103.

Tewari, S., and Noble, E. P., 1971, Ethanol and brain protein synthesis, *Brain Res.* **26**:469–474.

Tibblin, G., Wilhelmsen, L., and Werko, L., 1975, Risk factors for myocardial infarction and death due to ischemic heart disease and other causes, *Am. J. Cardiol.* **35**:514–522.

Tuma, D. J., and Sorrell, M. F., 1977, Acetaldehyde selectively impairs glycoprotein metabolism, *Gastroenterology* **73**:1250–1252A.

Viel, B., Donoso, S., Salcedo, D., Rojas, P., Varela, N., and Alessandri, R., 1966, Alcoholism and socioeconomic status, hepatic damage, and arteriosclerosis, *Arch. Intern. Med.* **117**:84–91.

Wilens, S. L., 1947, The relationship of chronic alcoholism to atherosclerosis, *J. Am. Med. Assoc.* **135**:1136–1139.

Wolfe, B. M., Havel, J. R., Marliss, E. B., Kane, J. P., Seymour, J., and Ahuja, S. P., 1976, Effects of 3-day fast and ethanol on splanchnic metabolism of FFA, amino acids, and carbohydrates in healthy young men, *J. Clin. Invest.* **57**:329–340.

Wooles, W. R., 1966, Depressed fatty acid oxidation as a factor in the etiology of acute ethanol-induced fatty liver, *Life Sci.* **5**:267–276.

Yano, K., Rhoads, G. G., and Kagan, A., 1977, Coffee, alcohol and risk of coronary heart disease among Japanese men living in Hawaii, *N. Engl. J. Med.* **297**:405–409.

Disorders of Lipid and Lipoprotein Metabolism

DeWitt S. Goodman

3.1. Introduction

This chapter will review the major advances that occurred during 1977 and early 1978 with regard to our knowledge of the major plasma lipids and lipoproteins, and about clinical abnormalities in lipid transport, with particular emphasis on the hyperlipidemias. The chapter will build on, and in part briefly summarize, the information and ideas reviewed during the past two years (Goodman, 1976, 1978). For excellent and in-depth reviews of familial disorders characterized by evidence of abnormal lipid metabolism, the reader is referred to the recent fourth edition of the textbook by Stanbury *et al.* (1978).

3.2. Lipoprotein Structure and Metabolism

3.2.1. General Review

Lipids are not soluble in water and circulate in plasma in association with certain specific proteins (apolipoproteins) in the form of plasma

DEWITT S. GOODMAN • Department of Medicine, College of Physicians and Surgeons of Columbia University, New York, New York 10032.

lipoproteins. Four classes of specific lipoproteins circulate in plasma, namely, chylomicrons, very-low-density lipoproteins (VLDL), low-density lipoproteins (LDL), and high-density lipoproteins (HDL). Two of these, chylomicrons and VLDL, are composed mainly of triglyceride and represent, respectively, the transport form of exogenous (dietary) and of endogenous triglyceride. Chylomicrons are normally not present in postabsorptive plasma after an overnight fast. LDL contain cholesterol as the major component and normally represent the circulating form of most of the plasma cholesterol. HDL are comprised of approximately half protein and half lipid, and will be discussed in more detail in Section 3.2.3.

During the past few years, a very great amount of information has been obtained about the structure and function of the apolipoproteins, and it has become clear that these proteins are central to many aspects of normal as well as abnormal lipid transport. At least eight distinct apolipoproteins have been described (Jackson *et al.*, 1976; Eisenberg and Levy, 1975). They are grouped into five families (designated apoA, apoB, apoC, apoD, and apoE) on the basis of their chemical, immunologic, and metabolic characteristics. During 1977, an excellent and in-depth review of the plasma lipoproteins and apolipoproteins was presented by Osborne and Brewer (1977).

The primary structure (amino acid sequence) is now known for all members of the human apoA (apoA-I and apoA-II) and apoC (apoC-I, apoC-II, and apoC-III) families. ApoA-I (mol. wt. 28,331) and apoA-II (mol. wt. 17,380) comprise about 90% of the protein mass of the HDL, where they are usually present in a weight ratio of about 3 : 1. Very recent studies have shown that apoA-I is also a component of newly formed intestinal lymph chylomicrons. ApoA-I plays a functional role as the activator protein for lecithin-cholesterol acyltransferase (LCAT), the enzyme responsible for the esterification of plasma cholesterol in man. It is rather loosely bound to HDL and can be separated from the rest of HDL by relatively mild procedures. ApoA-II is associated with lipid more tightly; its physiological role remains to be defined.

ApoB comprises more than 90% of the protein of LDL. It is also a major protein of chylomicrons and VLDL, and comprises, on the average, about 25–35% of VLDL protein. Severe problems of solubilization and association–dissociation of apoB have greatly retarded the characterization of this protein. ApoB is considered the fundamental structural protein of LDL, VLDL, and chylomicrons, and is thought to play a crucial role in the transport of triglycerides from the intestine and liver into the plasma. This is particularly well illustrated by the rare genetic disease abetalipoproteinemia, characterized by the genetic deficiency of apoB (Stanbury *et al.*, 1978).

The C apoproteins are major constituents of the protein of VLDL, where they comprise an average of about 40–50% of the protein mass; they are also minor constituents (about 10% of protein mass) of HDL. However, because of the larger amount of HDL protein normally present in plasma, the total mass of apoC is usually distributed roughly equally between VLDL and HDL. The proportion of the protein mass of VLDL comprised of the apoC proteins varies with particle size, so that the larger, less dense, "younger" particles contain relatively more apoC, while the smaller particles have relatively more apoB (Kane *et al.*, 1975). ApoC-I (mol. wt. 6631) has been shown to be capable of activating LCAT (as is apoA-I). ApoC-II comprises 5–10% of total VLDL protein, and has been shown to be a potent activator of lipoprotein lipase from human and rat postheparin plasma, and from bovine milk. ApoC-III (mol. wt. approximately 8750) is present in man in three polymorphic forms that are thought to differ with regard to sialic acid content. ApoC-III is the most abundant of the C apoproteins, accounting for 25–30% of VLDL protein.

Only limited information is available about apoD. As discussed last year (Goodman, 1978), apoE, also known as the "arginine-rich" apoprotein, has been of particular recent interest because it is found in elevated concentrations in several hypercholesterolemic, atherogenic states, both in man (type III hyperlipoproteinemia) and in experimental animals (cholesterol-fed rabbits, swine, dogs, and monkeys). ApoE occurs as a major component in VLDL, where it usually accounts for 6–12% of VLDL protein, and as a minor one in HDL. ApoE has a molecular weight of about 33,000. In a recent report (Shelburne and Quarfordt, 1977), it was demonstrated that apoE has a substantial binding affinity for heparin, and that this property could be used to isolate apoE, by chromatography on a heparin affinity column. It is hoped that this new and relatively simple procedure will enable more extensive studies to be developed on the structure and metabolic roles of apoE.

As summarized last year (Goodman, 1978), considerable information is now available about the metabolism of the different lipoproteins and apoproteins. Both VLDL and HDL are produced by the liver. The intestine also participates in VLDL and in HDL (Green *et al.*, 1978) production, as well as being the site of chylomicron formation. VLDL catabolism involves removal of most of VLDL triglyceride from the blood by a lipolytic process, mainly involving the enzyme lipoprotein lipase. During this process, the bulk of the apoC proteins are removed, mainly by transfer to HDL. This leads to the formation of intermediate-density lipoproteins (IDL), which in turn are further catabolized to LDL. Current evidence indicates that normally in man most, if not all, plasma LDL represents a catabolic product resulting from VLDL degradation.

More detailed and extended information about the metabolism of the B and C apolipoproteins was recently provided by Berman *et al.* (1978).

The kinetics of the B and C apoproteins were studied in 14 normal and hyperlipidemic subjects after injection of exogenously radioiodinated VLDL. The data were analyzed by the use of a complex multicompartmental model, developed mostly from this work. The model satisfied the data for all individuals studied, including four normal subjects and ten patients with four different patterns of hyperlipoproteinemia (types I, IIa, III, and IV). The results show that the VLDL particle undergoes a series of incremental density changes, most likely due to a number of delipidation steps, during which apoB stays with the particle until its density reaches the IDL range (1.006–1.019). There is, however, a loss of apoC associated with these delipidation steps. In the normal subjects, all IDL apoB eventually became LDL apoB. In the hyperlipidedmic subjects, some of the apoB on IDL was also degraded directly. The apoC lost by VLDL and IDL recycled to HDL, and most of it was picked up again by newly synthesized VLDL. In addition, there was a slowdown of the stepwise delipidation process in all hyperlipidemic subjects studied. Since the hyperlipidemic subjects were mainly patients with uncommon lipoprotein phenotypes (type I, three patients, and type III, five patients), conclusions about the effects of hyperlipidemia can be regarded only as very tentative. As pointed out by the authors, however, the model presented provides a quantitative tool for examining the metabolic derangements found in the different types of hyperlipoproteinemia, and the effects of diet and drugs on normal and abnormal lipoprotein metabolism.

3.2.2. Apolipoprotein C-II

Considerable interest has focused on apoC-II recently because of its demonstrated role as the activator protein for lipoprotein lipase. Since this enzyme plays a critical role in triglyceride removal from plasma, apoC-II serves an important function in the metabolism of triglyceride-rich lipoproteins (chylomicrons and VLDL).

The complete amino acid sequence of human apoC-II was reported recently (Jackson *et al.*, 1977). The protein has 78 amino acid residues and a molecular weight of 8837. Of interest in the structure of this apoprotein are the findings that apoC-II contains no cysteine, cystine, or histidine, and that 3 of the 4 prolines are contained within the first 12 amino-terminal residues.

Studies were also conducted to try to determine the minimal amino acid sequence requirements in apoC-II for activation of lipoprotein lipase (Kinnunen *et al.*, 1977). Both native and synthetic fragments of the apoC-II molecule were prepared and then tested for their ability to activate lipoprotein lipase isolated from bovine milk. A relatively small carboxy-terminal fragment, comprising amino acid residues 55–78, was found to provide maximal activation of the lipase. In contrast, a smaller fragment containing only residues 66–78 did not activate the enzyme. It was suggested that the amino-terminal two thirds of apoC-II might be mainly involved with binding apoC-II to the chylomicron and VLDL surface, leaving the carboxy-terminal residues available for interaction with the enzyme on the capillary wall.

In a recent report, a specific radioimmunoassay for human apoC-II was described, and was used to study apoC-II levels in normal and in hypertriglyceridemic subjects (Kashyap *et al.*, 1977). The mean (± S.E.M.) plasma apoC-II level in 47 normotriglyceridemic subjects was 52 ± 3 μg/ ml. ApoC-II levels were elevated in 28 hypertriglyceridemic patients, with values of 90 ± 5, 85 ± 7, and 133 ± 21 μg/ml being found, respectively, for patients with the type IIb, type IV, or type V lipoprotein patterns. The concentrations of plasma apoC-II and triglyceride correlated significantly in both normo- and hypertriglyceridemics; in addition, plasma triglycerides correlated inversely with the fraction of total apoC-II in VLDL-free plasma. Thus, as plasma triglycerides and apoC-II increase, apoC-II is redistributed from HDL to VLDL, presumably contributing to VLDL removal. However, it was noted also that the amount of apoC-II per milligram of VLDL protein, and its lipoprotein lipase activator potency per milligram of VLDL protein, appeared to be reduced in the hypertriglyceridemic patients, possibly contributing to impaired VLDL catabolism. Further studies on apoC-II metabolism can be expected to add to our understanding of the pathophysiology of the hypertriglyceridemias.

3.2.3. High-Density Lipoproteins

High-density lipoproteins are often subdivided into fractions of density 1.063–1.120 (called HDL_2) and 1.120–1.210 (called HDL_3). HDL_2 have molecular weights of about 375,000; HDL_3, of about 200,000. HDL are spherical molecules with diameters of about 9.5–10 nm for HDL_2, and about 7.0–7.5 nm for HDL_3. Several structural models have been proposed for HDL (Stanbury *et al.*, 1978; Jackson *et al.*, 1976).

Recent studies have provided valuable information about the metabolism of HDL in man. Detailed studies of the turnover of the two major apoproteins of HDL (apoA-I and apoA-II) were carried out by Blum *et al.* (1977) in a series of eight normal volunteers. All subjects were first studied under conditions of an isocaloric balanced diet. Four of the subjects were then studied while on a high (80%) carbohydrate diet, and two were studied while taking nicotinic acid (3 g/day). It was found that the turnover of apoA-I was completely parallel to that of apoA-II in all studies. Thus, these two apoproteins are catabolized together under both normal and perturbed conditions. The mean half-life of the terminal portion of the turnover curves was 5.8 days during the studies with a balanced diet. Mathematical modeling showed that the data were consistent with a simple two-compartment model. One compartment is within the plasma and exchanges with a nonplasma component. Catabolism occurs from both of these compartments.

With the balanced diet, the mean synthetic rate for HDL protein was 8.51 mg/kg per day. Carbohydrate feeding resulted in a smaller mean HDL particle size, a lower ratio of apoA-I to apoA-II in HDL, and a larger portion of the total plasma HDL present in the smaller HDL_3 fraction. In all these respects, reciprocal changes were seen with nicotinic acid treatment. Both perturbations had very little or no effects on the synthetic rates of HDL protein. Major effects were, however, seen on HDL catabolic pathways. Thus, the high-carbohydrate diet significantly increased the rate of HDL protein catabolism from the plasma compartment (and lowered plasma HDL levels), whereas nicotinic acid treatment had reciprocal effects.

Studies on the relationships between the plasma concentrations of apoA-I and apoA-II in men and women were reported recently by Cheung and Albers (1977). Specific immunoassays for each apoprotein were used to measure apoprotein levels in 172 men and 188 women varying in age from early 20's to mid-60's. ApoA-II levels did not increase with age in men, but showed a slight increase with age in women. ApoA-II levels correlated significantly with the levels of both apoA-I and HDL cholesterol. The plasma apoA-I to apoA-II mean weight ratio was approximately 3.6–3.8. In the density 1.10–1.21 (mainly HDL_3) subfraction, both males and females had similar apoA-I, apoA-II, and HDL cholesterol levels (means of approximately 100, 28, and 34 mg/dl, respectively). Women had approximately twice the amount of apoA-I, apoA-II, and HDL cholesterol that men had in the lighter (mainly HDL_2) (density 1.063–1.10) fraction (men: mean, 10, 2, and 10 mg/dl, respectively). The two HDL subfractions differed from each other in composition, with the lighter HDL fraction showing relatively more cholesterol (than total apoprotein) and a higher apoA-I/apoA-II ratio than did the more dense HDL fraction; similar findings were made for both men and women. The results suggest that the differences in HDL between men and women are due primarily to differences in the relative proportions of HDL subclasses rather than to intrinsic differences in HDL structure.

Detailed physical chemical studies on HDL from four normolipidemic males and from four females were reported by D. W. Anderson *et al.* (1977). The techniques employed included density gradient and analytic ultracentrifugation, gradient gel electrophoresis, electron microscopy, and various chemical analyses. The data obtained suggest that there are three major components in the HDL particle-size distribution of normal males and females instead of two (HDL_2 and HDL_3). Material within each of the three size ranges was characterized by considerable particle density and size homogeneity. The approximate densities for the three components (banding position densities in g/ml) were 1.090, 1.110, and 1.145, respectively. Clearly, more information is needed on the metabolic interrelationships and regulation of these HDL subfractions.

A comprehensive evaluation of the heparin–manganese precipitation procedure for estimating HDL cholesterol levels was recently carried out by Warnick and Albers (1978). Because of the implication of HDL as a negative risk factor in cardiovascular disease (discussed in detail in Section 3.5), a need exists for an accurate but convenient quantitative method. This paper explores in detail the strengths and limitations of the currently used heparin–manganese precipitation procedure, and suggests modifications to improve both convenience and accuracy.

3.2.4. The Lp(a) Lipoprotein

The Lp(a) lipoprotein, as discussed last year (Goodman, 1978), was studied originally as a possible human genetic marker. This lipoprotein is found in the density range 1.05–1.09, has pre-β mobility on electrophoresis, and is composed of 27% protein, 65% lipid (mainly esterified cholesterol), and 8% carbohydrate. Its protein has been found to contain 65% apoB, 15% albumin, and 20% of a unique apoprotein called apo-Lp(a).

An extensive clinical and immunological study of the Lp(a) lipoprotein was carried out by Albers *et al.* (1977a). Previous studies from this group, using a quantitative radial immunodiffusion assay, demonstrated measurable Lp(a) lipoprotein levels in 91% (911 of 1000) of subjects studied. To extend these observations, a sensitive and specific radioimmunoassay for Lp(a) lipoprotein was developed. All but one of the previously Lp(a) "negative" subjects (by immunodiffusion) had detectable levels of Lp(a) lipoprotein by radioimmunoassay; the levels in these subjects were mainly in the range of 2–5 mg/dl. The only subject without detectable Lp(a) had abetalipoproteinemia (without detectable apoB by radioimmunoassay). It was concluded that Lp(a) is present in all subjects with apoB, and that apoB appears necessary for the plasma transport of the Lp(a) lipoprotein.

Lp(a) levels varied widely in the overall population studied, from less than 1 to more than 50 mg/dl. The level of Lp(a) should therefore be considered as a quantitative or metric characteristic, rather than as a qualitative genetic trait. Lp(a) levels were not significantly correlated with the plasma levels of apoB, apoA-I, apoA-II, triglyceride, or net cholesterol [total cholesterol minus Lp(a) cholesterol].

Quantitation of Lp(a) levels in 90 male myocardial infarct survivors and their spouses showed that the distribution of Lp(a) levels of infarct survivors was significantly higher above the 50th percentile cutoff point, and exceeded that of the spouses. Furthermore, the younger (less than age 50) myocardial infarct survivors had an even further shift of Lp(a) levels to higher values. The data suggest that high Lp(a) levels may be positively associated with coronary disease, and demonstrate that this association is even stronger for subjects with premature coronary heart disease. Since it is possible that the onset of coronary heart disease may cause an increase in Lp(a) levels, the predictive value of Lp(a) levels for premature heart disease needs to be evaluated. The genetic and metabolic regulation of Lp(a) levels remain to be defined.

3.2.5. Lipoprotein-X and Liver Disease

The characteristic elevation of free (unesterified) cholesterol and phospholipid in patients with cholestasis is due to the presence of an abnormal lipoprotein, lipoprotein-X or LP-X, in the LDL density range (density 1.006–1.063). This lipoprotein appears to be formed when a lipoprotein normally excreted with the bile refluxes into the plasma stream and is converted to LP-X (see Goodman, 1978). An in-depth review of the structure and metabolism of LP-X appeared in German in 1977 (Seidel, 1977).

During 1977, new information about the structure and properties of LP-X was reported. In one study (Hauser *et al.*, 1977), the structure and morphology of LP-X was investigated by gel filtration, electron microscopy, and nuclear magnetic resonance spectroscopy. The studies showed that LP-X is a spherical lipoprotein particle with an average diameter of about 40 nm, and a wide size distribution ranging from 20 to 70 nm. Different from all other lipoproteins, LP-X is a hollow particle (= vesicle) with a water-filled internal cavity surrounded by a continuous single bilayer that is impermeable to cations. Detailed information was obtained about the packing of the lipid components that comprise the bilayer (and LP-X).

In another study, three different but related species of LP-X (called LP-X_1, LP-X_2, and LP-X_3) were isolated from cholestatic plasma by ethanol precipitation and zonal ultracentrifugation (Patsch *et al.*, 1977a). All three species of lipoprotein were rich in phospholipids (mainly lecithin, 64.9–67.5%) and cholesterol (23–27%), but poor in cholesteryl esters (0.4–1.9%), triglycerides (1.8–3.2%) and protein (3.2–6.7%). The three species of LP-X differed in buoyant densities (1.038, 1.049, and 1.058, respectively), due to differences in chemical composition. All three LP-X species contained human serum albumin and the C apoproteins as major protein constituents. In addition, LP-X_2 and LP-X_3 (but not LP-X_1) contained detectable amounts of apoA-I and apoE. It was pointed out that the metabolic significance and interrelationships of the three LP-X species are not known, but that this description of their physical and chemical properties represents a first step in efforts to understand better the pathophysiology in the disease states in which they occur.

3.3. Type III Hyperlipoproteinemia

The characteristics of this disorder, which is also referred to as "dysbetalipoproteinemia" and as "broad-beta disease," were reviewed in the past two years (Goodman, 1976, 1978). Type III hyperlipoproteinemia is a familial disorder of lipoprotein metabolism associated with xanthomatosis and early onset of severe atherosclerotic disease. The prevalence of this disorder has been estimated as approximately 1 in 5000 persons in the Western developed countries. A defect in the catabolism of triglyceride-rich lipoproteins apparently underlies the accumulation of an atypical lipoprotein in the VLDL fraction of affected subjects. This atypical VLDL has β (instead of pre-β) mobility on electrophoresis, and is rich in cholesterol and in apolipoprotein E (Havel and Kane, 1973).

3.3.1. Diagnosis

Methods for the diagnosis of type III hyperlipoproteinemia have been based on the abnormal mobility or abnormal chemical composition of the VLDL present in plasma in these patients. Thus, the diagnosis is usually based on either (1) the demonstration of VLDL with β mobility on paper or agarose gel electrophoresis ("floating-β lipoproteins" or "β-VLDL") or (2) the demonstration of the presence of cholesterol-rich VLDL. The former method is now generally considered to be insufficiently specific or precise as a diagnostic criterion. A widely used criterion for the second method has employed the ratio of VLDL cholesterol to plasma total triglyceride; ratios of 0.30 or greater are considered diagnostic of type III. Other chemical ratios have also been suggested, such as an index ratio of VLDL cholesterol to VLDL triglyceride of 0.42 or greater as diagnostic of this disorder.

Several reports appeared in 1977 dealing with the diagnosis of type III hyperlipoproteinemia. In one report, the currently available methods for the diagnosis of this disorder were evaluated (Patsch *et al.*, 1977b). In particular, the diagnostic value of the two methods described above ("floating-β lipoprotein" vs. chemical index definition) was compared. Limitations in both methods were noted that arose from the commonly used angle-head rotor (compared to zonal ultracentrifugation) in the ultracentrifuge. It was concluded that the chemical index method is the more reliable method for the diagnosis of type III disease.

An extensive study of several compositional (chemical index) criteria for the diagnosis of type III hyperlipoproteinemia was conducted by Albers *et al.* (1977b). Plasma triglyceride concentration-dependent cut-lines for the compositional criteria reduced false positives at low triglyceride levels and false negatives at high triglyceride levels. Furthermore, an agarose electrophoresis heparin–manganese precipitation technique was found effective for screening for a possible type III pattern in plasma, whereas the combination agarose–polyacrylamide gel electrophoresis system was not effective.

A new approach to the diagnosis of type III hyperlipoproteinemia was developed by Kushwaha *et al.* (1977a), based on the fact that the atypical VLDL in these patients is distinctively enriched in apoE. A radial immunodiffusion assay for apoE in whole plasma was first developed. Its diagnostic usefulness was then tested in randomly selected ($n = 174$) and hyperlipidemic ($n = 61$) subsets of an adult employee population. The assay was also tested in a hyperlipidemic clinic referral group ($n = 63$) that included 18 patients with well-documented type III hyperlipoproteinemia. ApoE levels were normally distributed among the random population subset, were equal between the two sexes, and increased little with age. The mean and 99th-percentile values were 24.6 and 40.1 mg/dl, respectively. Hyperlipidemic subjects with the type IIa, IIb, or IV lipoprotein pattern showed apoE levels that were fairly close to those of normolipidemic subjects. In contrast, all subjects with type III patterns as assigned by standard criteria from both population ($n = 4$) and referral sources exceeded the above-99th-percentile value. The apoE levels in the type III patients were 54.7 ± 9.7 mg/dl (mean $\pm$ S.D.). It was concluded that a plasma apoE concentration exceeding 40 mg/dl appears diagnostic of type III hyperlipoproteinemia. It was also pointed out, however, that this criterion might not prove to be absolutely diagnostic in all circumstances, e.g., in a patient with type III who responds well to therapy.

3.3.2. Apolipoprotein E

New insights into the metabolism of apoE and the abnormality in type III disease have come from the exciting recent studies of Utermann and his colleagues in Marburg, West Germany. In 1975, these investigators reported that apoE from VLDL is heterogenous on isoelectric focusing, and shows three main components on analytical isoelectric focusing in the presence of 6 M urea (Utermann *et al.*, 1975). The three apoE isoproteins were called apoE-I, apoE-II, and apoE-III. Patients with type

III hyperlipoproteinemia were deficient in the component apoE-III, and it was suggested that this might be the underlying defect in this hereditary dyslipoproteinemia.

This work was extended by studies of the apoprotein composition of the main lipoprotein fractions of 15 patients with type III hyperlipoproteinemia (Utermann *et al.,* 1977a). Analytical isoelectric focusing of urea-soluble apo-VLDL and apo-IDL demonstrated a variant pattern of the polymorphic apoE, with a deficient apoE-III band in all patients. The apoE-III deficiency pattern was seen in only 6 of 304 hyperlipidemic controls. These 6 apoE-III-deficient controls had characteristic signs of broad-beta disease and thus represented patients not previously recognized as having the disorder. The apoE focusing patterns were found to be constant on repeated examinations and were stable under different metabolic conditions. It was concluded that the apoE-III deficiency in VLDL may be a specific qualitative marker for broad-beta disease, and it was suggested that apoE-III deficiency may be the basic lipoprotein abnormality underlying this disorder.

More recent and extensive population and familial studies have demonstrated that this simple conclusion is apparently not valid, and that the apoE and type III story is much more complex than had first been appreciated (Utermann *et al.,* 1977b). This work has demonstrated that apoE shows a genetic polymorphism determined by two codominant alleles, *Apo E ^{n}* and *Apo E ^{d}*. Thus, when apoE patterns of urea-soluble apo-VLDL were determined in 490 blood donors, three distinct phenotypic patterns were observed. The three phenotypes, called Apo E-N, Apo E-ND, and Apo E-D (E-III deficiency pattern) were differentiated on the basis of the ApoE-II/III ratios. The ratio was 0.40 ± 0.07 for phenotype Apo E-N, 1.02 ± 0.25 for phenotype Apo E-ND, and 9.07 ± 4.48 for phenotype Apo E-D. No overlap was observed among the three distinct groups in this study. The frequencies of these three apoE phenotypes were 83.3, 15.7, and 1.0% for Apo E-N, E-ND, and E-D, respectively. Kindred studies were consistent with a simple Mendelian mode of transmission in which two alleles determine the three phenotypes. The frequency of the allele *Apo E^d* was 0.0888; thus, about 1% of the German population is homozygous for this allele and shows apoE-III deficiency.

Since the frequency of apoE-III deficiency is much higher than that of type III hyperlipoproteinemia, serum lipid and lipoprotein analyses were carried out on probands with the phenotype Apo E-D. It was found that all these persons had dysbetalipoproteinemia, in that they manifested both "floating-β" VLDL, and VLDL enriched in cholesterol. However, none of these persons had hypercholesterolemia, and in fact total serum cholesterol levels were abnormally low in some of the probands. Accordingly, it is clear that apoE-III deficiency is not a specific marker for type

III hyperlipoproteinemia, and in fact that most persons with this apoE pattern do not have hyperlipidemia. Future work will be needed to define the interrelationships among the different apoE patterns, dysbetalipoproteinemia, hyperlipoproteinemia, and atherosclerotic vascular disease. In the meantime, Utermann has suggested as a working hypothesis that type III disease might occur when the Apo E-D phenotype coexists with genes for familial hyperlipidemia, perhaps for familial combined hyperlipidemia.

3.3.3. Pathophysiology; Treatment

Evidence was summarized previously (Goodman, 1976, 1978) that the atypical VLDL that is found in type III hyperlipoproteinemia represents the abnormal accumulation of intermediates in the metabolism of triglyceride-rich lipoproteins (chylomicrons and VLDL). Additional evidence for reduced clearance of VLDL apoB in plasma has been reported from turnover studies with radioiodinated VLDL (Berman *et al.*, 1978; Chait *et al.*, 1977). These studies have also shown a considerably elevated production (synthesis) rate of VLDL apoB in type III patients. Treatment with clofibrate and nicotinic acid resulted in a sharp decrease in the VLDL apoB synthesis rates (Berman *et al.*, 1978). In contrast, estrogen treatment of a single type III patient increased VLDL production rate, yet resulted in a decrease in plasma lipid levels, normalization of lipoprotein composition, and correction of the defect in VLDL catabolism (Chait *et al.*, 1977). It was concluded, in this latter study, that the primary defect in this disorder seems to be impaired catabolism of VLDL, which is corrected with estrogen therapy.

The effects of estrogens (ethinyl estradiol, 1 μg/kg body weight per day) were further explored in 6 patients (5 women, 1 man) with type III hyperlipoproteinemia (Kushwaha *et al.*, 1977b). Estrogen, which stimulates triglyceride production in normal women and those with endogenous hypertriglyceridemia, was found to exert a paradoxical, hypolipidemic effect in the type III patients. Moreover, VLDL lipid and apoprotein composition became normal during estrogen treatment. Estrogen withdrawal promptly restored the type III pattern and the VLDL compositional abnormalities. It was suggested that estrogens facilitate the assimilation of chylomicron and VLDL remnants, a defect that appears likely to represent the metabolic abnormality underlying type III hyperlipoproteinemia.

A detailed report of the effects of clofibrate, nicotinic acid, and diet on the concentrations and characteristics of the plasma lipoproteins in a patient with type III hyperlipoproteinemia was presented by Patsch *et al.* (1977c). It was pointed out that drug and diet treatment of this disorder not only lowers the levels of plasma VLDL, IDL, and LDL, but also increases HDL, which are considered protective against atherosclerosis (see the discussion in Section 3.5).

3.4. Tangier Disease

Tangier disease (familial HDL deficiency) is a rare disorder of plasma lipid transport characterized by the absence of normal HDL and storage of cholesteryl esters in foam cells in many tissues. Twenty-six patients, representing many different kindreds, in several different countries have been described (Stanbury *et al.*, 1978). The condition is characterized clinically by hyperplastic orange tonsils, splenomegaly, corneal opacities, and relapsing neuropathy. Heterozygotes have HDL levels approximately half normal, but do not develop neuropathy or prominent cholesteryl ester storage. Homozygotes accumulate cholesteryl esters in reticuloendothelial cells in tonsils, spleen, lymph nodes, bone marrow, skin, thymus, intestinal mucosa, and probably Schwann cells and cornea. The profound HDL deficiency results in the generation of abnormal chylomicron remnants, and these, after phagocytosis, may account for the accumulation of cholesteryl esters in histiocytes. ApoA-I and apoA-II are found in Tangier plasma and, to the extent examined, appear normal. The basic metabolic defect in this disorder is not known, but may involve a defect in the regulation of HDL synthesis or catabolism (Stanbury *et al.*, 1978).

During 1977, several studies were reported that explored the lipoprotein abnormalities in Tangier disease. A detailed quantitative study of the A apoproteins in three adult patients with Tangier disease was carried out by Assmann *et al.* (1977a). In the Tangier plasma, the total amounts of both A apoproteins, and particularly apoA-I, were markedly decreased, with total apoA-I levels being less than 1% (0.4–0.9%) of normal, and total apoA-II levels 5–7% of normal. When Tangier plasma was ultracentrifuged at a density of 1.21, more than 90% of the apoA-I sedimented, whereas more than 95% of apoA-II floated. These data, plus immunologic studies, indicate that complete dissociation of the two A apoproteins occurs in Tangier plasma. Despite the exceedingly low apoA-I levels in these patients, immunochemical and other experiments did not provide evidence for a structural abnormality of apoA-I. It was concluded that normal HDL are absent from Tangier plasma, but that the nature of the basic metabolic defect remains to be defined.

Studies were also carried out recently on a large family group (kindred) affected with Tangier disease (Assmann *et al.*, 1977b). Besides two homozygous (and affected) propositi, several heterozygous patients were identified. With the use of a variety of quantitative immunologic methods, the amounts of apoA-I and apoA-II in plasma and the distribution of these A apoproteins among serum lipoproteins were determined. The molar ratio of apoA-I to apoA-II in HDL of Tangier heterozygotes did not differ significantly from that of normal controls, although the total concentration (mass) of HDL was reduced by approximately 50% in the Tangier heterozygotes. The elution profile of HDL from agarose columns and their morphological appearance by electron microscopy were similar to those of control preparations. In addition, lipid storage in histiocytes of rectal mucosa obtained from heterozygous patients was documented. Thus, patients heterozygous for Tangier disease appear to have normal HDL in the circulation, the total mass of which is reduced by approximately 50%.

The properties of VLDL and LDL in patients with Tangier disease were examined by Heinen *et al.* (1978). Tangier VLDL migrated more slowly than normal VLDL on paper electrophoresis, yet their morphology, gross chemical composition, and qualitative apoprotein content were similar. There were, however, quantitative abnormalities in composition, with a paucity of C apoproteins in Tangier VLDL. This abnormality may be related to the absence of normal HDL from Tangier plasma. LDL from Tangier plasma had a composition quite different from that of normal LDL. Triglyceride accounted for a mean of 29% of Tangier LDL mass (control = 6%), and the cholesteryl ester content was reduced by about 50%. Thus, HDL may be required for the generation of chemically normal LDL. The possibility was also raised that some or all of the lipoprotein abnormalities documented may be related to an unrecognized but fundamental defect affecting all lipoprotein classes in Tangier disease.

In addition to these studies involving plasma lipoproteins in Tangier disease, a study was reported recently describing the physical states and phase behavior of the lipids of the spleen, liver, and splenic artery from a 38-year-old man with Tangier disease (Katz *et al.*, 1977). This physical chemical study demonstrated the following: (1) Most of the storage lipids in the liver and spleen were in the liquid crystalline state at body temperature. (2) The phase behavior of the storage lipids conformed to that predicted by lipid model systems. (3) Lipid droplets within individual cells had similar compositions, whereas droplet composition varied from cell to cell. (4) Cholesteryl ester did not accumulate in the splenic artery. Since macrophages are the major site of lipid accumulation in Tangier disease, it was considered that macrophages may require HDL to remove cholesterol from the cells.

3.5. High-Density Lipoprotein Levels and Coronary Heart Disease

3.5.1. Epidemiologic Studies

During the past two years, a wealth of information has been published demonstrating the important role of HDL level as a protective factor against coronary heart disease. It is now clearly established that there is a strong negative correlation between HDL concentration and coronary risk, in contrast to the positive correlations that exist between coronary risk and total plasma cholesterol or LDL concentrations. Some of this evidence was summarized last year (Goodman, 1978).

The relationships between coronary heart disease prevalence and fasting lipid and lipoprotein levels were assessed by a case–control study in the Cooperative Lipoprotein Phenotyping Study (Castelli *et al.*, 1977b). The overall study involved a total of 6859 men and women of black, Japanese, and white ancestry, drawn from subjects aged 40 years and older from five populations, in Albany, Framingham, Evans County, Honolulu, and San Francisco. Each of these populations has been participating in ongoing prospective studies of cardiovascular disease. In each major study group, the mean levels of HDL cholesterol were lower in persons with coronary heart disease than in those without the disease. The average difference was small (typically 3–4 mg/dl) but statistically significant. It was found in most age–race–sex groups. Thus, this report, describing a wide diversity of populations and using modern quantitative techniques for measuring lipoproteins, shows that the inverse association between HDL and coronary heart disease is characterized by a high degree of generality and strength.

The inverse association between HDL cholesterol and coronary heart disease was not appreciably diminished when adjusted for levels of total plasma cholesterol, triglyceride, or LDL. LDL, total cholesterol, and triglycerides were all directly related to coronary heart disease prevalence; surprisingly, these findings were less uniformly present in the various study groups than the inverse association between HDL cholesterol and coronary heart disease.

Analysis for possible correlations between HDL cholesterol and other lipid and lipoprotein fractions demonstrated a moderately strong negative correlation between HDL cholesterol and triglyceride, which was consistent across populations. Triglyceride also had a small negative correlation with LDL cholesterol (except for women) and a moderate positive correlation with total cholesterol. As expected, there was a very strong positive correlation between LDL and total cholesterol. Statistical analysis (discriminant and multivariate analysis) indicated that HDL and LDL cholesterol levels were independent and significant factors in coronary heart disease prevalence. Because of the inverse correlation between HDL cholesterol and triglyceride levels, the role of triglyceride as an independent risk factor was not found to be statistically significant on multivariate analysis.

Prospective data from the Framingham Study have demonstrated the potent role of HDL as a protective factor against coronary heart disease (Gordon, T., *et al.*, 1977). Lipid and lipoprotein values, including fasting triglycerides, and HDL, LDL, and total cholesterol levels, were obtained on 2815 men and women aged 49–82 years chiefly between 1969 and 1971. In the approximately four years following the lipid analyses, coronary heart disease developed in 79 of the 1025 men and 63 of the 1445 women free of coronary heart disease. At these older ages, the major potent lipid risk factor was HDL cholesterol, which had an inverse association with the incidence of coronary heart disease ($p < 0.001$) in either men or women. HDL levels were inversely associated with each major manifestation of coronary heart disease. These associations were equally significant even when other lipids and other standard risk factors for coronary heart disease were taken into consideration. A weaker and positive association with the incidence of coronary heart disease was observed for LDL cholesterol. Triglycerides were associated with the incidence of coronary heart disease only in women, and then only when the level of other lipids was not taken into account.

Evidence for the protective role of HDL in coronary heart disease was also obtained in a prospective case–control study in Tromsø, Norway (Miller *et al.*, 1977a). This study involved a two year case–control follow-up study of 6595 men aged 20–49 years. Discriminant function analysis showed that coronary risk was inversely related to HDL cholesterol concentration and directly related to density less than 1.063 cholesterol. These relationships were independent of each other and of the other measured variables, which included other lipids and other coronary risk factors. HDL cholesterol made the strongest contribution to the prediction of future coronary heart disease in this cohort of young men. Thus, these findings support the conclusion that a low HDL concentration is a common antecedent of clinical coronary heart disease, and is important in accelerating the progression of coronary atherosclerosis.

Evidence that there may be an inverse association between HDL levels and atherosclerotic vascular disease generally, and not only with coronary heart disease, was reported from a study in young (under age 55) male and female patients who had survived an attack of ischemic cerebrovascular disease (Rössner *et al.*, 1978). Serum lipid and lipoprotein levels were measured in the cerebrovascular disease patients, and the results compared with findings in healthy controls. In the patients, total serum triglyceride and cholesterol levels were not increased. However, the mean HDL cholesterol level in the patients was 18% lower than in controls. Clearly, more data are needed to assess the possibility that low HDL may be a strong risk factor for cerebrovascular disease.

Studies are in progress in many institutions to determine the distribution of HDL (and other lipoprotein) levels in various populations, and to explore the associations among HDL levels and other variables. Information has been reported recently about HDL levels in families in Norway (the Tromsø Heart Study) (Mjøs et al., 1977), in children in Louisiana (the Bogalusa Heart Study) (Srinivasan et al., 1976), in neonates in Ohio (Glueck et al., 1977c), and in New Zealand adolescents (Stanhope et al., 1977). These studies and others have provided useful information about HDL levels in different population groups.

Extensive and definitive information about the levels of serum lipids and lipoproteins in several different populations was reported recently from the Cooperative Lipoprotein Phenotyping Study (Castelli et al., 1977a). Data were collected on men and women age 40 and older in six study populations (the five described above, plus Puerto Rico). Blood samples and lipid measurements were obtained after overnight fast by a common protocol as part of a cooperative study of lipoprotein phenotyping. Average cholesterol levels ranged from under 200 mg/dl (Puerto Rican men) to over 240 mg/dl (Framingham women). Average triglyceride levels also covered a wide range, from less than 100 mg/dl in Evans County to over 175 mg/dl in Honolulu and San Francisco. Variation by age and sex was evident not only for total cholesterol and triglyceride, but also for LDL and HDL cholesterol. For men, the peak total cholesterol level was generally at age 50–59; for women, at age 60–69. Estimates of the 95th-percentile values for each variable are also presented in this report. These values are useful in assessing the range of usual values for the various lipids and for the characterization of lipid abnormalities. The 95th-percentile values for LDL cholesterol differed relatively little by age and ranged from 196 to 209 mg/dl for men and from 221 to 228 mg/dl for women. The 95th-percentile values for triglycerides, however, varied greatly by age and population, mainly being in the range 205–350 mg/dl. This wide variation for triglyceride 95th-percentile values reflected the well-established highly skewed distribution of triglyceride values in a population. It was pointed out that appropriate general standards for hypertriglyceridemia would appear, therefore, to be difficult to establish.

Correlations among the various lipids and lipoproteins were explored. There was a high positive correlation between LDL and total cholesterol; this was not surprising, since, on the average, about two thirds of total cholesterol is in LDL. The high correlation implies that total cholesterol will ordinarily serve as a reasonable guide to LDL cholesterol levels. In contrast, there was a very low correlation between HDL and total cholesterol levels, so that HDL cholesterol supplies another separate piece of lipid information. As indicated above, there was a moderately strong negative correlation between HDL cholesterol and total triglyceride levels.

3.5.2. Alcohol, High-Density Lipoproteins, and Coronary Risk

Intriguing evidence has been obtained that alcohol, drunk in moderation, is associated with an increase in plasma HDL levels and with a reduced coronary risk status. Earlier studies, such as one carried out in chronic alcoholics after acute abuse (Johansson and Medhus, 1974), demonstrated an association between increased HDL levels and alcohol ingestion. More recently, data on the relationships between alcohol consumption and lipid and lipoprotein levels were reported from the Cooperative Lipoprotein Phenotyping Study (Castelli *et al.*, 1977c). Alcohol consumption was positively associated with HDL cholesterol level in all five study populations analyzed. Moreover, the HDL cholesterol level appeared to be a graded response even over the low levels of alcohol consumption reported. Less strong, but consistently negative, correlations were found with LDL cholesterol. Plasma triglyceride level showed a modest positive correlation with alcohol consumption. Because of the possibility that lipid response varied with the kind of alcoholic beverage used, separate correlations were computed for beer, wine, and spirits. Wine was generally a trivial source of alcohol in these populations. Little difference was found between beer and spirits in their association with the various blood lipids.

Epidemiologic evidence for a protective effect of moderate alcohol consumption in coronary heart disease was reported from the Honolulu Heart Study (Yano *et al.*, 1977). In this report, the relationship of coffee and alcohol consumption to the risk of coronary heart disease was examined during a six-year period in a cohort of 7705 Japanese men living in Hawaii. The analysis was based on 294 new cases of coronary heart disease. There was a positive association between coffee intake and risk, but it became statistically not significant when cigarette smoking was taken into account. There was a strong negative association between moderate alcohol consumption (up to 60 ml/day), mainly from beer, and the risk of nonfatal myocardial infarction and death from coronary heart disease. This association remained significant in multivariate analysis, taking into account smoking and other risk factors. It was pointed out that the correlation of alcohol consumption with the level of HDL cholesterol (positive) and LDL cholesterol (negative) may partly account for the observed negative association between alcohol and coronary heart disease.

3.5.3. Other Clinical Studies

It is well established that patients with severe chronic renal disease manifest accelerated atherosclerosis and a high risk of cardiovascular disease (see the discussion in Section 3.5.4). To explore whether HDL might be related to this phenomenon, HDL cholesterol levels were measured in patients with chronic renal disease, and compared with levels measured in 430 adult controls (Bagdade and Albers, 1977). The renal disease patients included 13 not on dialysis, 14 being maintained on hemodialysis, and 23 patients who had undergone successful renal transplantation. HDL cholesterol concentrations were significantly lower than control values in both the transplant and the nontransplant patients. The ratios of LDL to HDL cholesterol were significantly higher in the patients than those observed in both randomly selected controls and in controls matched for plasma lipid levels. Thus, the possibility exists that these lipoprotein findings are related to the premature morbidity and mortality from cardiovascular causes that exist in patients with chronic renal failure.

Evidence was summarized last year (Goodman, 1978) that the two conditions of hyperalpha lipoproteinemia and hypobeta lipoproteinemia are associated with increased life expectancy and decreased prevalence of coronary heart disease. Additional evidence supporting this conclusion was reported from studies carried out in octogenarian kindreds (Glueck *et al.*, 1977a, 1978). The kindreds were self-referred by virtue of having either two siblings or a parent and child living to age 80 or over. In 22 such kindreds, there was evidence for familial hyperalpha lipoproteinemia in 7, for familial hypobeta lipoproteinemia in 3, and for primary hyperalpha or hypobeta lipoproteinemia in an additional 2 and 2 kindreds. First-degree relatives of probands with hyperalpha or hypobeta lipoproteinemia had sharply reduced morbidity and mortality from myocardial infarction when compared with population controls ($p <$ 0.005). Longevity analysis in the 14 kindreds with hyperalpha or hypobeta lipoproteinemia revealed an average life expectancy for males and females, respectively, of 82 and 86 years, as compared with 71 and 75 years ($p < 0.001$) for males and females in the general population (U.S. Life Tables). Mean ± S.E.M. ratios of LDL to HDL cholesterol in 14 hypobeta and 23 hyperalpha subjects were 1.12 ± 0.18 and 1.50 ± 0.10, respectively, notably lower than the ratio in 124 free living controls (2.41 ± 0.10). Thus, these observations provide further support for the concept that high HDL or low LDL or both are associated with longevity.

Detection of a family with hypobeta lipoproteinemia in the course of screening cord blood samples for total and LDL cholesterol was reported recently (Stein, 1977).

Further information about the relationship between HDL levels and physical exercise was obtained in a study of 220 trained men, examined the day before participation in a cross-country ski race (Enger *et al.*, 1977). HDL cholesterol in the trained men was significantly higher than that in untrained men, but did not differ significantly from untrained women. HDL cholesterol was significantly higher in skiers above 60 years than in skiers of younger age. Tobacco smokers had lower HDL cholesterol and HDL/total cholesterol ratio than nonsmokers, but the differences were significant only in skiers, not in controls. Thus, the trained athletes had lipoprotein characteristics associated with a lower risk of coronary heart disease. It should be noted that longitudinal data are needed, determining the effect of physical conditioning in a given cohort, before more extensive interpretations regarding the effects of exercise on HDL levels can be made.

3.5.4. Pathophysiology

In view of the protective effect of HDL on the development of atherosclerotic cardiovascular disease, considerable interest exists among investigators in this field in trying to elucidate the factors involved in the regulation of plasma HDL levels and metabolism. The metabolic turnover studies described earlier in this chapter were in part directed toward this goal. At present, the regulatory factors are not known. One of the major lines of speculation and investigation, however, involves the demonstrated interrelationships between the levels of the two classes of lipoproteins, HDL and VLDL. As described above, epidemiologic studies have clearly shown a consistent inverse relationship between VLDL (as estimated from plasma triglyceride) levels and HDL levels in a number of different populations. Various forms of hypertriglyceridemia (types I, IV, and V hyperlipoproteinemic phenotypes) are associated with low HDL levels, and the homozygote and heterozygote states of Tangier disease (with nearly zero and half-normal HDL levels, respectively) are associated with elevated VLDL. Chronic renal failure is associated with elevated VLDL and low HDL levels. Furthermore, HDL and VLDL levels respond in reciprocal fashion to a number of perturbations of lipoprotein metabolism. Thus, weight loss, nicotinic acid treatment, clofibrate treatment, and tibric acid treatment all lower VLDL levels and raise HDL levels. Diets high in carbohydrate have the opposite effects on the levels of these two lipoproteins. In all these conditions, a reciprocity appears to be present between HDL and VLDL levels; the only known exceptions to this generalization are alcohol consumption and estrogen treatment, both of which raise both VLDL and HDL levels. Thus, it appears that the determinants of VLDL and HDL levels may be linked in some way, although the mechanisms involved in such a possible interrelationship remain to be defined.

Some of the possible mechanisms whereby HDL may exert a protective role toward the development of atherosclerosis were discussed last year (Goodman, 1978). These possible mechanisms included: (1) inhibition by HDL of the uptake of LDL by cells; (2) modulation by HDL of the transendothelial transport of LDL; and (3) transport of cholesterol by HDL from peripheral tissues, including the arterial wall.

Experiments dealing with the first of these possible mechanisms were reported in detail recently by Miller *et al.* (1977b). With the use of normal human fibroblasts in cell culture *in vitro,* the effect of HDL on the binding, internalization, and degradation of radioiodinated LDL was examined. Addition of HDL to the culture medium inhibited all these parameters of cell LDL metabolism. At HDL/LDL molar ratios of 25:1 (protein ratios about 5 : 1), these parameters were reduced by about 25%. Unlabeled LDL was about 25 times more effective in reducing labeled LDL binding. Preincubation of fibroblasts wtih HDL reduced the subsequent binding of labeled LDL during a second incubation. In other experiments, HDL reduced the net increase in cell cholesterol content induced by incubation with LDL. HDL alone had no net effect on cell cholesterol content. The authors conclude that these findings suggest that HDL reduces both the high-affinity and low-affinity binding of LDL to human fibroblasts, and that this in turn reduces the internalization and degradation of LDL. It was thought that these effects of HDL *in vitro* might be relevant to the negative correlation between HDL levels and the prevalence of clinically manifest atherosclerosis.

More recently, however, questions have arisen concerning the validity of these conclusions about the effects of HDL on LDL binding and uptake by cells. These questions have arisen from the work of Mahley and co-workers (Mahley and Innerarity, 1977; Mahley *et al.,* 1977), which has shown that cholesterol feeding in experimental animals results in the appearance of an unusual lipoprotein called HDL_c, in the HDL density range. HDL_c is particularly enriched in cholesterol and has apoE as its major protein component. HDL_c was shown to be able to bind to the high-affinity cell-surface receptor for LDL on cultured human fibroblasts, and to compete with LDL for binding to the receptor. Normal HDL (not cholesterol-induced) did not display this property. The possibility therefore exists that the effects of HDL on LDL binding and metabolism by fibroblasts discussed above may reflect effects of a human counterpart to HDL_c. If this were the case, and since HDL_c is thought to be atherogenic in experimental animals, it would cast doubt on the relevance of the results of the fibroblast studies to the protective role of HDL in atherosclerotic disease.

3.5.5. Implications

The rapidly increasing body of information about the clinical significance of HDL has provided physicians with several cogent reasons for measuring HDL levels in patients. Accordingly, these measurements are now being made available to clinicians in a large number of clinical chemistry laboratories throughout this country. The major clinical usefulness of HDL determinations lies in the assessment of overall coronary risk. This can be of particular use in the patient in whom the decision whether to initiate drug therapy of hyperlipidemia is a borderline one, such as in patients with marginally high levels of serum cholesterol. In addition, as pointed out above, the evidence available suggests that the excess risk of coronary heart disease associated with hypertriglyceridemia may reflect in large part the inverse relationship between triglyceride and HDL levels. Accordingly, information about the HDL level in a patient with moderately high triglyceride might be of value in deciding whether the patient's risk status warrants therapy beyond diet. Furthermore, measurement of HDL is of value for the rare patient in whom elevation of serum cholesterol reflects solely an elevated HDL. Thus, knowledge of the HDL level may obviate unnecessary therapy. HDL is usually quantitated as HDL cholesterol by measurement of the residual cholesterol in plasma after removal of VLDL and LDL by precipitation with a solution of heparin and manganese chloride. As discussed in Section 3.3.1, improvements in methodology are under investigation.

A final implication concerns therapy. In view of the findings with HDL, it would seem worthwhile to encourage measures that increase the concentration of HDL in plasma and avoid those that have the opposite effect. Only limited information is, however, available regarding the effects of various interventions and approaches on plasma HDL levels. A useful approach to the treatment of individual patients can, however, be developed by using the information summarized above regarding the known reciprocity between plasma VLDL (triglyceride) and HDL levels. Thus, many factors are now well known to reduce plasma triglyceride levels (e.g., weight loss, dietary and drug interventions). It can be anticipated that these interventions will raise HDL levels in many patients, and can therefore be adopted clinically as a therapeutic approach toward the reduction of coronary risk. In addition, as pointed out last year (Goodman, 1978), efforts are under way in the pharmaceutical industry and elsewhere to look for drugs that would particularly raise HDL levels, or raise the HDL/LDL ratio. An agent that would both raise HDL and lower LDL levels, if such an agent could be developed, would have considerable potential as preventive therapy for atherosclerotic vascular disease.

3.6. Cholesterol Metabolism and Its Regulation

3.6.1. In Intact Humans

Information about total body cholesterol metabolism *in vivo* in humans was discussed last year (Goodman, 1978). Considerable information is now available about the parameters of body cholesterol metabolism in man, and about the effects of different types of hyperlipidemia on these parameters.

One of the parameters of cholesterol metabolism of considerable interest to investigators is that of cholesterol absorption. In the past, methods for estimating cholesterol absorption in man have been highly laborious and time-consuming. As a much simpler approach, a dual isotope ratio method was developed by Zilversmit (1972) to measure cholesterol absorption in rats. The validity of this method was recently explored in humans (Samuel *et al.*, 1978). In this study, cholesterol absorption as measured by the isotope ratio method was compared with that simultaneously measured by a more laborious fecal radioactivity method. In 12 experiments in 11 patients, there was good to excellent agreement between the two methods in the same patient, except for one experiment. Statistical analysis indicated that one could be 95% confident that the two absorption methods will produce results within 5% of each other, and 99% confident that the differences are less than 7%. This method offers considerable promise of being able to be widely used to obtain information about cholesterol absorption in different kinds of patients under a variety of conditions.

3.6.2. In Cultured Cells

Cholesterol metabolism in fibroblasts and certain other cells in culture *in vitro* has been shown to be a highly regulated process. There is evidence, moreover, that similar regulatory mechanisms also operate *in vivo*. As discussed previously (Goodman, 1976, 1978), cholesterol metabolism in fibroblasts appears to be controlled mainly by a pathway involving specific cell-surface receptors for LDL. This LDL pathway constitutes a mechanism by which the cells take up plasma LDL and consequently regulate their cellular cholesterol. Binding of LDL to the receptor is the first step in this pathway, followed by internalization of the LDL by endocytosis, and intralysosomal hydrolysis of the protein and cholesteryl ester components of the lipoprotein. The resulting free cholesterol is then available for use by the cell for membrane synthesis. When sufficient cholesterol has accumulated, three regulatory events occur: (1) cholesterol synthesis is suppressed, through reduction in the activity of the enzyme β-hydroxy-β-methylglutaryl-CoA reductase; (2) excess free cholesterol is reesterified for storage as cholesteryl esters through an activation of an acyl-CoA:cholesterol acyltransferase enzyme; and (3) synthesis of the LDL receptor is diminished, therefore preventing further entry of LDL cholesterol into the cell. By regulating the number of cell-surface LDL receptors, cells are able to control the rate of entry of cholesterol, thereby assuring themselves an adequate supply of sterol while preventing its overaccumulation. Since plasma LDL is derived ultimately from lipoproteins synthesized in the liver or intestine, the LDL pathway constitutes a mechanism *in vivo* by which cholesterol can be delivered to peripheral tissues from the liver (the main site of cholesterol synthesis) or the intestine (the site of cholesterol absorption). A genetic defect in the LDL receptor or its function appears to be the biochemical lesion in familial hypercholesterolemia (FH).

The information available about the LDL receptor pathway and its relationship to atherosclerosis was effectively reviewed in 1977 by Goldstein and Brown (1977a,b), in whose laboratories much of this work was developed.

Our understanding of these phenomena was advanced during 1977 and early 1978 by a number of reports. Information on the role of the coated endocytic vesicle in the uptake of receptor-bound LDL was obtained by electron-microscopy studies using ferritin-labeled LDL (Anderson, R. G. W., *et al.*, 1977). The results demonstrated that the coated regions of the plasma membrane are specialized structures of rapid turnover that function to carry receptor-bound LDL, and perhaps other receptor-bound molecules, into the cell.

Further evidence has been reported that the LDL pathway and the LDL receptor-mediated regulation of cholesterol metabolism operates in a variety of mammalian cells maintained in culture, in addition to fibroblasts. Recent reports have included studies with freshly isolated human lymphocytes (Ho *et al.*, 1977), human aortic smooth muscle cells (Brown *et al.*, 1977), and cultured mouse adrenal cells (Faust *et al.*, 1977). In the latter study, it was found that receptor-mediated uptake of LDL was importantly involved in the provision of substrate (cholesterol) for steroid hormone biosynthesis.

Evidence that the LDL pathway operates *in vivo* in many tissues has been obtained in studies in the rat and in man. Studies in the rat have suggested that *in vivo* cholesterol metabolism in a large number of extrahepatic tissues is regulated by way of the LDL pathway (Andersen and Dietschy, 1977). Studies in humans with lymphocytes have also strongly suggested that the LDL pathway functions *in vivo*. Thus, normal human lymphocytes isolated freshly from the body exhibit a very low rate of cholesterol synthesis, presumably because they have just been removed from a medium with abundant LDL (Ho *et al.*, 1977). When these cells were incubated in the absence of lipoproteins, cholesterol synthesis increased markedly. This increase was prevented when LDL was included in the incubation medium, and was suppressed when LDL was later added back to the system. As expected, lymphocytes from FH homozygotes were resistant to LDL-mediated suppression of cholesterol synthesis. On the other hand, the rate of cholesterol synthesis was 2–4 times normal in freshly isolated lymphocytes from two subjects with abetalipoprotein-emia. These data all support the conclusion that the LDL pathway was functioning *in vivo*.

The LDL receptor pathway provides a sophisticated control mechanism that protects cells from overaccumulating cholesterol *in vitro*. As discussed last year (Goodman, 1978), however, the LDL receptor can be bypassed by chemically modifying LDL with the addition of a large number of positive charges to the molecule. Addition of such cationized LDL to human fibroblasts (Basu *et al.*, 1977), or to human aortic smooth muscle cells (Goldstein *et al.*, 1977), produced a massive increase in the content of both free and esterified cholesterol within the cell. The accumulation of this large amount of sterol gave rise to a biochemical and morphological picture resembling the alterations that occur within smooth muscle cells *in vivo* during the process of atherosclerosis. Thus, it has been suggested that these cells may provide a useful model system for study of the pathological consequences at the cellular level of massive deposition of cholesteryl ester.

The relationship of these observations to the development of atherosclerosis remains speculative. It has been suggested that arterial smooth muscle cells, particularly in atherosclerotic lesions, may be able to take up and digest LDL by a process that does not involve the LDL receptor (Goldstein and Brown, 1977b). In this hypothesis, increased LDL entering the arterial intima would lead to an overaccumulation of cholesterol within the cells, similar to the events that occur *in vitro* when cells are presented with cationized LDL. In both cases, the cells accumulate massive amounts of cholesteryl esters until toxicity results. This hypothesis is consistent with the known atherogenic potential of LDL from epidemiologic and experimental animal studies.

Other than blood cells and endothelial cells, most body cells cannot obtain LDL from plasma directly, but rather must obtain it from the interstitial fluid. Because of the large size of the LDL molecule, the capillary endothelium serves as a major barrier to its passage into the interstitial fluid. Data on the concentration of LDL in interstitial fluid were reported recently, from studies in which the concentration of apoB in human serum and peripheral lymph was measured immunologically (Reichl *et al.*, 1977). In 4 normal and 6 hyperlipidemic subjects, total lymph apoB levels were 5–15% of serum apoB levels in the same subject. These ratios were equivalent to lymph apoB levels of about 60–120 μg/ml (equivalent to LDL cholesterol of the order of 200 μg/ml). Since the data suggest that the LDL receptor functions optimally at LDL levels of about 25 μg LDL cholesterol/ml, it has been suggested that the usual mean plasma LDL cholesterol level in normal man is about 5- to 10-fold higher than the level required for plasma LDL to deliver cholesterol effectively to body cells (Goldstein and Brown, 1977b). This has, furthermore, led to the suggestion (Goldstein and Brown, 1977b) that Western populations are so prone to atherosclerosis because their "normal" (i.e., usual) concentration of plasma LDL is so unphysiologically high that when plasma leaks into the artery wall through areas of endothelial damage, the smooth muscle cells are presented with a load of LDL that exceeds the clearance capacity of the receptor-mediated process.

3.7. Familial Hypercholesterolemia

Familial hypercholesterolemia (FH), a single-gene disorder that produces hypercholesterolemia, xanthomatosis, and premature atherosclerosis, was discussed in some detail in two earlier reviews (Goodman, 1976, 1978). This section will consider briefly the major developments that were reported in 1977 and early 1978.

3.7.1. Epidemiologic and Clinical Studies

It is well established that FH is transmitted as an autosomal dominant trait in humans. The prevalence of the disorder is approximately 1 in 500 persons in the general American population.

A combined Norwegian and British study was carried out on the age at death from coronary heart disease of FH heterozygotes (Heiberg and Slack, 1977). The correlation coefficient within families for 43 sib pairs was 0.70 and for 14 first cousin pairs 0.61. There was no significant correlation between the age at death and serum cholesterol concentration in either series. The intrafamilial correlations suggest that information about the age at death from coronary heart disease in heterozygotes within families may have some prognostic value, and may also be interpreted as evidence for genetic heterogeneity in FH.

A recent report from Japan described serum lipid levels and prevalence of coronary heart disease in 122 FH heterozygotes in the Hokuriku district of Japan (Mabuchi *et al.*, 1977b). The occurrence of ischemic heart disease in 83 patients was 43%, and that of myocardial infarction was 21%. It was concluded that FH is as highly atherogenic in Japan as in Western countries, despite the low incidence of coronary heart disease in the general population in Japan, which has been attributed to the low level of serum cholesterol.

Useful clinical information was provided by the same Japanese investigators on the discrimination of FH and secondary hypercholesterolemia by Achilles tendon thickness (Mabuchi *et al.*, 1977a). The Achilles tendon thickness in normal subjects was 6.3 ± 0.2 mm (mean ± S.E.M.). The thickness was significantly correlated with age and with serum cholesterol level, but not with serum triglyceride concentration. Achilles tendon thickness in patients with secondary hypercholesterolemia (hypothyroidiam and nephrotic syndrome, particularly) was only slightly greater than that in normal subjects. In contrast, tendon thickness in FH heterozygotes was greatly increased, to 11.8 ± 1.0 mm (mean ± S.E.M.). In these patients, Achilles tendon thickness was strongly correlated with age ($r = 0.72$). Thus, measurement of Achilles tendon thickness may make it possible to discriminate FH from other hypercholesterolemic conditions in patients whose family histories are lacking or incomplete.

3.7.2. Pathophysiology

As discussed above, the pathogenetic defect in FH has been shown to be a defect in LDL receptor activity. This defect leads to hyperbetalipoproteinemia (and hypercholesterolemia), which then, in turn, leads to accelerated atherosclerosis via mechanisms involving excessive proliferation of arterial smooth muscle cells (Ross and Glomset, 1976; Ross and Harker, 1976). The defect in the LDL receptor pathway has been extensively examined in fibroblasts from patients with FH, and has also been shown to be present in other cells as well (Ho *et al.*, 1977).

Three types of genetic defects have been demonstrated in fibroblasts from patients with homozygous FH. One class of mutant cells, termed "receptor-negative," completely lacks the LDL receptor. The second class, termed "receptor-defective," exhibits a low but detectable ability to bind LDL at the receptor site, such that 5–20% of normal binding activity is expressed. Third, one patient has been identified whose fibroblasts are able to bind normal amounts of LDL at the receptor site, but are unable to internalize the LDL after it has bound to the receptor.

An extensive study of the genetics of the LDL receptor in lymphocytes from FH heterozygotes was reported recently (Bilheimer *et al.*, 1978). Circulating mononuclear cells were used as a readily available tissue, and the rate of high-affinity degradation of radioiodinated LDL was used as an index of LDL receptor activity. Receptor activity was measured in cells from 32 normals, 15 FH heterozygote patients, and 7 patients with other kinds of hyperlipidemic disorders. LDL receptor activity was assayed in purified lymphocytes that had been incubated for 3 days in the absence of lipoproteins so as to induce a high level of receptor activity. Labeled LDL degradation was also measured in mixed mononuclear cells (85–90% lymphocytes) immediately after their isolation from the bloodstream. Under both sets of conditions, cells from the FH heterozygotes expressed an average of about one half the normal number of LDL receptors. Thus, these findings further support the conclusion that

FH heterozygotes possess only one functional allele at the LDL receptor locus, and that the consequent deficiency of LDL receptors produces the clinical syndrome.

Studies on the turnover of LDL apoprotein (apoB) in the nonsteady state were carried out in four patients with FH, three of them homozygotes (Thompson *et al.*, 1977). LDL apoB synthesis was much higher in the three homozygotes than in the one heterozygote, in whom the synthetic rate was normal. The LDL apoB fractional catabolic rate remained relatively constant, even after marked reduction in LDL pool size by means of plasma exchange. It was concluded that this confirms the existence of an intrinsic defect in LDL catabolism in FH.

The fecal excretion of total bile acids was measured in two normal subjects and in seven patients with FH (four heterozygotes and three homozygotes), both in the untreated state and during treatment with near-maximal doses of cholestyramine resin (Moutafis *et al.*, 1977). There were no significant differences among the three groups. The increase in bile acid excretion in response to cholestyramine was as great in the homozygotes as in the normal subjects. It was concluded that FH is not generally due to an inherited defect in the mechanisms for catabolizing cholesterol to bile acids.

3.7.3. Therapy

Treatment of FH usually involves dietary therapy plus treatment with a bile acid sequestrant resin (cholestyramine or colestipol hydrochloride). A moderately good response to therapy is often achieved in FH heterozygotes. Homozygotes are generally much more resistant to treatment. Accordingly, a number of new approaches to therapy for homozygotes have been explored in recent years. These approaches have included portacaval shunt surgery, plasma exchange with a continuous-flow blood-cell separator, and intravenous hyperalimentation, and were discussed previously (Goodman, 1976, 1978). In addition, as discussed last year (Goodman, 1978), partial ileal bypass surgery has also been used as an approach to the treatment of hypercholesterolemia, particularly in FH heterozygotes.

The effects of dietary therapy in 23 children, aged 2–7 years, with heterozygous FH were reported recently (Glueck *et al.*, 1977d). Of these 23 children, 16 showed 10.5 and 11.3% reductions in total and LDL cholesterol, respectively, after 6 months on diet. After 1 year on diet, 3 of 11 children had normal values for total and LDL cholesterol. Of the 23 children, 6 (all 2 years old) had been maintained previously on low-cholesterol diets since age 1 or earlier. Dietary therapy appeared to be most effective when instituted in very young children (e.g., between ages 1 and 2).

A number of reports appeared in 1977 dealing with the effects of cholestyramine resin in patients with FH. In one study (Glueck *et al.*, 1977e), 16 children with heterozygous FH were treated with diet and cholestyramine for 2–3 years. For children with good drug adherence, mean cholesterol level was lowered 11–13% below that achieved with diet alone. Reduction in cholesterol was no greater with 16 than with 12 g cholestyramine/day. It was concluded that cholestyramine, added to diet, effects a significant reduction in total and LDL cholesterol in about 60% of children with heterozygous FH, but that continued reinforcement of both diet and drug adherence is essential for this effect.

Considerable information was provided in a study of 20 children and young adults with heterozygous FH treated with cholestyramine (added to previous dietary therapy) in a metabolic unit (Farah *et al.*, 1977). When the dose of resin was increased in 13 patients by 1 g/day up to 16 g/day, given twice daily, total and LDL cholesterol fell within the normal range in 11 patients (average dose, 7 g/day), and the response was directly proportional to the pretreatment concentrations of total and LDL cholesterol, but did not correlate with body weight. Cholesterol levels continued to fall and reached a plateau after which additional cholestyramine had no further effect (average dose 11 g/day). It was concluded that the minimum effective dose of cholestyramine in young FH patients can be predicted from the plasma total and LDL cholesterol, and may be given twice daily.

Somewhat different findings were reported by West and Lloyd (1977), who found that there was a positive correlation between reduction in serum cholesterol and the dose of cholestyramine expressed on a body-weight basis. In their experience, the plateau value after which further dosage increments of resin were without effect was about 0.7 g/kg, with a maximum reduction in serum cholesterol approaching 50% of the pretreatment level.

The effects of cholestyramine (16 g/day) and nicotinic acid (3 g/day) were compared in 11 patients heterozygous for FH (Mann *et al.*, 1977). During 3-month treatment periods, cholestyramine resulted in a mean decrease in cholesterol of 26% and nicotinic acid of 21%. The slow-release preparation of nicotinic acid used was found acceptable to the majority of patients studied.

A study was reported on the effects of complete bile diversion, by common-duct ligation and cholecystectomy, in two homozygous FH patients refractory to medical therapy (Deckelbaum *et al.*, 1977). This procedure was undertaken in an attempt to arrest the progression of their xanthomatosis and atherosclerosis by depletion of body cholesterol. Clofibrate was given after operation to one patient, and cholic acid to both, in an effort to enhance further the negative sterol balance. Bile diversion produced a 6- to 8-fold increase in gastrointestinal sterol output, which was not increased further by either clofibrate or cholic acid therapy. Despite a calculated sterol loss of 560 g over 14 months in one patient, and 400 g over 10 months in the other, neither plasma cholesterol nor xanthoma size decreased. Continuity of the biliary tree was therefore restored. The data suggest that patients with homozygous FH respond to even massive gastrointestinal sterol depletion with equal increases in sterol synthesis. It was concluded that treatment regimens, either medical or surgical, that aim for cholesterol depletion by interruption of the normal enterohepatic circulation are likely to be ineffective in patients with homozygous FH. Thus, further therapeutic efforts in homozygotes should aim at prevention and removal of cholesterol deposition by interference at other sites of cholesterol metabolism.

3.8. Chronic Renal Failure and Hyperlipidemia

Patients with chronic renal failure manifest a high prevalence of hyperlipidemia, accelerated atherosclerosis, and a high risk of premature cardiovascular disease; these phenomena were discussed previously (Goodman, 1976, 1978).

3.8.1. Pathophysiology

Hypertriglyceridemia (and a type IV lipoprotein pattern) is present in a large proportion of patients with chronic uremia and in renal failure patients on hemodialysis therapy. The mechanism in these patients appears to be defective triglyceride removal (clearance) from plasma (see Goodman, 1978).

Further information about the pathogenesis of hypertriglyceridemia in patients with renal disease was reported recently (Mordasini *et al.*, 1977). Three groups of patients were studied: (1) conservatively treated chronic uremia (13 patients); (2) patients on maintenance hemodialysis (39 patients); and (3) renal transplant recipients (23 patients). Plasma lipoprotein composition was determined, and the activities of lipoprotein lipase and of hepatic triglyceride lipase were assayed in postheparin plasma. A selective decrease of hepatic triglyceride lipase with normal lipoprotein lipase was found in uremic patients and in patients on hemodialysis. Elevated levels of VLDL and increased triglycerides in LDL occurred in these patients. In contrast, hepatic triglyceride lipase and lipoprotein lipase were both normal in patients after renal transplantation, who commonly had the type II lipoprotein pattern with increased LDL cholesterol and decreased HDL cholesterol levels. It was suggested that a defect in VLDL catabolism caused by the low hepatic triglyceride lipase activity is in part responsible for the accumulation of VLDL and of triglyceride-rich LDL in the chronic renal failure patients, and that this may be involved in their high risk of premature atherosclerotic disease.

Evidence supporting the conclusion that uremic patients on hemodialysis accumulate intermediates in VLDL catabolism in plasma (such as IDL and "remnants"), presumably reflecting defective VLDL catabolism, was also reported by Minamisono *et al.* (1978).

The occurrence of low plasma levels of HDL in patients with severe chronic renal disease, and its possible relationship to accelerated atherosclerosis in these patients, was discussed in Section 3.5.3 (Bagdade and Albers, 1977).

3.8.2. Therapy

The response of plasma triglyceride levels to changes in the composition of formula diets was studied in 12 patients with chronic renal failure (Sanfelippo *et al.*, 1977). Fasting plasma triglyceride levels (mean 256 mg/ dl) decreased in all subjects (to a mean of 169 mg/dl) in response to a reduction in the proportion of carbohydrate (from 50 to 35% of calories) and an increase in the polyunsaturated/saturated fat ratio (from 0.2 to 2.0) in an isocaloric diet. Thus, patients with renal failure and hypertriglyceridemia do respond to diet therapy; a longer-term study will be needed to determine whether the observed effects can be maintained.

Earlier work (see Goodman, 1976) demonstrated that renal failure patients are prone to toxicity when treated with clofibrate to lower plasma triglyceride levels. Detailed studies of clofibrate effects and pharmacokinetics were reported recently (Goldberg *et al.*, 1977). Plasma clofibrate disappearance was found to be prolonged as much as 7 times normal in severely uremic patients. A marked reduction in the usual 14 g/week clofibrate dose to a total dose of 1–1.5 g/week effectively lowered serum triglyceride level (−28%) in hypertriglyceridemic hemodialysis patients without toxicity. The serum clofibrate level at this dose was comparable to that in hypertriglyceridemic nonuremic patients receiving 2 g/day (14 g/ week) of clofibrate. Thus, the dose of clofibrate administered to hemodialysis patients can be adjusted to avoid toxicity and provide the desired therapeutic effect by monitoring serum creatine phosphokinase and triglyceride levels.

Similar findings were also reported recently by Di Giulio *et al.* (1977). Hyperlipidemic uremic patients were effectively treated with clofibrate at a daily oral maintenance dose of 5 mg/kg body weight after a short loading period. This dose led to plasma clofibrate levels of 75–100 μg/dl, and did not result in toxicity as monitored by plasma creatine kinase levels.

Finally, in a somewhat different but related area, a provocative study was reported wherein serum lipid levels were found to be increased during diuretic therapy of hypertension (Ames and Hill, 1976). In this study, 39 patients with mild primary hypertension were treated with diet and then with a diuretic drug. The use of diuretics was accompanied by an average increase of 11 mg/dl in serum cholesterol and of 34 mg/dl in triglyceride level. In a subgroup of 21 patients with greatest elevations in lipid levels during the administration of diuretics, little improvement in coronary risk status occurred because the increase in cholesterol balanced the decrease in systolic blood pressure. These observations warrant further exploration by and attention from clinicians.

3.9. Hypertriglyceridemia

3.9.1. Pathophysiology

Circulating triglyceride, in chylomicrons and VLDL, is normally catabolized mainly through the activity of the triglyceride hydrolase called lipoprotein lipase (LPL). This enzyme functions at the vascular endothelial surface. It is released into the circulation (solubilized) by heparin, and makes up a major part of the lipolytic activity of postheparin plasma. LPL is highly reactive only with protein-bound triglyceride, and is mainly (and almost entirely) activated by apoC-II. LPL activity is also present in extracts of tissues that utilize the fatty acid products of lipase activity for oxidative metabolism or storage. Thus, it is found at high levels in adipose tissue, muscle (especially heart and red skeletal muscles), lactating mammary gland, and lung. Human hypertriglyceridemias are not uncommonly associated with disorders of LPL activity. A good review of LPL appeared in 1977 (Fielding, C. J., and Havel, 1977). In addition to LPL, a triglyceride lipase from liver with properties distinct from those of LPL contributes significantly to postheparin lipolytic activity in plasma.

Recent studies in the rat have provided new information on the molecular heterogeneity of LPL activity in postheparin plasma (Fielding, P. E., *et al.*, 1977), and about the pattern and the regulation of LPL and hepatic triglyceride lipase activities during pre- and postnatal development (Chajek *et al.*, 1977).

Since apoC-II activates and apoC-III inhibits LPL, it has been suggested that the relative amounts of these C peptides may regulate VLDL triglyceride removal *in vivo* and contribute to certain forms of endogenous hypertriglyceridemia. Information about the relative levels of apoC-II and C-III during and following pregnancy was reported by Montes and Knopp (1977). Hypertriglyceridemia, with increased levels of VLDL and

IDL, usually occurs during pregnancy. It was found that the apoC-II/C-III ratio decreased during pregnancy and returned to normal postpartum. The pathophysiological implications of these observations need further exploration.

A study was reported on the postheparin plasma activities of LPL and hepatic triglyceride lipase in patients with alcoholic or viral hepatitis (Freeman *et al.*, 1977). Hepatic triglyceride lipase activity was considerably decreased in the liver disease patients (mean 21–24% of controls), whereas LPL was not affected. It was suggested that hepatic triglyceride lipase deficiency may partially account for the accumulation of a triglyceride-rich LDL in liver disease.

Studies were conducted to explore in more detail the metabolic heterogeneity of human VLDL triglyceride (Streja *et al.*, 1977). VLDL triglyceride kinetics were examined in three ultracentrifugally separated VLDL subfractions, and in a combined IDL–LDL fraction. VLDL triglyceride turnover was fastest for large VLDL and slowest for small VLDL. It seems clear that the entire spectrum of VLDL particles is not metabolized in a homogeneous fashion. It was concluded that the data do not exclude a cascade from large VLDL to small VLDL, and thence to IDL and LDL, but also suggest that this may not be the only route of VLDL metabolism.

A new method was developed for the measurement of fractional clearance rates of chylomicrons in man (Grundy and Mok, 1976). In 21 patients with normal triglyceride levels, clearance rates for chylomicrons were extremely rapid, with the half-life for chylomicron triglyceride being 4.5 ± 2.9 min (mean $\pm$ S.D.). In 30 patients with endogenous hypertriglyceridemia, clearance was generally prolonged (half-life 23 ± 5.5 min). This delay in chylomicron clearance could have been due either to a defect in removal of all triglyceride-rich lipoproteins or to competition for removal between endogenous and exogenous particles. A generalized defect in clearance capacity for plasma triglyceride was ruled out for most patients by showing that reduction of endogenous triglyceride by caloric restriction caused chylomicron removal to return to normal. It was also pointed out that endogenous triglyceride is removed much less efficiently than chylomicron triglyceride, and in some patients this discrepancy is particularly marked.

3.9.2. Diabetes Mellitus; Other Clinical Studies

An extensive study was reported on postheparin plasma LPL and hepatic triglyceride lipase activities in patients with diabetes mellitus, in relation to plasma triglyceride metabolism (Nikkilä *et al.*, 1977a). Mean LPL activity was decreased by 44% in patients with untreated ketotic diabetes, and by 20% in patients with untreated mild to moderate nonketotic early-onset diabetes. Insulin treatment of ketotic diabetes resulted in a rapid increase in LPL activity and decrease in serum triglyceride level, whereas sulfonylurea treatment of non-insulin-requiring diabetics did not significantly affect enzyme activity. In normolipidemic maturity-onset diabetics, LPL activity was within normal range, but in those with hypertriglyceridemia, the average LPL activity was decreased by 26%. LPL activity showed a significant negative correlation with log triglyceride level, and a positive correlation with VLDL triglyceride or intralipid fractional turnover. The hepatic lipase activity was not decreased in diabetics. It was concluded that a deficiency of LPL accounts for a great deal of the elevation of serum triglyceride in insulin-deficient human diabetes, but has a smaller role in the pathogenesis of hypertriglyceridemia associated with maturity-onset diabetes. The latter abnormality may be caused mainly by an increased secretion of triglyceride into the blood, even though a decreased LPL may contribute to hyperlipemia when marked.

Observations were reported on three young siblings with familial hyperchylomicronemia (type 1 hyperlipoproteinemia) (Sternowsky *et al.*, 1977), in an otherwise normal Turkish family of 10 members. The three affected children were very small, below the 3rd percentile, and the possible relationship between the hypertriglyceridemia and growth retardation was discussed.

3.9.3. Treatment Effects: Diet, Drugs, Exercise

A detailed study was reported on the dietary management of 44 children with familial hypertriglyceridemia (Glueck *et al.*, 1977b). Primary hypertriglyceridemia becomes apparent in approximately 20% of children (under age 21) born to parents with familial hypertriglyceridemia. Substantial obesity is associated with the pediatric expression of this condition in 30–60% of affected children. In the prospective study carried out, weight reduction for obese children, plus a diet program including 20% of calories as protein, 40% as carbohydrate, and 40% as fat with a polyunsaturate/saturate ratio of 1.5, was instituted. After 6 months on treatment, the group mean decrement in weight was not significant, and decrements in weight failed to correlate with decreases in plasma triglyceride. Despite this, after 6 months on diet, plasma triglyceride levels were reduced to normal (< 140 mg/dl) in 32 of 43 children, having been at mean levels above 250 mg/dl before therapy. With longer time intervals, the proportion of children maintaining the lowered triglyceride levels was reduced. It was concluded that amelioration of familial hypertriglyceridemia by diet is a realizable goal in children, but requires persistent, repetitive reexamination and reinstruction. Dietary management of pediatric familial hypertriglyceridemia may be important as a primary, longitudinal approach to reduction of the increased atherosclerotic risk associated with this condition.

A study was reported on the effectiveness of dietary counseling in the treatment of patients with endogenous hypertriglyceridemia and the type IV lipoprotein pattern (Gotto *et al.*, 1977). Over a period of 2 years, 103 patients who received instructions for a therapeutic diet and regular dietary counseling by a physician and dietician had a large decline in serum triglyceride level, as compared with 175 patients with the same diagnosis who received similar diets but little dietary counseling. Over the period of the study, the median plasma triglyceride level decreased from 302 to 210 mg/dl, and the mean weight from 84 to 80 kg, in the group receiving dietary counseling.

The effects of clofibrate on postheparin plasma triglyceride lipase activities were studied in 17 patients with primary hypertriglyceridemia (Nikkilä *et al.*, 1977b). The drug caused a significant reduction of serum cholesterol (mean 11%) and triglyceride (mean 45%) levels. LPL activity rose in all subjects, the average rise being 46%. The increase of LPL was positively correlated with the pretreatment LPL activity. During clofibrate treatment, the LPL activity of the hypertriglyceridemic patients was significantly higher than the corresponding value of untreated healthy normoglyceridemic subjects of similar age. The postheparin plasma hepatic triglyceride lipase activity was not influenced by clofibrate.

Data were also reported showing that clofibrate treatment of hypertriglyceridemic patients led to decreased plasma triglyceride levels, increased heparin-releasable LPL activity, and an increase in extractable LPL from biopsy samples of adipose tissue (Taylor *et al.*, 1977). It was concluded that an important effect of clofibrate may be to increase the levels of adipose tissue LPL and thereby improve the clearance of plasma triglycerides.

The effects of estrogen on the two different lipases (LPL and hepatic triglyceride lipase) present in postheparin plasma were examined in 13 normal women before and after 2 weeks of treatment with ethinyl estradiol (Applebaum *et al.*, 1977). Estrogens and estrogen-containing oral contraceptives are known to elevate triglyceride levels in normal women, and may aggravate preexisting hypertriglyceridemia. Estrogen treatment did not significantly change extrahepatic LPL activity in postheparin plasma, or in buttock fat biopsies. In contrast, estrogen led to a significant decrease in hepatic triglyceride lipase, and this was responsible for and correlated with a significant decrease in plasma postheparin lipolytic activity (PHLA). Thus, the decrease in PHLA during estrogen results from a selective decline in hepatic triglyceride lipase activity.

In summary, these reports on clofibrate and estrogen, and other studies commented on above, demonstrate that a number of metabolic and pharmacologic perturbations are now known that selectively affect either LPL or hepatic triglyceride lipase. It can be hoped and anticipated that in the future these kinds of studies will lead to more precise classification of patients according to pathophysiological mechanisms, and more specific approaches to therapy.

The comparative effects of a physical training program and diet were examined in 46 men with hypertriglyceridemia and a type IV pattern (Lampman *et al.*, 1977). Either modest alterations in dietary composition (even without caloric restriction), or a physical training program of modest intensity, or both, were found to be effective measures for lowering serum triglyceride levels. It appeared that patients needed to participate regularly in formal programs in order to maintain adherence to these interventions. It was felt that a program of diet and physical training appears to be a reasonable clinical approach to management.

In an extension of this project, the effects of high-intensity physical training, conducted in an unsupervised group or a supervised setting, were studied in 23 middle-aged men with hypertriglyceridemia and a type IV pattern (Lampman *et al.*, 1978). After 10 weeks, there were significant reductions in serum triglyceride and insulin levels in both groups, but no significant differences between the two groups. Thus, such physical training programs can be conducted in either an unsupervised or a supervised setting, provided the subjects are highly motivated.

The question arises as to what extent the triglyceride-lowering effect of exercise might be due to a negative caloric balance resulting from the energy expenditure of the exercise. To address this question, detailed studies were conducted in five hypertriglyceridemic (type IV) subjects, exercised (I) while maintaining usual caloric intake and (2) while increasing caloric intake to compensate for the exercise-induced increase in energy expenditure (Gyntelberg *et al.*, 1977). Reduction in plasma triglyceride levels, average 120 mg/dl, occurred regardless of whether or not the increase in caloric expenditure was compensated for by an increase in food intake. These data suggest that the triglyceride-lowering effect of exercise is not dependent on or mediated by a negative caloric balance.

3.10. Hyperlipidemia and Its Treatment

3.10.1. Epidemiologic Studies

In Section 3.5, there was a discussion of the recent epidemiologic reports that have provided extensive new information about the levels of serum lipids and lipoproteins in populations, and about the relationships between these levels and coronary heart disease. Two other recent reports on serum lipid or lipoprotein levels, or both, warrant comment. In the first report, plasma cholesterol and triglyceride levels were determined in 6775 school children, ages 6–17, in a biethnic school district in Ohio (Morrison *et al.*, 1977). Associations of age, sex, and race with the levels and distributions of lipids were studied. This paper, by providing useful age-, sex-, and race-specific cholesterol and triglyceride distributions, may allow more meaningful clinical assessment of plasma lipid levels in any individual child.

In the second report, serum lipid and lipoprotein concentrations in 1604 men and women in working populations in northwest London were studied (Slack *et al.*, 1977). In men, the best fit between serum cholesterol, triglycerides, and phospholipids, on the one hand, and age, on the other, was given by a curvilinear relationship expressed as a quadratic regression. In women, the best fit was given by a linear regression. Differences between whites and blacks were found in men, but not in women. The problem of trying to define "normal" limits of serum lipid and lipoprotein levels was discussed.

3.10.2. Definition and Classification

The definition and classification of the hyperlipidemias were reviewed previously (Goodman, 1976, 1978). It was pointed out in these previous reviews that hyperlipidemia is usually defined arbitrarily as being present when the plasma cholesterol or triglyceride level or both are above the 95th-percentile value (for a given age, sex, race, and community).

This approach is widely used for the definition and detection of hypercholesterolemia. The recent epidemiologic studies have, however, indicated that it is very difficult to apply the 95th-percentile cutoff approach to the definition of hypertriglyceridemia. Questions have, moreover, been raised as to the clinical desirability of applying this approach for the detection and management of hypertriglyceridemia, as it is for hypercholesterolemia. Thus, the Cooperative Lipoprotein Phenotyping Study found that the 95th-percentile values for triglyceride varied greatly by age and population, from values close to 200 to as high as 451 mg/dl (Castelli *et al.*, 1977a). Furthermore, the recent studies have found very little, if any, association between triglyceride levels and coronary risk, when triglycerides are considered as an independent risk factor.

These issues will, one hopes, be resolved by future studies. In the meantime, from a clinical and public health point of view, it seems reasonable to continue to try to find persons with high triglyceride levels and enroll them in intervention programs—as is done for persons with hypercholesterolemia. This approach is warranted because detection of a high-triglyceride population does detect a population with higher than average coronary risk. The increased risk may not be due to elevated triglyceride level as an independent variable, but rather to the association of elevated triglyceride with other variables (e.g., with low HDL level). In some instances (e.g., genetic disorders such as familial combined hyperlipidemia), the risk may be more directly dependent on the hyperlipoproteinemia. An attempt to reduce coronary risk in such persons would, however, seem appropriate.

It is difficult to decide at the present time when to consider triglyceride levels as elevated and warranting clinical attention. Different experts currently recommend cutoff values from 200 to 300 mg/dl, recognizing that these are "soft" values. Another approach has been to try to use the 90th-percentile cutoff values instead of the 95th-percentile ones. Clinically, it is probably desirable to review a patient's total coronary risk profile if the triglyceride level is 200 mg/dl or higher, but to not be too concerned about triglyceride level alone, if no other coronary risk factor is present, unless the triglyceride level is distinctly above the 200 mg/dl level.

3.10.3. Diet

As discussed previously (Goodman, 1976, 1978), treatment of hyperlipidemia is based on the assumption that the lowering of the coronary risk factor (hyperlipidemia) will result in a commensurate lowering of coronary risk itself. Definitive evidence that lowering serum lipids will reduce coronary risk is not yet available. Large-scale clinical trials designed to test this assumption are in progress.

Management of hyperlipidemia first involves modifying the diet so as to lower serum cholesterol or triglyceride level, or both. The most generally recommended diet is the American Heart Association fat-controlled diet, limited in cholesterol and saturated animal fat, with caloric intake appropriate for the patient to achieve and maintain an ideal body weight. Weight reduction is stressed in overweight patients. Dietary cholesterol is limited to less than 300 mg/day, the fat content to 35% of total calories, and the saturated fat to less than 10% of calories. This single diet approach is generally valid (with occasional, individual exceptions) for all the common types of hyperlipidemia. With such a diet, one can anticipate a 10–20% reduction in serum cholesterol concentration, and significant reductions in serum triglyceride levels (particularly in patients who are both hypertriglyceridemic and overweight).

Recent studies on the dietary treatment of patients with hypertriglyceridemia were discussed above.

A long-term study of the effects of diets prescribed in coronary prevention programs was conducted in 150 middle-aged men prone to coronary disease (Farinaro et al., 1977). To be accepted in the study, patients had to have two or more of the following risk factors: hypercholesterolemia, obesity, hypertension, cigarette smoking, ECG changes; a few men were accepted with severe hypercholesterolemia alone. Every man was followed for at least 5 years, as part of the Chicago Coronary Prevention Evaluation Program. The diet prescribed was similar to the fat-controlled diet described above, but with a total fat intake aimed at around 30% of calories. The reduced fat intake was mainly replaced by carbohydrate. An extensive nutritional education, counseling, and behavior modification program was employed to develop compliance and adherence to the prescribed diet.

Substantial changes in the pattern of nutrient intake were observed after both 2 and 4 years of study. These changes were associated with weight reduction and significant reductions in the serum cholesterol level. In addition, considerable data were obtained about plasma glucose levels and glucose tolerance. These data were collected to address the question of whether the diet, with an increased percentage of calories from carbohydrate, might have an adverse effect on glucose tolerance. In general, decreases in plasma glucose levels and improvement in glucose tolerance were observed. Decreases in plasma glucose were significantly related to decreases in body weight. Thus, no evidence of impairment of glucose tolerance with years-long consumption of this diet was observed.

A study was carried out to explore whether supplemental vitamin E would be of value in conjunction with diets rich in polyunsaturated fatty acids (Leonhardt, 1978). In 17 patients with hyperlipidemia on long-term treatment with a polyunsaturated-fat diet and clofibrate, no significant effect of vitamin E was seen on serum cholesterol or triglyceride levels.

Fiber has recently aroused interest as a major dietary component that may affect the incidence of coronary heart disease in Western societies. To investigate possible effects of dietary fiber on cholesterol metabolism in man, a detailed metabolic ward study was conducted in six adult volunteers fed eucaloric diets with or without cholesterol (from egg yolk), with or without a large quantity of added dietary fiber (Raymond et al., 1977). The results demonstrated that a large quantity of dietary fiber from diverse sources had little or no effect on the plasma lipid levels or the sterol balance in man, even though intestinal transit time and stool bulk changed greatly.

3.10.4. Drugs

Many patients will remain hyperlipidemic despite dietary therapy, and in these patients, the question of the desirability of drug treatment to lower serum lipid levels must then be considered. As discussed previously (Goodman, 1976, 1978), it is often difficult to decide whether a given patient warrants treatment with lipid-lowering drugs. In general, intervention—whether and how to treat hyperlipidemia—needs to be individualized, according to the patient's lipid and lipoprotein levels and total coronary risk profile. Most experts would agree that drug therapy is warranted for hyperlipidemic patients with greatly increased coronary risk status. This category would include patients with multiple risk factors, with one of the strongly familial forms of hyperlipidemia, or with very high lipid levels (e.g., above the 98th- or 99th-percentile values). The desirability of drug therapy for hyperlipidemic persons with lesser overall coronary risk status is much less clear.

Only a very limited number of lipid-lowering drugs are currently available for general medical practice in the United States. The drugs available were reviewed last year (Goodman, 1978). Two of the available drugs, colestipol hydrochloride and probucol, received approval for general use by the Food and Drug Administration in 1977.

The bile acid sequestrant resins, cholestyramine and colestipol, are considered by many experts the drug of choice for the treatment of hypercholesterolemia alone. These drugs have the theoretical advantage of producing a high fecal output of sterol derivatives (bile acids) without being absorbed by the body. In a recent study, the effects of colestipol treatment in patients with diet-resistant hypercholesterolemia were explored (Mishkel and Crowther, 1977). The mean fall in plasma cholesterol for 29 patients treated for 12 or more months was 21%. The drug was fairly well accepted and relatively free of side effects.

The most widely used drug during the past few years has been clofibrate, generally considered the drug of choice for patients with hypertriglyceridemia, with or without hypercholesterolemia. Recent studies on effects of clofibrate in patients with hypertriglyceridemia were discussed in Section 3.9. A great deal of information about clofibrate was obtained during the Coronary Drug Project (see Goodman, 1976).

One of the findings in the Coronary Drug Project was the occurrence of a statistically significant increase in clinically apparent gallstones among patients taking clofibrate. In a recent report, a more extensive analysis of data obtained during the Coronary Drug Project relating to gallbladder disease was presented (Gordon, R.S., et al., 1977). The project involved male survivors of myocardial infarction from 30 to 64 years of age. Of 2680 placebo-treated men, gallbladder disease developed in 69, or 2.6%, during a 6-year period. For men treated with estrogen or clofibrate, the corresponding incidence rates were 4.3% and 4.0%, respectively, for the 6-year period. Each treatment group differed from placebo by over twice the standard error of the difference, with $p < 0.05$ for each drug–placebo comparison. A total of 45 variables, including age, body weight, blood pressure, serum lipids, and blood sugar were evaluated as risk factors for gallbladder disease. Age correlated significantly with prevalance of known gallbladder disease at entry. No variable yielded a strong and consistent correlation with the incidence of subsequent new gallbladder disease. Thus, gallstone formation must be considered a risk whenever clofibrate or estrogen is prescribed.

Limited information is available about probucol, which appears to lower serum cholesterol levels with little or no effects on triglyceride levels. A study of the effects of probucol in 30 patients with familial hypercholesterolemia was reported recently (LeLorier *et al.*, 1977). The patients were treated first with diet, and then with the drug. Addition of probucol to diet resulted in a significant (mean approximately 12–13%) reduction in serum cholesterol levels. There were no effects on the plasma triglyceride concentrations, and the drug was well tolerated. More experience is needed to effectively evaluate the potential of this agent.

A study was conducted on the effects of plant sterols as cholesterol-lowering agents in 46 patients with hypercholesterolemia (Lees *et al.*, 1977). The plant sterol preparations were from two different sources (soya oil or tall oil), and were given in two different physical forms (a suspension and a powder), in addition to appropriate diet therapy. The maximal mean cholesterol-lowering response to any preparation was 12%, although it was much greater in some individual patients. Sterol balance studies, conducted in 7 patients, showed that plant sterols inhibit cholesterol absorption with maximal negative cholesterol balance in adults at a dose of 3 g/day of a tall oil sterol suspension. Interestingly, maximal plasma cholesterol reduction on this preparation was seen at the same dose level. It was concluded that since the tall oil sterol suspension is relatively palatable and is poorly absorbed, it has potential value as an adjunct to dietary therapy in patients with mild hypercholesterolemia for whom long-term drug therapy is deemed advisable.

3.10.5. Prevention of Ischemic Heart Disease

Evidence that regression of coronary atherosclerosis can occur with hyperlipidemic treatment has been obtained in studies with rhesus monkeys (Armstrong *et al.*, 1970), and more extensive studies in subhuman primates directed at this question are currently in progress. In a recent clinical study, evidence was provided that regression of early femoral atherosclerosis can occur in hyperlipidemic patients under treatment with diet and drugs (Barndt *et al.*, 1977). In this study, femoral angiograms were taken in 12 hypertriglyceridemic (type IV) and in 13 hypercholesterolemic (type II) patients. Repeat angiograms after a 13-month period of treatment showed regression of atherosclerosis in 9 patients, no change in 3, and progression in 13. Treatment significantly reduced the serum lipid and blood pressure levels in the group with lesion improvement, but not in the group with lesion progression. Thus, this study provides encouraging data that early human atherosclerosis associated with hyperlipidemia can show improvement when patients are effectively treated.

As discussed previously (Goodman, 1976, 1978), the question of whether treatment of hyperlipidemia with lipid-lowering drugs can prevent the development of ischemic heart disease is being addressed by major collaborative clinical trials. The ongoing and recent trials were summarized previously. In addition, a secondary intervention study is in progress to explore whether maximal cholesterol reduction by means of a combination of diet therapy and partial ileal bypass surgery, in hypercholesterolemic men who have survived a myocardial infarction, will reduce the subsequent rate of occurrence of new cardiovascular events and of mortality (Buchwald *et al.*, 1977). It is hoped that these studies may, in time, provide definitive evidence that intervention programs directed at known coronary risk factors, and specifically at hyperlipidemia, can indeed prevent coronary disease.

References

Albers, J. J., Adolphson, J. L., and Hazzard, W. R., 1977a, Radioimmunoassay of human plasma Lp(a) lipoprotein, *J. Lipid Res.* **18**:331–338.

Albers, J. J., Warnick, G. R., and Hazzard, W. R., 1977b, Type III hyperlipoproteinemia: A comparative study of current diagnostic techniques, *Clin. Chim. Acta* **75**:193–204.

Ames, R. P., and Hill, P., 1976, Elevation of serum lipid levels during diuretic therapy of hypertension, *Am. J. Med.* **61**:748–757.

Andersen, J. M., and Dietschy, J. M., 1977, Regulation of sterol synthesis in 15 tissues of rat. II. Role of rat and human high and low density plasma lipoproteins and of rat chylomicron remnants, *J. Biol. Chem.* **252**:3652–3659.

Anderson, D. W., Nichols, A. V., Forte, T. M., and Lindgren, F. T., 1977, Particle distribution of human serum high density lipoproteins, *Biochim. Biophys. Acta* **493**:55–68.

Anderson, R. G. W., Brown, M. S., and Goldstein, J. L., 1977, Role of the coated endocytic vesicle in the uptake of receptor-bound low density lipoprotein in human fibroblasts, *Cell* **10**:351–364.

Applebaum, D. M., Goldberg, A. P., Pykälistö, O. J., Brunzell, J. D., and Hazzard, W. R., 1977, Effect of estrogen on post-heparin lipolytic activity: Selective decline in hepatic triglyceride lipase, *J. Clin. Invest.* **59**:601–608.

Armstrong, M. L., Warner, E. D., and Connor, W. E., 1970, Regression of coronary atheromatosis in rhesus monkeys, *Circ. Res.* **27**:59–67.

Assmann, G., Smootz, E., Adler, K., Capurso, A., and Oette, K., 1977a, The lipoprotein abnormality in Tangier disease: Quantitation of A apoproteins, *J. Clin. Invest.* **59**:565–575.

Assmann, G., Simantke, O., Schaefer, H.-E., and Smootz, E., 1977b, Characterization of high density lipoproteins in patients heterozygous for Tangier disease, *J. Clin. Invest.* **60**:1025–1035.

Bagdade, J. D., and Albers, J. J., 1977, Plasma high-density lipoprotein concentrations in chronic-hemodialysis and renal-transplant patients, *N. Engl. J. Med.* **296**:1436–1439.

Barndt, R., Jr., Blankenhorn, D. H., Crawford, D. W., and Brooks, S. H., 1977, Regression and progression of early femoral atherosclerosis in treated hyperlipoproteinemic patients, *Ann. Intern. Med.* **86**:139–146.

Basu, S. K., Anderson, R. G. W., Goldstein, J. L., and Brown, M. S., 1977, Metabolism of cationized lipoproteins by human fibroblasts: Biochemical and morphologic correlations, *J. Cell Biol.* **74**:119–135.

Berman, M., Hall, M., III, Levy, R. I., Eisenberg, S., Bilheimer, D. W., Phair, R. D., and Goebel, R. H., 1978, Metabolism of apoB and apoC lipoproteins in man: Kinetic studies in normal and hyperlipoproteinemic subjects, *J. Lipid Res.* **19**:38–56.

Bilheimer, D. W., Ho, Y. K., Brown, M. S., Anderson, R. G. W., and Goldstein, J. L., 1978, Genetics of the low density lipoprotein receptor: Diminished receptor activity in lymphocytes from heterozygotes with familial hypercholesterolemia, *J. Clin. Invest.* **61**:678–696.

Blum, C. B., Levy, R. I., Eisenberg, S., Hall, M., III, Goebel, R. H., and Berman, M., 1977, High density lipoprotein metabolism in man, *J. Clin. Invest.* **60**:795–807.

Brown, M. S., Anderson, R. G. W., and Goldstein, J. L., 1977, Mutations affecting the binding, internalization, and lysosomal hydrolysis of low density lipoprotein in cultured human fibroblasts, lymphocytes, and aortic smooth muscle cells, *J. Supramol. Struct.* **6**:85–94.

Buchwald, H., Moore, R. B., and Varco, R. L., 1977, Maximum lipid reduction by partial ileal bypass: A test of the lipid–atherosclerosis hypothesis, *Lipids* **12**:53–58.

Castelli, W. P., Cooper, G. R., Doyle, J. T., Garcia-Palmieri, M., Gordon, T., Hames, C., Hulley, S. B., Kagan, A., Kuchmak, M., McGee, D., and Vicic, W. J., 1977a, Distribution of triglyceride and total, LDL and HDL cholesterol in several populations: A cooperative lipoprotein phenotyping study, *J. Chron. Dis.* **30**:147–169.

Castelli, W. P., Doyle, J. T., Gordon, T., Hames, C. G., Hjortland, M. C., Hulley, S. B., Kagan, A., and Zukel, W. J., 1977b, HDL cholesterol and other lipids in coronary heart disease: The cooperative lipoprotein phenotyping study, *Circulation* **55**:767–772.

Castelli, W. P., Gordon, T., Hjortland, M. C., Kagan, A., Doyle, J. T., Hames, C. G., Hulley, S. B., and Zukel, W. J., 1977c, Alcohol and blood lipids: The cooperative lipoprotein phenotyping study, *Lancet* **2**:153–155.

Chait, A., Albers, J. J., Brunzell, J. D., and Hazzard, W. R., 1977, Type-III hyperlipoproteinaemia ("remnant removal disease"): Insight into the pathogenetic mechanism, *Lancet* **1**:1176–1178.

Chajek, T., Stein, O., and Stein, Y., 1977, Pre- and post-natal development of lipoprotein lipase and hepatic triglyceride hydrolase activity in rat tissues, *Atherosclerosis* **26**:549–561.

Cheung, M. C., and Albers, J. J., 1977, The measurement of apolipoprotein A-I and A-II levels in men and women by immunoassay, *J. Clin. Invest.* **60**:43–50.

Deckelbaum, R. J., Lees, R. S., Small, D. M., Hedberg, S. E., and Grundy, S. M., 1977, Failure of complete bile diversion and oral bile acid therapy in the treatment of homozygous familial hypercholesterolemia, *N. Engl. J. Med.* **296**:465–470.

Di Giulio, S., Boulu, R., Drüeke, T., Nicolaï, A., Zingraff, J., and Crosnier, J., 1977, Clofibrate treatment of hyperlipidemia in chronic renal failure, *Clin. Nephrol.* **8**:504–509.

Eisenberg, S., and Levy, R. I., 1975, Lipoprotein metabolism, in: *Advances in Lipid Research*, Vol. 13 (R. Paoletti and D. Kritchevsky, eds.), pp. 1–89, Academic Press, New York.

Enger, S. V., Herbjørnsen, K., Erikssen, J., and Fretland, A., 1977, High density lipoproteins (HDL) and physical activity: The influence of physical exercise, age and smoking on HDL-cholesterol and the HDL–total cholesterol ratio, *Scand. J. Clin. Lab. Invest.* **37**:251–255.

Farah, J. R., Kwiterovich, P. O., Jr., and Neill, C. A., 1977, Dose–effect relation of cholestyramine in children and young adults with familial hypercholesterolaemia, *Lancet* **1**:59–63.

Farinaro, E., Stamler, J., Upton, M., Mojonnier, L., Hall, Y., Moss, D., and Berkson, D. M., 1977, Plasma glucose levels: Long-term effect of diet in the Chicago coronary prevention evaluation program, *Ann. Intern. Med.* **86**:147–154.

Faust, J. R., Goldstein, J. L., and Brown, M. S., 1977, Receptor-mediated uptake of low density lipoprotein and utilization of its cholesterol for steroid synthesis in cultured mouse adrenal cells, *J. Biol. Chem.* **252**:4861–4871.

Fielding, C. J., and Havel, R. J., 1977, Lipoprotein lipase, *Arch. Pathol. Lab. Med.* **101**:225–229.

Fielding, P. E., Shore, V. G., and Fielding, C. J., 1977, Lipoprotein lipase: Isolation and characterization of a second enzyme species from postheparin plasma, *Biochemistry* **16**:1896–1900.

Freeman, M., Kuiken, L., Ragland, J. B., and Sabesin, S. M., 1977, Hepatic triglyceride lipase deficiency in liver disease, *Lipids* **12**:443–445.

Glueck, C. J., Gartside, P. S., Steiner, P. M., Miller, M., Todhunter, T., Haaf, J., Pucke, M., Terrana, M., Fallat, R. W., and Kashyap, M. L., 1977a, Hyperalpha- and hypobeta-lipoproteinemia in octogenarian kindreds, *Atherosclerosis* **27**:387–406.

Glueck, C. J., Mellies, M. J., Tsang, R. C., Kashyap, M. L., and Steiner, P. M., 1977b, Familial hypertriglyceridemia in children: Dietary management, *Pediatr. Res.* **11**:953–957.

Glueck, C. J., Mellies, M. J., Tsang, R. C., and Steiner, P. M., 1977c, Low and high density lipoprotein cholesterol interrelationships in neonates with low density lipoprotein cholesterol ≤ the 10th percentile and in neonates with high density lipoprotein cholesterol ≥ the 90th percentile, *Pediatr. Res.* **11**:957–959.

Glueck, C. J., Tsang, R. C., Fallat, R. W., and Mellies, M. J., 1977d, Diet in children heterozygous for familial hypercholesterolemia, *Am. J. Dis. Child.* **131**:162–166.

Glueck, C. J., Tsang, R. C., Fallat, R. W., and Mellies, M. J., 1977e, Therapy of familial hypercholesterolemia in childhood: Diet and cholestyramine resin for 24 to 36 months, *Pediatrics* **60**:433–441.

Glueck, C. J., Gartside, P. S., Miller, L., Steiner, P. M., Todhunter, T., Terrana, M., Haaf, J., and Kashyap, M. L., 1978, Octogenarian kindred: Hyper-α-lipoproteinemia, *Prev. Med.* **7**:1–14.

Goldberg, A. P., Sherrard, D. J., Haas, L. B., and Brunzell, J. D., 1977, Control of clofibrate toxicity in uremic hypertriglyceridemia, *Clin. Pharmacol. Ther.* **21**:317–325.

Goldstein, J. L., and Brown, M. S., 1977a, The low-density lipoprotein pathway and its relation to atherosclerosis, *Annu. Rev. Biochem.* **46**:897–930.

Goldstein, J. L., and Brown, M. S., 1977b, Atherosclerosis: The low-density lipoprotein receptor hypothesis, *Metabolism* **26**:1257–1275.

Goldstein, J. L., Anderson, R. G. W., Buja, L. M., Basu, S. K., and Brown, M. S., 1977, Overloading human aortic smooth muscle cells with low density lipoprotein-cholesteryl esters reproduces features of atherosclerosis *in vitro*, *J. Clin. Invest.* **59**:1196–1202.

Goodman, D. S., 1976, Disorders of lipid and lipoprotein metabolism, in: *The Year in Metabolism 1975–1976* (N. Freinkel, ed.), pp. 153–180, Plenum Medical Book Company, New York.

Goodman, D. S., 1978, Disorders of lipid and lipoprotein metabolism, in: *The Year in Metabolism 1977* (N. Freinkel, ed.), pp. 183–218, Plenum Medical Book Company, New York.

Gordon, R. S., Jr., Forman, S., Canner, P., Berge, K., and Miller, D., 1977, Gallbladder disease as a side effect of drugs influencing lipid metabolism: Experience in the Coronary Drug Project, *N. Engl. J. Med.* **296**:1185–1190.

Gordon, T., Castelli, W. P., Hjortland, M. C., Kannel, W. B., and Dawber, T. R., 1977, High density lipoprotein as a protective factor against coronary heart disease: The Framingham Study, *Am. J. Med.* **62**:707–714.

Gotto, A. M., Jr., DeBakey, M. E., Foreyt, J. P., Scott, L. W., and Thornby, J. I., 1977, Dietary treatment of type IV hyperlipoproteinemia, *J. Am. Med. Assoc.* **237**:1212–1215.

Green, P. H. R., Tall, A. R., and Glickman, R. M., 1978, Rat intestine secretes discoid high density lipoprotein, *J. Clin. Invest.* **61**:528–534.

Grundy, S. M., and Mok, H. Y. I., 1976, Chylomicron clearance in normal and hyperlipidemic man, *Metabolism* **25**:1225–1239.

Gyntelberg, F., Brennan, R., Holloszy, J. O., Schonfeld, G., Rennie, M. J., and Weidman, S. W., 1977, Plasma triglyceride lowering by exercise despite increased food intake in patients with type IV hyperlipoproteinemia, *Am. J. Clin. Nutr.* **30**:716–720.

Hauser, H., Kostner, G., Muller, M., and Skrabal, P., 1977, The structure and morphology of the abnormal serum lipoprotein-X, *Biochim. Biophys. Acta* **489**:247–261.

Havel, R. J., and Kane, J. P., 1973, Primary dysbetalipoproteinemia: Predominance of a specific apolipoprotein species in triglyceride-rich lipoproteins, *Proc. Natl. Acad. Sci. U.S.A.* **70**:2015–2019.

Heiberg, A., and Slack, J., 1977, Family similarities in the age at coronary death in familial hypercholesterolaemia, *Br. Med. J.* **2**:493–495.

Heinen, R. J., Herbert, P. N., Frederickson, D. S., Forte, T., and Lindgren, F. T., 1978, Properties of the plasma very low and low density lipoproteins in Tangier disease, *J. Clin. Invest.* **61**:120–132.

Ho, Y. K., Faust, J. R., Bilheimer, D. W., Brown, M. S., and Goldstein, J. L., 1977, Regulation of cholesterol synthesis by low density lipoprotein in isolated human lymphocytes: Comparison of cells from normal subjects and patients with homozygous familial hypercholesterolemia and abetalipoproteinemia, *J. Exp. Med.* **145**:1531–1549.

Jackson, R. L., Morrisett, J. D., and Gotto, A. M., Jr., 1976, Lipoprotein structure and metabolism, *Physiol. Rev.* **56**:259–316.

Jackson, R. L., Baker, H. N., Gilliam, E. B., and Gotto, A. M., Jr., 1977, Primary structure of very low density apolipoprotein C-II of human plasma, *Proc. Natl. Acad. Sci. U.S.A.* **74**:1942–1945.

Johansson, B. G., and Medhus, A., 1974, Increase in plasma α-lipoproteins in chronic alcoholics after acute abuse, *Acta Med. Scand.* **195**:273–277.

Kane, J. P., Sata, T., Hamilton, R. L., and Havel, R. J., 1975, Apoprotein composition of very low density lipoproteins of human serum, *J. Clin. Invest.* **56**:1622–1634.

Kashyap, M. L., Srivastava, L. S., Chen, C. Y., Perisutti, G., Campbell, M., Lutmer, R. F., and Glueck, C. J., 1977, Radioimmunoassay of human apolipoprotein CII: A study in normal and hypertriglyceridemic subjects, *J. Clin. Invest.* **60**:171–180.

Katz, S. S., Small, D. M., Brook, J. G., and Lees, R. S., 1977, The storage lipids in Tangier disease: A physical chemical study, *J. Clin. Invest.* **59**:1045–1054.

Kinnunen, P. K. J., Jackson, R. L., Smith, L. C., Gotto, A. M., Jr., and Sparrow, J. T., 1977, Activation of lipoprotein lipase by native and synthetic fragments of human plasma apolipoprotein C-II, *Proc. Natl. Acad. Sci. U.S.A.* **74**:4848–4851.

Kushwaha, R. S., Hazzard, W. R., Wahl, P. W., and Hoover, J. J., 1977a, Type III hyperlipoproteinemia: Diagnosis in whole plasma by apolipoprotein-E immunoassay, *Ann. Intern. Med.* **87**:509–516.

Kushwaha, R. S., Hazzard, W. R., Gagne, C., Chait, A., and Albers, J. J., 1977b, Type III hyperlipoproteinemia: Paradoxical hypolipidemic response to estrogen, *Ann. Intern. Med.* **87**:517–525.

Lampman, R. M., Santinga, J. T., Hodge, M. F., Block, W. D., Flora, J. D., Jr., and Bassett, D. R., 1977, Comparative effects of physical training and diet in normalizing serum lipids in men with type IV hyperlipoproteinemia, *Circulation* **55**:652–659.

Lampman, R. M., Santinga, J. T., Bassett, D. R., Mercer, N., Block, W. D., Flora, J. D., Jr., Foss, M. L., and Thorland, W. G., 1978, Effectiveness of unsupervised and supervised high intensity physical training in normalizing serum lipids in men with type IV hyperlipoproteinemia, *Circulation* **57**:172–180.

Lees, A. M., Mok, H. Y. I., Lees, R. S., McCluskey, M. A., and Grundy, S. M., 1977, Plant sterols as cholesterol-lowering agents: Clinical trials in patients with hypercholesterolemia and studies of sterol balance, *Atherosclerosis* **28**:325–338.

LeLorier, J., DuBreuil-Quidoz, S., Lussier-Cacan, S., Huang, Y.-S., and Davignon,

J., 1977, Diet and probucol in lowering cholesterol concentrations: Additive effects on plasma cholesterol concentrations in patients with familial type II hyperlipoproteinemia, *Arch. Intern. Med.* **137**:1429–1434.

Leonhardt, E. T. G., 1978, Effects of vitamin E on serum cholesterol and triglycerides in hyperlipidemic patients treated with diet and clofibrate, *Am. J. Clin. Nutr.* **31**:100–105.

Mabuchi, H., Ito, S., Haba, T., Ueda, K., Ueda, R., Tatami, R., Kametani, T., Koizumi, J., Ohta, M., Miyamoto, S., Takeda, R., and Takegoshi, T., 1977a, Discrimination of familial hypercholesterolemia and secondary hypercholesterolemia by Achilles' tendon thickness, *Atherosclerosis* **28**:61–68.

Mabuchi, H., Haba, T., Ueda, K., Ueda, R., Tatami, R., Ito, S., Kametani, T., Koizumi, J., Miyamoto, S., Ohta, M., Takeda, R., Takegoshi, T., and Takeshita, H., 1977b, Serum lipids and coronary heart disease in heterozygous familial hypercholesterolemia in the Hokuriku district of Japan, *Atherosclerosis* **28**:417–423.

Mahley, R. W., and Innerarity, T. L., 1977, Interaction of canine and swine lipoproteins with the low density lipoprotein receptor of fibroblasts as correlated with heparin/manganese precipitability, *J. Biol. Chem.* **252**:3980–3986.

Mahley, R. W., Innerarity, T. L., Pitas, R. E., Weisgraber, K. H., Brown, J. H., and Gross, E., 1977, Inhibition of lipoprotein binding to cell surface receptors of fibroblasts following selective modification of arginyl residues in arginine-rich and B apoproteins, *J. Biol. Chem.* **252**:7279–7287.

Mann, J. I., Harding, P. A., Turner, R. C., and Wilkinson, R. H., 1977, A comparison of cholestyramine and nicotinic acid in the treatment of familial type II hyperlipoproteinaemia, *Br. J. Clin. Pharmacol.* **4**:305–308.

Miller, N. E., Thelle, D. S., Førde, O. H., and Mjøs, O. D., 1977a, The Tromsø Heart Study—High-density lipoprotein and coronary heart-disease: A prospective case-control study, *Lancet* **1**:965–968.

Miller, N. E., Weinstein, D. B., Carew, T. E., Koschinsky, T., and Steinberg, D., 1977b, Interaction between high density and low density lipoproteins during uptake and degradation by cultured human fibroblasts, *J. Clin. Invest.* **60**:78–88.

Minamisono, T., Wada, M., Akamatsu, A., Okabe, M., Handa, Y., Morita, T., Asagami, C., Naito, H. K., Nakamoto, S., Lewis, L. A., and Mise, J., 1978, Dyslipoproteinemia (a remnant lipoprotein disease) in uremic patients on hemodialysis, *Clin. Chim. Acta* **84**:163–172.

Mishkel, M. A., and Crowther, S. M., 1977, Long-term therapy of diet-resistant hypercholesterolemia with colestipol, *Curr. Ther. Res.* **22**:398–412.

Mjøs, O. D., Thelle, D. S., Førde, O. H., and Vik-Mo, H., 1977, Family study of high density lipoprotein cholesterol and the relation to age and sex: The Tromsø Heart Study, *Acta Med. Scand.* **201**:323–329.

Montes, A., and Knopp, R. H., 1977, Lipid metabolism in pregnancy. IV. C apoprotein changes in very low and intermediate density lipoproteins, *J. Clin. Endocrinol. Metab.* **45**:1060–1063.

Mordasini, R., Frey, F., Flury, W., Klose, G., and Greten, H., 1977, Selective deficiency of hepatic triglyceride lipase in uremic patients, *N. Engl. J. Med.* **297**:1362–1366.

Morrison, J. A., deGroot, I., Edwards, B. K., Kelly, K. A., Rauh, J. L., Mellies, M. J., and Glueck, C. J., 1977, Plasma cholesterol and triglyceride levels in 6775 school children, ages 6–17, *Metabolism* **26**:1199–1211.

Moutafis, C. D., Simons, L. A., Myant, N. B., Adams, P. W., and Wynn, V., 1977, The effect of cholestyramine on the faecal excretion of bile acids and neutral steroids in familial hypercholesterolaemia, *Atherosclerosis* **26**:329–334.

Nikkilä, E. A., Huttunen, J. K., and Ehnholm, C., 1977a, Postheparin plasma lipoprotein lipase and hepatic lipase in diabetes mellitus: Relationship to plasma triglyceride metabolism, *Diabetes* **26**:11–21.

Nikkilä, E. A., Huttunen, J. K., and Ehnholm, C., 1977b, Effect of clofibrate on postheparin plasma triglyceride lipase activities in patients with hypertriglyceridemia, *Metabolism* **26**:179–186.

Osborne, J. C., Jr., and Brewer, H. B., Jr., 1977, The plasma lipoproteins, *Adv. Protein Chem.* **31**:253–337.

Patsch, J. R., Aune, K. C., Gotto, A. M., Jr., and Morrisett, J. D., 1977a, Isolation, chemical characterization, and biphysical properties of three different abnormal lipoproteins: LP-X$_1$, LP-X$_2$, and LP-X$_3$, *J. Biol. Chem.* **252**:2113–2120.

Patsch, J. R., Jackson, R. L., and Gotto, A. M., Jr., 1977b, Evaluation of the classical methods for the diagnosis of type III hyperlipoproteinemia, *Klin. Wochenschr.* **55**:1025–1030.

Patsch, J. R., Yeshurun, D., Jackson, R. L., and Gotto, A. M., Jr., 1977c, Effects of clofibrate, nicotinic acid and diet on the properties of the plasma lipoproteins in a subject with type III hyperlipoproteinemia, *Am. J. Med.* **63**:1001–1009.

Raymond, T. L., Connor, W. E., Lin, D. S., Warner, S., Fry, M. M., and Connor, S. L., 1977, The interaction of dietary fibers and cholesterol upon the plasma lipids and lipoproteins, sterol balance, and bowel function in human subjects, *J. Clin. Invest.* **60**:1429–1437.

Reichl, D., Myant, N. B., and Pflug, J. J., 1977, Concentration of lipoproteins containing apolipoprotein B in human peripheral lymph, *Biochim. Biophys. Acta* **489**:98–105.

Ross, R., and Glomset, J. A., 1976, The pathogenesis of atherosclerosis, *N. Engl. J. Med.* **295**:369–377, 420–425.

Ross, R., and Harker, L., 1976, Hyperlipidemia and atherosclerosis: Chronic hyperlipidemia initiates and maintains lesions by endothelial cell desquamation and lipid accumulation, *Science* **193**:1094–1100.

Rössner, S., Mettinger, K. L., Kjellin, K. G., Sidén, A., and Söderström, C. E., 1978, Normal serum-cholesterol but low H.D.L.-cholesterol concentration in young patients with ischaemic cerebrovascular disease, *Lancet* **1**:577–579.

Samuel, P., Crouse, J. R., and Ahrens, E. H., Jr., 1978, Evaluation of an isotope ratio method for measurement of cholesterol absorption in man, *J. Lipid Res.* **19**:82–93.

Sanfelippo, M. L., Swenson, R. S., and Reaven, G. M., 1977, Reduction of plasma triglycerides by diet in subjects with chronic renal failure, *Kidney Int.* **11**:54–61.

Seidel, D., 1977, Studien zur Charakterisierung und zum Stoffwechsel des Lipoprotein-X (LP-X), des abnormen Lipoproteins der Cholestase, *Klin. Wochenschr.* **55**:611–623.

Shelburne, F. A., and Quarfordt, S. H., 1977, The interaction of heparin with an apoprotein of human very low density lipoprotein, *J. Clin. Invest.* **60**:944–950.

Slack, J., Noble, N., Meade, T. W., and North, W. R. S., 1977, Lipid and lipoprotein concentrations in 1604 men and women in working populations in north-west London, *Br. Med. J.* **2**:353–356.

Srinivasan, S. R., Frerichs, R. R., Webber, L. S., and Berenson, G. S., 1976, Serum lipoprotein profile in children from a biracial community: The Bogalusa Heart Study, *Circulation* **54**:309–318.

Stanbury, J. B., Wyngaarden, J. B., and Fredrickson, D. S., 1978, *The Metabolic Basis of Inherited Disease*, 4th ed., pp. 544–865, McGraw-Hill, New York.

Stanhope, J. M., Sampson, V. M., and Clarkson, P. M., 1977, High-density-lipoprotein cholesterol and other serum lipids in a New Zealand biracial adolescent sample: The Wairoa College Survey, *Lancet* **1**:968–970.

Stein, E. A., 1977, Familial hypo-β-lipoproteinemia: A family detected by cord blood tests, *Am. J. Dis. Child.* **131**:1363–1365.

Sternowsky, H. J., Gaertner, U., Stahnke, N., and Kaukel, E., 1977, Juvenile familial hypertriglyceridemia and growth retardation: Clinical and biochemical observations in three siblings, *Eur. J. Pediatr.* **125**:59–70.

Streja, D., Kallai, M. A., and Steiner, G., 1977, The metabolic heterogeneity of human very low density lipoprotein triglyceride, *Metabolism* **26**:1333–1344.

Taylor, K. G., Holdsworth, G., and Galton, D. J., 1977, Clofibrate increases lipoprotein-lipase activity in adipose tissue of hypertriglyceridaemic patients, *Lancet* **2**:1106–1107.

Thompson, G. R., Spinks, T., Ranicar, A., and Myant, N. B., 1977, Non-steady-state studies of low-density-lipoprotein turnover in familial hypercholesterolaemia, *Clin. Sci. Mol. Med.* **52**:361–369.

Utermann, G., Jaeschke, M., and Menzel, J., 1975, Familial hyperlipoproteinemia type III: Deficiency of a specific apolipoprotein (apo E-III) in the very-low-density lipoproteins, *FEBS Lett.* **56**:352–355.

Utermann, G., Canzler, H., Hees, M., Jaeschke, M., Mühlfellner, G., Schoenborn, W., and Vogelberg, K. H., 1977a, Studies on the metabolic defect in broad-β disease (hyperlipoproteinaemia type III), *Clin. Genet.* **12**:139–154.

Utermann, G., Hees, M., and Steinmetz, A., 1977b, Polymorphism of apolipoprotein E and occurrence of dysbetalipoproteinaemia in man, *Nature (London)* **269**:604–607.

Warnick, G. R., and Albers, J. J., 1978, A comprehensive evaluation of the heparin–manganese precipitation procedure for estimating high density lipoprotein cholesterol, *J. Lipid Res.* **19**:65–76.

West, R., and Lloyd, J. K., 1977, Cholestyramine in hypercholesterolaemia, *Lancet* **1**:488–489.

Yano, K., Rhoads, G. G., and Kagan, A., 1977, Coffee, alcohol, and risk of coronary heart disease among Japanese men living in Hawaii, *N. Engl. J. Med.* **297**:405–409.

Zilversmit, D. B., 1972, A single blood sample dual isotope method for the measurement of cholesterol absorption in rats, *Proc. Soc. Exp. Biol. Med.* **140**:862–865.

Nutrition and Cellular Growth of the Brain

Myron Winick and Brian L. G. Morgan

4.1. Methods for Producing Early Malnutrition

The most common method employed in altering the nutritional status of neonatal rats is to vary the number of pups nursing from a single mother. The normal rat litter consists of from 8 to 12 pups; a nursing group of 10 animals has arbitrarily been considered normal. Malnutrition is imposed by increasing the size of the nursing group to 18 animals and overnutrition by decreasing the size to 3 animals. But in addition to altering the nutrition, this changes the amount of maternal stimulation available to each pup. More recently, other methods of inducing undernutrition have been employed. Protein restriction in the lactating mother reduces the quantity of milk produced without altering its composition. Allowing the animals to nurse for only a single 8-hr period per day also reduces the quantity of milk consumed. In a combination of these approaches, protein-restricted mothers have been given an increased number of animals to nurse. All these methods produce a total caloric restriction as well as a restriction in individual nutrients, the most important of which is probably protein. So far, all the methods have had comparable effects on brain growth, and we will therefore examine them together.

MYRON WINICK and BRIAN L. G. MORGAN • Institute of Human Nutrition, College of Physicians and Surgeons of Columbia University, New York, New York 10032.

4.2. Malnutrition and Brain Size

Using the "large and small litter" technique, Widdowson and McCance (1960) demonstrated a number of years ago that the growth rate of nursing pups was proportionately slowed down as the number of pups nursing from a single mother was increased. Moreover, they demonstrated that the weight of the brain was less in undernourished animals and more in overnourished animals relative to controls. Perhaps their most important finding was that no matter what the state of nutrition after weaning, the undernourished animals never attained normal size and their brains never reached normal adult weight. Other experiments with neonatal pigs confirmed these results. Undernutrition caused profound growth retardation in pigs during the neonatal period, and neither body nor brain size ever reached normal adult standards, even when maximum nutritional rehabilitation was attempted (Dickerson *et al.*, 1966–1967). Previous studies had indicated that undernutrition rehabilitation could restore normal body weight and brain weight (Jackson and Steward, 1920). What determined whether the animal recovered seemed to be the time at which malnutrition occurred. The earlier the undernutrition, the less likely was recovery. The same difference between early and later growth was described in dogs (Platt, 1962). In pups born of malnourished mothers and fed a low-protein diet, brain weight relative to the age of the animal was either below or in the lower part of the normal range; this lower average brain size persisted in the adult (Platt, 1962). From these studies, it would appear that in dogs and pigs, just as in rats, early malnutrition will result in permanent impairment of body and brain growth, whereas later malnutrition will produce reversible changes.

4.3. Malnutrition and Cellular Growth of the Brain

Studies of normal cellular growth during the past decade suggested a possible explanation for this difference in response between early and late malnutrition. Early organ growth is mainly due to cell division and an increase in the number of cells. Later organ growth is due to hypertrophy, with existing cells becoming larger (Winick and Noble, 1966). When the original McCance and Widdowson experiments were repeated and compared with experiments on animals undernourished at two later times during the growing period, it became clear that if malnutrition were imposed during the proliferative phase of growth, the rate of cell division as measured by the increase in total DNA content was slowed, and the ultimate number of cells was reduced. Moreover, this change was permanent and could not be reversed once the normal time for cell division had passed. In contrast, undernutrition imposed during the period of hypertrophy will curtail the cellular enlargement as measured by the increase in the protein/DNA ratio, but on subsequent rehabilitation, the cells will regain their normal size. These experiments demonstrated that total brain cell number could be permanently reduced by undernourishing the rat during the first 21 days of life; no matter what feeding regimen was attempted thereafter, this reduction in cell number persisted (Winick and Noble, 1966).

When animals were reared in litters of 3, these overnourished animals had an increased number of brain cells when compared with animals nursed in normal-size litters. In fact, the rate of cell division can actually be manipulated in either direction by changing the state of nutrition during the proliferative phase. Undernutrition for the first 9 days of life produces a deficit in brain cell number that can be entirely overcome by overnutrition during the next 12 days (Winick et al., 1968). It should be noted, however, that we cannot differentiate one cell type from another using these methods. It is quite possible that the deficit is made up by the proliferation of a different type of cell than was inhibited during the earlier restriction.

Thus, the number of cells present in any organ at maturity is only partially under genetic control. Environmental variables during the proliferative phase of cellular growth also have a part in determining the ultimate number of cells, not by altering the time during which cells can divide but rather by altering the rate at which cell division occurs during the time prescribed by the genetic makeup of the animals. Thus, malnutrition slows the rate of cell division, but cells continue to divide for the same period of time in the malnourished animal as in the normal animal.

4.4. Malnutrition and Myelination

In rats, malnutrition during the first 3 weeks of life was shown to interfere with the synthesis of lipids (Davison and Dobbing, 1966, 1968; Culley and Lineberger, 1968). Total brain cholesterol and cholesterol concentration are reduced (Dickerson et al., 1966–1967). In pigs malnourished during the first year of life, total brain cholesterol and phospholipid content are markedly reduced and cholesterol concentration is slightly reduced (Dickerson et al., 1966–1967). These changes, in both rats and pigs, persist even when the animals are rehabilitated for a long time. In addition, it has been demonstrated that the incorporation of sulfatide into the myelin of rat brain is reduced both in vivo and in vitro by malnutrition during the first 3 weeks of life (Chase et al., 1967). Moreover, brain activity of galactocerebroside sulfokinase, the enzyme responsible for this incorporation, is also reduced (Chase *et al.,* 1967). Although the lower lipid content could be due to a reduction in the number of oligodendroglia, the enzymatic effect suggests that lipid synthesis per cell may also be reduced.

Measuring lipid deposition to study myelination gives us two types of data: lipid concentration and total lipid content. The increase in total lipid concentration that occurs during normal development, which is mainly due to reduction in water content, represents a progressive increase in sheath thickness and has therefore been regarded as a "maturity index" (Winick, 1976). In contrast, the increase in total lipid content represents the growth in length or number of axons and either the elongation of existing myelin sheaths or the laying down of new sheaths. Malnutrition prior to weaning in the rat results not only in fewer or shorter myelin sheaths, as assessed by reduced total brain cholesterol, but also in thinner sheaths, since the concentration of cholesterol is also reduced. In the pig, although the number or length of the sheaths is reduced, the thickness would appear to be nearly normal, since there is very little effect on cholesterol concentration.

During the past few years, studies have been initiated in an attempt to determine whether qualitative changes can be induced in the myelin of the central nervous system as reflected by changes in the concentration of the constituent fatty acids. The dietary manipulation most used is the production of an essential fatty acid (EFA) deficiency in the nursing mother or the weanling pup. When this is done, a number of changes in the composition of brain lipids have been reported. $C_{16:1}$ and $C_{20:3}$ fatty acids increase, whereas arachidonic acid specifically decreases, and a general trend toward increased saturation occurs. These changes, however, appear to be reversible at any time, so that restoration of a normal diet will result in a redistribution of fatty acids within the lipid components of the brain and ultimately in a normal fatty acid content of brain lipids (Galli, 1973).

Recent experiments have been carried out in which beagle pups were raised from birth using hyperalimentation with dextrose and amino acids but no lipids. These animals were compared with animals receiving dextrose alone and with animals receiving bitch milk. The animals receiving the amino acids grew at a normal rate but showed the most marked changes in brain lipids. The fatty acid composition was abnormal, showing a reversal of the triene–tetraene ratio. The animals who received only dextrose grew poorly but had fewer changes within the brain. The data suggest that in a rapidly growing animal, EFA deficiency will develop rapidly and result in the deposition of an abnormal myelin. Whether these changes are reversible in dogs is unknown at present (Bieber *et al.,* 1976).

4.5. Other Effects of Malnutrition on the Growing Brain

Malnutrition during the first 21 days of life in the rat has been shown to affect the synthesis of certain proteins, the synthesis of certain neurohormones, and the activity of certain enzymes involved in both protein and RNA metabolism. There is a reduced synthesis of norepinephrine and serotonin in the brains of malnourished animals (Shoemaker and Wurtman, 1971). Activity of the enzyme acetylcholinesterase increases, and this increase persists into adulthood (Im *et al.*, 1972). These findings have come from studies of whole brain, so that it is impossible to know whether or not there are any regionally specific changes in these processes. It is impossible at this time to ascribe functional significance to any of these changes. However, these alterations in neurotransmitter metabolism will no doubt eventually be correlated with neurophysiologic changes under their control. The mechanisms by which some of these changes in neurohormone secretion may be induced are at present under intensive investigation. Serotonin concentration in the brain is directly proportional to the concentration of brain tryptophan, which in turn is proportional to the concentration of tryptophan in the blood. The concentration of tryptophan in the blood will vary directly with the concentration of this amino acid in the diet. Thus, dietary intake of tryptophan influences secretion of serotonin in the brain. This is the first demonstration of direct control of hormone secretion, in this case a brain hormone, by a single dietary constituent. Recent experiments suggest that secretion of acetylcholine in brain may similarly be influenced by the intake of choline in the diet (Wurtman and Fernstrom, 1976; Ulus and Wurtman, 1976).

Another area of brain biochemistry that has received a good deal of attention is the synthesis and deposition of sialoglycocompounds—glycoproteins and gangliosides. Gangliosides and other glycolipids usually constitute a small portion of the glycoconjugates that form an integral part of all cell surfaces. However, in the mammalian central nervous system, 65% of the total N-acetylneuraminic acid (NANA) is present bound to gangliosides and only 32% is bound to glycoproteins, while the rest is free NANA (Brunngraber *et al.*, 1972). Furthermore, the brain has the highest concentration of gangliosides of any tissue in the body, with that of gray matter being 15 times as high as that of liver (Svennerholm, 1970), which represents 5–10% of the total lipid content of some nerve tissue cell membranes (Ledeen, 1978).

Although small quantities of these glycolipids are found in all cellular and subcellular fractions including myelin (Suzuki, 1967), the majority is localized in the neurons (Ledeen, 1978). Similarly, while sialoglycoproteins may be present in glial cells in small amounts, the bulk seem to be bound to neurons (Dekirmenjian *et al.*, 1969). However, the precise location of both gangliosides and glycoproteins within neurons has not been resolved.

Early studies suggested that neuronal cell bodies accounted for only a small fraction of total gray matter gangliosides (Norton and Poduslo, 1971; Hamberger and Svennerholm, 1971). Later studies showed that by far the majority of gangliosides were located in the dendritic and axonal plexuses (Hess *et al.*, 1976). However, the way in which gangliosides are distributed within the processes is a controversial issue. On the basis of the results of studies involving the measurement of ganglioside levels in isolated synaptosomes, it was widely postulated that the synaptic plasma membranes are the major loci of gangliosides (Lapetina *et al.*, 1968; Dekirmanjian *et al.*, 1969). These studies were recently critically reviewed by Ledeen (1978), who concluded that gangliosides are probably evenly distributed over the entire neuronal surface with nerve endings contributing less than 12% of total cerebral cortical gangliosides in the rat. Hence, the location of gangliosides within the nerve cell is still a matter of great controversy.

Several investigators have studied the ganglioside content of the developing rat brain. Pritchard and Cantin (1962) found a linear increase in the concentration of gangliosides in the gray matter up to 25 years of age. James and Fotherby (1963) observed a similar linear increase in ganglioside NANA in the whole brain between 3 and 16 days of age, while Suzuki (1965) found a rapid increase in the amount of gangliosides at about 10 days after birth, with no increase after approximately 22 days. Merat and Dickerson (1973) found that the concentration of ganglioside NANA in the forebrain rose rapidly during the interval of 1–21 days after birth, fell to 3 months, and subsequently rose to the mature value at 6 months. In the cerebellum, the peak concentration was reached by 2 months of age and the lowest at 9 months (the adult value), while in the brainstem, the concentration rose more slowly and had a broad peak from 15 days to 2 months.

There are also definite changes in the patterns of the presence of the different gangliosides (G_{M1}, G_{D1a}, G_{D1b}, and G_{T1b} being the main types present in mammalian brain) from one area of the brain to another and from one developmental period to another. Holm and Svennerholm (1972), utilizing rat brains, suggested that some monosialogangliosides (G_{M1}) are converted to disialogangliosides (G_{D1a} and G_{D1b}) and trisialogangliosides (G_{T1b}) during development, and that the turnover of gangliosides in the immature animal was more than in the adult.

The timing of the developmental pattern of brain gangliosides established by chemical analysis is similar to that found by histological techniques for the development of neuronal processes. Eayrs and Goodhead

(1959) found that the density of axons increases at a maximal rate between the ages of 6 and 18 days in the rat, while dendritic denity increases maximally between 18 and 24 days. Roukema *et al.* (1970) found a close correlation between the development of gangliosides and sialogly-coproteins and the period corresponding to the rapid growth of axonal membranes.

It has been shown that the concentration of gangliosides is markedly reduced in the brains of neonatally malnourished rats and pigs (Dickerson and Jarvis, 1970; Merat and Dickerson, 1973). This would suggest that the number of axonal and dendritic arborizations is reduced by malnutrition, since the concentration of gangliosides is an indication of the number of such arborizations.

Recent studies also strongly suggest that malnutrition imposed on rats shortly after birth will reduce the content of both soluble and insolu-ble glycoproteins (DiBenedetta and Cioffi, 1972). Moreover, the electro-phoretic patterns derived from the brains of these malnourished animals would suggest that qualitative changes in the kinds of glycoproteins present also occur after neonatal malnutrition.

Several authorities have shown that axonal and dendritic develop-ment is extremely sensitive to nutritional deprivation. As early as 1955, Eayrs and Horn (1955) reported that undernutrition during the first 21 days of postnatal life interfered with the production of these processes. More recent studies (Salas *et al.,* 1974) confirmed that early undernutri-tion reduces the total number of dendritic spines, the density of the basilar dendritic network, and the thickness of the dendritic prolongations of the large pyramidal cells in both frontal and occipital cortical regions of animals sacrificed at days 7, 9, 12, and 15.

Histological studies have shown that synaptic fine structure also seems to be susceptible to the effects of undernutrition. Dyson and Jones (1976a) showed a decrease in the height and an increase in the base width of the dense projections in 20-day-old undernourished rat cerebral cor-tex. Further, the same authors (Dyson and Jones, 1976b) detected an apparent general retardation in development of synapses, which may be partially compensated for if the animals are nutritionally rehabilitated. Yu and Yu (1977) noted "degenerative" ultrastructural changes in the pre-synaptic terminals and axons in the cerebellum of chronically malnour-ished rats.

Using a slightly different approach, Morgan and Naismith (1979) examined the effects of undernutrition imposed during the growth spurt on the activities of enzymes that are known to regulate lipid synthesis and metabolism in the brain. The enzymes selected were components of the two glycolipid synthesizing systems, namely, that responsible for cerebro-side synthesis located in the myelin sheath and that causing ganglioside synthesis. UDP-galactosyltransferase is a key enzyme in cerebroside synthesis. UDP-glucosyltransferase is thought to be the rate-limiting enzyme in ganglioside synthesis, and cytidine monophosphate N-acetylneuraminic acid synthetase (CMP-NANA-synthetase) also participates in ganglioside synthesis. An additional enzyme involved in ganglioside metabolism was also studied, namely, sialidase. This converts di- and trisialogangliosides to G_{M1}, the N-acetylneuraminic acid of which is resistant to this enzyme under physiologic conditions.

A comparison of the profiles of these enzymes between well-nourished and poorly nourished pups showed that in each case, malnutrition delayed attainment of peak activity and lowered the mature levels attained. The differences in UDP-glucosyltransferase and CMP-NANA-synthetase activities between the two groups suggest that the production of glycoproteins and gangliosides in the undernourished pups would be retarded and reduced in amount. Likewise, the lower activity of UDP-galactosyltransferase found throughout the period of the growth spurt, and the delay in timing of peak activity in the malnourished animals, would postpone the onset and reduce the extent of myelination. The delayed development of peak activity and the lower mature sialidase activity in the malnourished rats provided further evidence of disturbed maturation of the brain.

It has been suggested that gangliosides play an important role in neuronal transmission. Theoretical models have been proposed in which sialo compounds are viewed as important constituents in the functional units of neuronal membranes in that they exert an ion-binding and -releasing function (Burton *et al.*, 1964; Lehninger, 1968; Rahmann *et al.*, 1976). Bretscher (1973) postulates that the hydrophilic carbohydrate chains of glycoproteins and glycolipids extend away from the lipid bilayer of the cell membranes, effecting a certain specific conformation and orientation of the glycomolecules in the membrane environment. In this way, the negative charge associated with the NANA moieties on the terminal portion of the carbohydrate chains may cause binding of the positively charged neurotransmitters to the synaptic membranes. However, very little evidence has come forth to support these hypotheses.

Synaptogenesis includes the growth of the presynaptic axon, contact with and "recognition" of the appropriate postsynaptic neuron, replacement of growth cone organelles, and assembly at the active zone of pre- and postsynaptic dense material, complete with ion channels and transmitter receptor molecules. There is some evidence to implicate surface glycoproteins incorporated into the synaptic membrane in the recognition process (Rees, 1978). Dette and Weseman (1978) demonstrated that NANA is required for the synaptosomal uptake of 5-hydroxytryptamine. Schengrund and co-workers (Schengrund and Rosenberg, 1970; Schengrund and Nelson, 1975) postulated a role for sialidase, which is located in the synaptic membranes, in which it causes a change in the local density of negative charge about the membrane by releasing NANA from the membrane and so possibly affects the movement of positively charged neurotransmitters. Gangliosides were also shown to help retain the excitability of isolated cerebral tissue (McIlwain, 1961).

Thus, NANA is mainly a constituent of gangliosides and glycoproteins. Hence, it increases in concentration during the period of rapid dendritic arborization, which corresponds to the latter part of the so-called "brain growth spurt." Malnutrition during early development reduces the magnitude of this increase. Morgan and Winick (1979a) investigated the possibility that the reduced concentration of NANA secondary to malnutrition was related to the behavioral defects induced by early malnutrition, using two approaches.

In the first approach, they designed an experiment using a two-by-two design in which the nutritional and early stimulation conditions of rat pups were manipulated during the first 3 weeks of life. It was demonstrated that early stimulation reduced the abnormalities in behavior caused by malnutrition, as well as resulted in a smaller number of larger cells with a higher ganglioside and glycoprotein NANA content in both the cerebrum and cerebellum of the malnourished rats at 21 days postnatally. Animals similarly treated were tested at 6 months, at which time it was found that these changes persisted into adulthood after 21 weeks of refeeding on rat chow.

In the second approach (Morgan and Winick, 1979b), rats similarly malnourished were injected with 1 mg NANA/50 g body weight daily during days 14–21 postnatally. The administration of NANA was associated with an increase in NANA concentrations in cerebral and cerebellar gangliosides and glycoproteins at 21 days and prevention of the expected behavioral abnormalities. NANA injections had similar but reduced effects on the parameters in well-fed control rats. At 21 days of age, similarly treated animals were weaned onto rat chow and behaviorally tested at 6 months of age, at which time these effects were again found to be permanent.

Intraperitoneal injection of [^{14}C]-NANA into malnourished and control animals during the same period (Morgan and Winick, 1979b) showed that it was readily incorporated into the brain ganglioside and glycoprotein fractions. These results suggest that the concentrations of brain ganglioside or glycoprotein NANA or both have an effect on behavior. This is the first demonstration that an agent normally found in the brain, if injected intraperitoneally, can both specifically be incorporated at or near its site of action and prevent behavioral abnormalities that would be expected to occur.

4.6. Regional Changes Induced by Malnutrition

Regional patterns of cellular growth in rat brain are modified by malnutrition during the nursing period (Fish and Winick, 1969). The cerebellum, where the rate of cell division is most rapid, is affected earliest (by 8 days of life) and most markedly (Fish and Winick, 1969). The cerebrum, where cell division occurs at a slower rate, is affected later (at 14 days of life) and less markedly. The effects include a reduced rate of cell division in both areas, as well as a reduction in overall protein synthesis and in the synthesis of various lipids. In addition to these effects on areas of rapid cell division, the increase in DNA content that normally occurs in the hippocampus between the 14th and 17th days, and that is due to a migration of cells from under the lateral ventricle, is delayed and perhaps even partially prevented (Fish and Winick, 1969). It would thus appear that those regions in which the rate of cell division is highest are affected earliest and most markedly. Whether the reduced cell number in the hippocampus represents interference with the migratory patterns or an inhibition of cell division at the source below the lateral ventricle is not fully known, but the available data (Winick, 1970) strongly suggest that inhibition of cell division accounts, at least in part, for the reduction.

Regional patterns of lipid synthesis and the effects of malnutrition on these patterns have not been clearly established. The available data suggest, however, that areas where myelination is most rapid are most vulnerable to the effects of early malnutrition (Culley, 1971).

More recent studies in rat and pig brain have shown that malnutrition reduces the content of gangliosides in the cerebellum more than that of other lipids, suggesting selective reduction in the quantity of this lipid and hence limitation of dendritic arborization in the cerebellum (Dickerson, personal communication).

In a recent investigation of the spinal cords of rats malnourished from birth, alterations in lipid content and concentrations were observed. After 1 week of malnutrition, the total spinal cord content of galactolipids, cholesterol, and phospholipids was reduced. However, only galactolipids were reduced in concentration. By 3 weeks, all three compounds were reduced in both content and concentration. Thus, in the spinal cord, axonal number and length are affected first, with the thickness affected later and to a lesser extent. These changes are similar to those previously described by these authors and others for the rat brain. In contrast, galactolipids that may reflect dendritic arborization are reduced early in both content and concentration, which again suggests selective effects on dendritic arborization within the spinal cord (Rajalakshmi and Nakhasi, 1976).

4.7. Malnutrition and Cellular Growth of the Peripheral Nerves

All the work outlined thus far has been concerned with changes induced in the developing central nervous system. Recently, there have been studies of the effect of early malnutrition on the development of peripheral nerves in young rats (Sima, 1974). Careful analysis has revealed that undernutrition initiated early in life reduces the caliber of nerve fibers in the sciatic nerve and its roots. This reduction is most marked in the thicker fibers. Myelin deposition is also impaired in the ventral and dorsal root fibers and in the fibers of other peripheral nerves such as the optic nerve. The quantitative effect of early malnutrition varies with the particular nerve being examined. In the ventral root fibers, myelin deposition is curtailed more than axonal expansion. In the dorsal root fibers, the reduction in myelination and radial axonal growth is proportional. In the optic nerve, the effect on axonal growth is greater than the effect on myelination.

Rehabilitation will also produce different changes depending on the nerve or root studied. The reduction of the caliber and myelin content in the dorsal root fibers persisted even after a long period of nutritional rehabilitation. In the ventral root, all the changes were completely reversible. In both the sciatic and optic nerves, partial recovery took place. These studies demonstrate that malnutrition early in life can induce changes in peripheral nerves similar to those described in the central nervous system. Some of the changes are reversible, whereas others are not. Certain nerves and roots are more susceptible than others. This work is only beginning but could yield important findings that might help in our understanding of some of the deficits produced by early malnutrition.

4.8. Malnutrition and Cellular Growth of the Human Brain

DNA content and, hence, cell number in the human brain increases linearly until birth, when it begins to level off, reaching a plateau at about 12–18 months of life (Winick and Rosso, 1969). This sequence is the same for cerebrum, cerebellum, and brainstem, the only three regions studied (Winick et al., 1970). Prenatally, there are two peak rates of cell division: one at 26 weeks' gestation (probably neuronal) and one at birth (probably glial) (Dobbing and Sands, 1973). Myelination of the human brain proceeds for at least the first 3 years of life, but adult myelin composition is achieved during the first 6 months (Winick, 1976). Arborization of dendrites continues well beyond 3 years. The exact time at which adult numbers are reached is still undetermined.

Studies of the effects of malnutrition on cellular growth of the human brain have been limited. In marasmic infants who died of malnutrition during the first year of life, wet weight, dry weight, total protein, total RNA, total cholesterol, total phospholipid, and total DNA content are proportionally reduced (Winick and Rosso, 1969; Rosso *et al.*, 1970). Thus, the rate of DNA synthesis is slowed and cell division is curtailed, reducing the total number of cells. Since the reduction in the other elements is proportional to the reduction in DNA content, the ratios are unchanged, and the size of cells as well as the lipid or RNA content of the individual cell are not altered. Again, it should be emphasized that we are describing "average" cells; it is quite possible that certain cells, i.e., those in which lipid is being actively deposited, are affected differently. If the malnutrition persists beyond about 8 months of age, not only the number of cells but also their size is reduced. In addition, the lipid per cell is also reduced (Winick, 1976).

Thus, in the human brain, there is a type of response to malnutrition similar to that which has been described in lower animals. During proliferative growth, cell division is curtailed; during hypertrophic growth, the normal enlargement of cells is prevented. We can interpret the effects of malnutrition on the human brain as affecting myelination in a manner more analogous to the effects on the pig than to those on the rat brain. Total cholesterol or phospholipid content is reduced; hence, the number or length of myelin sheaths is reduced; but because both phospholipid and cholesterol concentration are unaffected, the thickness of those myelin sheaths that are present is unaffected. One could then argue that the major effect of malnutrition is to interfere with cellular growth. During the first 8 months of life, this interference reduces the number of glia, specifically oligodendroglia, and myelination is proportionally reduced. Continued malnutrition reduces cell size. In neurons, this would probably be associated with a reduction in the number or length of processes, and myelination would be proportionally curtailed. However, the deposition of myelin around those processes that are present and that do grow proceeds normally. Note that this interpretation is based on limited observations.

Recently, it has been shown that ganglioside *concentrations* are reduced in the brains of human infants who died of severe malnutrition (Dickerson, personal communication). This would indicate that, as in rats and pigs, early undernutrition will selectively reduce the concentration of certain gangliosides in the human brain. If ganglioside concentration reflects the number of dendritic arborizations, then the process of dendritic branching may be retarded by early undernutrition.

Malnutrition in the human reduces the rate of cell division as estimated by DNA content in all three areas of the brain studied to date:

cerebrum, cerebellum, and brainstem. As in experimental animals, malnutrition will thus curtail cell division in any brain region undergoing hyperplastic growth.

It now seems clear that early postnatal malnutrition will affect both cell division and myelination in the developing rat and human brain. In both species, it would appear that the vulnerable periods coincide with the maximum rate of synthesis of DNA and of myelin. All brain regions seem to be vulnerable, but the timing of their vulnerability will vary, again depending on the maximum rate of synthesis in the particular region. All cell types studied so far are affected if they are dividing at the time the undernutrition occurs. Finally, there is a selective reduction in the number of dendritic arborizations in the rat, pig, and human brain subjected to early undernutrition. In the rat, recovery appears to be possible only if the nutritional status is changed during these vulnerable periods. In the human, although we cannot prove it, presumably the same is true.

References

Bieber, M. A., Pulito, A. R., Brasel, J. A., and Heird, W. C., 1976, Effect of total parenteral nutrition on serum and tissue essential fatty acid status, *Fed. Proc. Fed. Am. Soc. Exp. Biol.* **35**:262 (abstract).

Bretscher, M. S., 1973, Membrane structure: Some general principles, *Science* **181**:622–629.

Brunngraber, E. G., Witting, L. A., Haberland, C., and Brown, B., 1972, Glycoproteins in Tay–Sachs disease: Isolation and carbohydrate composition of glycopeptides, *Brain Res.* **38**:151–162.

Burton, R. M., Howard, R. E., Baer, S., and Balfour, Y. M., 1964, Gangliosides and acetylcholine of the central nervous system, *Biochim. Biophys. Acta* **84**:441–447.

Chase, H. P., Dorsey, J., and McKhann, G. M., 1967, The effect of malnutrition on the synthesis of a myelin lipid, *Pediatrics* **40**:551–559.

Culley, W. J., and Lineberger, R. O., 1968, Effect of undernutrition on the size and composition of the rat brain, *J. Nutr.* **96**:375–381.

Davison, A. N., and Dobbing, J., 1966, Myelination as a vulnerable period in brain development, *Br. Med. Bull.* **22**:40–44.

Davison, A. N., and Dobbing, J., 1968, The developing brain, in: *Applied Neurochemistry* (A. N. Davison and J. Dobbing, eds.), p. 253, F. A. Davis, Philadelphia.

Dekirmenjian, H., and Brunngraber, E. G., 1969, Distribution of protein-bound *N*-acetylneuraminic acid in subcellular particulate fractions prepared from rat whole brain, *Biochim. Biophys. Acta* **177**:1–10.

Dekirmenjian, H., Brunngraber, E. G., Lemkey-Johnston, N., and Larramendi, L. M. H., 1969, Distribution of gangliosides, glycoprotein-NANA and acetylcholinesterase in axonal and synaptosomal fractions of cat cerebellum, *Exp. Brain Res.* **8**:97–104.

Dette, G. A., and Weseman, W., 1978, On the significance of sialic acid in high affinity 5-hydroxytryptamine uptake by synaptosomes, *Hoppe-Seyler's Z. Physiol. Chem.* **359**:399–406.

DiBenedetta, C., and Cioffi, L. A., 1972, Early malnutrition, brain glycoproteins and behavior in rats, *Bibl. Nutr. Dieta* **17**:69–82.

Dickerson, J. W. T., and Jarvis, J., 1970, The effect of undernutrition and subsequent rehabilitation on the growth and chemical composition of the cerebellum, brain stem and forebrain of the rat, *Proc. Nutr. Soc.* **29**:4A.

Dickerson, J. W. T., Dobbing, J., and McCance, R. A., 1966–1967, The effect of undernutrition on the postnatal development of the brain and cord in pigs, *Proc. R. Soc. London Ser. B* **166**:396–407.

Dobbing, J., and Sands, J., 1973, Quantitative growth and development of human brain, *Arch. Dis. Child.* **48**:757–767.

Dyson, S. E., and Jones, D. G., 1976a, The morphological characterization of developing synaptic junctions, *Cell Tissue Res.* **167**:363–371.

Dyson, S. E., and Jones, D. G., 1976b, Some effects of undernutrition on synaptic development—A quantitative ultrastructural study, *Brain Res.* **114**:365–378.

Eayrs, J. T., and Goodhead, B., 1959, Postnatal development of the cerebral cortex in the rat, *J. Anat.* **93**:385–402.

Eayrs, J. T., and Horn G., 1955, The development of cerebral cortex in hypothyroid and starved rats, *Anat. Rec.* **121**:53–61.

Fish, I., and Winick, M., 1969, Effect of malnutrition on regional growth of the developing rat brain, *Exp. Neurol.* **25**:534–540.

Galli, C., 1973, Dietary lipids and brain development, in: *Dietary Lipids in Postnatal Development* (C. Galli, G. Jacini, and A. Pecile, eds.), pp. 191–202, Raven Press, New York.

Hamberger, A., and Svennerholm, L., 1971, Composition of gangliosides and phospholipids of neuronal and glial cell enriched fractions, *J. Neurochem.* **18**:1821–1829.

Hess, H. H., Bass, N. H., Thalheimer, C., and Devarakonda, R., 1976, Gangliosides and the architecture of human frontal and rat somatosensory isocortex, *J. Neurochem.* **26**:1115–1121.

Holm, M., and Svennerholm, L., 1972, Biosynthesis and biodegradation of rat brain gangliosides studied *in vivo*, *J. Neurochem.* **19**:609–622.

Im, H. S., Barnes, R. H., Levitsky, D., Krook, L., and Pond, W. G., 1972, Postnatal malnutrition and regional cholinesterase activities in brain of pigs, *Fed. Proc. Fed. Am. Soc. Exp. Biol.* **31**:697 (abstract).

Jackson, C. M., and Steward, C. A., 1920, The effects of inanition in the young upon the ultimate size of the body and of the various organs in the albino rat, *J. Exp. Zool.* **30**:97–128.

James, F., and Fotherby, K., 1963, Distribution in brain of lipid bound sialic acid and factors affecting its concentration, *J. Neurochem.* **10**:587–592.

Lapetina, E. G., Soto, E. F., and DeRobertis, E., 1968, Lipids and proteolipids in isolated subcellular membranes of rat brain cortex, *J. Neurochem.* **15**:437–445.

Ledeen, R. W., 1978, Ganglioside structure and distribution: Are they localized at the nerve ending?, *J. Supramol. Struct.* **8**:1–17.

Lehninger, A. L., 1968, The neuronal membrane, *Proc. Natl. Acad. Sci. U.S.A.* **60**:1069–1080.

McIlwain, H., 1961, Characterization of naturally occurring materials which restore excitability to isolated cerebral tissues, *Biochem. J.* **78**:24–32.

Merat, A., and Dickerson, J. W. T., 1973, The effect of development on the gangliosides of rat and pig brain, *J. Neurochem.* **20**:873–880.

Morgan, B. L. G., and Naismith, D. J., 1979, The effect of early post-natal undernutrition on the growth and development of the rat brain, *Br. J. Nutr.* (in press).

Morgan, B. L. G., and Winick, M., 1979a, Effects of environmental stimulation on brain ganglioside *N*-acetylneuraminic acid content in relation to behavior (submitted for publication).

Morgan, B. L. G., and Winick, M., 1979b, Effects of administration of *N*-acetylneuraminic acid (NANA) on brain ganglioside NANA in relation to behavior (submitted for publication).

Norton, W. T., and Poduslo, S. E., 1971, Neuronal perikarya and astroglia of rat brain: Chemical composition during myelination, *J. Lipid Res.* **12**:84–90.

Platt, B. S., 1962, Proteins in nutrition, *Proc. R. Soc. London Ser. B* **156**:337–344.

Pritchard, E. T., and Cantin, P. L., 1962, Gangliosides in maturing rat brain, *Nature (London)* **193**:580–581.

Rahmann, H., Rosner, H., and Breer, H., 1976, A functional model of sialoglycomacromolecules in synaptic transmission and memory formation, *J. Theor. Biol.* **57**:231–237.

Rajalakshmi, R., and Nakhasi, H. L., 1976, Effects of neonatal undernutrition on the lipid composition of the spinal cord in rats, *Exp. Neurol.* **51**:330–336.

Rees, R. P., 1978, The morphology of interneuronal synaptogenesis: A review, *Fed. Proc. Fed. Am. Soc. Exp. Biol.* **37**:2000–2009.

Rosso, P., Hormazabal, J., and Winick, M., 1970, Changes in brain weight, cholesterol, phospholipid and DNA content in marasmic children, *Am. J. Clin. Nutr.* **23**:1275–1279.

Roukema, P. A., VanDenEijnden, D. H., Heijlman, J., and Van DerBerg, G., 1970, Sialoglycoproteins, gangliosides and related enzymes in developing rat brain, *FEBS Lett.* **9**:267–270.

Salas, M., Diaz, S., and Nieto, A., 1974, Effects of neonatal food deprivation on cortical spines and dendritic development of the rat, *Brain Res.* **73**:139–144.

Schengrund, C. L., and Nelson, J. T., 1975, Influence of cation concentration on the sialidase activity of neuronal synaptic membranes, *Biochem. Biophys. Res. Commun.* **63**:217–223.

Schengrund, C. L., and Rosenberg, A., 1970, Intracellular location and properties of bovine brain sialidase, *J. Biol. Chem.* **245**:6196–6200.

Shoemaker, W. J., and Wurtman, R. J., 1971, Perinatal undernutrition: Accumulation of catecholamines in rat brain, *Science* **171**:1017–1019.

Sima, A., 1974, Studies on fibre size in developing sciatic nerve and spinal roots in normal, undernourished, and rehabilitated rats, *Acta Physiol. Scand.* (Suppl.) **406**:1–55.

Suzuki, K., 1965, The pattern of mammalian brain gangliosides. II. Evaluation of the extraction procedures, postmortem changes and the effect of formalin preservation, *J. Neurochem.* **12**:629–638.

Suzuki, K., 1967, Formation and turnover of the major brain gangliosides during development, *J. Neurochem.* **14**:917–925.

Svennerholm, L., 1970, Deamination of nucleotides and the role of their deamino forms in ammonia formation from amino acids, in: *Handbook of Neurochemistry*, Vol. 3 (A. Lajtha, ed.), pp. 425–452, Plenum Press, New York.

Ulus, I. H., and Wurtman, R. J., 1976, Choline administration: Activation of tyrosine hydroxylase in dopaminergic neurons of rat brain, *Science* **194**:1060–1061.

Widdowson, E. M., and McCance, R. A., 1960, Some effects of accelerating growth. I. General somatic development, *Proc. R. Soc. London Ser. B* **152**:188–206.

Winick, M., 1970, Cellular growth in intrauterine malnutrition, *Pediatr. Clin. North Am.* **17**:69–78.

Winick, M., 1976, Nutrition and cellular growth of the brain, in: *Malnutrition and Brain Development*, p. 67, Oxford University Press, New York.

Winick, M., and Noble, A., 1966, Cellular response in rats during malnutrition at various ages, *J. Nutr.* **89**:300–306.

Winick, M., and Rosso, P., 1969, The effect of severe early malnutrition on cellular growth of human brain, *Pediatr. Res.* **3**:181–184.

Winick, M., Fish, I., and Rosso, P., 1968, Cellular recovery in rat tissues after a brief period of neonatal malnutrition, *J. Nutr.* **95**:623–626.

Winick, M., Rosso, P., and Waterlow, J., 1970, Cellular growth of cerebrum, cerebellum, and brain stem in normal and marasmic children, *Exp. Neurol.* **26**:393–400.

Wurtman, R. J., and Fernstrom, J. D., 1976, Control of brain neurotransmitter synthesis by precursor availability and nutritional state, *Biochem. Pharmacol.* **25**:1691–1696.

Yu, M. C., and Yu, W. A., 1977, Ultrastructural changes in the developing rat cerebellum in chronic undernutrition, *Neuropathol. Appl. Neurobiol.* **3**:391–401.

Metabolic Aspects of Renal Stone Disease

Edwin L. Prien, Jr., and Hibbard E. Williams

5.1. Introduction

In previous editions of this chapter, the spectrum of metabolic stone disease was reviewed and updated. Over the past year, most work was devoted to the problem of calcium stone disease. Certain aspects of this disease were pursued with great fervor. In addition, the first double-blind trials of therapy were carried out and yielded unexpected results. Therefore, it seems appropriate in this edition to scrutinize these areas and confine our comments to calcium stone disease, the most common and still the most enigmatic of stone diseases.

5.2. Renal Stone Disease Secondary to Increased Crystalloid Excretion

5.2.1. Hypercalciuria

It is generally agreed that hypercalciuria is an important factor in calcium stone disease. The consensus is that the syndrome of idiopapathic

EDWIN L. PRIEN, JR. • Arthritis Unit, Medical Services, Massachusetts General Hospital, Boston, Massachusetts 02114; Harvard Medical School, Boston, Massachusetts 02115. HIBBARD E. WILLIAMS • Department of Medicine, Cornell University Medical College, New York, New York 10021.

hypercalciuria can be identified in at least half the patients with calcium stone disease. However, the definition and mechanism of idiopathic hypercalciuria continue to be fervently debated, and intense investigation continues to yield conflicting results. Furthermore, the importance of idiopathic hypercalciuria in the recurrence of calcium stone formation while the patient is on a low-calcium diet is not clear.

It appears that the term hypercalciuria, although useful in some ways, does not accurately define the phenomenon in relation to stone formation. Furthermore, the upper limit of the normal range for calcium excretion (300 mg/day for men and 275 mg/day for women) is somewhat arbitrary (Hodgkinson and Pyrah, 1958). Careful statistical analysis and probit transformation of the cumulative frequency distributions show that urinary excretion of calcium by stone-formers is not consistently in the upper portion of the normal range; instead, these patients form stones at all levels of urinary calcium excretion, although the levels are about 20% higher than would be expected when compared with the stone-free population (Robertson and Morgan, 1972; Ljunghall, 1977). Thus, hypercalciuria in stone-formers is really relative hypercalciuria occurring throughout the normal range and represents one of the many "risk factors" for calcium stone formation.

However, retention of the notion that hypercalciuria is urinary excretion of calcium in excess of 300 mg/day for men and 275 mg/day for women results in studies of patients who should demonstrate clear-cut abnormalities of calcium metabolism. This "extra" urinary calcium can come from the diet, the bones, or both. As noted in previous editions, the majority of patients with true idiopathic hypercalciuria have intestinal hyperabsorption of dietary calcium that is generally proportional to the degree of hypercalciuria. This hypercalciuria returns to or toward normal values when the dietary calcium intake is restricted and thus has become known as *absorptive* hypercalciuria (Nordin, 1973; Pak *et al.*, 1974). The mechanism of the augmented absorption is unknown, but some patients have elevated levels of $1\alpha,25$-$(OH)_2$-vitamin D_3 (Haussler *et al.*, 1976). At this point, the consensus disintegrates: is the intestinal hyperabsorption the primary defect or is it secondary to a primary abnormality elsewhere, either in the kidney or the bone, resulting in urinary loss of calcium and perhaps mildly negative calcium balance with consequent secondary stimulation of intestinal absorption? This has become an issue of considerable subtlety, and the answers are proving to be most elusive.

Before these questions are pursued, a second type of hypercalciuria should be mentioned. A minority of patients with hypercalciuria (less than 10% depending on screening techniques) have well-defined disorders of calcium metabolism, often with frank hypercalcemia, except for renal tubular acidosis. The list of such disorders is well known, but the point here is that the associated hypercalciuria can be shown to be due wholly or in part to increased bone resorption. In these patients, urinary calcium excretion does not decline significantly during a low-calcium diet or in the fasting state (morning urinary calcium/creatinine ratio greater than 0.15). This type of hypercalciuria has become known as *resorptive* hypercalciuria (Nordin, 1973; Pak *et al.*, 1974). In such patients, it is important to recognize the underlying disease and treat it directly.

The possibility of a third type of hypercalciuria, namely, renal hypercalciuria, has been suggested, and its existence is ardently debated. It would be characterized as a primary renal loss or leak of calcium (although even this could be secondary to some very subtle primary bone disorder) resulting in negative calcium balance, secondary stimulation of the parathyroid glands, and consequent loss of calcium from bone. Urinary calcium excretion would not decline during low-calcium diets, and therefore the disorder would mimic resorptive hypercalciuria. It has been claimed that the majority of patients with idiopathic hypercalciuria have a primary renal leak of calcium (Edwards and Hodgkinson, 1965) and elevated plasma parathyroid hormone levels (Coe *et al.*, 1973). However, a significant negative calcium balance and particularly elevated parathyroid hormone levels have been difficult to confirm in the majority of patients. Recently, Pak *et al.* (1975) described these features in about 10% of stone-formers and documented decreased bone densitometry in some. Other investigators have not been able to detect such patients using similar techniques, but they no doubt exist. Although this disorder is quite uncommon, such patients are probably those described in chapters on osteoporosis as having been hypercalciuric for many years. It is important not to miss such patients because their hypercalciuria and presumably negative calcium balance are correctable with thiazide therapy.

Within the past year, two studies have shown that the majority of stone-formers with hypercalciuria have normal urinary calcium levels during a low-calcium diet (Bordier *et al.*, 1977) or fasting (Ljunghall, 1977). Patients with persistent hypercalciuria (40% of the total) while on a low-calcium diet were categorized according to their plasma parathyroid hormone level with comments on their bone biopsies. Of these patients, 19 (27% of the total) had elevated parathyroid hormone levels but normal blood levels of calcium; these patients were categorized as Type 2. In half these patients, the elevated parathyroid hormone levels were suppressible with either methylchlorothiazide or vitamin D administration. Their bone biopsies showed increased osteoblastic and osteoclastic surfaces consistent with hyperparathyroidism. This group (Type 2a) was considered to have secondary hyperparathyroidism presumably due to a primary renal loss of calcium i.e., renal hypercalciuria. The other half had nonsuppressible parathyroid hormone levels and were found surgically to have parathyroid adenomas. Remarkably, these patients remained hypercalciuric in the postoperative state in contrast to the usual patient with surgically cured primary hyperparathyroidism. This led Bordier et al. (1977) to hypothesize that these patients (Type 2b) had renal loss of calcium as a primary abnormality with hyperparathyroidism as a secondary effect that because of chronic stimulation had ultimately become autonomous, resulting in tertiary hyperparathyroidism.

The remaining 25 patients with persistent hypercalciuria (21% of the total) had low or undetectable parathyroid hormone levels during a low-calcium diet; these patients were classified as Type 3. Chemical analyses of blood and urine of Type 3 patients did not differ significantly from those of Type 2 patients, but bone biopsies of Type 3 patients showed uncoupling of skeletal homeostasis with increased osteoclastic surfaces and decreased osteoblastic surfaces. These bony changes were partially reversed after 4–6 weeks of oral orthophosphate therapy. The hypothesis was offered that Type 3 patients have a primary renal phosphate leak. The hypercalciuria and osteopenia would be the natural consequence of chronic phosphate deficiency. Although the data in support of this hypothesis are sketchy, Bordier et al. (1977) raised some interesting issues and discussed them critically. Perhaps the weakest part of this study is the categorization of patients using the notoriously problematic parathyroid hormone assay. What is needed is assessment by some physiologic derivative of parathyroid function such as urinary cyclic adenosine monophosphate (cAMP) assay.

Ljunghall (1977) assayed urinary cAMP in 34 hypercalciuric stone-formers during fasting. This assay is quite useful in identifying hypercalcemic cases of primary hyperparathyroidism. Urinary cAMP was comparable in stone-formers and control subjects. He showed that stone-formers have relative hypercalciuria and that it is proportional to intestinal hyperabsorption of calcium. Furthermore, the degree of hypercalciuria was *inversely* proportional to the amount of cAMP present in the urine, suggesting that factors other than increased parathyroid function are related to the hypercalciuria. Five stone-formers had fasting urinary calcium levels greater than 2 standard deviations above the mean, but there was no associated increase in urinary levels of hydroxyproline. This raises the possibility that in a few such stone-formers, a mild abnormality of bone metabolism (resorption) may coexist with primary intestinal hyperabsorption of calcium.

Recently, objections have been made that urinary cAMP correlates poorly with the hyperparathyroid state and that it should be expressed as a function of glomerular filtration rate (Broadus et al., 1977). Whether or not evaluation of nephrogenous cAMP will help resolve the dilemma in categorization of stone-formers remains to be seen.

One remaining aspect of idiopathic hypercalciuria warrants comment. Hypophosphatemia, originally thought to be one of the hallmarks of the disorder, continues to intrigue and perplex most investigators. It is certainly not universally present and is inconstant in many patients in whom it is present. There is little question that the majority of hypercalciuric stone-formers have intestinal hyperabsorption of calcium. In many, it may be secondary to elevated (documented) plasma levels of $1\alpha,25$-$(OH)_2$-vitamin D_3. Two stimuli for the production of this active vitamin D metabolite are parathyroid hormone and hypophosphatemia. The difficulties in assessing parathyroid hormone excess in stone-formers have already been mentioned. The possible role of hypophosphatemia in hypercalciuric stone-formers has recently been investigated. In one study (Gray *et al.*, 1977), significant hypophosphatemia was found among patients, and the degree of $1\alpha,25$-$(OH)_2$-vitamin D_3 elevation correlated with the degree of hypophosphatemia and not with any elevations in plasma parathyroid hormone. Interestingly, these same observations applied to patients with primary hyperparathyroidism. However, in another study (Kaplan *et al.*, 1977), similar elevations of $1\alpha,25$-$(OH)_2$-vitamin D_3 were observed in hypercalciuric stone-formers and patients with primary hyperparathyroidism, but hypophosphatemia was not found and no correlations could be made between the vitamin levels and plasma levels of calcium or phosphorus or urinary levels of cAMP or parathyroid hormone. Although there is no doubt that the clinical syndrome of phosphate deficiency can result in hypercalciuria and bone loss, it would be premature to conclude at present that this disorder serves as a model for any of the hypercalciuric stone diseases.

5.2.2. Hyperuricosuria

As mentioned in previous editions, hyperuricemia and hyperuricosuria are related to calcium oxalate stone disease. This association of hyperuricemia and calcium stones (and other stones as well) was first noted by Smith *et al.* (1969) in 1969 and extended to hyperuricosuria by Coe and Kavalach (1974) in 1974. Both these groups conducted clinical trials of allopurinol for calcium stone prophylaxis and both claimed significant success (Smith and Boyce, 1969; Coe and Kavalach, 1974). Such results were surprising and are difficult to explain. One hypothesis suggested that small crystals of either uric acid or sodium urate were nucleating stones that were otherwise pure calcium oxalate or calcium phosphate or both. Recent studies have shown that the urine of stone-formers is often supersaturated with sodium urate (Pak *et al.*, 1977), and that both uric acid crystals and sodium urate crystals can accelerate the precipitation of calcium oxalate crystals to some extent from solutions that are supersaturated with calcium oxalate (Meyer *et al.*, 1976; Coe *et al.*, 1975). Another possible explanation arises from the fact that xanthine oxidase is one of the three enzymes capable of oxidizing glyoxalate to oxalate, and that its inhibition by allopurinol might result in suppression of urinary excretion of oxalate. This needs to be reexamined closely, because an important earlier study found no such effect of allopurinol (Gibbs and Watts, 1966). Recent evidence has raised the possibility that the excess uric acid or urate (perhaps in colloidal form) might be interfering with a naturally occurring urinary inhibitor of calcium oxalate crystallization (Robertson, 1976). A final possibility is that the clinical trials showed only a placebo effect.

Perhaps the most exciting event of the year was the publication of the first double-blind controlled trial of any drug for calcium stone prophylaxis (Smith, 1977). The efficacy of allopurinol was compared with a placebo in stone-formers. The study appears well designed on the whole. The results clearly showed that when the criterion for success is simply improvement or fewer stones, then both the placebo and allopurinol are equally effective. However, if the criterion for success is no recurrence of stones, then allopurinol had a persistent 60% success rate compared with only 5–10% for the placebo. The patients were not strictly selected for the degree of hyperuricosuria at the outset because this abnormality was not fully appreciated at the time of the inception of the study. Nevertheless, the results are quite provocative. They also raise serious questions about the validity of clinical treatment studies undertaken without a concurrent control group and also the therapeutic effect of close supervision by a physician, the so-called "remission artifact."

5.2.3. Hyperoxaluria

During the past year, interest in the hyperoxaluric states has focused mainly on the syndrome of enteric hyperoxaluria. This syndrome continues to be reported with increasing frequency in patients with a wide variety of chronic intestinal disorders (Ogilvie *et al.*, 1976) and after jejunoileal bypass procedures for obesity (Stauffer, 1977a). The actual incidence of renal stone disease in these groups of patients varies remarkably (Earnest, 1977; McDonald *et al.*, 1977; Quaade, 1977) for reasons that are not entirely clear, although hypocalciuria in many of these patients may reduce the saturation of urine relative to calcium oxalate. Clinical manifestations of the hyperoxaluria have largely been confined to recurrent nephrolithiasis, but one fatal case of oxalosis and chronic renal failure after intestinal bypass was reported (Gelbart *et al.*, 1977).

Hyperoxaluria in patients with intestinal disorders clearly results from increased oxalate absorption, largely from the colon (Dobbins and Binder, 1976, 1977; Fairclough *et al.*, 1977), although in one *in vitro* study using isolated intestinal segments from rats, oxalate absorption was found to be greatest in the jejunum (Madorsky and Finlayson, 1977). The mechanism for the increased oxalate absorption remains the subject of debate. Several studies have demonstrated an excellent correlation between fecal fat excretion and the degree of hyperoxaluria (Andersson and Gillberg, 1977; Earnest, 1977; McDonald *et al.*, 1977; Stauffer, 1977b), but other investigators have not been able to confirm this (Dobbins and Binder, 1977). The finding of a negative correlation between the degree of hyperoxaluria and calcium excretion (Stauffer, 1977b), together with the effect of oral calcium on lowering urinary oxalate (Earnest, 1977; Stauffer, 1977b), led to the so-called *competition theory* to explain the hyperoxaluria. According to this theory, unabsorbed fatty acids in the lumen of the intestinal tract compete with oxalate for intraluminal calcium ion. In the presence of steatorrhea, calcium is bound largely to fatty acids, leaving more soluble oxalate available for absorption. Factors that lower intraluminal fatty acid and oxalate concentrations and raise intraluminal calcium concentration have been shown to correct the hyperoxaluria (Earnest, 1977). In addition, binding oxalate to other cations such as aluminum can also reduce absorption of oxalate and decrease the hyperoxaluria in these patients (Earnest, 1977). A second mechanism was proposed to explain the increased oxalate absorption in patients with enteric hyperoxaluria (Dobbins and Binder, 1976, 1977; Fairclough *et al.*, 1977). This theory (the *permeability theory*) proposes that unabsorbed fatty acids and certain bile acids increase the permeability of the colon to calcium oxalate. This is supported by the absence of hyperoxaluria in ileostomy patients, by the effect of cholestyramine in lowering oxalate excretion in some patients, and by several *in vivo* and *in vitro* studies in animals and humans that have shown an effect of ricinoleic acid and chenodeoxycholate and deoxycholate on oxalate permeability in the colon (Dobbins and Binder, 1976, 1977; Fairclough *et al.*, 1977). The high concentration of fatty acids and bile acids used in the *in vitro* studies and the failure of orally administered ricinoleic acid to raise urinary oxalate in some patients have raised some questions about the relative importance of this proposed mechanism (Earnest, 1977).

As is so often the case in medical research, two theories often prompt investigators to take sides as though they were in opposition, which may not necessarily be the case. In fact, it seems likely that both theories to explain the increased oxalate absorption are applicable in most patients with enteric hyperoxaluria, although differences in relative importance undoubtedly exist in individual patients. Probably both mechanisms are operative in patients with severe steatorrhea, but one mechanism may be dominant in patients with lesser degrees of steatorrhea or differing causes of the malabsorptive state. In any case, the importance of the studies that have elucidated these mechanisms is that they have led to rational and effective means of treatment of the hyperoxaluria in these patients. A low-oxalate diet and control of fat malabsorption lower urinary excretion of oxalate. If this is sufficient to eliminate the hyperoxaluria, nothing further needs to be done. If oxalate levels remain elevated, then addition of oral calcium (750–1000 mg/day) to the regimen may be tried, but with very careful monitoring of urinary excretion of calcium. If this is unsuccessful or if urinary calcium increases substantially, cholestyramine may be tried. In most patients, this sequential combined approach is nearly always effective, assuming good patient compliance. If this approach is unsuc-cessful in patients with hyperoxaluria after an intestinal bypass procedure, restoration of normal intestinal contiguity must be considered in view of the potential for the appearance of chronic renal failure in such patients (Gelbart et al., 1977).

5.3. Treatment of Renal Stone Disease

Treatment of the various stone diseases has been outlined in previous editions. Yet the treatment of calcium stone disease in general continues to be problematic. This is a result of at least two phenomena: the inability to properly categorize individual patients and the general lack of con-trolled therapeutic trials.

Coe (1977) published his results of therapy in 202 patients with idiopathic hypercalciuria, hyperuricosuria, or both. He used thiazides, allopurinol, or both, and achieved apparent good results in uncontrolled trials. The hypocalciuric effect of thiazides seems to be persistent and desirable. As mentioned previously, the efficacy of allopurinol appears substantiated. Although the mechanism of allopurinol's action is not yet clear, the use of this drug at least on a provisional basis seems warranted, especially in problem patients, until more data become available on proper classification of patients.

The situation with orthophosphate therapy is less clear. A double-blind trial was conducted in patients with calcium stone disease with three treatment categories: orthophosphate, low-calcium diet, and placebo (Ettinger, 1976). The patients receiving phosphate therapy had no fewer stone episodes than those receiving the placebo or low-calcium diet. However, the dose of phosphate was generally 1.4 g/day, which is lower than the often-recommended 2.0-g dosage. Also, the drug used was acid phosphate rather than neutral phosphate. The former has been shown to have a less potent hypocalciuric effect (Lau et al., 1977). Although ortho-phosphate may well be an effective medicine, it would be helpful if this were known with some certainty before committing patients to long-term therapy with a medicine that could raise urinary oxalate and stimulate parathyroid hormone secretion.

References

Andersson, H., and Gillberg, R., 1977, Urinary oxalate on a high-oxalate diet as a clinical test of malabsorption, *Lancet* **2**:677–679.

Bordier, P., Ryckewart, A., Gueris, J., and Rasmussen, H., 1977, On the pathogenesis of so-called idiopathic hypercalciuria, *Am. J. Med.* **63**:398–409.

Broadus, A. E., Mahaffey, J. E., Bartter, F. C., and Neer, R. M., 1977, Nephrogenous cyclic adenosine monophosphate as a parathyroid function test, *J. Clin. Invest.* **60**:771–783.

Coe, F. L., 1977, Treated and untreated recurrent calcium nephrolithiasis in patients with idiopathic hypercalciuria, hyperuricosuria, or no metabolic disorder, *Ann. Intern. Med.* **87**:404–410.

Coe, F. L., and Kavalach, A. G., 1974, Hypercalciuria and hyperuricosuria in patients with calcium nephrolithiasis, *N. Engl. J. Med.* **291**:1344–1350.

Coe, F. L., Canterbury, J. M., Firpo, J. J., and Reiss, E., 1973, Evidence for secondary hyperparathyroidism in idiopathic hypercalciuria, *J. Clin. Invest.* **52**:134–142.

Coe, F. L., Lawton, R. L., Goldstein, R. B., and Tembe, V., 1975, Sodium urate accelerates precipitation of calcium oxalate *in vitro*, *Proc. Soc. Exp. Biol. Med.* **149**:926–929.

Dobbins, J. W., and Binder, H. J., 1976, Effect of bile salts and fatty acids on the colonic absorption of oxalate, *Gastroenterology* **70**:1096–1100.

Dobbins, J. W., and Binder, H. J., 1977, Importance of the colon in enteric hyperoxaluria, *N. Engl. J. Med.* **296**:298–301.

Earnest, D. L., 1977, Perspectives on incidence, etiology, and treatment of enteric hyperoxaluria, *Am. J. Clin. Nutr.* **30**:72–75.

Edwards, N. A., and Hodgkinson, A., 1965, Studies of renal function in patients with idiopathic hypercalciuria, *Clin. Sci.* **29**:327–338.

Ettinger, B., 1976, Recurrent nephrolithiasis: Natural history and effect of phosphate therapy. A double-blind controlled study, *Am. J. Med.* **61**:200–206.

Fairclough, P. D., Feest, T. G., Chadwick, V. S., and Clark, M. L., 1977, Effect of sodium chenodeoxycholate on oxalate absorption from the excluded human colon—a mechanism for "enteric" hyperoxaluria, *Gut* **18**:240–244.

Gelbart, D. R., Brewer, L. L., Fajardo, L. F., and Weinstein, A. B., 1977, Oxalosis and chronic renal failure after intestinal bypass, *Arch. Intern. Med.* **137**:139–143.

Gibbs, D. A., and Watts, R. W. E., 1966, An investigation of the possible role of xanthine oxidase in the oxidation of glyoxalate to oxalate, *Clin. Sci.* **31**:285–297.

Gray, R. W., Wilz, D. R., Caldas, A. E., and Lemann, J., Jr., 1977, The importance of phosphate in regulating plasma 1,25-$(OH)_2$-vitamin D levels in humans:

Studies in healthy subjects, in calcium-stone formers and in patients with primary hyperparathyroidism, *J. Clin. Endocrinol. Metab.* **45**:299–306.

Haussler, M. R., Baylink, D. J., Hughes, M. R., Brumbaugh, P. F., Wergedal, J. E., Shen, F. H., Nielsen, R. L., Counts, S. J., Bursac, K. M., and McCain, T. A., 1976, The assay of 1α,25-dihydroxyvitamin D₃: Physiologic and pathologic modulation of circulating hormone levels, *Clin. Endocrinol.* **5**:151–165s.

Hodgkinson, A., and Pyrah, L. N., 1958, The urinary excretion of calcium and inorganic phosphate in 344 patients with calcium stone of renal origin, *Br. J. Surg.* **46**:10–18.

Kaplan, R. A., Haussler, M. R., Deftos, L. J., Bone, H., and Pak, C. Y. C., 1977, The role of 1α,25-dihydroxyvitamin D in the mediation of intestinal hyperabsorption of calcium in primary hyperparathyroidism and absorptive hypercalciuria, *J. Clin. Invest.* **59**:756–760.

Lau, K., Wolf, C., Nussbaum, P., Agus, Z., and Goldfarb, S., 1977, Acid vs. neutral phosphate therapy in idiopathic hypercalciuria (IHC): Effects on calcium and acid excretion, *Kidney Int.* **12**:457 (abstract).

Ljunghall, S., 1977, Renal stone disease: Studies of epidemiology and calcium metabolism, *Scand. J. Urol. Nephrol. Suppl. 41,* 96 pp.

Madorsky, M. L., and Finlayson, B., 1977, Oxalate absorption from intestinal segments of rats, *Invest. Urol.* **14**:274–277.

McDonald, G. B., Earnest, D. L., and Admirand, W. H., 1977, Hyperoxaluria correlates with fat malabsorption in patients with sprue, *Gut* **18**:561–566.

Meyer, J. L., Bergert, J. H., and Smith, L. H., 1976, The epitaxially induced crystal growth of calcium oxalate by crystalline uric acid, *Invest. Urol.* **14**:115–119.

Nordin, B. E. C., 1973, Urinary tract calculi, in: *Metabolic Bone and Stone Disease,* pp. 206–243, Williams and Wilkins, Baltimore.

Ogilvie, D., McCollum, J. P., Packer, S., Manning, J., Oyesiku, J., Muller, D. P. R., and Harries, J. T., 1976, Urinary outputs of oxalate, calcium, and magnesium in children with intestinal disorders: Potential cause of renal calculi, *Arch. Dis. Child.* **51**:790–795.

Pak, C. Y. C., Ohata, M., Lawrence, E. C., and Snyder, W., 1974, The hypercalciurias: Causes, parathyroid functions, and diagnostic criteria, *J. Clin. Invest.* **54**:387–400.

Pak, C. Y. C., Kaplan, R., Bone, H., Townsend, J., and Waters, O., 1975, A simple test for the diagnosis of absorptive, resorptive and renal hypercalciurias, *N. Engl. J. Med.* **292**:497–500.

Pak, C. Y. C., Waters, O., Arnold, L., Holt, K., Cox, C., and Barilla, D., 1977, Mechanism for calcium urolithiasis among patients with hyperuricosuria: Supersaturation of urine with respect to monosodium urate, *J. Clin. Invest.* **59**:426–431.

Quaade, F., 1977, Studies of operated and nonoperated obese patients: An interim report on the Scandinavian Obesity Project, *Am. J. Clin. Nutr.* **30**:16–20.

Robertson, W. G., 1976, Physical chemical aspects of calcium stone-formation in the urinary tract, in: *Urolithiasis Research* (H. Fleisch, W. G. Robertson, L. H. Smith, and W. Vahlensieck, eds.), pp. 25–39, Plenum Press, New York.

Robertson, W. G., and Morgan, D. B., 1972, The distribution of urinary calcium excretions in normal persons and stone-formers, *Clin. Chim. Acta* **37**:503–508.

Smith, M. J. V., 1977, Placebo versus allopurinol for renal calculi, *J. Urol.* **117**:690–692.

Smith, M. J. V., and Boyce, W. H., 1969, Allopurinol and urolithiasis, *J. Urol.* **102**:750–753.

Smith, M. J. V., Hunt, L. D., King, J. S., Jr., and Boyce, W. H., 1969, Uricemia and urolithiasis, *J. Urol.* **101**:637–642.

Stauffer, J. Q., 1977a, Hyperoxaluria and calcium oxalate nephrolithiasis after jejunoileal bypass, *Am. J. Clin. Nutr.* **30**:64–71.

Stauffer, J. Q., Hyperoxaluria and intestinal disease: The role of steatorrhea and dietary calcium in regulating intestinal oxalate absorption, *Am. J. Dig. Dis.* **22**:921–928.

Hormone Receptors, Cyclic Nucleotides, and Control of Cell Function

Gerald D. Aurbach and Edward M. Brown

6.1. Introduction

The general scope established with the first chapter in this series (Aurbach, 1976) is developed further in this chapter. Since the writing of that first chapter, considerable further progress has been made in identification by direct binding studies of receptors with novel ligands for β-adrenergic, α-adrenergic, and dopaminergic receptors. The latter are discussed here for the first time in this series. New knowledge has been gained concerning the biosynthesis of the ACTH precursor molecule, which, remarkably, has now been discovered to contain the opiate-receptor-active polypeptide endorphin as well. There is further understanding of the interrelationships at the receptor level of somatomedins (now renamed IGF-I and IGF-II, insulinlike growth factors), multiplication-stimulating activity (MSA), and proinsulin. The structures of these molecules, it is now recognized, share extensive amino acid sequence homologies and additional similarities in secondary structure.

GERALD D. AURBACH and EDWARD M. BROWN • Metabolic Diseases Branch, National Institute of Arthritis, Metabolism, and Digestive Diseases, National Institutes of Health, Bethesda, Maryland 20014.

Progress in the understanding of how adenylate cyclase enzyme is regulated has also broadened our understanding of the pathophysiology of cholera. Cholera toxin activates adenylate cyclase in cells apparently through inhibition of a GTPase normally involved in the deactivation of adenylate cyclase enzyme. It is becoming ever more apparent that calcium can control cyclic nucleotide concentrations through interactions with a · regulatory protein that influences adenylate cyclase as well as cyclic nucleotide phosphodiesterase activity. Of further importance to clinical medicine is the detailed quantitative analysis of cyclic AMP (cAMP) clearance now available. This type of careful analysis allows segregation of urinary cAMP into the nephrogenous fraction as distinct from the fraction cleared from the plasma via glomerular filtration. Nephrogenous cAMP is of particular utility in diagnosing parathyroid disorders. These topics and others concerning receptor regulation and localization as well as control of cyclic nucleotide concentration are discussed herein.

6.2. Receptor Systems

6.2.1. Physiological Regulation of Receptors

A variety of mechanisms have been described whereby receptor number or affinity or both may be modulated *in vivo* and *in vitro*. Regulation of a receptor by the hormone normally binding to it in a number of systems was reviewed earlier (Aurbach, 1976). This regulation may be effected through a decrease in affinity of unbound sites with partial receptor occupancy ["negative cooperativity" (Demeyts *et al.*, 1973; Limbird and Lefkowitz, 1976)] or actual loss of receptors following exposure to the hormone ["desensitization" or "down regulation" (Roth *et al.*, 1975; Mickey *et al.*, 1975)]. Thus, pharmacologically defined tachyphylaxis (decreased sensitivity of a tissue following prolonged exposure to a drug) may be explained in some cases by alterations at the level of the receptor. Similarly, the phenomenon of denervative hypersensitivity is also associated with alterations in receptor number. Berg *et al.* (1972) showed an increase in acetylcholine receptors in denervated muscle. Harden *et al.* (1977a) also recently demonstrated an increase in β-adrenergic receptors in rat cerebral cortex following depletion of endogenous catecholamines with 6-hydroxydopamine.

There are now many examples of regulation of receptor to one hormone by a second hormone. Several instances of this type of regulation will be given in the section on catecholamine receptors (Section 6.2.4), including alterations in β-receptor number by adrenal and thyroid hormones and α-receptor number by estrogens. Such heterologous regulation (not discussed further in this review) has also been described for other hormone systems: dihydrotestosterone appears to increase the number of prolactin receptors (Charreau *et al.,* 1977), while follicle-stimulating hormone is capable of inducing human chorionic gonadotropin receptors in rat granulosa cells *in vitro* (Nimrod *et al.,* 1977). Undoubtedly, further examples of this type are yet to be described.

Although possibly not physiological in nature, several types of receptor alterations have also been described with neoplastic and viral transformation. "Ectopic" β-receptors have been found on plasma membranes from an adrenal carcinoma (Williams *et al.,* 1977a). Cultured 3T3 mouse cell lines transformed with simian virus (SV40) show increased numbers of β-receptors as well as a shift from β_1 to β_2 subtype (Sheppard, 1977). It is possible that alterations of this type might serve as "tumor markers" and thus become clinically useful.

6.2.2. Relationship of Receptors to Adenylate Cyclase

Dramatic progress has been made in the past two years in defining the relationship of receptors to adenylate cyclase. The problem has been studied through several approaches: cell fusion and genetic and biochemical studies. Schramm's group (Orly and Schramm, 1976) showed that a receptor from one cell type can be coupled with adenylate cyclase from another. They fused turkey erythrocytes with β-receptors that were intact (but lacked a functional adenylate cyclase) with Friend erythroleukemia cells containing the enzyme but lacking β-receptors, and obtained hybrid cells with β-agonist-sensitive adenylate cyclase. This elegant approach demonstrated directly that receptor and enzyme are separate entities, presumably capable of lateral diffusion within the plane of the membrane to yield functionally coupled receptor–adenylate cyclase complex.

Bourne, Coffino, Insel, Gilman, and their colleagues (Insel *et al.,* 1976) used the genetic approach and isolated mutants of S49 mouse lymphoma cells lacking various components of the receptor–adenylate cyclase complex. In some instances, adenylate cyclase activity appears to be lacking ("cyclase-negative"). In others, mutant cells (the UNC or "uncoupled" mutant) contain receptors and adenylate cyclase but do not manifest hormone-stimulable adenylate cyclase because they lack a "coupling factor" (Haga *et al.,* 1977). The loss of adenylate cyclase independent of receptor is highly suggestive of the fact that they are separate gene products. This approach also promises to be valuable in dissecting out other components in the receptor–adenylate cyclase complex (see Section 6.3).

Finally, it has also been possible to separate physically receptor–adenylate cyclase as distinct entities. Limbird and Lefkowitz (1977) were able to show that the solubilized frog erythrocyte β-adrenergic receptor and adenylate cyclase migrated separately on gel exclusion columns. These three approaches provide cogent evidence that receptors are distinct from adenylate cyclase and support the notion that receptors or adenylate cyclase or both are relatively free to diffuse within the plane of the plasma membrane (Bennett et al., 1975). Although most of these studies relate to the β-adrenergic receptor, already these methods are being employed to provide similar conclusions about the relationship of other receptors to adenylate cyclase.

6.2.3. Opiate Receptors and Endorphins

Progress in the area of opiate receptors, endorphins, and biosynthesis of ACTH continues to produce new revelations concerning secretion and function. The earlier chapter (Aurbach, 1976) summarized information indicating that enkephalin, a peptide in the brain, represents a portion of the amino acid sequence of the recognized peptide β-lipotropin. More recently, larger fragments of β-lipotropin equally active in opiate receptor activity were isolated from the pituitary gland and named α- and β-endorphins, respectively (see Guillemin et al., 1977). The work of Mains and co-workers (Mains et al., 1977; Mains and Eipper, 1976) and Crine et al. (1977) suggests that β-lipotropin and ACTH as well as β-melanocyte-stimulating hormone are all derived from a large 31,000-dalton precursor protein synthesized in pituitary cells. ACTH represents a region near the amino-terminal end of the precursor molecule, and β-lipotropin containing β-endorphin represents regions more C-terminal in the precursor molecule. Studies on biosynthesis were based on incorporation of radioactive amino acids into protein in vitro. Crine et al. (1977) found incorporation of [^{35}S]methionine and [^{3}H]lysine into isolated peptides that gave Edman degradation patterns similar to those known for endorphins. Mains and co-workers (Mains and Eipper, 1976; Mains et al., 1977) utilized antibodies directed to ACTH to identify a high-molecular-weight protein precursor of ACTH.

The studies suggesting that a common high-molecular-weight prohormone is the precursor of both β-lipotropin, and consequently β-endorphin as well as ACTH, are supported by the findings of Rossier and co-workers (Rossier et al., 1977; Guillemin et al., 1977). These studies showed that the opiate-active peptide β-endorphin and ACTH are secreted concomitantly in vivo in response to acute stress (tibial fracture or electric shock) as well as in vitro in response to corticotropin-releasing factor, other secretagogues, or long-term adrenalectomy. It was also shown that dexamethasone inhibits concomitantly secretion of both ACTH and β-endorphin. Of further interest is their finding that elevated endogenous secretion *in vitro* of ACTH by fragments of pituitary taken from a patient with Nelson's syndrome is also accompanied by correspondingly high secretory rates for β-endorphin (Guillemin *et al.*, 1977). Illustrated in Fig. 1 is the response *in vivo* of rats to stress caused by electric shock to the foot. Note the parallel increases in β-endorphin and ACTH in the plasma of the test animals. Although β-endorphin accompanied ACTH in release from the pituitary in response to stress, there was no accumulation of β-endorphin in the brain. In fact, hypothalamic concentrations of β-endorphin were slightly reduced in response to 30-min exposure to electric shock to the foot. These results differ from the findings of Madden *et al.* (1977), who found apparent increases in opiate-reactive material in the brain after stress. They, however, used radioreceptor assay procedures that would not necessarily detect β-endorphin determined by radioimmunoassay by the Guillemin group. Indeed, it is possible that enkephalinlike material could accumulate in the brain and be detected by radioreceptor assay but not be recognized by radioimmunoassay. In any event, it is still unclear whether endogenous opiatelike material released under stress conditions can actually induce analgesia by accumulation in the brain.

6.2.4. Catecholamine Receptors

Since the studies of the early-20th-century physiologists, there has been a continuing interest in the effects of catecholamines on a variety of

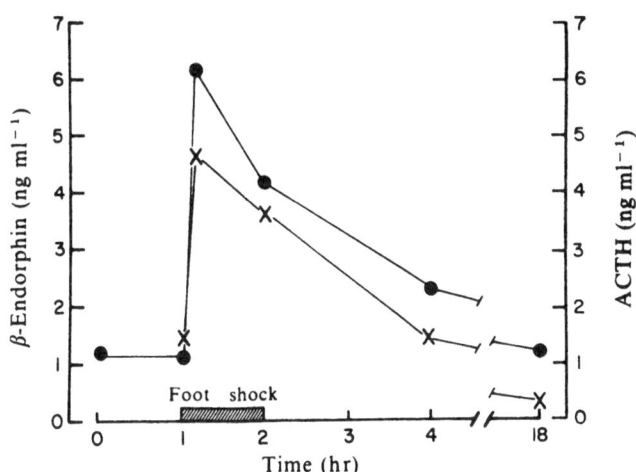

Fig. 1. Parallel increase in plasma ACTH and β-endorphin content in response to electric shock to the foot. ($\bullet$) β-Endorphin; (X) ACTH. From Rossier *et al.* (1977).

tissues. Dale (1906) was the first to suggest the presence of specific receptor sites ("the receptive mechanism for adrenaline") on smooth muscles. He also recognized that the stimulatory properties of epinephrine were specifically blocked by ergot alkaloids, while its inhibitory effects were unaltered. Cannon and Rosenbleuth (1937) had proposed that excitatory and inhibitory sympathetic effects could be attributed to distinct mediatory substances. Ahlquist (1948) first clearly enunciated the concept of distinct adrenergic receptor sites—α and β—based on the order of potency of a series of sympathomimetic amines. It has also been recognized in the past 15 years that a third catecholamine, dopamine, is an important neurotransmitter in the central nervous system. Since dopaminergic receptors and α-adrenergic receptors were not reviewed in *The Year in Metabolism 1975–1976* or *The Year in Metabolism 1977*, a general overview of this area will be given. The intense interest in the β-adrenergic receptor, which was reviewed in the former volume, has continued, and new developments will be described.

6.2.4.1. β-Adrenergic Receptors

Since the last review of this subject by Aurbach (1976), the availability of the well-characterized radiolabeled β-adrenergic antagonists [³H]dihydroalprenolol ([³H]-DHA) (Lefkowitz *et al.*, 1974) and [¹²⁵I]iodohydroxybenzylpindolol ([¹²⁵I]-HYP) (Brown *et al.*, 1976; Maguire *et al.*, 1976b) has resulted in a profusion of studies directly identifying β-adrenergic receptors (Table I). Several excellent reviews are available on this rapidly expanding field (Lefkowitz *et al.*, 1976; Wolfe *et al.*, 1977; Maguire *et al.*, 1977). There has been reasonable uniformity in numbers of receptors observed with both [³H]-DHA and [¹²⁵I]-HYP, varying over approximately a 10-fold range, with the exception of HeLa cells, which have about 500,000 receptors per cell. Studies on the same tissue (e.g., rat cerebral cortex) with both ligands generally have given good agreement for receptor number. The affinities obtained with [³H]-DHA have been relatively constant (from 1.3 to 30 mM), but there has been considerable variability in affinity for [¹²⁵I]-HYP (15–2400 pM). The reasons for these differences are not yet clear.

In addition to radiolabeled antagonists, several intriguing ligands have been developed by Atlas and Levitzki. A brominated β-blocker was developed (Atlas *et al.*, 1976), which appears to bind irreversibly and covalently to the β-adrenergic receptor. In addition, two fluorescent derivatives of propranolol were synthesized (Atlas and Levitzki, 1977), which compete with [¹²⁵I]-HYP for binding to the turkey erythrocyte β-receptor. These authors have already employed these ligands to detect β-adrenergic receptors in the rat central nervous system. Apparently spe-

Table I. Tissues in Which β-Adrenergic Receptors Have Been Directly Identified[a]

Tissue	Ligand	K_d (nM)	Receptor concentration (fmol/mg)	Receptors/cell	Reference
Frog erythrocyte	[¹H]-DHA	7	300	1500	Maguire et al. (1977)
Dog heart	[¹H]-DHA	11	350	—	Maguire et al. (1977)
Rat pineal	[¹H]-DHA	18	600	—	Maguire et al. (1977)
Human lymphocyte	[¹H]-DHA	10	75	2000	Maguire et al. (1977)
Rat cerebral cortex	[³H]-DHA	7	250	—	Maguire et al. (1977)
Rat cerebral cortex	[¹H]-DHA	1.3	300	—	Maguire et al. (1977)
Rat adipocyte	[³H]-DHA	15	240	—	Maguire et al. (1977)
HeLa cells	[³H]-DHA	12		500,000	Tallman et al. (1977)
Balb 3T3 cells	[³H]-DHA	30	300	17,000	Sheppard (1977)
Turkey erythrocyte	[¹²⁵I]-HYP	0.025	250	500	Maguire et al. (1977)
Rat glioma	[¹²⁵I]-HYP	0.250	75	4000	Maguire et al. (1977)
Human fibroblast	[¹²⁵I]-HYP	0.015	100	—	Maguire et al. (1977)
Mouse lymphoma	[¹²⁵I]-HYP	0.090	25	500	Maguire et al. (1977)
Rat heart	[¹²⁵I]-HYP	1.4	160	—	Maguire et al. (1977)
Rat liver	[¹²⁵I]-HYP	2.4	40	—	Maguire et al. (1977)
Rat cerebral cortex	[¹²⁵I]-HYP	1.3	300	—	Maguire et al. (1977)
Bovine parathyroid	[¹²⁵I]-HYP	0.040	100	5000	Brown et al. (1977a)
Rat reticulocyte	[¹²⁵I]-HYP	0.200	90	—	Bilezikian et al. (1977)

[a] Primary references not cited may be found in the review of Maguire et al. (1977), from which this table is reproduced with modifications.

cific localization of fluorescence could be inhibited by prior injection of the animals with L- but not D-propranolol. This type of approach might offer a means of visualizing and mapping β-adrenergic receptors both *in vivo* and *in vitro*.

A significant advance in the study of β-adrenergic receptors was reported by Lefkowitz's group (Lefkowitz and Williams, 1977). The same approach with tritiation to develop radiolabeled blockers was applied to achieve a high-affinity β-adrenergic agonist, [³H]hydroxybenzylisoproterenol ([³H]-HBI) (Fig. 2); the latter interacts with a class of binding sites on frog erythrocyte membranes having the properties expected of β-adrenergic receptors. High concentrations of ascorbic acid and catechol

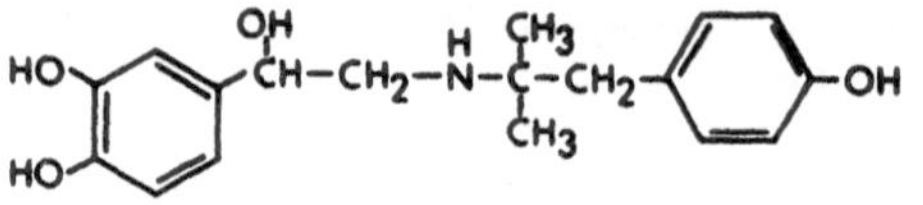

Fig. 2. Structure of hydroxybenzyl-isoproterenol. From Lefkowitz and Williams (1977).

were employed to inhibit nonspecific binding, apparently due to oxidation of the catechol portion of the molecule. Employing this ligand, Lefkowitz and Hamp (1977) were able to show that sites identified by radiolabeled agonists were essentially identical to those previously studied with the radiolabeled antagonist [³H]-DHA. This result contrasted with that found in certain other receptor systems (Snyder and Bennett, 1976) in which agonist and antagonist appear to bind to distinct sites. Considerable care must be taken, however, in using identical conditions for studying binding of agonist and antagonist. The radiolabeled agonist has also been useful in studying the phenomenon of desensitization by agonists (see the following section).

6.2.4.1a. Regulation of β-Adrenergic Receptors. Since the last discussion of this topic in *The Year in Metabolism 1975–1976,* progress has been rapid in defining factors controlling β-adrenergic receptor concentration in many different systems. In addition to β-adrenergic agonists, other hormones and neoplastic and developmental changes may alter β-receptors.

6.2.4.1b. Subsensitivity. The development of the radiolabeled β-adrenergic agonist [³H]-HBI has shed further light on the phenomenon of subsensitivity of β-adrenergic receptors. With the frog erythrocyte membrane system, Williams and Lefkowitz (1977a) showed that the degree of subsensitivity induced by preincubation with [³H]-HBI correlated closely with the amount of residual slowly dissociable [³H]-HBI bound to the β-adrenergic receptor. "Resensitization" of the receptor could be brought about by guanine nucleotides [Gpp(NH)p] and was associated with rapid dissociation of the residual-labeled agonist. It is probable that this effect of guanine nucleotides on dissociation rate is related to the agonist-specific decrease in β-adrenergic affinity brought about by these agents (Maguire *et al.,* 1976a). Antagonists, whose affinity is unaltered by Gpp(NH)p, do not cause desensitization. It remains to be determined whether this phenomenology *in vitro* can account for *in vivo* subsensitivity.

6.2.4.1c. Adrenal Steroids. Wolfe *et al.* (1976) recently described a 3- to 5-fold increase in the number of β-adrenergic receptors on rat liver membranes following adrenalectomy as assessed by [¹²⁵I]-HYP binding. There was no change in receptor affinity, and administration of glucocorticoids was associated with a return to the normal number of receptors. It is possible that this increase in receptors is a "compensatory" response to the impaired gluconeogenesis seen with glucocorticoid deficiency.

6.2.4.1d. Thyroid Hormones. Williams *et al.* (1977b) demonstrated that administration of exogenous triiodothyronine to rats causes a 2-fold increase in cardiac plasma membrane β-adrenergic receptors. Thus, the signs of β-adrenergic excess in thyrotoxicosis may have a direct counterpart in an increased complement of β-adrenergic receptors in peripheral tissues.

    6.2.4.1e. Sodium Butyrate. Tallman *et al.* (1977) showed that incubation of HeLa cells with sodium butyrate resulted in a 2- to 3-fold increase in β-adrenergic receptors without alterations in fluoride-stimulated adenylate cyclase, suggesting the induction of new receptor synthesis.

    6.2.4.1f. Ectopic β-Adrenergic Receptors. Unlike the normal adrenal, certain adrenal tumors have a catecholamine-sensitive adenylate cyclase. These tumors have been shown to contain β-adrenergic receptors (Williams *et al.*, 1977a) by [^{3}H]-DHA binding, thus apparently constituting an example of an ectopic β-adrenergic receptor.

    6.2.4.1g. Viral Transformation. Another type of β-adrenergic receptor alteration associated with neoplasia was described by Sheppard (1977). SV40 viral transformation of 3T3 mouse cells in culture resulted not only in an increase in numbers of β-adrenergic receptors, but also in a change in receptor subtype from β_1 to β_2. Whether the appearance of the distinct receptor subtype results from expression of a separate gene or from alterations in the environment of the receptor has not been determined.

    6.2.4.1h. Developmental Changes. Two groups (Charness *et al.*, 1976; Bilezikian *et al.*, 1977) showed that the number of β-adrenergic receptors and the degree of catecholamine-sensitive adenylate cyclase vary as a function of the age of rat reticulocytes. While mature rat erythrocytes contain almost no isoproterenol-stimulated adenylate cyclase, a significant number of β-adrenergic receptors remain. Harden *et al.* (1977b) studied the presence of β-receptors in rat brain as a function of age. There are relatively few receptors during the first week after birth, but the density of β-receptors increases rapidly from days 7 to 14 and remains at adult levels from that time on. Undoubtedly, numerous other examples will appear of changes in many receptors that occur with development of the organism.

6.2.4.2. α-Adrenergic Receptors

    6.2.4.2a. Direct Identification of α-Adrenergic Receptors. Although a vast pharmacological literature, beyond the scope of this review, exists on the effects of α-adrenergic agonists on a wide variety of tissues, it was not until 1976 that the α-receptor could be directly identified. Employing the same principles that were successfully applied to the development of radiolabeled β-adrenergic antagonists, Williams and Lefkowitz (1976) reported the use of [^{3}H]dihydroergocryptine ([^{3}H]-DHE) to directly identify α-adrenergic receptors. The binding of this potent α-adrenergic antagonist to uterine plasma membrane preparations was saturable and was inhibited stereospecifically by α-adrenergic agonists and antagonists (Fig. 3). The order of potency of a series of α-agonists was the same as anticipated from previous physiological studies. Moreover, β-adrenergic antagonists and physiologically inactive catecholamines did not compete for [³H]-

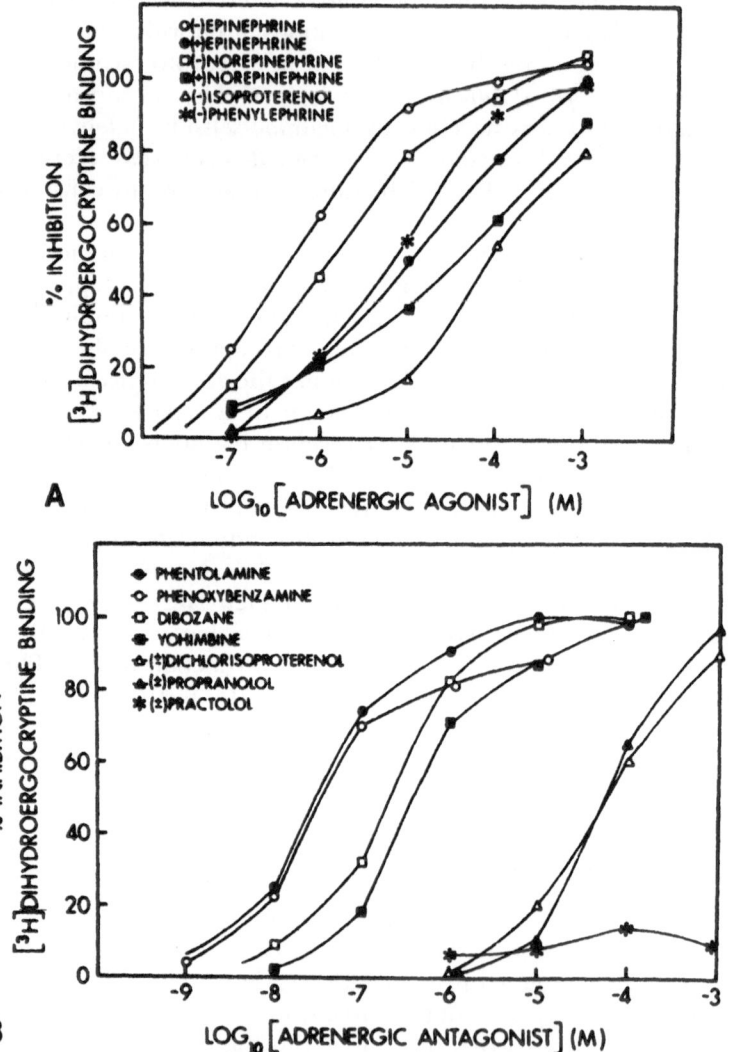

Fig. 3. Inhibition of [³H]-DHE binding to uterine plasma membrane α-adrenergic receptors by selected α-adrenergic agonists (A) and antagonists (B). From Williams *et al.* (1976).

DHE binding. Thus, the criteria for interaction with true α-adrenergic receptors appear to have been satisfied.

Greenberg and Snyder (1977) also employed [³H]-DHE to identify α-adrenergic receptors in the central nervous system. The same group also found that [³H]clonidine, an α-adrenergic agonist, and [³H]-WB101, a potent α-adrenergic antagonist, are useful ligands to study binding to brain receptors (U'Prichard *et al.*, 1977). Evidence has been marshaled that α-adrenergic agonists bind more avidly to [³H]clonidine binding sites, while antagonists show a preference for [³H]-WB101 binding sites. This pattern is similar to that which has been observed for binding to the opiate, glycine, serotonin, and dopamine receptors (Snyder and Bennett, 1976) and suggests the possibility of a "two-site" model for the α-adrenergic receptor. It should be pointed out, however, that the specific activity of these ligands is relatively low (compared with ¹²⁵I), that brain membrane preparations represent a heterogeneous population of cell types, and that "nonspecific" binding is relatively high. In addition, no direct correlations of binding with biological effects have been made in these brain preparations. Confirmation by other groups, employing additional ligands, preferably with a homogeneous cell population, will help to establish the generality of the two-site model for the α-adrenergic receptor.

6.2.4.2b. Regulation of α-Adrenergic Receptors. Little work has been carried out in this area, but Lefkowitz and colleagues observed two types of control with α-adrenergic receptors that have been observed previously with other receptor types. Strittmatter *et al.* (1977a) observed that desensitization of both [³H]-DHE binding and α-adrenergic stimulation of potassium efflux (see below) occurred with prolonged exposure to α-adrenergic agonists. This effect was not observed with antagonists and could be reversed by incubation without agonist. Williams and Lefkowitz (1977b) also observed that progesterone-primed rabbits have only one third as many [³H]-DHE binding sites per milligram of uterine membrane as estrogen-treated controls. This observation suggests that the previously observed reduced sensitivity of the uterus to α-adrenergic stimulation during pregnancy may result in part from reduction in α-receptors. Similar findings were reported by Roberts *et al.* (1977), who found, in addition, that sex steroids had very little effect on rabbit uterine β-receptors as assessed by [¹²⁵I]-HYP binding.

6.2.4.2c. Mediators of α-Adrenergic Effects. Although a second messenger(s) for the α-adrenergic receptor has not been definitely identified as yet, changes in concentration of several putative intracellular mediators (e.g., cAMP, cGMP, Ca^{2+}) have been described with α-adrenergic stimulation. Lowering of cAMP was first reported by Turtle and Kipnis (1967) in pancreatic islets. A similar reduction in cellular cAMP, particularly that stimulated by a variety of agonists, has now been observed in a number of other tissues. Jakobs *et al.* (1976) recently demonstrated an α-adrenergic reduction in adenylate cyclase activity in human platelet lysates, consistent with a direct effect on the enzyme. The mechanistic details of this effect, however, remain obscure.

In contrast to the effect just mentioned, α-adrenergic stimulation *increases* cAMP content in brain slices (Chasin *et al.*, 1971; Perkins and Moore, 1973). This increase is blocked by α-adrenergic antagonists and appears to fulfill the expected criteria for a direct α-adrenergic effect. In some instances, adenosine appears to be necessary for the stimulatory effects of norepinephrine on cAMP (Sattin *et al.*, 1975). In addition, the heterogeneity of cell and receptor types in these preparations makes it difficult to rule out indirect effects mediated through other neurotransmitters. The reasons for the difference in α-adrenergic effects on cAMP in the central nervous system as compared with peripheral tissues remain obscure.

α-Adrenergic agonists cause increased cyclic GMP (cGMP) concentrations in human plasma (Ball *et al.*, 1972). More recently, a similar effect was observed *in vitro* (Schultz *et al.*, 1973). This increase in cGMP appears to require extracellular Ca^{2+}, as does the effect of other agents that increase concentrations of this cyclic nucleotide. The effect may be mimicked by calcium ionophores such as A23187, suggesting that alterations in Ca^{2+} flux might mediate α-adrenergic effects (Butcher, 1975).

α-Adrenergic agonists increase potassium efflux from a variety of tissues and result in depolarization of the cells involved (Batzri *et al.*, 1973; Ellis and Beckett, 1963). In the parotid gland, this efflux is dependent, at least in part, on extracellular calcium, again suggesting a relationship between Ca^{2+} flux and more distal α-adrenergic effects (Batzri *et al.*, 1973). Strittmatter *et al.* (1977b) recently employed this alteration in K flux to directly compare for the first time the binding of [^{3}H]-DHE to a biological effect of α-adrenergic stimulation.

The mechanism whereby α-adrenergic effects are mediated is still not clear. It is possible that mechanisms may vary from tissue to tissue and that there may be a complex interaction between cAMP, cGMP, free cytosolic calcium, and membrane potential. Further studies in this area are awaited with interest.

6.2.4.3. Dopamine

Steady progress has been made over the past 15 years in elucidating the biochemical and clinical significance of dopamine receptors in man. Particularly exciting work has been carried out in understanding the pathogenesis of Parkinson's disease and the role of dopamine analogues in its therapy. The possible role of dopaminergic pathways in schizophrenia has also generated intense interest, and dopaminergic agonists and antagonists have found increasing use both diagnostically and therapeutically in endocrinology.

Three principal dopaminergic pathways exist in the central nervous system (Fig. 4). *Nigrostriatal* neurons arise in the substantia nigra of the brainstem and terminate in the basal ganglia (striatum). The *mesolimbic* and *mesocortical* systems arise in the interpeduncular region of the brainstem and terminate in several areas of the limbic system. The *tuberoinfundibular* neurons arise in the area of the arcuate nucleus of the hypothalamus and terminate on the median eminence and infundibular stem of the pituitary. Dopaminergic pathways have also been found in the retina. Outside the central nervous system, dopamine is found in some species in the cervical sympathetic ganglia and in mast cells.

The work of Greengard, Kebabian, Iversen, Makman, and their colleagues has been of fundamental importance in elucidating the probable biochemical mechanisms of dopaminergic synaptic transmission. Studies in the superior cervical ganglion have demonstrated that the nerve transmission through a morphologically defined dopaminergic pathway is associated with elevations of total ganglion cAMP (Greengard and Kebabian, 1974). This effect may be mimicked by exogenously applied dopamine, and is accompanied by the so-called "slow inhibitory postsynaptic potential." Subsequent studies with homogenates of superior cervical ganglion identified a dopaminergic-sensitive adenylate cyclase inhibited by low concentrations of dopamine antagonists of the phenothiazine class

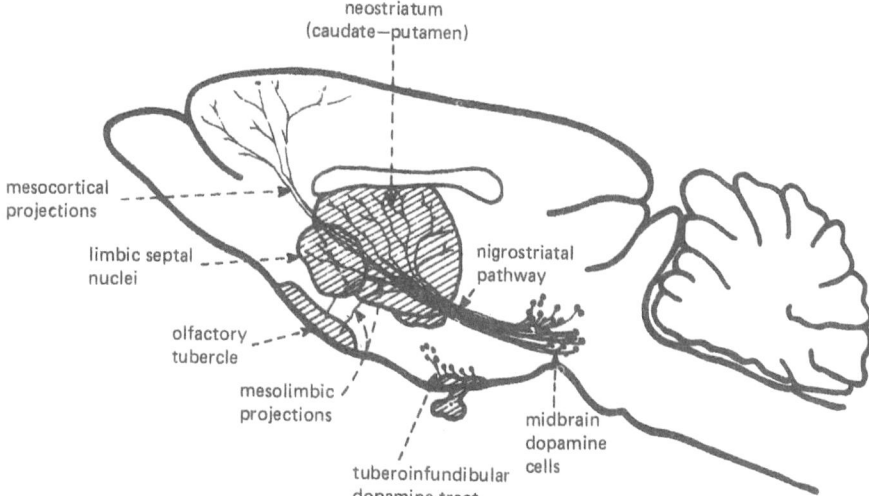

Fig. 4. Dopaminergic pathways in the rat central nervous system. From Baldessarini (1977).

(e.g., fluphenazine or chlorpromazine) or higher concentrations of the butyrophenones (haloperidol) (Clement-Cormier *et al.*, 1974). A similar dopamine-sensitive adenylate cyclase has been found in those areas of the brain known to contain dopaminergic nerve endings (Kebabian, 1977; Miller *et al.*, 1974). These data have suggested that release of dopamine from nerve endings activates adenylate cyclase through interaction with a specific dopamine receptor. cAMP generated by this interaction is presumed to account for the neurophysiological effects of the neurotransmitter, possibly by phosphorylation of specific membrane proteins (Ueda *et al.*, 1973).

Several groups (Seeman *et al.*, 1975; Burt *et al.*, 1975) have developed radiolabeled ligands to identify dopaminergic receptors in the central nervous system. In contrast to the β-adrenergic receptor (see above), somewhat different results have been obtained when radiolabeled agonists, as opposed to antagonists, have been utilized. Studies with [^{3}H]dopamine have demonstrated a high affinity for agonists with a relatively lower affinity for antagonists, while the converse was true when [^{3}H]haloperidol was employed. These data have been interpreted according to a "two-site" model for hormone receptors (Snyder and Bennett, 1976). In this formulation, a receptor may exist in two discrete configurations having high affinity for either agonists or antagonists, respectively. Whether these two putative receptor configurations are separate entities or interconvertible forms of a single receptor has not been established. There are several discrepancies, moreover, between dopamine receptors as defined by binding studies and those defined by the activation and inhibition of adenylate cyclase. The potency of dopamine in inhibiting binding of [^{3}H]dopamine is 2–3 orders of magnitude higher than its potency in activating adenylate cyclase. Moreover, the butyrophenone haloperidol has a K_i of about 10^{-6} M for effects on adenylate cyclase as compared with its very high affinity ($K_d \approx 10^{-9}$ M) in the binding assay (Kebabian, 1977). The source of these discrepancies has not been elucidated to date, and the relationship between adenylate cyclase and dopamine and haloperidol binding sites remains uncertain.

There are several well-documented examples of dopaminergic receptors outside the central nervous system. L. I. Goldberg *et al.* (1968) carried out extensive studies on the effects of dopamine on the renal vasculature. Recently, Brown *et al.* (1977b) showed that dispersed bovine parathyroid cells have dopaminergic receptors that may be distinguished from the β-adrenergic receptors also present on this cell type. This system may be particularly useful as a model system, for the effects of dopamine on increasing cAMP accumulation are closely linked to the enhanced release of parathyroid hormone, thus permitting studies of the relationship among dopamine receptors, cAMP, and a well-defined biological response.

6.2.4.3a. Clinical Aspects of Dopamine Receptors. In Parkinson's disease, there is selective loss of dopamine-containing neurons in the nigrostriatal pathway (Bernheimer *et al.,* 1973). Cotzias *et al.* (1967), in particular, demonstrated the dramatic clinical efficacy of L-dopa in treatment of this disorder. Biochemical studies have shown an increase in dopamine and its metabolites in the basal ganglia of treated patients. The effectiveness of L-dopa arises through decarboxylation to dopamine by the remaining neurons of the nigrostriatal pathway. More recently, the long-acting dopamine agonist bromergocryptine (2-bromo-ergocryptine) has also proved useful in Parkinson's disease, particularly in cases that have become refractory to L-dopa alone (Calne *et al.,* 1974).

Antipsychotic agents of the phenothiazine and butyrophenone classes have revolutionized the therapy of schizophrenia. The description of the mesolimbic dopamine pathway, the realization of the importance of the limbic system in memory and emotion, and the demonstration of the dopamine-blocking effects of the antipsychotic drugs have been fascinating clues to a possible pathogenetic role of dopamine in schizophrenia (Baldessarini, 1977). These associations as well as the widely recognized parkinsonian side effects of many of the antipsychotic drugs have led to the "dopamine hypothesis" for the cause of schizophrenia. In this formulation, overactivity of the mesolimbic dopamine pathways is of pathogenetic importance, and the therapeutic effects of the antipsychotic agents result from blockade of these pathways. The striking correlation between clinical potency of these drugs and their ability to compete for [^{3}H]haloperidol binding sites (Fig. 5) has been taken as evidence in favor of this hypothesis. As pointed out in a recent review on schizophrenia, however, much of the evidence for the "dopamine hypothesis" is pharmacological and indirect (Hornykiewicz, 1977). The intense research interest in this area may help to further elucidate this problem in the next few years.

Dopamine has a tonic inhibitory effect on prolactin release and probably represents the actual prolactin inhibitory factor. Dopamine may also be involved in the regulation of several other pituitary hormones [e.g., enhanced human growth hormone (hGH) release with L-dopa]. It seems likely that endogenous dopaminergic control of pituitary function relates to activity of the tuberoinfundibular pathways. In the case of prolactin, dopamine released from nerve endings appears to traverse the hypophyseal portal system and exert a direct inhibitory effect on the pituitary. Although there are no well-documented syndromes due to functional abnormalities of this system, several tests of pituitary function have taken advantage of the neuroendocrinological effects of dopamine. Moreover, the use of ergot alkaloids such as bromergocryptine with dopaminergic properties shows great promise in the therapy of several endocrine abnormalities. Galactorrhea, menstrual abnormalities, hypogo-

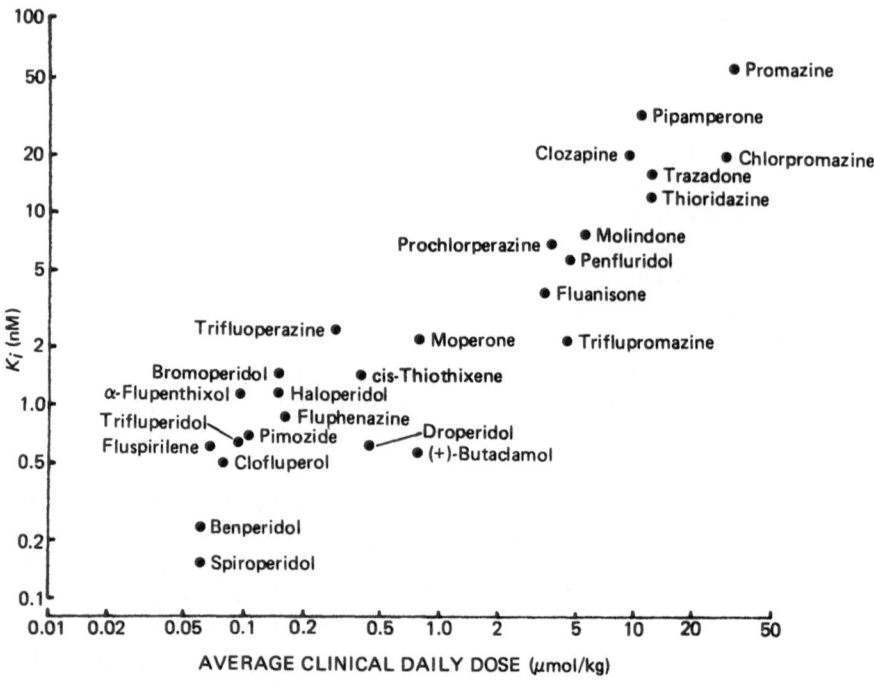

Fig. 5. Correlation between clinical potency of selected antipsychotic agents and binding affinity (represented as inhibitor constant, K_i) for dopaminergic receptors in the brain. From Baldessarini (1977).

nadism, and infertility associated with hyperprolactinemia appear to be particularly amenable to the prolactin-lowering effects of bromergocryptine (Besser *et al.*, 1972). An extensive literature has accumulated in the past five or six years on the use of the drug for this purpose. Ergots have also shown early promise in the therapy of acromegaly (Thorner *et al.*, 1975), following the observation (Liuzzi *et al.*, 1974) that (unlike the effect in normal man, where dopaminergic agonists stimulate growth hormone release) bromergocryptine inhibits secretion of hGH in most acromegalics. Improvement in acromegalic features has been reported in several studies on this use of the drug. The report of possible side effects, however, such as digital vasospasm and gastrointestinal bleeding, will merit continued caution in the clinical use of these drugs.

6.2.5. Hormone Receptors in the Kidney

Chabardes, Morel, and associates (Chabardes *et al.*, 1976, 1978) have studied further the distribution of parathyroid-hormone (PTH) and calcitonin-sensitive adenylate cyclase in microdissected segments of the renal tubule. Sites for PTH action were found in the proximal cortical tubule and in the granular portion of the distal cortical tubule of the rabbit kidney. Two areas of the proximal tubule of the rabbit responded to PTH: the convoluted and the straight portions. Salmon calcitonin, on the other hand, showed a different distribution of activation of adenylate cyclase. The major effect was in the "bright" region of the distal convoluted tubule and also the medullary portions of the thick ascending limb of the nephron (Chabardes et al., 1976). The nephron of the mouse is somewhat different in distribution of PTH- and calcitonin-sensitive adenylate cyclase. PTH receptors in mouse kidney appeared to be localized not only in the proximal cortical tubule and in the distal convoluted tubule but also in the cortical ascending limb. Calcitonin receptors in the mouse kidney are distributed more distally and appear in the granular portions of the distal convoluted tubule and the cortical collecting tubule ("light" region). Further information on distribution of PTH receptors was obtained by Chambers et al. (1978), who developed an ultrasensitive (1–1000 fg/ml) cytochemical assay for PTH using microtome sections of guinea pig kidney. They found that glucose-6-phosphate dehydrogenase activity is stimulated in the distal convoluted tubule and that alkaline phosphatase activity as well as carbonic anhydrase activity are stimulated in the proximal convoluted tubules of the guinea pig kidney. These findings tend to confirm the localizations found by Chabardes and collaborators for PTH-sensitive sites. It is assumed that cAMP generated in these areas of the nephron is the intermediary for activation of these enzymes. However, experimental evidence for this has not yet been reported.

Effects of PTH or calcitonin on calcium flux in sensitive tissues have been reported recently. Biddulph and Wrenn (1977) found that PTH causes increased rates of calcium flux from isolated renal cortical tubules from the golden hamster. cAMP increased rapidly in this preparation, becoming maximal within 2 min. Calcium efflux increased to maximal rates at 6 min, and in parallel with this response, there was an increase in cGMP concentration. Calcitonin was shown to influence calcium flux in perfused preparations of the salmon gill (Milhaud et al., 1977). Calcitonin decreased the influx of water and calcium from Ringer's solution across the gill into the circulation. It also decreased the influx of water in this preparation. Norepinephrine was found to have an opposite effect—causing an increase in calcium influx from the bathing medium across the perfused gill preparation. The effect of calcitonin in inhibiting influx of calcium appears to be of physiological significance in maintaining normal calcium concentration, 2 mM, in the fish plasma against the higher calcium content of sea water, 8.4 mM. After spawning, there is a remarkable change in sensitivity of the gills to the two hormone preparations. Sensitivity to calcitonin increases and sensitivity to norepinephrine decreases markedly. These responses presumably reflect a marked decrease in circulating calcitonin and an increase in circulating catechol-amine concentration. Ineffective secretion of calcitonin may be the explanation for the death of fish experimentally returned from fresh water to sea water after spawning. These recent reports are significant in that they offer experimental evidence for the possibility that both PTH and calcitonin are capable of regulating calcium transport through the intermediation of cAMP in physiological receptor tissues.

6.2.6. Somatomedin Receptors, Multiplication-Stimulating Activity, and Other Growth Factors

Peptides with growth-promoting and insulinlike activity have been described and are known as somatomedins, nonsuppressible insulinlike activity (NSILA), and multiplication-stimulating activity (MSA). These peptides share certain chemical properties and biological interactions with specific receptors on cells *in vitro*. It is also known that insulin and proinsulin bind specifically but with decreased potency to the growth-promoting receptors. The amino acid sequence of NSILA, now renamed IGF-I (insulinlike growth factor I) has been determined, and a very high degree of homology was found with the A and B chains of insulin (Rinderknecht and Humbel, 1976). The region of IGF-I corresponding to the connecting peptide of proinsulin is shorter than that of human proinsulin (12 residues rather than 35). IGF-II shares a similar isoelectric point and amino acid composition with IGF-I. Somatomedin-C also shows an isoelectric point similar to that of the IGF factors. The latter, then, are quite analogous to proinsulin, but with shortened connecting peptide chains. This observation helps explain the fact that proinsulin shows a higher affinity for growth-promoting receptors than does insulin (Nissley *et al.*, 1977). Moreover, although proinsulin shows only 3–5% of the activity of insulin in stimulating glucose oxidation in fat cells or interaction with insulin receptors, it shows considerably greater relative potency in stimulating DNA synthesis in cultured fibroblasts *in vitro* and in interacting with the MSA receptor on chicken embryo fibroblasts (Nissley *et al.*, 1977). The latter group purified MSA to virtual homogeneity from culture media of buffalo rat liver cells *in vitro*. The purified MSA was labeled with ^{125}I and used as the ligand in the receptor studies (Rechler *et al.*, 1977). Rechler and Nissley (1977) summarized results of a recent workshop on the growth factors. Although the extensive structural homology between IGF-I and II and somatomedin-C as well as MSA is apparent from chemical or biological/receptor studies, or both, two of the factors, somatomedin-A and nonsuppressible insulinlike protein (NSILP), are not sufficiently similar to the other growth factors to be certain about homology. It has been proposed that NSILP may represent a form of NSILA bound to a plasma-binding protein.

6.2.7. Insulin Receptors

Further studies have been carried out on autoantibodies to insulin receptors. The work of Flier, Roth, Kahn, and their collaborators, outlined in the earlier chapter (Aurbach, 1976), has been extended considerably. Such antibodies cause severe insulin resistance. It is now apparent that antibodies directed to the insulin receptor can actually produce insulinlike activity *in vitro* and perhaps *in vivo* as well (Kahn *et al.*, 1977). Sera from three patients with severe insulin resistance stimulated glucose oxidation by fat cells *in vitro* (Kahn *et al.*, 1977). The terminal phase of the illness of one of these cases was marked by intractable hypoglycemia coupled with low concentrations of insulin in the circulation. In this instance, it appeared as though anti-insulin-receptor antibody had agonist activity and was the cause of the hypoglycemia. This would be entirely analogous to the agonistlike effects of the immune globulin fractions obtained from patients with Graves's disease. Autoantibodies against the insulin receptor also apparently are capable of blocking binding of [^{125}I]-MSA to somatomedin receptors (Rechler and Nissley, 1977).

6.3. Regulation of Adenylate Cyclase

6.3.1. Guanine Nucleotide Control

Guanine nucleotides are important in modulating hormone-regulated adenylate cyclase activity through formation of a guanine nucleotide–enzyme complex, producing an activated state of the enzyme as outlined in the earlier chapter in this series (Aurbach, 1976). Interaction of agonist with receptor allows more rapid access of GTP with a specific guanine nucleotide site on the enzyme (Aurbach, 1976).* The concerted actions of hormonal agonist and GTP produce a highly active state of adenylate cyclase. Indeed, under appropriate assay conditions, it can be proved that a guanine nucleotide is absolutely essential for adenylate cyclase activity. Commerical ATP preparations may contain sufficient GTP to allow significant adenylate cyclase activity without added guanine nucleotide (Kimura and Nagata, 1977).

New information developed through use of nucleotide analogues has provided some further understanding of how guanine nucleotides influence adenylate cyclase activity. Guanosine triphosphatases have been found in cell homogenates and cell membrane preparations. Guanosine

---

*Rendell *et al.* (1977) propose that hormone interaction with receptor does not influence rate of occupation of guanine nucleotide site with GTP, but rather accelerates the transition of an inactive enzyme GTP complex to an active one. In any event, attempts to determine directly specific binding of guanine nucleotides to a site strictly influenced by hormone have so far been unsuccessful.

triphosphatase (GTPase) activity could explain how the active state of adenylate cyclase in the presence of GTP can readily degrade (or "turn off") toward the inactive state by hydrolyzing GTP. Analogues such as guanylylimidodiphosphate [Gpp(NH)p] that contain poorly hydrolyzable bonds allow development of a persistently activated state of adenylate cyclase (Aurbach, 1976). Observations on the efficacy of Gpp(NH)p led some (Cuatrecasas *et al.*, 1975) to propose that activation of adenylate cyclase involves a pyrophosphorylation of the enzyme. The effects of Gpp(NH)p as well as Gpp(CH₂)p already had excluded monophosphory-lation via the gamma phosphate of GTP. Spiegel *et al.* (1977) showed that another analogue, Gp(CH₂)pp, with a methylene bond in the α-β position, is equally capable of allowing development of the active form of the enzyme stimulated by isoproterenol in turkey erythrocyte membranes or rat reticulocyte membranes. The methylenediphosphonate analogue was also effective in producing a high activity state of adenylate cyclase in rat liver membranes (Londos *et al.*, 1977). The efficacy of Gp(CH₂)pp in forming the active state of adenylate cyclase seems to eliminate the pyrophosphorylation mechanism proposed by Cuatrecasas *et al.* (1975). The stable diphosphonate configuration in the α-β position exemplified by Gp(CH₂)pp is not susceptible to pyrophosphorylytic cleavage. Another analogue capable of maintaining adenylate cyclase in the fully active state is GTPγS (Pfeuffer, 1977). The structures of the several GTP analogues are illustrated in Fig. 6.

The activated state of adenylate cyclase was studied further by Pfeuffer (1977). Interaction of the hormone with receptor appears to occur first

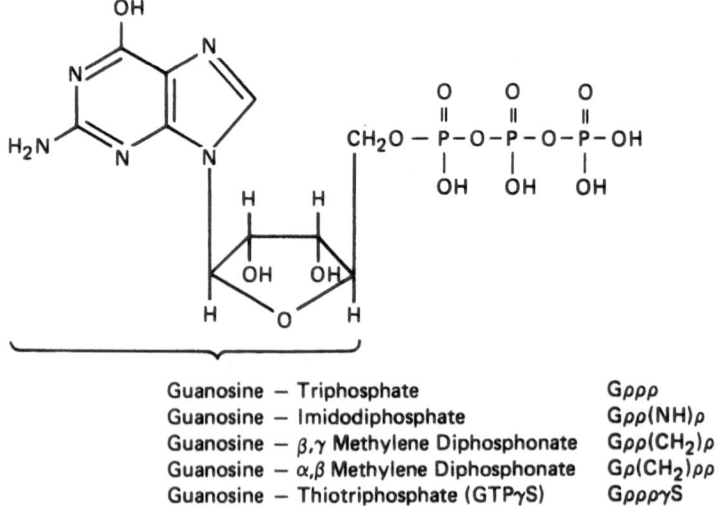

Guanosine – Triphosphate	Gppp
Guanosine – Imidodiphosphate	Gpp(NH)p
Guanosine – β,γ Methylene Diphosphonate	Gpp(CH₂)p
Guanosine – α,β Methylene Diphosphonate	Gp(CH₂)pp
Guanosine – Thiotriphosphate (GTPγS)	GpppγS

Fig. 6. Structure of guanosine nucleotide analogues capable of modulating hormone-regulated adenylate cyclase.

and allows more ready access of guanine nucleotides to a specific guanine nucleotide binding (G-binding) site. Pfeuffer (1977) showed that 5'-guanylic acid can maintain the G-binding site in an accessible state on activation of the hormone receptor with agonist. The latter nucleotide, 5'-GMP, however, is not capable of inducing the active state of the enzyme, but on addition of guanylylimidodiphosphate (see Fig. 8), formation of the activated state of the enzyme can occur without further addition of agonist. The G-binding protein can be isolated by affinity chromatography after solubilizing membranes pretreated with isoproterenol plus GMP (Pfeuffer, 1977).

6.3.2. Guanosine Triphosphatase

Cassel and Selinger (1976, 1977a,b), and Cassel *et al.* (1977) found that β-adrenergic catecholamines added to turkey erythrocyte membranes cause not only activation of adenylate cyclase but also stimulation of an apparently specific GTPase. The effect of catecholamines on the GTPase was stereospecific and inhibited by β-adrenergic blockers. The nonhydrolyzable guanine nucleotide analogue GTPγS caused inhibition of the specific GTPase (Cassel and Selinger, 1977b). Cassel and Selinger conclude that the specific GTPase is involved in the inactivation of the active form of adenylate cyclase. So far, hormone-stimulated GTPase has been observed only with turkey erythrocyte membranes and catecholamines. However, the concept of hormonally stimulated GTPase activity is compatible with the kinetics observed by Rendell *et al.* (1977) on glucagon-activated adenylate cyclase of the rat liver.

6.3.3. Guanine Nucleotides and Agonist Affinity

Rodbell *et al.* (1971) were the first to observe that guanine nucleotides could influence binding of hormones to receptor as well as the adenylate cyclase enzyme stimulated by hormones. This effect of guanine nucleotides has been observed with a number of hormone receptor–adenylate cyclase systems in membranes, but not in all instances (Spiegel *et al.*, 1976a). Gilman and his collaborators (Maguire *et al.*, 1976a) investigated this phenomenon further and found that in certain β-adrenergic-regulated systems, guanine nucleotide influence on receptor activity is observed only with binding of agonist. Williams and Lefkowitz (1977a) investigated this phenomenon using a ^{3}H-labeled agonist. They found that several guanine nucleotides as well as high concentrations of ATP were able to decrease specific binding of the agonist. Gpp(NH)p, however, was by far the most potent of the nucleotide analogues in reducing binding of the agonist. Guanine nucleotides do not influence receptor affinity for antagonists (Maguire *et al.*, 1976a; Williams and Lefkowitz, 1977a). Indeed, it is apparent that a change in affinity induced by guanine nucleotide for ligand binding to a receptor could be a criterion to establish the agonist nature of a β-adrenergic catecholamine. Such a test system obviously would be dependent on utilization of receptors from cell membrane sensitive to the guanine-nucleotide-induced shift in agonist affinity. Ross *et al.* (1977) also observed that mutant cells that contain no detectable adenylate cyclase activity but retain receptor show agonist binding similar to that of wild-type cells in the presence of guanine nucleotide. Affinity of soluble receptor for agonist is not reduced by guanine nucleotide (Williams and Lefkowitz, 1977a). These observations suggest that high affinity of receptor for agonist requires close coupling within the membrane to adenylate cyclase units. Conversely, when the adenylate cyclase unit is fully activated in the presence of guanine nucleotide, a low-affinity state of the receptor develops.

6.3.4. Cholera Toxin and Adenylate Cyclase

Interaction of cholera toxin with cell membranes leads to activation of adenylate cyclase and sensitizes adenylate cyclase responsiveness of cells to effects of hormonal agonists. Rudolph *et al.* (1977) reported that cholera toxin-activated turkey erythrocytes are more sensitive to epinephrine in accumulation of cAMP as well as in responsiveness determined by measuring potassium transport, a function known to be mediated by cAMP in these cells. They also showed that this sensitization to β-adrenergic catecholamines is produced without changing the number or affinity of β-adrenergic receptors on the cells. In membranes isolated from cells treated with cholera toxin, there is enhanced sensitivity of adenylate cyclase activation to isoproterenol when GTP is added. This enhanced sensitivity to GTP is very similar to the enhanced isoproterenol sensitivity of untreated membranes when exposed to guanylylimidodiphosphate or other nonhydrolyzable GTP analogues. The analogy between effects of guanylylimidodiphosphate on untreated membranes and the effects of cholera toxin in intact cells was discussed in the earlier chapter (Aurbach, 1976). Cassel and Selinger (1977b) extended the analysis of cholera toxin effects to GTPase activity. They showed that effects of cholera toxin on turkey erythrocyte membranes is associated not only with enhanced sensitivity of isoproterenol/GTP, but also with concomitant inactivation of GTPase. Indeed, they point out that the toxin-treated adenylate cyclase was maximally activated in the presence of isoproterenol by either GTP or guanylylimidodiphosphate, while adenylate cyclase not treated with toxin was stimulated by hormone plus GTP to only one fifth the activity achieved with hormone plus guanylylimidodiphosphate. They also observed that the toxin-treated enzyme remained active after stimulation by isoproterenol plus GTP for an extended period, and this active state was not inhibitable by the β-adrenergic blocker propranolol. Again, this was analogous to refractoriness to propranolol of the "holocatalytic"

(Aurbach, 1976) state of the enzyme (preactivated with isoproterenol plus guanylylimidodiphosphate, the nonhydrolyzable analogue of GTP). Levinson and Bloom (1977) also concluded that altered guanine nucleotide hydrolysis was the basis for enhanced adenylate cyclase activity in response to cholera toxin added to mouse neuroblastoma cells. They also made the analogy between effects of guanylylimidodiphosphate on the normal enzyme and that of GTP on the cholera toxin-treated enzyme. Still another analogy between the action of cholera toxin and guanylylimidodiphosphate is an apparent inhibition of the activation produced by fluoride.

Moss and Vaughan and their collaborators (Moss and Vaughan, 1977a,b; Moss et al., 1976, 1977) studied further the biochemical mechanism for choleragen activation of adenylate cyclase. It had been known earlier that a thiol and NAD were among the factors necessary for choleragen activation of adenylate cyclase. The thiol is necessary for release of the A-1 active subunit of the toxin. Vaughan and her colleagues (Moss and Vaughan, 1977a; Moss et al., 1977) found suggestive evidence that NAD is a substrate for enzymatic activity of the toxin A-1 subunit that possibly catalyzes ADP ribosylation of a protein important in the adenylate cyclase enzyme activity. ADP ribosylation is a reaction (Fig. 7) that had been observed earlier in connection with the mechanism of action of diphtheria toxin (Kandel et al., 1974). In addition to a thiol and NAD, M. Gill (1976) and Wodnar-Filipowicz and Lai (1976) had found that there were still other factors in cell supernatants required for choleragen activation of adenylate cyclase. Moss and Vaughan (1977b) investigated further

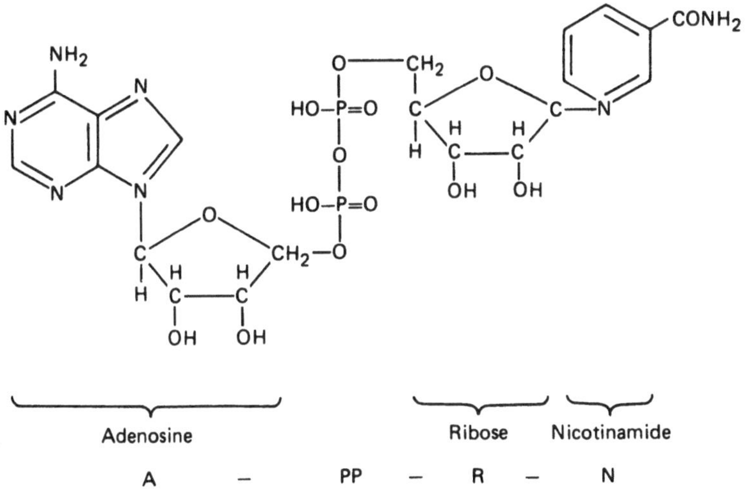

APPRN + PROTEIN ⇌ APPR − PROTEIN + NICOTINAMIDE

Fig. 7. Mechanism for ADP ribosylation of protein.

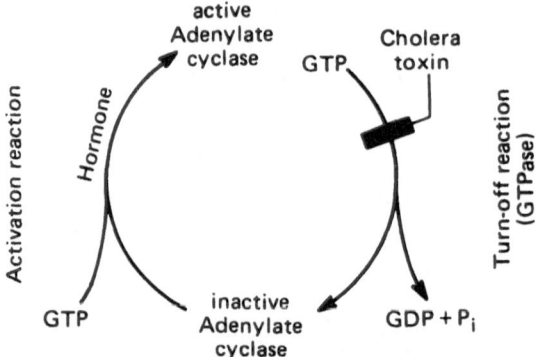

Fig. 8. Model for control of adenylate cyclase activity by guanine nucleotides. GTPase activity is the apparent mechanism allowing deactivation of the active form of adenylate cyclase enzyme. Activation of the enzyme by cholera toxin appears to be mediated by inhibiting GTPase action. From Cassel and Selinger (1977b).

the requirement for additional cofactors in toxin activation of adenylate cyclase. They showed that with brain adenylate cyclase, the following factors are necessary in addition to NAD and thiol for choleragen activation of enzyme: (1) GTP, (2) adenylate cyclase activator protein, (3) calcium, and (4) another protein as yet unidentified that is found in the boiled supernatant fraction from brain. This work is of significance in that it may lead to purification of all the factors required and allow complete understanding of how cholera toxin activates adenylate cyclase.* This information obviously will be important in helping to understand how hormones activate the adenylate cyclase system. This work also suggests that a complex series of proteins as well as cofactors are required for the choleragen effect, and if the latter is mediated entirely by inhibition of GTPase, then the inactivation of the latter enzyme will also prove to be a complex series of reactions. A highly simplified model for control of adenylate cyclase activity is illustrated in Fig. 8.

6.4. Protein Kinases

Further information accumulates indicating that the action of cAMP in controlling a variety of metabolic processes is mediated through interaction with specific protein kinases. The earlier review (Aurbach, 1976) cited the primary work of Krebs and several other investigators in this

*Cassel and Pfeuffer (1978), Gill and Meren (1978), and Johnson *et al.* (1978) recently reported that the 42,000-dalton guanine nucleotide (G-binding) protein is the specific substrate affected by cholera toxin in activating adenylate cyclase. The G-binding protein is specifically labeled by α-^{32}P-NAD (to form ADP-ribose-GN protein) and, labeled as such, can also be purified on a GTP-affinity matrix.

area that established the biochemical sequence of events for cAMP activation of protein kinases. In general, cAMP-sensitive kinases are composed of two types of subunits—the receptor (R) subunit and the catalytic (C) subunit. On interaction with cAMP, the R subunit dissociates from the C subunit and the latter is thereby activated. The activated C subunit in the free form is no longer subject to cAMP regulation. Reconstitution of the R and C subunits restores cAMP dependence. Each subunit, the R and the C component, respectively, is a dimer. The entire complex (R_2C_2) exists as a 186,000-dalton complex. On interaction with 2 mol cAMP, it dissociates into a R_2–$cAMP_2$ (110,000 daltons) plus 2-C (catalytic units) of 38,000 daltons each. cGMP kinases also exist as dimers with a molecular weight of the inactive complex being 165,000. On interaction with 2 mol cGMP, a complex of the nature of E_2–$cGMP_2$ is formed without dissociation of R subunit. Thus, although both cAMP- and cGMP-regulated kinase complexes each interact with 2 mol of the corresponding cyclic nucleotide, there is no induced separation of R subunit from the cGMP-dependent kinase. Recent reports (Gill, G. N., 1977; Lincoln and Corbin, 1977) suggest, however, that cAMP and cGMP kinase complexes are similar in overall physical property, are predicted to be similar in overall steric configurations, and show similar amino acid composition. Moreover, it has been shown that substrate specificities of cAMP and cGMP kinases overlap. Both cGMP-dependent and cAMP-dependent kinases are capable of catalyzing phosphorylation of histone, pyruvate kinase, glycogen synthase, and phosphorylase-b kinase (Lincoln and Corbin, 1977). Studies from Rosen's laboratory (Rangel-Aldao and Rosen, 1976, 1977) established that autophosphorylation of cardiac-muscle-cAMP-dependent protein kinase can be an important regulatory mechanism. The dissociated enzyme (i.e., cAMP-activated) C subunit can catalyze the transfer of phosphate from the gamma phosphate of ATP to two specific serine residues in R_2. In the absence of cAMP, the phosphorylated R_2 reassociates with the C unit much more slowly (about 20% the rate) than does the nonphosphorylated R_2 (Rangel-Aldao and Rosen, 1977). Thus, phosphorylation of the R_2 unit would tend to prolong the biological effect of a given concentration of cAMP intracellularly. Conversely, a protein phosphatase, identified by Chou *et al.* (1977), that specifically dephosphorylates the phosphorylated R_2 unit would tend to allow more rapid reassociation of R_2 and C subunits and thereby reduce the period of activation in the biological system *in vivo*. Because the phosphatase acts specifically on the dissociated phospho-R subunit, the phosphatase can appear to be cAMP-dependent (Chou *et al.*, 1977). All this work on phosphorylated R_2 components and its phosphatase has been shown primarily in bovine heart. To what extent this interesting regulatory phenomenon involving phospho-R subunits applies to other systems is unknown. It is of particular interest to cite in this regard the observation of DeLorenzo and

Greengard (1973) wherein activation of a membrane-bound phosphoprotein phosphatase was observed on addition of cAMP to a toad bladder membrane preparation.

Coffino and his associates (Lemaire and Coffino, 1977) pursued studies on cAMP-resistant S-49 mouse lymphoma cells and found mutants that possess abnormal protein kinases as the explanation for resistance to cAMP (Coffino *et al.*, 1976). Three subclasses of kinase mutants have been found: (1) one that requires increased concentrations of cAMP for activation (K_m type mutant), (2) a V_{max} type mutant wherein maximal rates of enzyme activity are much reduced below wild type, and (3) mutants in which no enzymatic activity is detectable (Lemaire and Coffino, 1977). The mutation involves the R subunit of the protein kinase.

6.4.1. Cell Regulation by Occupied Cyclic AMP Receptors

There are several instances wherein discrepancies between cAMP formation and biological activity have been observed. Dufau *et al.* (1977) investigated this phenomenon in the testis, wherein low concentrations of gonadotropin can cause stimulation of steroidogenesis without detectable change in cAMP production. Dufau *et al.* (1977) found, however, that there was a chorionic gonadotropin dose-dependent increase in occupancy of cAMP receptors by endogenous cAMP with a preparation of isolated Leydig cells *in vitro*. The gonadotropin dose–response effect on testosterone production corresponded very closely to the dose–response effect on receptor-bound cAMP. There was a concomitant decrease in free cAMP receptors. Schwoch and Hilz (1977) carried out a similar type of analysis on the liver of rats treated with glucagon. They found a sharp increase in bound cAMP within minutes after injecting glucagon into the animals. There was a corresponding increase in liver protein kinase activity that became maximal within the same 2-min period as the increase in bound cAMP. Keely and Corbin (1977) examined further the involvement of cAMP-dependent kinase in regulation of contractile force of the heart. They studied cAMP concentrations, force of contraction, phosphorylase activity, and protein kinase activity in perfused rat heart. Epinephrine caused an increase in all these parameters, but doses of epinephrine lower than those producing a detectable increase in cAMP caused increases in force of contraction. The increased force, however, correlated well with the increase in activity of protein kinase. Results of this work with the heart are similar to results of the same group in studying the active form of protein kinase in fat tissue *in vivo* (Corbin *et al.*, 1975). These several reports give important descriptions of useful methods painstakingly worked out to analyze for activated protein kinase and bound cAMP. The results presented in these reports lead to the conclusion that the amount of bound cAMP (and consequently the fraction of active kinase) is the function that correlates best and thus presumably is causal in effecting the biological response.

6.5. Calcium Regulation of Cyclic Nucleotide Concentration

Calcium-binding proteins found in brain and other tissues seem to be important in regulating adenylate cyclase as well as cyclic nucleotide phosphodiesterase. These proteins appear to represent one mechanism whereby calcium can control cyclic nucleotide concentrations *in vivo*.

Ho *et al.* (1977) purified calcium-activatable cyclic nucleotide phosphodiesterase from bovine heart utilizing DEAE chromatography in buffers containing alternately calcium or EGTA plus calcium-dependent modulator protein. These procedures take advantage of the fact that in the presence of calcium, the modulator protein binds to phosphodiesterase and thereby changes its elution pattern in DEAE cellulose chromatography. Klee (1977) reported on a conformational transition occurring in cAMP-phosphodiesterase on binding of the protein activator in the presence of calcium. Both the latter groups indicate that activation of the phosphodiesterase proceeds in two steps. First, calcium is bound to the protein activator, then the calcium activator complex binds to the cyclic nucleotide phosphodiesterase. The studies of Klee were carried out on pig brain phosphodiesterase. The apparent dissocation constant for calcium in activating the phosphodiesterase complex from bovine heart was approximately 2 μM (Ho *et al.*, 1977). Highly purified calcium-activatable cyclic nucleotide phosphodiesterase in the latter study was prepared taking advantage of the DEAE cellulose chromatography maneuver described above. Gnegy *et al.* (1977) described supersensitivity of striatal dopaminergic adenylate cyclase activity in rats treated with dopaminergic inhibitors, e.g., haloperidol, clozapine, or butaclamol. In the preparations made from supersensitized rats, there appeared to be an increased content of particulate-bound adenylate cyclase activator protein. This work suggests that another mechanism for control of cell metabolism could be brought about by governing the compartmentalization of calcium-binding protein regulator.

Kretsinger (1976) reviewed the literature on calcium-binding proteins with particular emphasis on chemistry and physical properties. In general, it is the carboxylate ions of aspartate and glutamate residues in proteins that coordinate with calcium. There is no obvious correlation between the affinity of the protein for calcium and the number of carboxylate ligands in the protein. Kretsinger also summarized amino acid composition data and affinity constants for a variety of calcium-binding proteins from diverse sources.

6.6. Cyclic Nucleotides in the Extracellular Fluids

cAMP and cGMP have been detected in most of the body fluids including plasma, urine, cerebrospinal fluid, saliva, pancreatic, biliary, and gastric secretions (Aurbach and Chase, 1976; Aurbach, 1976; Broadus, 1977; Murad and Aurbach, 1977). So far, clinical measurements of cyclic nucleotide metabolism have been most clearly of utility in terms of parathyroid function. The initial observations of Chase and Aurbach (Chase and Aurbach, 1967, 1968; Chase et al., 1969) indicated that parathyroid gland secretory activity was a major influence on generation of cAMP within the kidney and excretion of the cyclic nucleotide into the urine, and that urinary cAMP determinations could be of clinical diagnostic utility. These observations have been confirmed in a number of laboratories and utility of urinary cAMP determination has been established as a diagnostic parameter for parathyroid disorders. Broadus (1977) presented an excellent review of cyclic nucleotide clearance and discussion of factors affecting plasma cAMP and nephrogenous cAMP and their clearance into the urine. Since urinary excretion of cAMP reflects that cleared from plasma as well as directly contributed by the kidney and since PTH regulates predominantly nephrogenously generated cAMP, it is important in certain instances to be able to segregate nephrogenous cAMP from that cleared from the plasma. For this purpose, it is necessary to develop methods for measuring plasma cAMP. Babka et al. (1976) utilized radioimmunoassay for cAMP in plasma filtrates prepared by ultrafiltration. Broadus et al. (1977) utilized the competitive binding assay of Gilman, but were careful to purify the cyclic nucleotides from plasma by chromatography to remove interfering substances in this assay. The problems of interfering substances in radioimmunoassays or competitive binding assays for cAMP in biological fluids were reviewed by Broadus (1977). M. Goldberg (1977) found that the sensitive radioimmunoassay of Harper and Brooker (1975), which depends on acetylation of the sample, can be validly applied to plasma samples after dilution of plasma with an equal volume of 0.1 N HCl. Spiegel, Windeck, and Aurbach (unpublished) confirmed the latter findings but found that addition of an equal volume of 0.01 N HCl gives uniform and reproducible results. Addition of 0.1 N HCl, as recommended in the report of M. Goldberg (1977), causes precipitation of plasma components and interferes with recovery. Appropriate procedures should be instituted in collecting plasma for cAMP determinations to ensure inhibition of endogenous cyclic nucleotide phosphodiesterase (discussed by Broadus, 1977). An effective method is to collect plasma directly into EDTA (Broadus, 1977).

6.6.1. Nephrogenous Cyclic AMP in Parathyroid and Related Disorders

Broadus *et al.* (1977) carried out an extensive analysis of cAMP clearance in normal subjects and in subjects with hyperparathyroidism, hypoparathyroidism, and varying degrees of renal failure. Determinations of plasma and urinary cAMP and plasma and urinary creatinine allowed simultaneous calculations of urinary cAMP excretion expressed in a variety of parametric forms: cAMP excretion in nmol/min; cAMP excretion in nmol/mg creatinine; in nmol/100 ml glomerular filtrate (GF); cAMP clearance; clearance ratio cAMP/creatinine; and nephrogenous cAMP, nmol/100 ml GF. Presentation of the data as nephrogenous cAMP expressed in nmol/100 ml GF gave the sharpest differentiation among hypoparathyroid, normal, and hyperparathyroid groups and the least overlap. This determination obviously requires measurement of plasma cAMP. Almost as good discrimination among the groups was afforded by expressing total urinary cAMP as a function of GFR in terms of nmol cAMP/100 ml GF (Fig. 9). The latter parameter represents a simple correction of urinary cAMP/creatinine ratio for plasma creatinine ($U_{cAMP}/U_{Cr} \times P_{Cr}$). Broadus *et al.* (1977) discussed extensively the disadvantages of expressing urinary cAMP as simply a rate (per unit time or per mg creatinine). They found that sex differences (females excrete less creatinine and thus show higher cAMP/creatinine ratios than males) and any debilitating illness that decreases creatinine excretion would similarly spuriously increase the latter ratio. Artifactually high ratios of cAMP/creatinine excretion are also evidenced in hyperthyroidism [see also Carter and Heath (1977) and the discussion in the earlier chapter (Aurbach, 1976)], wherein there is also diminished excretion of creatinine. Although lithium interferes with activation of adenylate cyclase by certain hormones *in vitro*, doses of lithium that are effective in mental illness do not inhibit the clinical cAMP response to PTH (Spiegel *et al.*, 1976b).

The study of Broadus *et al.* (1977) indicates that urinary cAMP as a function of GFR (U_{cAMP} in nmol/100 ml GF) is a very satisfactory routine determination. Interpretation of this parameter would be affected, however, with significant degrees of chronic renal disease wherein plasma cAMP concentration can be elevated and total excretion of cAMP (nephrogenous as well as that cleared by glomerular filtration) can be

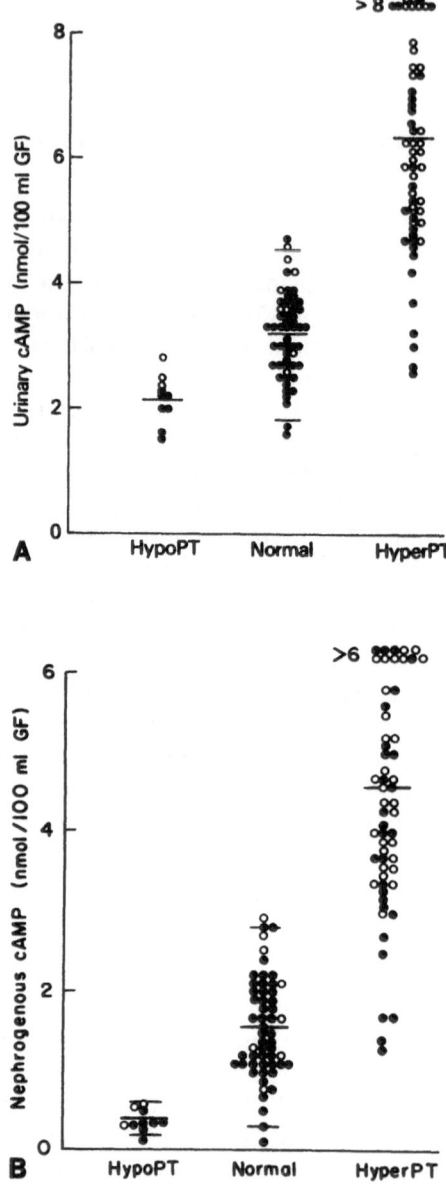

Fig. 9. Urinary excretion of cAMP in differing states of parathyroid function. (A) Urinary cAMP expressed as excretion per 100 ml glomerular filtrate; (B) urinary cAMP excretion expressed as nephrogenous cAMP excretion.

reduced.* Broadus *et al.* (1977) suggest, however, that this is not a serious problem in interpretation as long as GFR exceeds 20 ml/min. A recent preliminary report (Hong and Forrest, 1977) suggests that the increased plasma concentration in chronic renal disease is dependent on β-adrenergic catecholamines and can be abolished by administration of propranolol. Increased physical activity and stress are other potential causes for increases in plasma cAMP concentration (Broadus, 1977).

Brodows *et al.* (1976) examined further the effects of hypoglycemia on plasma cAMP. In normal subjects, plasma cAMP increased 2- to 3-fold, similar to the finding originally described by Hamet *et al.* (1975). Both groups conclude that the rise in plasma cAMP in response to hypoglycemia is mediated by β-adrenergic stimulation. The response does not occur in adrenalectomized subjects, in sympathectomized subjects, or when propranolol is administered.

References

Ahlquist, R. P., 1948, A study of the adrenotropic receptors, *Am. J. Physiol.* **153**:586–600.

Atlas, D., and Levitzki, A., 1977, Probing of β-adrenergic receptors by novel fluorescent β-adrenergic blockers, *Proc. Natl. Acad. Sci. U.S.A.* **74**:5290–5294.

Atlas, D., Steer, M. L., and Levitzki, A., 1976, Affinity label for beta-adrenergic receptor in turkey erythrocytes, *Proc. Natl. Acad. Sci. U.S.A.* **73**:1921–1925.

Aurbach, G. D., 1976, Hormone receptors, cyclic nucleotides, and control of cell function, in: *The Year in Metabolism 1975–1976* (N. Freinkel, ed.), pp. 1–43, Plenum Medical Book Company, New York.

Aurbach, G. D., and Chase, L. R., 1976, Cyclic nucleotides and biochemical actions of parathyroid hormone and calcitonin, in: *Handbook of Physiology* (R. O. Greep and E. B. Astwood, eds.), Section 7, *Endocrinology*, Vol. VII, *Parathyroid Gland* (G. D. Aurbach, ed.), pp. 353–381, American Physiological Society, Washington, D. C.

---

*Patients with chronic renal disease apparently also show diminished responsiveness to exogenous PTH as determined by urinary cAMP determinations (Monn *et al.*, 1976; Lilienfeld-Toal *et al.*, 1974). This defective response has been observed in children (Monn *et al.*, 1976) as well as in adults (Lilienfeld-Toal *et al.*, 1974). The apparent decrease in renal responsiveness to PTH presumably represents, in addition to the rise in cAMP in plasma in uremia, another abnormality that would decrease the diagnostic utility of urinary cAMP clearance measurements for determination of parathyroid function. So far, there is no definitive explanation for the decreased responsiveness in chronic renal failure. The defective response might reflect simply a decrease in number of functioning nephrons, a specific defect in transport of cAMP across the luminal border of the renal tubule, or possibly a reduction in numbers of PTH receptors (down regulation of receptors) attendant on prolonged excessive concentrations of PTH in the circulation. The latter possibility is suggested by a report by Forte *et al.* (1976) that rats made vitamin-D-deficient, a condition usually associated with excessive secretion of PTH, show decreased responsiveness to PTH in terms of phosphate and cAMP excretion into the urine.

Babka, J. C., Bower, R. H., and Sode, J., 1976, Nephrogenous cyclic AMP levels in primary hyperparathyroidism, *Arch. Intern. Med.* **136**:1140–1144.

Baldessarini, R. J., 1977, Schizophrenia, *N. Engl. J. Med.* **297**:988–995.

Ball, J. H., Kaminsky, N. I., Hardman, J. G., Broadus, A. E., Sutherland, E. W., and Liddle, G. W., 1972, Effects of catecholamines and adrenergic blocking agents on plasma and urinary cyclic nucleotides in man, *J. Clin. Invest.* **51**:2124–2129.

Batzri, S., Selinger, Z., Schramm, M., and Rubinovitch, M. R., 1973, Potassium release mediated by the epinephrine alpha-receptor in rat parotid slices, *J. Biol. Chem.* **248**:361–368.

Bennett, V., O'Keefe, E., and Cuatrecasas, P., 1975, Mechanism of action of cholera toxin and the mobile receptor theory of hormone receptor adenylate cyclase interactions, *Proc. Natl. Acad. Sci. U.S.A.* **72**:33–37.

Berg, D. K., Kelly, R. B., Sargent, P. B., Williamson, P., and Hall, Z. W., 1972, Binding of alpha-bungarotoxin to acetylcholine receptors in mammalian muscle, *Proc. Natl. Acad. Sci. U.S.A.* **69**:147–151.

Bernheimer, H., Birkmayer, W., Hornykiewicz, O., Jellinger, K., and Seitelberger, F. S., 1973, Brain dopamine and the syndromes of Parkinson and Huntington: Clinical, morphological and neurochemical correlations, *J. Neurol. Sci.* **20**:415–455.

Besser, G. M., Parkes, L., Edwards, C. R. W., Forsyth, I. A., and McNeilly, A. S., 1972, Galactorrhea: Successful treatment with reduction of plasma prolactin levels by brom-ergocryptine, *Br. Med. J.* **3**:669–672.

Biddulph, D. M., and Wrenn, R. W., 1977, Effects of parathyroid hormone on cyclic AMP, cyclic GMP, and efflux of calcium in isolated renal tubules, *J. Cyclic Nucleotide Res.* **3**:129–138.

Bilezikian, J. P., Spiegel, A. M., Brown, E. M., and Aurbach, G. D., 1977, Identification and persistence of beta-adrenergic receptors during maturation of the rat reticulocyte, *Mol. Pharmacol.* **13**:775–785.

Broadus, A. E., 1977, Clinical cyclic nucleotide research, *Adv. Cyclic Nucleotide Res.* **8**:509–548.

Broadus, A. E., Mahaffey, J. E., Bartter, F. C., and Neer, R. M., 1977, Nephrogenous cyclic adenosine monophosphate as a parathyroid function test, *J. Clin. Invest.* **60**:771–783.

Brodows, R. G., Ensinck, J. W., and Campbell, R. G., 1976, Mechanism of plasma cyclic AMP response to hypoglycemia in man, *Metabolism* **25**:659–663.

Brown, E. M., Aurbach, G. D., Hauser, D., and Troxler, F., 1976, Beta-adrenergic receptor interactions: Characterization of iodohydroxybenzylpindolol as a specific ligand, *J. Biol. Chem.* **251**:1232–1238.

Brown, E. M., Hurwitz, S., Woodard, C. J., and Aurbach, G. D., 1977a, Direct identification of beta-adrenergic receptors on isolated bovine parathyroid cells, *Endocrinology* **100**:1703–1709.

Brown, E. M., Carroll, R. J., and Aurbach, G. D., 1977b, Dopaminergic stimulation of cyclic AMP accumulation and parathyroid hormone release from dispersed bovine parathyroid cells, *Proc. Natl. Acad. Sci. U.S.A.* **74**:4210–4213.

Burt, D. R., Enna, S. J., Creese, I., and Snyder, S. H., 1975, Dopamine receptor binding in the corpus striatum of mammalian brain, *Proc. Natl. Acad. Sci. U.S.A.* **72**:4655–4659.

Butcher, F. R., 1975, The role of calcium and cyclic nucleotides in alpha-amylase release from slices of rat parotid: Studies with the divalent cation ionophore A23187, *Metabolism* **24**:409–418.

Calne, D. B., Teychenne, P. F., Claveria, L. E., Eastman, R., Greenacre, J. K., and Petrie, A., 1974. Bromocryptine in Parkinsonism, *Br. Med. J.* **4**:442–444.

Cannon, W. B., and Rosenbleuth, A., 1937, *Autonomic Neuroeffector Systems*, Macmillan, New York.

Carter, D. J., and Heath, D. A., 1977, The effect of treatment of hyper- and hypothyroidism on urinary excretion of cyclic adenosine 3′,5′-monophosphate, *Acta Endocrinol.* **84**:542–547.

Cassel, D., and Pfeuffer, R., 1978, Mechanism of cholera toxin action: Covalent modification of the guanyl nucleotide-binding protein of the adenylate cyclase system, *Proc. Natl. Acad. Sci. USA* **75**:2669–2673.

Cassel, D., and Selinger, Z., 1976, Catecholamine-stimulated GTPase activity in turkey erythrocyte membranes, *Biochim. Biophys. Acta* **452**:538–551.

Cassel, D., and Selinger, Z., 1977a, Activation of turkey erythrocyte adenylate cyclase and blocking of the catecholamine-stimulated GTPase by guanosine 5′-(gamma-THIO) triphosphate, *Biochem. Biophys. Res. Commun.* **77**:868–873.

Cassel, D., and Selinger, Z., 1977b, Mechanism of adenylate cyclase activation by cholera toxin: Inhibition of GTP hydrolysis at the regulatory site, *Proc. Natl. Acad. Sci. U.S.A.* **74**:3307–3311.

Cassel, D., Levkovitz, H., and Selinger, Z., 1977, The regulatory GTPase cycle of turkey erythrocyte adenylate cyclase of turkey erythrocyte membrane, *J. Cyclic Nucleotide Res.* **3**:393–406.

Chabardes, D., Imbert-Teboul, M., Montegut, M., Clique, A., and Morel, F., 1976, Distribution of calcitonin-sensitive adenylate cyclase activity along the rabbit kidney tubule, *Proc. Natl. Acad. Sci. U.S.A.* **73**:3608–3612.

Chabardes, D., Imbert-Teboul, M., Gagnan-Brunette, M., and Morel, F., 1978, Distribution of adenylate cyclase-linked hormone receptors in the nephron, in: *Endocrinology of Calcium Metabolism* (D. H. Copp and R. V. Talmage, eds.), pp. 209–215, Excerpta Medica, Amsterdam.

Chambers, D. J., Schafer, H., Laugharn, J. A., Jr., Johnstone, J., Zanelli, J. M., Parsons, J. A., Bitensky, L., and Chayen, J., 1978, Dose-related activation by PTH of specific enzymes in various regions of the kidney, in: *Endocrinology of Calcium Metabolism* (D. H. Copp and R. V. Talmage, eds.), pp. 216–220, Excerpta Medica, Amsterdam.

Charness, M. E., Bylund, D. B., Beckman, B. S., Hollenberg, M. D., and Snyder, S. H., 1976, Independent variation of beta-adrenergic receptor binding and catecholamine-stimulated adenylate cyclase activity in rat erythrocytes, *Life Sci.* **19**:243–249.

Charreau, E. H., Attramadal, A., Torjesen, P. A., Calandra, R., Purvis, K., and Hansson, V., 1977, Androgen stimulation of prolactin receptors in rat prostate, *Mol. Cell. Endocrinol.* **7**:1–7.

Chase, L. R., and Aurbach, G. D., 1967, Parathyroid function and the renal excretion of 3′,5′-adenylic acid, *Proc. Natl. Acad. Sci. U.S.A.* **58**:518–525.

Chase, L. R., and Aurbach, G. D., 1968, Renal adenyl cyclase: Anatomical separation of sites sensitive to parathyroid hormone and vasopressin, *Science* **159**:545–547.

Chase, L. R., Melson, G. L., and Aurbach, G. D., 1969, Pseudohypoparathyroidism: Defective excretion of 3′,5′-AMP in response to parathyroid hormone, *J. Clin. Invest.* **48**:1832–1844.

Chasin, M., Rivkin, I., Mamrak, F., Samaniego, S. G., and Hess, S. M., 1971, Alpha and beta-adrenergic receptors as mediators of accumulation of cyclic adenosine 3′,5′-monophosphate in specific areas of guinea pig brain, *J. Biol. Chem.* **246**:3037–3041.

Chou, C.-K., Alfano, J., and Rosen, O. M., 1977, Purification of phosphoprotein phosphatase from bovine cardiac muscle that catalyzes dephosphorylation of cyclic AMP-binding protein component of protein kinase, *J. Biol. Chem.* **252**:2855–2859.

Clement-Cormier, Y., Kebabian, J. W., Petzold, G. L., and Greengard, P., 1974, Dopamine-sensitive adenylate cyclase in mammalian brain: A possible site of action of antipsychotic drugs, *Proc. Natl. Acad. Sci. U.S.A.* **71**:1113–1117.

Coffino, P., Bourne, H. R., Friedrich, U., Hochman, J., Insel, P. A., Lemaire, I., Melmon, K. L., and Tomkins, G. M., 1976, Molecular mechanisms of cyclic AMP action: A genetic approach, *Recent Prog. Horm. Res.* **32**:669–684.

Corbin, J. D., Keely, S. L., Soderling, T. R., and Park, C. R., 1975, Hormonal regulation of adenosine 3′,5′-monophosphate-dependent protein kinase, *Adv. Cyclic Nucleotide Res.* **5**:265–279.

Cotzias, G. C., VanWoert, M. H., and Schiffer, L. M., 1967, Aromatic amino acids and modification of Parkinsonism, *N. Engl. J. Med.* **276**:374–379.

Crine, P., Benjannet, S., Seidah, N. G., Lis, M., and Chretien, M., 1977, *In vitro* biosynthesis of beta-endorphin, gamma-lipotropin, and beta-lipotropin by the pars intermedia of beef pituitary glands, *Proc. Natl. Acad. Sci. U.S.A.* **74**:4276–4280.

Cuatrecasas, P., Jacobs, S., and Bennett, V., 1975, Activation of adenylate cyclase by phosphoramidate and phosphonate analogs of GTP: Possible role of covalent enzyme–substrate intermediates in the mechanism of hormonal activation, *Proc. Natl. Acad. Sci. U.S.A.* **72**:1739–1743.

Dale, H. H., 1906, On some physiological actions of ergot, *J. Physiol.* **34**:163–206.

DeLorenzo, R. J., and Greengard, P., 1973, Activation by adenosine 3′,5′-monophosphate of a membrane-bound phosphoprotein phosphatase from toad bladder, *Proc. Natl. Acad. Sci. U.S.A.* **70**:1831–1835.

DeMeyts, P., Roth, J., Neville, D. M., Jr., Gavin, J. R., III, and Lesniak, M. A., 1973, Insulin interactions with its receptors: Experimental evidence for negative cooperativity, *Biochem. Biophys. Res. Commun.* **55**:154–161.

Dufau, M. L., Tsuruhara, T., Horner, K. A., Podesta, E., and Catt, K. J., 1977, Intermediate role of adenosine 3′,5′-cyclic monophosphate and protein kinase during gonadotropin-induced steroidogenesis in testicular interstitial cells, *Proc. Natl. Acad. Sci. U.S.A.* **74**:3419–3423.

Ellis, S., and Beckett, S. B., 1963, Mechanism of the potassium mobilizing action of epinephrine and glucagon, *J. Pharmacol. Exp. Ther.* **142**:318–326.

Forte, L. R., Nichols, G. A., and Anast, C. S., 1976, Renal adenylate cyclase and the interrelationship between parathyroid hormone and vitamin D in the regulation of urinary phosphate and adenosine cyclic monophosphate excretion, *J. Clin. Invest.* **57**:559–568.

Gill, D. M., 1976, Multiple roles of erythrocyte supernatant in the action of adenylate cyclase by *Vibrio cholerae* toxin *in vitro*, *J. Infect. Dis.* **133**:S55–S63.

Gill, D. M., and Meren, R., 1978, ADP-ribosylation of membrane proteins catalyzed by cholera toxin: Basis of the activation of adenylate cyclase, *Proc. Natl. Acad. Sci. USA* **75**:3050–3054.

Gill, G. N., 1977, A hypothesis concerning the structure of cAMP- and cGMP-dependent protein kinases, *J. Cyclic Nucleotide Res.* **3**:153–162.

Gnegy, M., Uzunov, P., and Costa, E., 1977, Participation of an endogenous calcium-binding activator in the development of drug-induced supersensitivity of striatal dopamine receptors, *J. Pharmacol. Exp. Ther.* **202**:558–564.

Goldberg, L. I., Sonneville, P. F., and McNay, J. L., 1968, An investigation of the structural requirements for dopamine-like renal vasodilatation: Phenylethylamines and apomorphine, *J. Pharmacol. Exp. Ther.* **163**:188–197.

Goldberg, M. L., 1977, Radioimmunoassay for adenosine 3′,5′-cyclic monophosphate and guanosine 3′,5′-cyclic monophosphate in human blood, urine and cerebrospinal fluid, *Clin. Chem.* **23**:576.

Greenberg, D. A., and Snyder, S. H., 1977, Selective labeling of alpha-noradrenergic receptors in rat brain with [^{3}H]dihydroergocryptine, *Life Sci.* **20**:927–931.

Greengard, P., and Kebabian, J. W., 1974, Role of cyclic AMP in synaptic transmission in the mammalian peripheral nervous system, *Fed. Proc. Fed. Am. Soc. Exp. Biol.* **33**:1059–1067.

Guillemin, R., Vargo, T., Rossier, J., Minick, S., Ling, N., Rivier, C., Vale, W., and Bloom, F., 1977, Beta-endorphin and adrenocorticotropin are secreted concomitantly by the pituitary gland, *Science* **197**:1367–1369.

Haga, T., Ross, E. M., Anderson, H. J., and Gilman, A. G., 1977, Adenylate cyclase permanently uncoupled from hormone receptors in a novel variant of S49 mouse lymphoma cells, *Proc. Natl. Acad. Sci. U.S.A.* **74**:2016–2020.

Hamet, P., Lowder, S. C., Hardman, J. G., and Liddle, G. W., 1975, Effect of hypoglycemia on extracellular levels of cyclic AMP in man, *Metabolism* **24**:1139–1144.

Harden, T. K., Wolfe, B. B., Sporn, J. R., Poulos, B. K., and Molinoff, P. B., 1977a, Effects of 6-hydroxydopamine on the development of the beta-adrenergic receptor/adenylate cyclase system in rat cerebral cortex, *J. Pharmacol. Exp. Ther.* **203**:132–143.

Harden, T. K., Wolfe, B. B., Sporn, J. R., Perkins, J. P., and Molinoff, P. B., 1977b, Ontogeny of beta-adrenergic receptors in rat cerebral cortex, *Brain Res.* **125**:99–108.

Harper, J. F., and Brooker, G., 1975, Femtomole sensitive radioimmunoassay for cyclic AMP and cyclic GMP after 2′O acetylation by acetic anhydride in aqueous solution, *J. Cyclic Nucleotide Res.* **1**:207–218.

Ho, H. C., Wirch, E., Stevens, F. C., and Wang, J. H., 1977, Purification of a Ca^{2+}-activatable cyclic nucleotide phosphodiesterase from bovine heart by specific interaction with its Ca^{2+}-dependent modulator protein, *J. Biol. Chem.* **252**:43–50.

Hong, C. R., and Forrest, J. H., 1977, Effects of ablations of plasma (pcAMP) and nephrogenous urinary cyclic AMP (NucAMP) in renal insufficiency, *Clin. Res.* **25**:435A (abstract).

Hornykiewicz, O., 1977, Psychopharmacological implications of dopamine and dopamine antagonists: A critical evaluation of current evidence, *Annu. Rev. Pharmacol. Toxicol.* **17**:545–559.

Insel, P. A., Maguire, M. E., Gilman, A. G., Bourne, H. R., Coffino, P., and Melmon, K. L., 1976, Beta-adrenergic receptors and adenylate cyclase: Products of separate genes, *Mol. Pharmacol.* **12**:1062–1069.

Jakobs, K. H., Saur, W., and Schultz, G., 1976, Reduction of adenylate cyclase activity in lysates of human platelets by the alpha-adrenergic component of epinephrine, *J. Cyclic Nucleotide Res.* **2**:381–392.

Johnson, G. L., Kaslow, H. R., and Bourne, H. R., 1978, Genetic evidence that cholera toxin substrates are regulatory components of adenylate cyclase, *J. Biol. Chem.* **253**:7120–7123.

Kahn, C. R., Baird, K., Flier, J. S., and Jarrett, D. B., 1977, Effects of autoantibodies to the insulin receptor on isolated adipocytes, *J. Clin. Invest.* **60**:1094–1106.

Kandel, J., Collier, R. J., and Chung, D. W., 1974, Interaction of fragment A from diphtheria toxin with nicotinamide adenine dinucleotide, *J. Biol. Chem.* **249**:2088–2097.

Kebabian, J. W., 1977, Biochemical regulation and physiological significance of cyclic nucleotides in the nervous system, *Adv. Cyclic Nucleotide Res.* **8**:421–508.

Keely, S. L., and Corbin, J. D., 1977, Involvement of cAMP-dependent protein kinase in the regulation of heart contractile force, *Am. J. Physiol.* **233**:H269–H275.

Kimura, N., and Nagata, N., 1977, The requirement of guanine nucleotides for glucagon stimulation of adenylate cyclase in rat liver plasma membranes, *J. Biol. Chem.* **252**:3829–3835.

Klee, C. B., 1977, Conformational transition accompanying the binding of Ca^{2+} to the protein activator of $3',5'$-cyclic adenosine monophosphate phosphodiesterase, *Biochemistry* **16**:1017–1024.

Kretsinger, R. H., 1976, Evolution and function of calcium-binding proteins, *Int. Rev. Cytol.* **46**:323–393.

Lefkowitz, R. J., and Hamp, M., 1977, Comparison of specificity of agonist and antagonist radioligand binding to beta-adrenergic receptors, *Nature (London)* **268**:453–454.

Lefkowitz, R. J., and Williams, L. T., 1977, Catecholamine binding to the beta-adrenergic receptor, *Proc. Natl. Acad. Sci. U.S.A.* **74**:515–519.

Lefkowitz, R. J., Mukherjee, C., Coverstone, M., and Caron, M. G., 1974, Stereospecific [³H] (−)alprenolol binding sites, beta-adrenergic receptors and adenylate cyclase, *Biochem. Biophys. Res. Commun.* **60**:703–709.

Lefkowitz, R. J., Limbird, L. E., Mukherjee, C., and Caron, M. G., 1976, The beta-adrenergic receptor and adenylate cyclase, *Biochim. Biophys. Acta* **457**:1–39.

Lemaire, I., and Coffino, P., 1977, Coexpression of mutant and wild type protein kinase in lymphoma cells resistant to dibutyryl cyclic AMP, *J. Cell. Physiol.* **92**:437–445.

Levinson, S. L., and Blume, A. J., 1977, Altered guanine nucleotide hydrolysis as basis for increased adenylate cyclase activity after cholera toxin treatment, *J. Biol. Chem.* **252**:3766–3774.

Lilienfeld-Toal, H. v., Hesch, R. D., Hufner, M., and McIntosh, C., 1974, Excretion of cyclic 3',5'-adenosine monophosphate in renal insufficiency and primary hyperparathyroidism after stimulation with parathyroid hormone, *Horm. Metab. Res.* **6**:314–318.

Limbird, L. E., and Lefkowitz, R. J., 1976, Negative cooperativity among beta-adrenergic receptors in frog erythrocyte membranes, *J. Biol. Chem.* **251**:5007–5014.

Limbird, L. E., and Lefkowitz, R. J., 1977, Resolution of beta-adrenergic receptor binding and adenylate cyclase activity by gel exclusion chromatography, *J. Biol. Chem.* **252**:799–802.

Lincoln, T. M., and Corbin, J. D., 1977, Adenosine 3',5'-cyclic monophosphate- and guanosine 3,5'-cyclic monophosphate-dependent protein kinases: Possible homologous proteins, *Proc. Natl. Acad. Sci. U.S.A.* **74**:3239–3243.

Liuzzi, A., Chiodini, P. G., Botalla, L., Cremascoli, G., Muller, E., and Silvestrini, F., 1974, Decreased plasma growth hormone (GH) levels in acromegalics following CB154 (2-Br-alpha-ergocryptine) administration, *J. Clin. Endocrinol.* **38**:910–912.

Londos, C., Lin, M. C., Welton, A. F., Lad, P. M., and Rodbell, M., 1977, Reversible activation of hepatic adenylate cyclase by guanyl-5'-yl-(alpha,beta-methylene) diphosphonate and guanyl-5'-yl imidodiphosphate, *J. Biol. Chem.* **252**:5180–5182.

Madden, J., IV, Akil, H., Patrick, R. L., and Barchas, J. D., 1977, Stress-induced parallel changes in central opioid levels and pain responsiveness in the rat, *Nature (London)* **265**:358–360.

Maguire, M. E., Van Arsdale, P. M., and Gilman, A. G., 1976a, An agonist-specific effect of guanine nucleotides on binding to the beta-adrenergic receptor, *Mol. Pharmacol.* **12**:335–339.

Maguire, M. E., Wiklund, R. A., Anderson, H. J., and Gilman, A. G., 1976b, Binding of [^{125}I]iodohydroxybenzylpindolol to putative beta-adrenergic receptors of rat glioma cells on other cell clones, *J. Biol. Chem.* **251**:1221–1231.

Maguire, M. E., Ross, E. M., and Gilman, A. G., 1977, Beta-adrenergic receptor: Ligand binding properties and the interaction with adenylyl cyclase, *Adv. Cyclic Nucleotide Res.* **8**:1–83.

Mains, R. E., and Eipper, B. A., 1976, Biosynthesis of adrenocorticotropic hormone in mouse pituitary tumor cells, *J. Biol. Chem.* **251**:4115–4120.

Mains, R. E., Eipper, B. A., and Ling, N., 1977, Common precursor to corticotropins and endorphins, *Proc. Natl. Acad. Sci. U.S.A.* **74**:3014–3018.

Mickey, J., Tate, R., and Lefkowitz, R. J., 1975, Subsensitivity of adenylate cyclase and decreased beta-receptor binding after chronic exposure to (−)isoproterenol *in vitro, J. Biol. Chem.* **250**:5727–5729.

Milhaud, G., Rankin, J. C., Bolis, L., and Benson, A. A., 1977, Calcitonin: Its hormonal action on the gill, *Proc. Natl. Acad. Sci. U.S.A.* **74**:4693–4696.

Miller, R. J., Horn, A. S., and Iversen, L. L., 1974, The action of neuroleptic drugs on dopamine-stimulated adenosine cyclic 3',5'-monophosphate production in rat neostriatum and limbic forebrain, *Mol. Pharmacol.* **10**:759–766.

Monn, E., Osnes, J. B., and Øye, I., 1976, Basal and hormone-induced urinary cyclic AMP in children with renal disorders, *Acta Paediatr. Scand.* **65**:739–745.

Moss, J., and Vaughan, M., 1977a, Choleragen activation of solubilized adenylate cyclase: Requirement for GTP and protein activator for demonstration of enzymatic activity, *Proc. Natl. Acad. Sci. U.S.A.* **74**:4396–4400.

Moss, J., and Vaughan, M., 1977b, Mechanism of action of choleragen: Evidence for ADP-ribosyltransferase activity with arginine as an acceptor, *J. Biol. Chem.* **252**:2455–2457.

Moss, J., Manganiello, V. C., and Vaughan, M., 1976, Hydrolysis of nicotinamide adenine dinucleotide by choleragen and its A protomer: Possible role in the activation of adenylate cyclase, *Proc. Natl. Acad. Sci. U.S.A.* **73**:4424–4427.

Moss, J., Osborne, J. C., Jr., Fishman, P. M., Brewer, H. B., Jr., Vaughan, M., and Brady, R. O., 1977, Effect of gangliosides and substrate analogues on the hydrolysis of nicotinamide adenine dinucleotide by choleragen, *Proc. Natl. Acad. Sci. U.S.A.* **74**:74–78.

Murad, F., and Aurbach, G. D., 1977, Cyclic GMP in metabolism: Interrelationship of biogenic amines, hormones, and other agents, in: *The Year in Metabolism 1977* (N. Freinkel, ed.), pp. 1–32, Plenum Medical Book Company, New York.

Nimrod, A., Tsafriri, A., and Lindner, H. R., 1977, *In vitro* induction of binding sites for hCG in rat granulosa cells by FSH, *Nature (London)* **267**:632–633.

Nissley, S. P., Rechler, M. M., Moses, A. C., Short, P. A., and Podskalny, J. M., 1977, Proinsulin binds to a growth peptide receptor and stimulates DNA synthesis in chick embryo fibroblasts, *Endocrinology* **101**:708–716.

Orly, J., and Schramm, M., 1976, Coupling of catecholamine receptor from one cell with adenylate cyclase from another cell by cell fusion, *Proc. Natl. Acad. Sci. U.S.A.* **73**:4410–4414.

Perkins, J. P., and Moore, M. M., 1973, Characterization of the adrenergic receptors mediating a rise in cyclic 3′,5′-adenosine monophosphate in rat cerebral cortex, *J. Pharmacol. Exp. Ther.* **185**:371–378.

Pfeuffer, T., 1977, GTP-binding proteins in membranes and the control of adenylate cyclase activity, *J. Biol. Chem.* **252**:7224–7234.

Rangel-Aldao, R., and Rosen, O. M., 1976, Dissociation and reassociation of the phosphorylated and nonphosphorylated forms of adenosine 3′,5′-monophosphate-dependent protein kinase from bovine cardiac muscle, *J. Biol. Chem.* **251**:3375–3380.

Rangel-Aldao, R., and Rosen, O. M., 1977, Effect of cAMP and ATP on the reassociation of phosphorylated and nonphosphorylated subunits of the cAMP-dependent protein kinase from bovine cardiac muscle, *J. Biol. Chem.* **252**:7140–7145.

Rechler, M. M., and Nissley, S. P., 1977, Somatomedins and related growth factors, *Nature (London)* **270**:665–666.

Rechler, M. M., Podskalny, J. M., and Nissley, S. P., 1977, Characterization of the binding of multiplication-stimulating activity to a receptor for growth polypeptides in chick embryo fibroblasts, *J. Biol. Chem.* **252**:3898–3910.

Rendell, M. S., Rodbell, M., and Berman, M., 1977, Activation of hepatic adenylate cyclase by guanyl nucleotides: Modeling of the transient kinetics suggests an "excited" state of GTPase is a control component of the system, *J. Biol. Chem.* **252**:7909–7912.

Rinderknecht, E., and Humbel, R. E., 1976, Amino-terminal sequences of two polypeptides from human serum with nonsuppressible insulin-like and cell growth-promoting activities: Evidence for structural homology with insulin B chain, *Proc. Natl. Acad. Sci. U.S.A.* **73**:4379–4381.

Roberts, J. M., Insel, P. A., Goldfien, R. D., and Goldfien, A., 1977, Alpha-adrenoreceptors but not beta-adrenoreceptors increase in rabbit uterus with oestrogen, *Nature (London)* **270**:624–625.

Rodbell, M., Krans, H. M. J., Pohl, S. L., and Birnbaumer, L., 1971, The glucagon-sensitive adenyl cyclase system in plasma membranes of rat liver. IV. Effects of guanyl nucleotides on binding of ^{125}I-glucagon, *J. Biol. Chem.* **246**:1872–1876.

Ross, E. M., Maguire, M. E., Sturgill, T. W., Biltonen, R. L., and Gilman, A. G., 1977, Relationship between the beta-adrenergic receptor and adenylate cyclase, *J. Biol. Chem.* **252**:5761–5775.

Rossier, J., French, E. D., Rivier, C., Ling, N., Guillemin, R., and Bloom, F. E., 1977, Foot-shock induced stress increases beta-endorphin levels in blood but not brain, *Nature (London)* **270**:618–620.

Roth, J., Kahn, C. R., Lesniak, M. A., Gorden, P., DeMeyts, P., Megyesi, K., Nerville, D. M., Jr., Gavin, J. R., III, Soll, A. H., Freychet, P., Goldfine, I. D., Bar, R. S., and Archer, J. A., 1975, Receptors for insulin, NSILA-s, and growth hormone: Applications to disease states in man, *Recent Prog. Horm. Res.* **31**:95–139.

Rudolph, S. A., Schafer, D. E., and Greengard, P., 1977, Effects of cholera enterotoxin on catecholamine-stimulated changes in cation fluxes, cell volume, and cyclic AMP levels in the turkey erythrocyte, *J. Biol. Chem.* **252**:7132–7139.

Sattin, A., Rall, T. W., and Zanella, J., 1975, Regulation of cyclic adenosine 3′,5′-monophosphate levels in guinea-pig cerebral cortex by interaction of alpha-adrenergic and adenosine receptor activity, *J. Pharmacol. Exp. Ther.* **192**:22–32.

Schultz, G., Hardman, J. G., Schultz, K., Davis, J. W., and Sutherland, E. W., 1973, A new enzymatic assay for guanosine 3′,5′-cyclic monophosphate and its application to the ductus deferens of the rat, *Proc. Natl. Acad. Sci. U.S.A.* **70**:1721–1725.

Schwoch, G., and Hilz, H., 1977, Protein-bound adenosine 3′,5′-monophosphate in liver of glucagon-treated rats, *Eur. J. Biochem.* **76**:269–276.

Seeman, P., Chau-Wong, M., Tedesco, J., and Wong, K., 1975, Brain receptors for antipsychotic drugs and dopamine: Direct binding assays, *Proc. Natl. Acad. Sci. U.S.A.* **72**:4376–4380.

Sheppard, J. R., 1977, Catecholamine hormone receptor differences identified on 3T3 and Simian virus-transformed 3T3 cells, *Proc. Natl. Acad. Sci. U.S.A.* **74**:1091–1094.

Snyder, S. H., and Bennett, J. P., Jr., 1976, Neurotransmitter receptors in the brain: Biochemical identification, *Annu. Rev. Physiol.* **38**:153–175.

Spiegel, A. M., Brown, E. M., Fedak, S. A., Woodard, C. J., and Aurbach, G. D., 1976a, Holocatalytic state of adenylate cyclase in turkey erythrocyte membranes: Formation with guanylylimidodiphosphate plus isoproterenol without effect on affinity of beta-receptor, *J. Cyclic Nucleotide Res.* **2**:47–56.

Spiegel, A. M., Gerner, R. H., Murphy, D. L., and Aurbach, G. D., 1976b, Lithium does not inhibit the parathyroid hormone-mediated rise in urinary cyclic AMP and phosphate in humans, *J. Clin. Endocrinol.* **43**:1390–1393.

Spiegel, A. M., Downs, R. W., Jr., and Aurbach, G. D., 1977, Guanosine 5', alpha-beta-methylene, triphosphate, a novel GTP analog, causes persistent activation of adenylate cyclase: Evidence against pyrophosphorylation mechanism, *Biochem. Biophys. Res. Commun.* **76**:758–764.

Strittmatter, W. J., Davis, J. N., and Lefkowitz, R. J., 1977a, Alpha-adrenergic receptors in rat parotid cells. I. Correlation of [³H]dihydroergocryptine binding and catecholamine-stimulated potassium efflux, *J. Biol. Chem.* **252**:5472–5477.

Strittmatter, W. J., Davis, J. N., and Lefkowitz, R. J., 1977b, Alpha-adrenergic receptors in rat parotid cells. II. Desensitization of receptor binding sites and potassium efflux, *J. Biol. Chem.* **252**:5478–5482.

Tallman, J. F., Smith, C. C., and Henneberry, R. C., 1977, Induction of functional beta-adrenergic receptors in HeLa cells, *Proc. Natl. Acad. Sci. U.S.A.* **74**:873–877.

Thorner, M. O., Chait, A., Aitken, M., Benker, G., Bloom, S. R., Mortimer, S. H., Sanders, P., Stuart-Mason, A., and Besser, G. M., 1975, Successful treatment of acromegaly, *Br. Med. J.* **1**:299–303.

Turtle, J. R., and Kipnis, D. M., 1967, An adrenergic receptor mechanism for the control of cyclic 3',5'-adenosine monophosphate synthesis in tissues, *Biochem. Biophys. Res. Commun.* **28**:797–802.

Ueda, T., Maeno, H., and Greengard, P., 1973, Regulation of endogenous phosphorylation of specific proteins on synaptic membrane fractions from rat brain by adenosine 3',5'-monophosphate, *J. Biol. Chem.* **248**:8295–8305.

U'Prichard, D. C., Greenberg, D. A., and Snyder, S. H., 1977, Binding characteristics of a radiolabeled agonist and antagonist at central nervous system alpha-noradrenergic receptors, *Mol. Pharmacol.* **13**:454–473.

Williams, L. T., and Lefkowitz, R. J., 1976, Alpha-adrenergic receptor identification by [³H]dihydroergocryptine binding, *Science* **192**:791–793.

Williams, L. T., and Lefkowitz, R. J., 1977a, Slowly reversible binding of catecholamine to a nucleotide-sensitive state of the beta-adrenergic receptor, *J. Biol. Chem.* **252**:7207–7213.

Williams, L. T., and Lefkowitz, R. J., 1977b, Regulation of rabbit myometrial alpha-adrenergic receptors by estrogen and progesterone, *J. Clin. Invest.* **60**:815–818.

Williams, L. T., Mullikin, D., and Lefkowitz, R. J., 1976, Identification of alpha-adrenergic receptors in uterine smooth muscle membranes by [³H]dihydroergocryptine binding, *J. Biol. Chem.* **251**:6915–6923.

Williams, L. T., Gore, T. B., and Lefkowitz, R. J., 1977a, Ectopic beta-adrenergic receptor binding sites: Possible molecular basis of aberrant catecholamine responsiveness of an adrenocortical tumor adenylate cyclase, *J. Clin. Invest.* **59**:319–324.

Williams, L. T., Lefkowitz, R. J., Watanabe, A. M., Hathaway, D. R., and Besch, H. R., 1977b, Thyroid hormone regulation of beta-adrenergic receptor number, *J. Biol. Chem.* **252**:2787–2789.

Wodnar-Filipowicz, A., and Lai, C. Y., 1976, Stimulation of adenylate cyclase in washed pigeon erythrocyte membrane with cholera toxin and its subunits, *Arch. Biochem. Biophys.* **176**:465–471.

Wolfe, B. P., Harden, T. K., and Molinoff, P. B., 1976, Beta-adrenergic receptors in rat liver: Effects of adrenalectomy, *Proc. Natl. Acad. Sci. U.S.A.* **73**:1343–1347.

Wolfe, B. P., Harden, T. K., and Molinoff, P. B., 1977, *In vitro* study of beta-adrenergic receptors, *Annu. Rev. Pharmacol. Toxicol.* **17**:575–604.

Diabetes Mellitus

Stefan S. Fajans and John C. Floyd, Jr.

7.1. Heterogeneity of Diabetes Mellitus

7.1.1. The Histocompatibility System (HLA) and Genetic Susceptibility to Diabetes Mellitus

In recent years, the close association of genes controlling the immune response with a variety of antigens of the major histocompatibility system (HLA) has been well established. Such an association was found mainly in those diseases in the pathogenesis of which immunological mechanisms are active. It seems likely that genes at loci closely linked to HLA loci are involved in susceptibility to diabetes. Whether these HLA-linked diabetic genes code for viral receptors, are associated with an immune response gene to pancreatic or viral antigens, or are linked to diabetes in some other ways is not known (Notkins, 1977).

Among Caucasians, a definite positive association of juvenile-onset type, insulin-dependent diabetes (JOD) with HLA-B8 and BW15, B18, DW3, and DW4 has been reported (see Fajans, 1976, 1978). This implies that a gene or genes predisposing to insulin-dependent diabetes, occurring at a locus closely linked to HLA, would be particularly associated in populations with haplotypes containing the types named above. The

STEFAN S. FAJANS and JOHN C. FLOYD, JR. • Division of Endocrinology and Metabolism, Metabolism Research Unit, and Michigan Diabetes Research and Training Center, The University of Michigan, Ann Arbor, Michigan 48109.

possibility remains that linkage disequilibrium of the HLA locus might be different among various races (Patel *et al.*, 1977). Since racial differences in HLA phenotypes have been observed, further studies are necessary to confirm the relationship between various HLA phenotypes and JOD in Caucasians and other populations. Studies have appeared within the last year that confirm the increased prevalence of certain HLA antigens in JOD and also suggest that there is marked genetic heterogeneity within groups of patients with insulin-dependent diabetes.

Barta and Simon (1977) found that in 180 insulin-dependent diabetic patients, diagnosed before age 18 years, there was a significant increase in HLA-B8, but not in BW15. HLA-BW8 and BW15 were also significantly increased, and the simultaneous prevalence of the two antigens led to the potentiation of their effects in the manifestation of diabetes.

In a study of 102 juvenile diabetic patients, Ludvigsson *et al.* (1977) found that HLA-B8 or BW15 or both were found with increased frequency. These patients did not differ significantly from other patients with regard to C-peptide levels, but the results suggested that when both alleles of the *B* locus are occupied by diabetes-predisposing genes, the relative risk of getting diabetes is higher, the onset of diabetes seems to be earlier, and beta cell damage seems more severe. The significantly increased incidence of measurable C-peptide in a small group of patients with HLA-B18 (and with HLA-B7) may imply that this HLA antigen is associated with a milder form or shorter duration of diabetes. BW15 alone was not increased significantly.

In 90 insulin-dependent diabetic patients age 2–20 years, Illeni *et al.* (1977) found that HLA-AW30 was significantly increased and HLA-BW35 significantly decreased. HLA-B8 was significantly increased only in the 0- to 5-year age group.

Barbosa *et al.* (1977) studied the HLA types in 24 nearly complete sibships with two or more cases of JOD and also studied their parents. This is the first study of HLA haplotypes in complete sibships of JOD multiplex families. It is an important extension of previous reports in that it allows a comparison between diabetic and nondiabetic siblings. The authors found a statistically significant association between the sharing of identical haplotypes and the frequency of development of JOD within the sibship, confirming earlier findings of Cudworth and Woodrow (1975). More than half the diabetics in these sibships with two or more diabetics were HLA-identical. The increased frequency of both HLA types identified among diabetic siblings and the relatively few siblings with different haplotypes suggest that there may be one or more genes closely associated with the HLA system that influence the development of diabetes. The authors' HLA studies of diabetic multiplex families support the theory of marked heterogeneity within JOD. One group of diabetic siblings had both haplotypes, while another group shared only one haplotype. Clinical differences between the two groups (concordance for age of onset and seasonal incidence) support this suggestion.

In another study (Jaworski *et al.*, 1977), 18 families with two or more siblings with JOD diabetes were haplotyped. In 9 of 13 families, the affected siblings were concordant for both HLA haplotypes, and in 3 of 13, the affected sibs were concordant for only one haplotype. One of 13 families had affected children with completely discordant haplotypes. It was concluded that HLA-linked genes are probably important but not the sole determinants of risk of developing diabetes mellitus.

Rubinstein *et al.* (1977) investigated the genetic predisposition to JOD in families of 31 index cases in relation to the inheritance of the HLA system. The diabetes-predisposing gene was thought to be recessive. Penetrance was estimated at 50%, because half the HLA-identical sibs and index cases were diabetic.

The authors proposed that in juvenile diabetics there is a gene traveling with the HLA segment that increases the frequency of intra-HLA recombinations, and this in turn is associated with the development of diabetes. In commenting on this report, Neel (1977) states in an editorial that there are alternative possibilities. Whenever incomplete penetrance is introduced into a genetic explanation, it is often impossible with the amount and kind of data available to distinguish clearly among multifactorial, dominant, recessive, simple one-locus additive, and over-dominance inheritance (the last two are not identical, as implied by Rubinstein and co-workers). Neel (1977) also stresses the possibility of etiological heterogeneity, and that there may be multiple genetic paths to the absence of insulin that characterizes diabetes, each with a different penetrance and occurring with different frequencies in different populations. Crossing over in the HLA region, as postulated by Rubinstein *et al.* (1977), was not confirmed by the studies of Barbosa *et al.* (1977), Jaworski *et al.* (1977), Nerup *et al.* (1977), and Hsu *et al.* (1977).

The distribution of 20 HLA antigens in 382 diabetics and 184 control subjects of white, Mexican-American, and black ancestry was studied by Patel *et al.* (1977). In all three populations, the incidence of antigens B8 and BW15 was higher in the insulin-dependent diabetics than in controls. The differences fell short of statistical significance when corrections were made for the number of antigens studied. Yet when the results of previous studies were combined with the authors', there was a highly significant association of insulin-dependent diabetes and the antigens B8 and BW15 in the white population. It seems likely that this association would also hold true for the Mexican-American and the black populations. These results need to be confirmed in larger studies.

A low order of magnitude of association between given HLA phenotypes and diabetes may be due to the fact that genes determining susceptibility to disease are situated at loci closely linked to HLA. This view is supported by the finding that the *HLA-D* alleles are more strongly associated with insulin-dependent diabetes than are *HLA-B* alleles, with which they are associated in linkage disequilibrium. Finding of an association of insulin-dependent diabetes with the same HLA phenotypes in three different populations is of considerable interest. It would favor a more direct involvement of the HLA genes rather than just relinked genes in promoting disease susceptibility.

On the other hand, in Japanese patients, JOD is associated with HLA-B12 and not HLA-B8 and BW15, as in Caucasians. Nakao *et al.* (1977) found HLA-B12 in 37.5% of 32 patients with JOD, in 13.5% of 52 patients with maturity-onset diabetes, and in 9.3% of 150 control subjects. The increase of HLA-B12 in JODs was significant. It is possible that *HLA-B8* and *B12* are situated close to some major pathogenic genes that may predispose to JOD. The data appeared to show again that HLA-B8 is not itself necessary to the development of JOD, but rather that there is a gene in linkage disequilibrium with *HLA-B8*. This study is of interest in that it shows that in a different race, a postulated immune response gene may be linked to a different HLA specificity in loci *A* and *B*. The authors also mention the possibility that the association between HLA antigens and diabetes is due, not to an abnormal immune response gene linked to HLA genes and specific for a given disease, but to the fact that *HLA-B8* and *HLA-B12* may be in linkage disequilibrium with the gene that enhances or facilitates immune responses generally. The study in Japanese patients suggests again that there are genetically at least two different types of diabetes, the juvenile-onset form being associated with histocompatibility antigens. This is evidence for heterogenetity of diabetes within the Japanese population, as has been demonstrated in Caucasian populations.

Cudworth *et al.* (1977) investigated, as early as possible after diagnosis, the interrelationship of genetic susceptibility, environmental influences, and immunological factors in 110 persons in whom insulin-dependent diabetes developed when they were less than 30 years old. Mean interval from diagnosis to interview and taking of samples for investigation was 5.5 days (range: 0–18 days). Of this group, 56% had symptoms for up to 4 weeks and 34% for 5–30 weeks before diagnosis. There was evidence for clustering of cases with BW15-positive phenotype during the winter peak, but not during the autumn peak. Subjects who were BW15-positive, and in particular those who were B8- and BW15-positive, had higher neutralizing antibody titers to Coxsackie virus type B1 to B4. Of the total 110 cases, 58% had islet cell antibodies (ICA), but the presence of ICA was not correlated with the HLA phenotypes, viral antibody titers, or history of antecedent infection. This prospective investigation further

suggests probable interdependent roles of HLA-linked genetic susceptibility, environmental influences, and immunological factors.

Although population studies have established the association of the
HLA factors B8, BW15, and B18 with insulin-dependent diabetes mellitus, a preliminary report by Nerup *et al.* (1977) establishes a significantly
stronger association with *D* alleles than with corresponding *B* alleles.
HLA-D typing was performed in 125 JODs and 17 diabetic families. DW3
and DW4 were found in 46 and 51%, respectively, of the JODs (vs. 82 and
25%, respectively, in controls). The relative risk for DW3, DW4, and
DW3/DW4 carriers of developing JOD was 3.7, 4.9, and 9.4, respectively.
Previous suggestions of the presence of two diabetogenic genes in the
HLA region were confirmed.

Other alloantigens (Ia-type antigens found on B lymphocytes) that
are identical to, or closely linked with, genes that code for immune
responsiveness to a variety of antigens must be explored in diabetes
mellitus. They may be related to HLA-D antigens. Schernthaner *et al.*
(1977) reported a significantly increased frequency of Ia-type alloantigen
DRW3, as being closely associated with insulin-dependent diabetes.

In a small series of JOD patients from five families with multiple cases
of JOD, Bodmer *et al.* (1977) also found an association with Ia antigen.
There was a very high frequency of WIA4, 73% in patients as compared
with 19% in controls. WIA3 was also found with an increased frequency
that can probably be explained by the presence of BW8. This small study
indicated the complex nature of the inheritance of diabetes.

These diverse results suggest that further studies of the histocompatibility system in man are necessary before one can evaluate which antigens
are most closely linked with diabetes and what their role is in the pathogenesis of JOD.

In last year's chapter (Fajans, 1978), a new model of experimental
diabetes mellitus in mice described by Like and Rossini (1976) was
reviewed. The pathogenesis suggested was a chemically initiated (multiple
injection of streptozotocin), cell-mediated immune reaction through activating a virus *in vivo* in susceptible hosts. The authors extended their
experiments to determine whether a relationship exists between the major
histocompatibility genes and the ability of streptozotocin to induce inflammatory islet lesions and hyperglycemia (Rossini *et al.,* 1977a). The present
study demonstrates differences in susceptibility to both the insulitis and
the hyperglycemic action of streptozotocin among different strains of
mice tested. However, the data are most consistent with the conclusion
that the major histocompatibility complex genes cannot be the sole regulators of insulitis or hyperglycemia or both in the streptozotocin-induced
insulitis model.

In another study, Rossini *et al.* (1977b) described findings that suggest that multiple injections of streptozotocin induce, in susceptible hosts, the triad of direct beta cell cytotoxicity, type C virus induction within beta cells, and a cell-mediated autoimmune reaction directed against pancreatic beta cells with lymphocytic infiltration. These factors, acting separately or in concert, appear to induce destructive insulitis and severe diabetes. Almost complete inhibition of the lymphocytic infiltration was accomplished by the administration of rabbit anti-mouse lymphocyte serum (ALS) together with 3-*O*-methyl-D-glucose (3-OMG). Neither insulitis nor hyperglycemia was observed in these mice during the period of 3-OMG and ALS injections. When these agents were discontinued, plasma glucose elevation occurred within 2–3 weeks.

Van Thiel *et al.* (1977) described a kindred of 43 in which three persons had variable expressions of a syndrome consisting of immunoglobin A deficiency, diabetes mellitus, malabsorption, and a common HLA haplotype, HLA-2, B8, and DW3. Other conditions present in the family include Graves's disease, vitiligo, hypocomplementemia, rheumatic fever, multiple sclerosis, and a high frequency of antibodies to multiple endocrine tissues. The authors believe that the inheritance of this family is of an association of diabetes mellitus, thyroiditis, and selective IGA deficiency with a single immune response gene or gene complex that is linked to *HLA-B8* and *HLA-DW3*. The genetic basis of these diseases may be the inheritance of a predisposition to respond immunologically in a potentially harmful manner.

7.1.2. Susceptibility to Viral Infection and Viral Infection in the Etiology of Diabetes Mellitus

A possible role of viral infection as the environmental agent superimposed on genetic susceptibility to such infection has been proposed to be involved in the pathogenesis of JOD. Human epidemiological evidence is indirect and still controversial.

Notkins (1977) reviews what has been learned from studies of animal models and tissue cultures that might be applicable to an understanding of JOD in man. In mice, there are viruses that are capable of attacking beta cells and producing a diabeteslike syndrome, but genetic factors control its development. The author presents a good review of replication of viruses in beta cell cultures, of viral infections in animals and humans, and of related genetic and immunological factors.

Webb *et al.* (1976) found a positive correlation between genetic predisposition to diabetes in the mouse and susceptibility to group B Coxsackie virus infection in the host. Pathological findings in the pancreas of three genotypes during the acute stage of infection were closely parallel to genotypically dependent susceptibility of the host.

Jansen *et al.* (1977) performed pilot experiments to examine the hypothesis that the diabetic syndrome provoked by encephalomyocarditis (EMC) virus in mice might be due to an immune reaction. Mice were inoculated with EMC virus with and without immunosuppression with sublethal X irradiation or administration of a cyclophosphamide derivative. Average glucose levels after X irradiation and infection remained normal, while virus-infected, otherwise untreated mice had significantly higher mean glucose levels. This indicates an important role of the cellular immune reaction, insulitis, in the destruction of the islets and in the development of virus-induced diabetes. Results obtained with X irradiation were not found with administration of the chemical immunosuppressant. Immunosuppression simultaneously decreases the host defense, favoring virus multiplication. This resulted in a high mortality in mice treated with virus plus immunosuppression. Preliminary histopathological examinations in irradiated mice suggested a complete lack of insulitis without lymphocytic infiltration but with islet cell necrosis indicating that the virus had been present.

Evidence is tenuous that viral infection participates in the etiology of human diabetes mellitus. MacMillan *et al.* (1977) studied the monthly incidence of onset and detection of diabetes in school-age children. Of 86 children, 59 (69%) over 6 years but under 17 years of age became symptomatic in the autumn and winter months, October through March. The monthly onset and detection pattern for children under 6 years of age bears little resemblance to that of those older children, although the number of patients studied was small. Thus, a seasonal incidence pattern in the onset of detection of diabetes mellitus among school age children is apparent. The authors themselves were cautious in the interpretation of these data. Whether the seasonal pattern reflects the influence of viral infection as an aggravating, a precipitating, or a true etiological factor in the onset of juvenile diabetes awaits further studies.

Wilson *et al.* (1977) reported on an 18-month-old boy with a 1-week history of acute-onset diabetes. The combination of lymphocytosis and high titers of Coxsackie B2 neutralizing antibody and Coxsackie B IgM suggested that the diabetes was associated with a recent Coxsackie B2 virus infection. Coxsackie B IgM and fibrillar anticellular IgM were not detected 14 months after onset, which shows that the acute phase of the viral infection had ended. Coxsackie B2 neutralizing antibody was also present in members of the family. The HLA types of the patient and his 6-year-old brother, who was 4 years old when he developed diabetes, were not those associated with JOD.

Yoon *et al.* (1977) examined the presence of neutralizing antibodies to members of the EMC virus in the sera from 41 patients with JOD and 66 nondiabetic controls. In this study, 12% of the JODs and 6% of the nondiabetic controls had elevated neutralizing antibody titers. The possibility that the rare case of JOD may be due to the infection by a member of the EMC virus group cannot be excluded. However, since most of the diabetic patients had no antibody to EMC virus, this virus does not appear to be a major cause of JOD. Since the medium length of time between the onset of diabetes and the collection of serum for testing was 2.68 years, these studies are inconclusive.

7.1.3. Autoimmunity in Diabetes Mellitus

Earlier evidence supporting a role of autoimmunity in the development of insulin-dependent diabetes (summarized in Fajans, 1976, 1978) has been supported by later reports, and a classification of idiopathic diabetes mellitus based on autoimmunity has been proposed (Irvine, 1977).

Irvine *et al.* (1977a) presented a detailed correlation between the prevalence of pancreatic islet cell antibodies (ICA) and the age of onset, duration and type of diabetes, sex, and coexistence of other evidence of organ-specific autoimmunity and the HLA type. This paper confirms with a much larger series of patients that ICA is associated with insulin-dependent diabetes.

In this study of 972 patients with diabetes mellitus, humoral ICA were more prevalent in insulin-treated diabetics with than without (38 vs. 22%; $p < 0.01$) organ-specific autoimmune disease (AID) when consideration was not given to the duration of diabetes. In insulin-treated diabetes of more than 5 years duration, prevalence of ICA was again higher in those patients with associated overt organ-specific AID (26%) than those without (7%), indicating that ICA persists longer in patients with AID. In insulin-treated diabetics tested for ICA within the year of diagnosis, the prevalence was no different in those who had associated AID than in those who did not. There was also an 8% prevalence of ICA in diabetics treated with oral hypoglycemic agents but not in diabetics requiring diet alone, and in only 0.5% of 434 control subjects. ICA also occurred in patients with AID without clinical diabetes (6%). ICA were present in the sera of 2.5% of 157 first-degree relatives of ICA-positive subjects.

The prevalence of ICA was strongly dependent on the duration of diabetes. It was 65% in newly diagnosed diabetes, 60% during the first year from diagnosis in the insulin-treated group, and fell to 20% at 2–5 years and to 5% at 10–20 years. When the duration of diabetes was taken into account, the prevalence of ICA in insulin-treated diabetics showed no correlation with the patient's age at the time of testing. Diabetics who did not require insulin for treatment but who were ICA-positive showed a significant tendency to require insulin subsequently and to have a higher prevalence of AID than insulin-independent diabetics who were ICA-negative.

Persistence of ICA for more than 5 years from diagnosis of diabetes was associated with coexistent overt organ-specific AID and with HLA-B8, A1 and A1+B8. There was no correlation between BW15 and persistence of ICA.

It appeared to the authors that diabetics requiring insulin treatment, whatever the age of onset, may have the same pathogenesis, and so may ICA-positive diabetics requiring insulin but having diabetes in a milder form. The concept of an autoimmune form of diabetes in contrast to other nonimmunological forms of the disease is supported by studies of the clinical association of insulin-treated diabetics with organ-specific auto-immunity, the higher prevalence of thyroid-gastric antibodies in insulin-treated diabetics, and the evidence of cell-mediated immunity to the endocrine pancreas in insulin-dependent but not in insulin-independent diabetics.

In another report, Irvine *et al.* (1977b) described in greater detail their finding of pancreatic ICA in patients with diabetes treated with oral hypoglycemic agents. Of 170 diabetics treated with oral hypoglycemic agents within 3 months of diagnosis, 20 had ICA in the sera at diagnosis or later. Of these 20, 13, compared with only 14 of the remaining 159, subsequently required insulin after mean follow-up of 2 years 10 months and 4 years 11 months, respectively. The 13 patients who required insulin had significant symptoms before changing from oral hypoglycemic agents to insulin. Of 7 ICA-positive diabetics still continuing on oral hypogly-cemic agents, 5 had a more severe diabetes manifested by requiring maximum or near-maximum combined oral therapy, while only 34 of 145 ICA-negative diabetics continuing on oral hypoglycemic agents did so.

A group of 81 diabetics treated initially with diet for a mean of 4 years 7 months before going onto oral hypoglycemic agents had a high preva-lence of history of organ-specific AID, thyroid-gastric antibodies, and family history of insulin-dependent diabetes and possibly of HLA-B8, comparable to patients with insulin-dependent diabetes. The authors believe that ICA-positive diabetes controlled by oral hypoglycemic agents is an earlier and less severe form of insulin-dependent diabetes.

Del Prete *et al.* (1977) carried out a study on a large series of patients to determine the incidence of ICA in different states and types of diabetes as well as the relationship between these antibodies and islet cell metabolic function.

ICA and organ-specific autoantibodies (OSA) were determined by the indirect immunofluourescence technique in 920 diabetics, 1159 non-diabetic patients, and 100 young and 100 adult healthy controls with normal glucose tolerance. In control subjects, ICA were not detected and only 20 miscellaneous patients with normal glucose tolerance tests showed ICA (1.7%). ICA were present in 45.4% of patients with juvenile insulin-dependent diabetes during the first 6 months of the disease and in 29% of patients between 6 and 12 months of disease onset; ICA presence decreased to 19.2 and 20.6% after 1 and 5 years of duration of diabetes.

In patients with maturity-onset insulin-dependent diabetes, ICA incidence was 19.4% in the first year, 20% between 1 and 5 years, and 12.2% after 5 years of disease. In this group, 64% of ICA-positive patients showed clinical or serological evidence, or both, of thyroid-gastric and adrenal autoimmune disorders.

In sera from young patients with non-insulin-dependent diabetes, ICA were not detected. In adult patients with the same type of diabetes, ICA were present in 9.8% and were not related to the duration of diabetes. ICA were found in 19% of patients with chemical diabetes under 35 years of age and in 13% of chemical diabetics over 35 years of age. In a great number of these patients, organ-specific autoimmune disorders were observed, suggesting a relationship between subclinical glucose intolerance and autoimmunity. Three patients with chemical diabetes developed insulin-dependent diabetes some months after demonstration of high and persistent ICA titers. Thus, diabetes related to organ-specific autoimmunity is not necessarily insulin-dependent at the time of diagnosis. In metabolic studies performed in a group of such patients, a severely depressed insulin secretory response following oral or intravenous glucose was found. On the basis of this observation, insulin dependency may in general be considered the natural evolution of ICA-positive patients even if it is sometimes delayed.

Tiengo et al. (1977) conducted a study to ascertain whether ICA positivity is always associated with functional islet cell damage and whether in such patients the lack of insulin secretion is associated with reduced glucagon secretion. A group of 39 diabetic patients with circulating ICA were studied and compared with nondiabetic and diabetic ICA-negative controls. Insulin and glucagon secretion after oral and intravenous glucose loading and with arginine infusions were evaluated. In the nondiabetic group, insulin and glucagon responses to glucose were similar in patients with and without ICA. In ICA-positive diabetic patients, the responses of these hormones to arginine infusion were reduced. Similar alterations in insulin and glucagon secretion were observed in ICA-positive and -negative patients with chemical or overt diabetes. Hormonal differences between diabetics with and without ICA could not be detected. Thus, in nondiabetics, the presence of ICA does not seem to be associated with diabeteslike alterations of beta cell function. The presence of autoantibodies may antedate the onset of endocrine impairment in diabetics. Only prospective studies will clarify whether the presence of

ICA should be considered a marker of a "prediabetic" condition. Neither overt nor chemical autoimmune diabetes showed beta or alpha cell alterations different from those generally reported in diabetes mellitus. Autoimmune diabetes cannot be classified among the diabetic conditions characterized by both beta and alpha cell functional damage.

Irvine (1977) has suggested a classification of idiopathic diabetes based on autoimmunity. He delineates two main types.

Type I includes classic insulin-dependent, juvenile-onset type diabetes and insulin-dependent diabetes presenting in later life. Also included in Type I are diabetic patients initially adequately controlled for at least 2 months on oral hypoglycemic agents but with ICA. As previously reviewed, such patients have a propensity to progress to insulin-dependent diabetes.

Type II includes classic maturity-onset type, insulin-dependent diabetes (MOD) as well as insulin-independent diabetes at a younger age (MODY), both types being negative for islet cell ICA.

Irvine (1977) subdivides Type I diabetes into three categories: Type Ia has a severe genetically determined islet cell autoimmune diathesis. Type Ic has islet cell damage by an appropriate viral infection or other agent in the absence of islet cell autoimmunity. In Type Ib, there is a combination of viral infection and autoimmunity in the pathogenesis of the disease. Thus, within Type I, Irvine postulates two genetically determined susceptibilities, one toward autoimmunity and one toward a viral infection. The common form of diabetes within Type I is the one in which there is a degree of susceptibility to both these factors. Although this is an attractive classification and should facilitate further experimental work to determine the significance of viral infection and autoimmunity in the pathogenesis of diabetes mellitus, it is clear that at our present stage of knowledge it is not possible to classify the majority of insulin-dependent diabetics into the groups suggested.

In another study, Irvine et al. (1977c) reported on familial studies of Type I and Type II idiopathic diabetes mellitus. Using their classification of diabetes as defined above and studying a total of 296 diabetic patients, these authors found a significant association between the type of diabetes in the propositi and that in their first degree relatives. This association was still maintained when only the propositi in whom the diabetes was diagnosed at the age of 30 years or later were considered. The authors concluded that the disease should be subdivided into types according to the treatment needed rather than by the age of onset. Although these findings do not establish a separate genetic inheritance of the two main types of idiopathic diabetes, they verify that they are not genetically identical. There are several limitations in the authors' study. The classification of the type of diabetes was based on the treatment prescribed (by one clinic for the propositi, by many clinics for the diabetic relatives); there were unavoidable inaccuracies in the family histories; information about the weight of the diabetic relative treated with oral hypoglycemic agents was not always available. In the absence of data on serum ICA, they equated diabetics requiring oral agents who were not obese at diagnosis with Type I, and diabetics who were obese at diagnosis but required oral agents with Type II. Classification of the disease based on the type of treatment needed (insulin) does not take into account that many true MODs or MODYs (Type II) require insulin for correction of fasting hyperglycemia, although they are nonketotic and do not have ICA or other evidence of related autoimmunity. Thus, we would not agree that diabetes can be divided into two types according to treatment needed. Nevertheless, the authors' findings indicate that in general the distinction can be made between Type I and Type II, or juvenile-onset-type (insulin-dependent) and maturity-onset-type (insulin-independent) diabetes.

Ludwig *et al.* (1977) detected ICA in 11 of 67 patients with JOD. ICA were found to be closely associated with HLA-B8. The authors concluded that the demonstration of ICA, particularly in HLA-B8-positive juvenile diabetics, constitutes further circumstantial evidence of a genetically determined autoimmune pathogenesis in some patients with JOD. As reviewed previously (Fajans, 1978), not all investigators have found a correlation between ICA and HLA-B8 positivity.

Based on the hypothesis that a loss of immune regulatory suppressor T cells could be important in the development of autoaggressive reactions, Horowitz *et al.* (1977) examined suppressor-T-cell function in nine children with insulin-dependent diabetes. Of 9 patients, 6 lacked suppressor-T-cell function, while none of 15 controls did. These preliminary data suggest that decreased suppressor-T-cell function should be considered in the pathogenesis of some forms of diabetes mellitus. For an excellent article on autoimmunity in endocrine disease, the reader is referred to the review of Volpé (1977).

7.2. Insulin Secretion

7.2.1. Experimental Results in Animals: Hypothalamic Influences

Evidence in rats that the early insulin and glucagon responses to food ingestion are of reflex origin was obtained by DeJong *et al.* (1977). They showed that plasma insulin and plasma glucagon increased simultaneously by the first minute after ingestion of food was begun, whereas no significant change of blood glucose occurred until after the third minute. Injection of norepinephrine into the lateral hypothalamus caused a large increase in plasma insulin, but no change in blood glucose or plasma glucagon. Injection into the ventromedial hypothalamus caused increases in plasma insulin, glucagon, and glucose that were not preventable by atropine. Saline injection into the hypothalamic areas was without effect. Earlier experiments suggested that receptors triggering the early insulin response to food ingestion are situated proximal to the stomach. Their results suggest that the early insulin and glucagon responses to food ingestion must be of reflex origin, and they postulated that the relay stations of the reflexes are situated in the lateral and ventromedial hypothalamus, respectively.

Another study has called attention to the possible role of the hypothalamus in regulating insulin release (Hill *et al.*, 1977). When perfusates of the ventrolateral hypothalamus of rhesus monkeys were added to isolated rat islets, insulin release was approximately doubled. Perfusates were also injected *in vivo* in monkeys; concentration of portal vein insulin and glucagon increased significantly from baseline and peaked within 30 min, while glucose concentrations did not change. In other studies, these workers have accomplished preliminary isolation of a small peptide from bovine hypothalamus that modulates insulin release. The authors concluded that a humoral factor originating in the region of the ventrolateral hypothalamus increases insulin release *in vivo* and *in vitro*.

Further evidence of neurogenic stimulation of insulin secretion was obtained by Hommel and Fischer (1977). When they administered glucose orally to dogs, portal venous insulin (chronic portal vein catheters) increased significantly after 5 min, whereas peripheral venous glucose increased significantly at 15 min. Portal vein glucose was significantly increased after 7½ min. The results suggested to the authors that the early increase in portal venous insulin reflects a pancreatic secretory reflex involving the autonomic nervous system.

7.2.2. Regulation in Man

7.2.2.1. Effects of Intraportal and Peripheral Infusions of Glucagon on Insulin Secretion

Sherwin *et al.* (1976) reported that infusions of glucagon to produce elevations of plasma glucagon concentrations of three to six times basal levels caused only transient and inconspicuous rises in blood glucose levels and were without effect on plasma insulin and glucose tolerance. This led them to conclude that glucagon itself is not diabetogenic. Holst *et al.* (1977) questioned whether the effects noted by Sherwin *et al.* (1976) might have been different had the glucagon been introduced into the portal vein as though it had been secreted by the pancreas. Therefore, they infused glucagon in patients for 120 min on one occasion through the portal vein (portal vein catheter had been placed via obliterated umbilical vein) and on a separate occasion through a peripheral vein. At 60 min of the infusion, 25 g glucose were given intravenously over 2 min. There were no differences in concentrations of insulin and glucose in peripheral venous blood whether the glucagon was given intraportally or into a peripheral vein. Nor were the results of intravenous glucose injection different under the two circumstances of glucagon administration. They interpreted their findings as supporting the conclusions of Sherwin and associates that the hyperglycemic activity of glucagon will not be displayed unless the insulin levels in blood are depressed, as in insulinopenic diabetes.

7.2.2.2. Effects of Secretin

Another gastrointestinal hormone, secretin, was studied for its effects on insulin release. Lerner (1977) administered isoproterenol, tolbutamide, arginine, glucagon, and secretin intravenously. Of all these stimuli, only prior secretin administration enhanced glucose-induced insulin release. The intravenous injection of 5 g glucose, following secretin administration, enhanced insulin release by 56% over that released prior to secretin injection. Although the effects of ingested nutrients, e.g., glucose, on release of endogenous secretin remains controversial, the findings were thought to be consistent with a possible role of secretin in the stimulation of insulin release in man.

7.2.2.3. Effects of Hypocalcemia and Theophylline

Glucose tolerance tests were performed in patients with hypoparathyroidism when they were hypocalcemic and again when they were eucalcemic after administration of vitamin D_2 (Gedik and Zileli, 1977). When there was hypocalcemia, there was markedly abnormal glucose tolerance and markedly reduced insulin release; these abnormalities disappeared after correction of hypocalcemia. Abnormal glucose tolerance in hypocalcemic patients does not necessarily indicate diabetes. In a second group of hypocalcemic patients, plasma insulin response, but not glucose tolerance, became normal during theophylline infusion. Overall, these findings were judged to support the importance of calcium in the mediation of insulin release.

7.2.2.4. Plasma Insulin in Early Diabetes

Pima Indians have relatively high circulating-insulin levels and the highest reported prevalence of diabetes in the world, and thus lend themselves to a study of prediabetes. Aronoff *et al.* (1977) studied 26 genetically normal Pimas (nondiabetic offspring of nondiabetic parents), 32 genetically prediabetic Pimas (normoglycemic monozygotic twin of a diabetic or offspring of two diabetic parents), 10 diabetic Pimas, and 29 normal Caucasians. Prediabetic Pimas with normal or abnormal cortisone-glucose tolerance tests had insulin levels similar to those of normal Indians during the intravenous glucose tolerance test, oral glucose tolerance test, and arginine infusion. Diabetic Pimas had no acute-phase insulin release during the intravenous glucose tolerance test. Both normal and prediabetic Indians had fasting and stimulated insulin levels during all the tests that were two- to threefold greater than in the Caucasians. Statistical analysis indicated that this could not be explained by any differences in glucose levels, age, or obesity. The hyperinsulinemia in these Indians was thought to have a genetic basis. The relationship of this hyperinsulinemia to the development of diabetes and/or obesity, both of which are extremely common among the Pima Indians, remains uncertain.

An examination of insulin-secretory dynamics in another population of "prediabetics" was made by Koncz *et al.* (1977). As a means of stressing beta cell function, they administered two intravenous injections of glucose 60 min apart and measured glucose and insulin responses. After the first injection, there were no significant differences in plasma glucose levels or in plasma insulin levels between the 9 prediabetics (offspring of two diabetic parents) and the 18 normal subjects. After the second injection, the time of the mean insulin peak response was delayed in the prediabetic subjects. In addition, after the second glucose injection, the 0- to 10-min and the 0- to 60-min blood glucose areas were significantly greater in the prediabetic subjects. Additional subtle differences were delineated. Thus, the double-stimulation technique amplified slight but statistically significant defects in insulin secretion. It was postulated that the prediabetics displayed a decrease in the responsiveness of a glucose sensor or relay mechanism to both increasing and decreasing glucose levels and that qualitative differences between insulin secretion in prediabetics and normals can be demonstrated if all aspects of dynamics of secretion of insulin and glucose response are carefully scrutinized.

In another investigation of insulin-secretory dynamics in diabetes-prone persons, Turner *et al.* (1977) studied nonpregnant mothers, grouped according to their nonpregnant percentage ideal body weight and to the birth weight of their infants. In addition, latent diabetic subjects (formerly with gestational diabetes) were studied. Normal-weight and obese women who had given birth to large-for-date babies, obese women who had given birth to normal-for-date (NFD) weight babies, and normal and obese latent-diabetic women had fasting plasma glucose concentrations (range 79–96 mg/dl) significantly higher than normal-weight women who had given birth to NFD babies (74 mg/dl). Among all mothers, there was a correlation of basal plasma glucose and basal plasma insulin ($r = 0.55$; $p < 0.001$). On the other hand, there was a negative correlation of basal plasma glucose concentrations with first-phase insulin secretion stimulated by a 25-mg/dl increment in glucose. The higher fasting plasma glucose levels in the majority of these patients who had normal or high basal plasma insulin levels were thought possibly to result from a decreased insulin-secretory response to small changes in plasma glucose levels encountered day to day in these patients.

Abnormalities in insulin responses to glucose ingestion were also reported in mild and definite diabetes by Kosaka et al. (1977). These authors studied 446 patients with definite diabetes (FBS > 140 mg/dl or diabetic retinopathy plus glucose intolerance) and 330 subjects with equivocal (mild) diabetes (presence of abnormal glucose tolerance test, fasting blood glucose never > 140, no retinopathy). During glucose tolerance tests, mean plasma insulin (immunoreactive insulin, IRI) curves were highest in normal subjects, lowest in definite diabetes, and intermediate in equivocal diabetes. The ratio, increment in IRI divided by increment in blood glucose ($\Delta IRI/\Delta BG$), was used as an index of early insulin release. In definite diabetes, it was almost invariably less than 0.5; in the controls, almost invariably above 0.5. In equivocal diabetes, it was consistently lower than 0.5 in 234 cases and higher than 0.5 in 68 cases. During a 3-month to 8-year follow-up, 40 patients with equivocal diabetes became diabetic; half had a family history of diabetes; and, in all, the ratio initially was less than 0.5 and, with only a few exceptions, remained consistently low during the entire follow-up. The findings suggested to the authors that impaired insulin release during the glucose tolerance test is a feature of true diabetes appearing during the stage of equivocal diabetes. In the absence of data concerning the ages of the patients, "equivocal diabetes" may, in part, represent the effect of age on glucose tolerance. Thus, the true incidence of subjects with equivocal diabetes developing overt diabetes may be underestimated. The finding that overt diabetes develops in those equivocal (mildly) diabetic patients who have low insulin responses is in keeping with the finding of Fajans et al. (1976).

DeNobel et al. (1977) studied patients who had a lag-storage type of oral glucose tolerance test (after 100 g glucose ingestion, plasma glucose is 200 mg/dl or more at 30–60 min but below 130 mg/dl at 2 hr) to determine whether such a test result has prognostic implication with respect to development of diabetes. A total of 2100 oral glucose tolerance tests were screened to find 31 subjects with lag-tests on at least two occasions within 1 month. In subjects in whom lag-storage-type glucose tolerance test was associated with a positive family history of diabetes, there was a subnormal early insulin response to glucose. The authors thought that in such subjects the possibility of diabetes developing was increased.

7.2.2.5. Plasma Insulin in Diabetes

Evidence for a role of endogenous prostaglandin synthesis in the defective insulin secretion and glucose intolerance of diabetes mellitus was obtained by Robertson and Chen (1977). Their earlier study demonstrated that prostaglandins (PGs) of the E series inhibit glucose-induced insulin secretion *in vivo* in dogs. The infusion of PGE_2 into healthy subjects inhibited the acute insulin response to a glucose pulse by about 50%. An infusion of sodium salicylate, an inhibitor of prostaglandin synthesis, was associated with a 100% increase of the acute insulin response to glucose. In patients with adult-onset diabetes (mean basal glucose about 200 mg/dl), the acute insulin response to glucose was an increase of 5% of basal; during sodium salicylate infusion, it was an increase of 97% of basal. During salicylate infusion, the diabetic patients had a significantly improved glucose disappearance rate (K_G was 0.56 without and 1.02 with sodium salicylate infusion, $p < 0.005$). In addition to the beneficial effects on acute-phase insulin release, there was a fourfold augmentation of second-phase insulin secretion during the sodium salicylate infusion in the diabetics. The authors hypothesized that an abnormality of endogenous PGE synthesis may play a role in defective insulin secretion and in glucose intolerance in diabetes mellitus.

McCarthy *et al.* (1977) reexamined the question of whether basal insulin secretion, as distinguished from stimulated insulin secretion, was abnormal in MOD and JOD patients. During glucose infusions sufficient to increase plasma glucose about 1 mmol/liter, plasma insulin increased less relative to basal level in diabetic patients than in control subjects (1.8 and 5.11 μU/ml, respectively). During an infusion of fish insulin, a significantly greater decrease in plasma glucose in the diabetic patients was accompanied by a decrease in insulin similar to that in healthy subjects (1.2 vs. 1.6 μU/ml). In a second study, 0.2 U fish insulin/kg was given intramuscularly. Again, the diabetics were found to suppress basal insulin relatively less than the controls, and the impairment was proportionate to the degree of their fasting hyperglycemia. The results were interpreted to show that the response of basal insulin secretion is impaired in diabetes, compared to the response of normal subjects. The possibility was entertained that if these diabetic patients had a decreased number of beta cells, those cells remaining would have to function toward their maximal capacity in order to maintain a basal plasma insulin concentration. This might result in a decreased capacity for them to respond to changes in plasma glucose, which would affect basal (and stimulated) insulin secretion.

Reynolds *et al.* (1977) identified abnormalities of insulin secretion and glucagon (immunoreactive glucagon, IRG) secretion in unstable diabetes. Stability was assessed from ascertainment of fluctuations of glucose and from measurement of glucose in the urine. When insulin was infused so as to produce comparable degrees of hypoglycemia, increases in plasma IRG were similar in stable diabetics and normal subjects, but were significantly less in unstable patients; during arginine infusions, increases in IRG were of similar magnitude in all three groups. In the unstable diabetic patients, there was no increase in C-peptide response to hyperglycemia or arginine. The degree of stability correlated with the magnitude of increase in C-peptide after oral glucose or after arginine and with the increase in glucagon during hypoglycemia. The conclusion was reached that unstable diabetes is characterized by virtually total endogenous insulin deficiency and abnormally regulated endogenous glucagon secretion; some persisting endogenous insulin-secretory capacity and persisting ability to increase glucagon secretion during hypoglycemia probably contribute importantly to increasing the stability of diabetes.

The findings and conclusions of Reynolds *et al.* (1977) were closely paralleled by those of Shima *et al.* (1977).

A further concomitant of deficiency of insulin secretion in diabetes mellitus was shown to be hypersecretion of gastric inhibitory polypeptide (GIP). Ross *et al.* (1977) showed that after ingestion of glucose, increases in GIP levels in plasma were greater and in plasma insulin were less in diabetic patients (mean fasting plasma glucose 145 mg/dl) than in control subjects. The groups did not differ in basal plasma GIP or insulin. Concomitantly, IRG levels not only failed to suppress but in fact rose in the diabetic patients. It was speculated that hypersecretion of GIP might be due to chronic insulin insufficiency and might have been in turn the cause, through its glucagonotropic effect, of the paradoxical rise in glucagon in the presence of defective insulin response to glucose ingestion. GIP is implicated in the metabolic derangements associated with diabetes mellitus.

7.2.2.6. Measurement of Other Beta Cell Secretory Products: Proinsulin and C-Peptide

In diabetic patients, the percentage of proinsulin, as well as the absolute level of proinsulin and insulin, were found to rise with increasing basal glucose concentrations (Mako *et al.*, 1977). At basal glucose levels greater than 200 mg/dl, however, IRI levels tended to fall, but proinsulin levels (absolute) continued to rise. Of 50 diabetic patients studied, 11 showed an increase in percentage (> 25%) of proinsulin in basal plasma, and in all but one of them, plasma glucose level was higher than 170 mg/dl. The findings were considered compatible with a secretion of less mature beta cell granules containing a higher proportion of unconverted proinsulin, or its intermediates, by more severely hyperglycemic diabetic patients.

A comprehensive review of proinsulin and C-peptide by Kitabchi (1977) cited measurements of proinsulin by a different technique than those of Mako *et al.* (1977). He reported that neither diabetes *per se* nor obesity *per se*, but a combination of obesity and diabetes in an individual was associated with increased percentage of proinsulinlike material in plasma. These conclusions were based on proinsulin levels during the entire glucose tolerance tests and not from basal levels. Differences in basal proinsulin levels were less apparent among the groups reported by Kitabchi (1977).

Residual beta cell function in 83 insulin-treated diabetics was estimated by Hendriksen *et al.* (1977). When fasting C-peptide was above 0.07 pmol/ml, all had an increase in C-peptide after injection of glucagon; in those with fasting C-peptide below 0.04 pmol/ml, none responded. Of 36 patients with a C-peptide response to glucagon, 30 had a response to ingestion of a standard breakfast; the responses correlated well. No patient with a negative response to glucagon responsed to the meal. Thus, the glucagon test appears to predict beta cell response during everyday life. Residual beta cell function was present most frequently in patients whose diabetes was of shortest duration. Metabolic importance of endogenous insulin secretion was apparent in that there was a lower insulin dosage requirement in those with residual beta cell function.

The metabolic importance of residual beta cell function was also pointed out by Faber and Binder (1977) in a study of 17 insulin-dependent diabetic patients within the first month of treatment. In blood samples before and after meals, mean C-peptide concentration (index of functional beta cell secretory capacity) and the mean amplitude of glycemic excursions (index of stability of blood glucose) were determined; these two parameters correlated negatively. Those patients with the highest insulin-secretory capacities had required the smallest insulin dose. These findings pointed to the importance of measures to restore or improve beta cell function when aiming at better control of diabetes.

Kuzuya *et al.* (1977a) outlined the details of methods for determination of free and total insulin and C-peptide in plasma of insulin-treated diabetics. The methods involved polyethylene glycol precipitation of anti-insulin antibodies and measuring free insulin in the supernate. After acidification of plasma to separate bound insulin from insulin antibody, followed by polyethylene glycol precipitation, the supernate contained total plasma insulin, which was measured by radioimmunoassay. It was shown that in JOD patients who received a single dose of NPH insulin before breakfast, the time of day in which serum free insulin reached its peak varied considerably from patient to patient, but that the peak free insulin correlated well with the maximal fall in plasma glucose. The authors thought that these findings added to the understanding of reasons for poor control in some of the patients, and suggested that these findings could indicate appropriate changes in the choice of insulin therapy.

The measurement of urinary C-peptide can provide a useful assessment of beta cell secretory capacity over time, and this can be especially advantageous when frequent blood sampling is not feasible, as in children. Horwitz *et al.* (1977) described a method for measuring urinary C-peptide. Healthy subjects excreted 36 μg C-peptide for 24 hr; adult-onset diabetic patients, 24 μg/24 hr; and juvenile-onset diabetic patients, 1.1 μg/ 24 hr. In two diabetic patients well controlled on small doses of insulin, urinary C-peptide increased to supernormal levels during acute infection; after amputations, C-peptide excretion fell markedly. Evidently, differences in C-peptide excretion reflect day-to-day variations in pancreatic C-peptide secretion. The findings indicate an absolute deficiency of insulin secretion in established juvenile-type diabetes, while the range of values for adult-onset diabetes is consistent with varying degrees of beta cell loss.

Kuzuya *et al.* (1977b) produced evidence of heterogeneity in circulating forms of C-peptide in human plasma. It had been observed with different assays from different laboratories that fasting concentrations of C-peptide in healthy subjects ranged from 0.9 to 3.5 ng/ml, with similar disparity in peak levels after oral glucose. Kuzuya *et al.* (1977b) found disparate results analyzing plasmas using two C-peptide antisera. These studies highlight the importance of validating each particular assay with respect to dilution curves, recoveries, and cross-reacting substances before using them for clinical studies.

Jaspan *et al.* (1977) confirmed that plasma levels of insulin and proinsulin were increased in patients with chronic renal failure, and further showed that C-peptide concentrations were also elevated. During glucose tolerance tests in renal failure, the usual close correlation between insulin and C-peptide levels is distorted in that C-peptide concentrations rise proportionately more than insulin. Jaspan and co-workers pointed out that the high C-peptide levels in renal failure could be mistakenly taken to indicate adequate beta cell reserve. Similarly, in patients with renal insufficiency and hypoglycemia, elevated C-peptide levels (and elevated proinsulin levels) might be erroneously taken to suggest endogenous hyperinsulinism. The disproportionate increase of C-peptide and proinsulin relative to insulin in chronic renal failure, the authors concluded, depends on the greater hepatic extraction and metabolism of insulin.

7.2.2.7. Effects of Control of Diabetes on Insulin Secretion

Genuth (1977) demonstrated in an obese diabetic patient that weight reduction induced a decrease in basal plasma glucose and insulin and a $2\frac{1}{2}$-times increase in meal-stimulated release of insulin. On regain of adiposity, and basal hyperglycemia (plasma glucose 130 mg/dl) and hyper-insulinemia, the heightened response of plasma insulin to breakfast persisted. However, with prolongation of hyperalimentation and obesity, beta cell function eventually deteriorated and returned to the original condition, in which there were fasting hyperglycemia, basal hyperinsulinemia, and a decreased and modest response of insulin to ingestion of a meal. The case demonstrates that reduction of hyperalimentation and adiposity can restore beta cell capacity to secrete insulin in response to food and emphasizes, as well, the importance of developing reliable methods of weight maintenance after successful weight reduction in obese diabetics to maintain beta cell function.

7.3. Insulin Resistance and Insulin Receptors

7.3.1. Insulin Resistance and Sensitivity

Harano *et al.* (1977) described a technique for determining insulin sensitivity that involved the simultaneous infusion of glucose, insulin, and somatostatin, the determination of steady-state glucose levels, and the calculation of an insulin sensitivity index. The authors thought the method was safe and reliable for estimating insulin sensitivity *in vivo*. As compared to control subjects, the index was subnormal in a group of insulin-treated diabetics, a group of untreated diabetics, and a group of borderline diabetics (1-hr blood glucose between 130 and 160 mg/dl or 2-hr value between 100 and 130 mg/dl). Of the 11 diabetic patients, only 2 exhibited normal insulin sensitivity. Ginsberg (1977a) found, however, that well-controlled subjects with ketosis-prone diabetes have normal insulin sensitivity. A group of 12 young adults who had recently experienced their first episodes of ketoacidosis near the onset of diabetes received insulin therapy for 2–8 weeks before receiving infusions containing glucose, insulin, epinephrine, and propranolol. A second group of patients received infusions containing insulin and glucose. In each group, neither steady-state plasma insulin levels nor steady-state plasma glucose levels were different in diabetic patients as compared to control subjects.

Only two of the 12 diabetic patients were judged to have insulin resistance and these two had had poor control of their diabetes at the time of study. All patients with ketosis-prone diabetes under control were shown to have normal insulin sensitivity.

Reaven and Olefsky (1977) confirmed the observation of Fajans *et al.* (1976) of considerable variation in insulin response to oral glucose among normal subjects and among patients with mild diabetes. They also showed that there exists variability of insulin resistance in the same subjects. They demonstrated a highly significant correlation between the height of the insulin response and the degree of insulin resistance in 75 nonobese subjects classified as normal, borderline glucose-intolerant, or chemically diabetic on the basis of an oral glucose tolerance test. The authors stated that this relationship seems to confirm the suggestion of Fajans *et al.* (1976) that there is heterogeneity in patients with chemical diabetes. The subdivision of chemical diabetes into those patients with both insulin resistance and a secondary increased insulin response, as contrasted to those with a primary defect of insulin release without insulin resistance, seems to account for both heterogeneity and the variable clinical course of these patients. Only patients with chemical diabetes who had a diminished insulin response to glucose showed progressive deterioration in glucose tolerance.

Olefsky *et al.* (1977) concluded that abnormality in plasma glucagon concentration does not play a role in the insulin resistance (determined by infusion technique) of adults with chemical diabetes or with nonketotic diabetes and fasting hyperglycemia. Fasting and steady-state plasma glucagon levels were not significantly different among the control patients and two groups of diabetic patients. Further, there was no significant correlation between fasting plasma glucagon level and fasting plasma glucose level. These authors thought that insulin resistance was probably due to an abnormality at the level of target tissue responsiveness to insulin.

Reaven *et al.* (1977), having shown that nonketotic diabetic patients with fasting hyperglycemia have insulin resistance and decreased insulin secretion in response to glucose, suggested that the insulin resistance develops as a consequence of insulin deficiency. To test this idea, they measured insulin resistance (propranolol–epinephrine–glucose–insulin infusion technique) and found it to be increased in the dog made severely diabetic with alloxan. Resistance was corrected when diabetes was controlled with insulin. They interpreted these findings to be compatible with the postulate that insulin deficiency is a primary cause of diabetes in nonketotic diabetic patients with fasting hyperglycemia and a subnormal insulin response to glucose, and that insulin resistance is a secondary consequence of the insulin-deficient state in these patients. They suggested that because insulin resistance could not be demonstrated in dogs with only a moderate degree of hyperglycemia secondary to alloxan, insulin resistance does not necessarily develop in man with milder degrees of diabetes.

7.3.2. Insulin Receptors

Beck-Nielsen *et al.* (1977) found a highly significant positive correlation between insulin-binding to mononuclear leukocytes and the monocyte content of isolated cell suspensions from normal persons. Removal of monocytes from mononuclear cell suspension reduced insulin-binding by approximately 80%. Granulocytes possessed about one-quarter and lymphocytes $\frac{1}{26}$ the binding ability of monocytes. Thrombocytes bound insulin, but erythrocytes did not. The mean number of receptors per monocyte was estimated to be 7000. Five percent of [^{125}I]insulin when dissociated from monocyte receptors was found to be degraded. From these findings, the authors concluded that monocytes *per se* were a useful model for insulin receptor studies in man.

The ingestion of glucose by normal volunteers was followed at 2 hr, but more prominently at 5 hr, by decreased affinity of insulin receptors for insulin on circulating monocytes (Muggeo *et al.*, 1977). The authors concluded that acute changes in receptor affinity occur normally as part of the physiological regulation of the sensitivity of target cells to hormone stimulation.

Davidson and Kaplan (1977) demonstrated that streptozotocin-induced diabetes in rats induced their hepatic plasma membranes to bind approximately twice as much insulin as did membranes from nondiabetic rats. There was no difference in glucagon binding, however. The increase in insulin-binding was attributed to enhanced binding capacity and was returned to normal by treating streptozotocin-diabetic rats with insulin. The results were considered compatible with the hypothesis that insulin concentration modulates the number of insulin receptors. Since evidence has been reported that fat, muscle, and hepatic tissue of rats made diabetic by alloxan are insensitive to insulin, it seemed apparent to the authors that sentitivity of the diabetic liver to insulin is determined, in part, by events subsequent to the binding of insulin to its receptor.

7.3.2.1. Insulin Receptors and Insulin Resistance in Diabetes

Olefsky and Reaven (1977) showed that diabetic patients with abnormal glucose tolerance tests (chemical diabetes) had a 45% decrease in insulin-binding to their circulating monocytes (reduced number of receptors per cell), were insulin-resistant, and as a group were hyperinsulinemic. Insulin resistance was demonstrated by elevated steady-state plasma glucose levels in response to infused glucose, insulin, epinephrine, and propranolol. In normal and chemical-diabetic subjects, there was a highly significant inverse correlation between the amount of insulin bound and (1) both the fasting plasma insulin level and the incremental insulin area during oral glucose tolerance test and (2) the degree of insulin resistance. Likewise, patients with fasting hyperglycemia had decreased insulin-binding, but the data suggested that insulin resistance in these subjects is independent of changes in insulin receptors. Considering all the diabetic patients, decreased binding to monocytes was found only in those with fasting hyperinsulinemia. The insulin resistance of patients with chemical diabetes may be related to a decrease in insulin receptors, but this did not appear to be the case for patients who had fasting hyperglycemia. Further, it appeared that basal, not the stimulated, insulin levels are associated with changes in insulin receptors.

7.3.2.2. Insulin-Binding in Other Clinical Conditions

Rosenbloom *et al.* (1977a) found no difference in the insulin-binding of cultured fibroblasts obtained from patients with lipoatrophic diabetes as compared to that of fibroblasts from control subjects. This suggested to the authors that resistance to exogenous insulin in this condition is not due to a genetic defeat in insulin receptors, but might be due to some secondary disruption of binding *in vivo*, possibly by a circulating factor.

Oseid *et al.* (1977) showed that the monocuclear leukocytes from patients with congenital generalized lipodystrophy bound significantly less insulin (mainly reduced binding affinity) than cells from normal subjects. A regain of insulin-binding following 60 hr of fasting suggested that the receptor defect might not be primary. The reduced binding affinity was thought to be due to the high concentrations of plasma insulin seen in such patients, whereas in other circumstances of hyperinsulinemia the number of insulin receptors is reduced. Oseid *et al.* (1977) thought that their findings suggested a defect of the insulin receptor. Roth *et al.* (1977), commenting on this report, note that insulin resistance associated with generalized lipodystrophy has been added to the list of diseases in which there is altered sensitivity to hormones and functional alterations in the hormone receptor.

7.3.3. Autoantibodies to Insulin Receptors

Flier *et al.* (1977) and Kahn *et al.* (1977) studied the sera of patients who had the syndrome of insulin-resistant diabetes and serum anti-insulin receptor antibodies to further characterize this disorder. The data were interpreted as showing binding of receptor autoantibodies to different determinants of the insulin receptor; these autoantibodies were said to be useful as unique probes of insulin receptor structure and function.

Blackard *et al.* (1977) documented clinical and serological remission of insulin-resistant diabetes mellitus caused by anti-receptor antibodies. A 37-year-old female with laboratory and physical stigmata of rheumatic disease was discovered to have insulin-resistant diabetes. A 1 : 10 dilution of the patient's serum inhibited binding of radiolabeled insulin to IM-9 lymphoblastoid cells by 50%. No circulating anti-insulin antibodies were present. Subsequently, there was spontaneous remission of insulin resistance, and insulin therapy was discontinued. Insulin antibodies were then present, but there was no evidence of antibodies to insulin receptors.

7.4. Diabetes and Exercise

7.4.1. Exercise and Diabetes Mellitus in Man

Berger *et al.* (1977) studied the metabolic and hormonal effects of muscular exercise in diabetic patients. One group of juvenile-diabetic patients were in moderate metabolic control, having had two thirds of their usual evening dose of insulin at 1800 hours on the day preceding the test. A second group had had insulin withheld for 18–48 hr and were in ketosis at the onset of the exercise test. The degree of exercise (bicycle ergometer) was estimated to be 30–40% of the subjects' maximal work capacity. In both groups of diabetic patients, blood lactate rose significantly higher than in control subjects; blood alanine rose transiently and significantly only in the patients. Glucose declined markedly in the moderately controlled patients; free fatty acids, ketone bodies, and glucagon increased in degree comparable to that of the normal controls. In the ketotic patients, however, glucose concentration rose; increases in ketone bodies, glucagon, and cortisol levels were significantly greater than in the moderately controlled patients and the control subjects. The results were thought to substantiate the clinical experience that in contrast to the possible beneficial effects of exercise in moderately well controlled juvenile-type diabetes, in ketotic, relatively insulin-deficient patients, even nonstrenuous exercise can have deleterious effects.

Zinman *et al.* (1977) and Murray *et al.* (1977) studied the effects of exercise on diabetic patients receiving intermediate-acting insulin subcutaneously or receiving insulin by infusion. In patients receiving insulin by infusion, the at-rest glucose production rate exceeded normal by 25% when plasma glucose was near normal. Subsequent exercise induced no change in blood glucose, but comparable to changes in control subjects, there was an increase in glucose production and disappearance. However, increases in lactate and pyruvate were supernormal, and glycerol and ketone body concentrations tended to increase. In the patients receiving insulin subcutaneously, at-rest glucose production exceeded normal by more than 100%; during exercise, glucose disappearance was normal, but there was a remarkable fall in plasma glucose and in glucose production. In these patients, the fall in plasma glucose during exercise was probably the result of decreased glucose production, due to the hepatic effects of insulin, the mobilization of which was increased by exercise. In two of these patients, concentration of plasma insulin rose during exercise. Thus, in the patients treated with subcutaneous insulin, there was insulin deficiency at rest (mean plasma glucose level 227 mg/dl) and increased insulin effect during exercise. These studies also demonstrate that in diabetic patients who are maintained near normal glycemia by intravenous infusion of insulin, exercise is not followed by a totally normal metabolic response.

7.4.2. Effect of Exercise in Depancreatized Dogs

Kawamori and Vranic (1977) exercised pancreatectomized dogs 8–9 hr after food intake and injection of crystalline insulin subcutaneously in the thigh. At 60 min after an hour's run, the dogs were fed, given subcutaneous injections of protamine zinc and crystalline insulin, and immediately begun on a second run. The authors produced evidence that exercise accelerates insulin mobilization from its injection site and that this is important in inducing the decrease in blood glucose that these dogs experienced. Glucose uptake by muscle was not greater than normal, but hepatic glucose production failed to meet the increased energy needs of the exercising dogs.

7.4.3. Effect of *in Vitro* Contracting Skeletal Muscle on Glucose Uptake

The question of whether increased glucose uptake by skeletal muscle during exercise is due to increased delivery of glucose to the exercising muscle or to that plus some exercise-induced change in glucose transport into muscle was explored by Schultz et al. (1977). These authors found that when flow to the rat hindlimb was increased glucose disappearance increased, but when flow was decreased glucose disappearance decreased, and when flow was kept constant, glucose disappearance remained unchanged. Further, the addition of electrical stimulation of muscle contraction during these three conditions of flow did not influence glucose disappearance. Insulin caused an increased disappearance of glucose, but the addition of exercise with flow held constant was without additional effect. Because blood flow to the muscle increases during exercise *in vivo*, they reasoned that increased glucose delivery may be a modulator of the augmented glucose consumption by muscle observed during exercise *in vivo*. The authors were unable to account for studies by others showing that glucose disappearance was increased during electrical stimulation, but was not further increased with the addition of a twofold increase in perfusate flow. Nor could they reconcile their findings with those of others demonstrating a two- to threefold increase in glucose uptake with electrical stimulation in similar isolated perfused rat hindlimb preparations.

7.5. Diabetes and Pregnancy

7.5.1. Special Considerations

Over 50 years of experience with pregnancy in diabetic women was reviewed by Hare and White (1977), focusing on 416 pregnancies in mothers who had either microvascular or macrovascular disease. Only in White Class H (mothers with arteriosclerotic heart disease) was there mortality; one mother died undelivered and two died within 4 weeks of delivery. Fetal survival improved steadily throughout the 50 years, there being an approximate 50% increase in suvival in the period 1963–1975, as compared to 1924–1962. Whereas fetal survival for infants of diabetic mothers as a whole has reached that of women without diabetes delivered in the same hospital in this series of patients, this was not true if the mother had vascular disease. Thus, maternal vascular disease adversely affects survival both of the mother and of the infant.

In a study of lipid metabolism in pregnancy, which included overtly diabetic women, women with gestational diabetes, and normal pregnant women, Warth and Knopp (1977) concluded that hypertriglyceridemia occurring during pregnancy was due to a different mechanism from that associated with atherosclerosis. This conclusion was based on their failure to find any effect of diabetes mellitus, body weight, or high carbohydrate ingestion on hypertriglyceridemia of pregnancy. They suggested that increased secretion of estrogen might be a factor in the hypertriglyceridemia of pregnancy.

7.5.2. Management of Pregnancy in Diabetic Patients

Brittle diabetes may become less brittle during the course of pregnancy (Lev-Ran and Goldman, 1977). These authors determined the variability of blood glucose at various times in the course of pregnancy. When the mean of daily differences (MDD) of blood glucose at 4 time points exceeded 100 mg/dl under optimal control circumstances, diabetes was defined as brittle. They found, in eight pregnant brittle-diabetic patients, that MDD which was 127 mg/dl before pregnancy was 46 mg/dl at 24 weeks and 55 mg/dl at 36 weeks. MDD in nondiabetic individuals was 12–16 mg/dl. In severe but nonlabile diabetic patients, it remained stable in the range of 49–53 mg/dl throughout pregnancy. Similarly, the mean within-day glycemic excursions dropped from 147 mg/dl before pregnancy in brittle diabetics to 85 mg/dl at 36 weeks; in the stable diabetics this was 55 and 72 mg/dl, and in nondiabetics 34 and 46 mg/dl, throughout the pregnancy. Thus, brittleness seemed to decrease near the end of pregnancy.

Ayromlooi *et al.* (1977) examined their experience with 56 pregnant diabetics managed during 1969–1971 with that gained with 76 pregnant diabetic patients managed during 1973–1975. Observations made were: amniotic fluid shake test as an estimate of the lecithin/sphingomyelin ratio (L/S ratio), 24-hr urinary estriol, serial ultrasonographic biparietal diameters, fetal stress testing with oxytocin infusion, electronic fetal heart rate–uterine contraction monitoring, and pH of fetal scalp blood. During the 1973–1975 period, the result of fetal lung maturity testing (shake test) and clinical condition were, in the authors' opinion, the most important factors that aided in the proper timing of delivery of the diabetic patient. Delivery was accomplished when evidence of fetal lung maturity by the shake test was attained, irrespective of whether the urinary estriol measurement was normal or the oxytocin challenge test negative. On the other hand, when the shake test was judged as representing immaturity, serial estriols, biparietal diameter, and oxytocin challenge test was positive, a decision to deliver the patient was made. Perinatal death, corrected for congenital malformation, was 14.3% in the earlier period and 7.9% in the 1973–1975 period. Total perinatal death, including malformation, decreased from 17.9 to 9.2% in the latter period. In the 1973–1975 period, seven neonates developed respiratory distress syndrome (RDS). Six of these had mild to moderate affectation and, of these, five had an intermediate result on the amniotic fluid shake test; the sixth, who developed mild RDS, had a shake test that suggested immaturity. In the authors' opinion, the modern management of diabetic pregnancy involves all the measurements indicated above, with special emphasis placed on the interpretation of the shake test.

An analogous experience was reported by Drury *et al.* (1977), who concluded that the use of the L/S ratio of amniotic fluid made a substantial contribution to decreasing the incidence of RDS and led to an improvement in perinatal mortality in their hands. They reported a perinatal mortality rate of 9.5% for the period 1951–1976. In the period 1963–1972, ten infants died of hyaline membrane disease (HMD), and half these deaths followed elective deliveries. On the other hand, the only case of RDS that they recognized in the past three years (1973–1976) was when spontaneous labor ensued at 38 weeks when the L/S ratio was 1.4. The infant succumbed to respiratory distress. It is the authors' current policy to effect delivery at 38 weeks only if the ratio is 1.8 or greater. In the past three years, 69 infants were delivered at 38 weeks. Delivery was deferred to 40 weeks in 10 and to 41 weeks in an additional 10. During this period, perinatal mortality was 6% compared to 9.5% for the entire period. In the authors' opinion, blind adherence to a policy of delivery at 38 weeks is neither necessary nor desirable, and the L/S ratio contributed far more than estrogen measurements or ultrasound measurements of biparietal diameter to the favorable outcomes of these diabetic pregnancies. They found that respiratory distress did not occur when the L/S ratio was 1.8 or more.

Sutton (1977) reported a rather remarkable reduction in perinatal mortality in a hospital in the South Seas with limited technological facilities and no experienced neonatal staff. Perinatal mortality had been 47% in 1963 and 45% in 1975, but was 0% in 1976. The new procedures introduced in 1976 were the use of 8 mg dexamethasone i.m. every 8 hr for 48 hr 1 week before delivery to increase surfactant production by the fetus, weekly amniocentesis and estimation of the L/S ratio by the shake test, and increased use of elective cesarean section for all patients over 35 and in those with poor obstetric history or with persistent or worsening preeclampsia. Severe preeclampsia was treated with diazepam infusion, intravenous hypotensives, and intensive nursing care. No patient was induced into labor until the shake test was unequivocally positive. The dramatic reduction in perinatal mortality was thought to be due principally to the use of the shake test and to the administration of dexamethasone. It should be noted that it has not been established whether such use of dexamethasone may affect other aspects of fetal development. NIH multicenter studies now in progress may help clarify these issues. Widespread use of dexamethasone must await the availability of more information.

Gabbe *et al.* (1977) also reported on the usefulness of the L/S ratio in the timing of delivery of infants of overtly diabetic women. A retrospective status confirmed that the L/S ratio increases with advancing gestational age. In this respect, no differences were noted among White Classes B,C, and D,F, and R. There was a 3% incidence of RDS and HMD in the 200 infants of diabetic women with L/S ratios of 2 or greater. This was not different from the incidence of 2.6% observed in 279 other nondiabetic patients. Ten women had L/S ratios of 1.5–1.9; seven infants had RDS.

These authors felt that infants of diabetic mothers delivered soon after the determination of a mature L/S ratio (≥ 2.0) are not at greater risk for RDS and HMD than infants of nondiabetic mothers in their hospital population. An L/S ratio of 2.0 or more appeared to be a reliable predictor of fetal pulmonary maturity even in pregnancies complicated by diabetes.

Whitelaw (1977) studied an additional well-known effect of maternal diabetes on the fetus. He discovered a significant correlation between the skin-fold thickness of infants and the mean blood glucose or the fasting blood glucose of mothers during their third trimesters. Furthermore, there was a significant correlation between the fasting blood glucose of the mothers and the adipose cell diameter in the neonates. These findings were judged consistent with the hypothesis that in diabetic pregnancy, fetal hyperglycemia, a result of maternal hyperglycemia, and fetal hyperinsulinism stimulate increased triglyceride synthesis in adipose cells and enlargement of adipose cells, and lead to increase in fetal subcutaneous fat. A corollary to be drawn is that reduction of maternal hyperglycemia should result in less adiposity of infants of diabetic mothers.

The infant of the diabetic mother has a propensity to develop hypoglycemia in the early hours after delivery. Kalhan *et al.* (1977) not unexpectedly found that in five infants of insulin-dependent diabetic mothers, mean plasma glucose concentration had decreased more at $3\frac{1}{2}$ hr of age than in infants of healthy mothers (40.0 vs. 50.6 mg/dl; $p <$ to .05). The glucose production rate was also significantly lower in the infants of diabetic mothers. The authors thought that the reduced glucose output for the most part was probably the result of inhibited glycogenolysis rather than decrease in gluconeogensis, since the finding was made very shortly after birth. They postulated that the cause of this was multifactorial and probably included the combined effects of increased insulin levels in these infants and diminished glucagon and catecholamine responsiveness to hypoglycemia.

7.6. Acidosis in Diabetes

7.6.1. Diabetic Ketoacidosis

Asplin and Hartog (1977) measured free insulin in plasma of patients in diabetic coma and precoma. One group had been previously treated with insulin and had circulating antibodies. The other group had not been treated with insulin. Treatment for ketoacidosis was intramuscular insulin, 10 U hourly. Initial serum free insulin levels in those with and without insulin antibodies were 13 and 9 μU/ml; at 1–2 hr after treatment was begun, levels were 23 and 22 μU/ml; and at 7–8 hr, 74 and 73 μU/ml, respectively. No relationship was found between concentrations of serum free insulin and the rate of decline of blood glucose. The highest values of free insulin were achieved only after several hours of treatment. The authors therefore felt that an initial dose of 20 U i.m., followed by 5 U i.m. hourly, or an intravenous infusion might be a more logical treatment protocol than the one they chose. Kanter *et al.* (1977) studied phosphate metabolism and 2,3-diphosphoglycerate (2,3-DPG) levels in diabetic ketoacidotic patients. Measurements were made in patients in ketoacidosis on admission and at 2-hr intervals for 6 hr and again at 24 hr and were compared with the results of measurements in patients under good control on insulin therapy. Red blood cell 2,3-DPG and total phosphate were significantly lower in the ketoacidotic patients at all intervals. Serum inorganic phosphate steadily declined during treatment. The work of others showing that intravenous phosphate administration normalized 2,3-DPG content of red cells within hours, rather than within days, was cited. In the face of evidence that low 2,3-DPG levels produce reduced oxygen delivery to tissues and that 2,3-DPG formation is increased when phosphate levels are increased, the authors reemphasized that the treatment of ketoacidosis should include replacement of phosphate.

Barnes *et al.* (1977a) were unable to detect glucagon in plasma of pancreatectomized patients who developed ketoacidosis on insulin withdrawal. They concluded that glucagon was not essential for the development of ketoacidosis. However, in nonpancreatectomized ketoacidotic patients in whom glucagon was present in plasma, 3-hydroxybutyrate and plasma glucose were higher. The authors felt, therefore, that glucagon may accelerate onset of ketonemia and hyperglycemia when there is insulin deficiency.

Schade and Eaton (1977) cited evidence that diabetic ketoacidosis is characterized by elevations in plasma levels of glucagon, catecholamines, cortisol, and growth hormone, and that these elevations can initiate excess production of ketone bodies in the presence of insulin insufficiency. They suggest that a rational therapy in preventing diabetic ketoacidosis would be the pharmacological control of excess secretion of these hormones.

Ginsberg (1977b) found during initial episodes of ketoacidosis that the steady-state plasma glucose level produced by infusion of glucose and insulin was significantly higher than it was 2–7 weeks after recovery from ketoacidosis. Cortisol and free fatty acid concentrations correlated significantly with steady-state plasma glucose levels during ketoacidosis and in the later recovery period. Ginsberg suggested that insulin resistance was a feature of diabetic ketoacidosis and that this might be attributed in part to elevated free fatty acids and cortisol in plasma.

Lufkin *et al.*(1977) reported a patient who survived presumed acute cerebral edema developing during treatment for diabetic ketoacidosis. These authors then reviewed all clinical records and necropsy findings of patients who died within 5 days of treatment of ketoacidosis at the Mayo Clinic from 1950 to 1974, or who had a clinical or postmortem diagnosis of cerebral edema. Of 14 cases reviewed who had histological examination of the brain, acute cerebral dysfunction had been diagnosed in three. In two of these, significant cerebral edema was seen at autopsy and, in the third case, was diagnosed on the basis of elevated CSF pressure. The authors were uncertain of the pathogenesis of the acute neurological manifestation in all cases studied.

7.6.1.1. Diabetic Ketoacidosis and Low-Dose Insulin Therapy

Fisher *et al.* (1977) concluded that low-dose treatment of diabetic ketoacidosis is quite effective regardless of the route of administration of insulin. A total of 45 subjects with ketoacidosis were grouped for receiving insulin by the intramuscular, subcutaneous, and intravenous routes. Each subject received initially 0.33 U insulin/kg body weight. Thereafter, 7 U was given hourly until plasma glucose reached 250 mg/dl. The treatments were similarly effective regardless of route with respect to changes in levels of plasma glucose, serum bicarbonate, blood pH, serum acetone, number of units of insulin given to achieve glucose of 250 mg/dl, and number of units of insulin used for total control. During the first 2 hr, those receiving intravenous insulin (bolus then infusion) had the most rapid decreases of plasma glucose and ketone bodies. These authors recommend an initial intravenous bolus of insulin followed immediately by hourly intramuscular insulin. They concluded that insulin resistance is not commonplace in diabetic ketoacidosis, and that fluid and electrolyte replacement and monitoring of the patient are the truly critical factors in treatment of ketoacidosis.

Alberti (1977) asserts that low-dose insulin therapy is proved to be effective as a treatment for diabetic ketoacidosis. An intramuscular insulin regimen, he believes, is safe and applicable in nonspecialist centers. When using low-dose intravenous therapy, a loading dose was said to be unnecessary; 4–5 U/hr is recommended in adults. When blood glucose has fallen to less than 250 mg/dl, the infusion rate can be reduced to 2 U/hr or subcutaneous insulin begun along with 5% dextrose. The importance of rehydration, early use of potassium, clinical care, and common sense, whatever treatment method is used, was emphasized. The use of hourly intravenous boluses rather than continuous infusion was said to be irrational because the effects of high concentration of insulin were said to be intermittent and associated with sharp increases in concentrations of cortisol, growth hormone, lactate, and pyruvate. If intramuscular insulin is used, a 20-U loading dose is followed by 4–5 U/hr. Difficulties with intermittent intramuscular therapy and with intravenous insulin infusions were cited.

Heber *et al.* (1977) found no difference in the result of treatment of ketoacidosis by low-dose infusion as compared to treatment with a combination of intravenous boluses and subcutaneous injections on a 2-hr schedule. The infusion group received a 6-U insulin bolus followed by 6 U/hr. The conventional therapy group received doses from 25 U i.v. plus 25 U s.c. to as high as 150 U by each route. Rates of fall of plasma glucose and plasma glucagon were similar in both groups; growth hormone rose transiently in both, and mild hypoglycemia occurred in one patient in the infusion group. Some advantages, however, were claimed for the low-dose intravenous therapy: (1) it eliminates varying initial and repeat insulin dosages to provide a more predictable rate of fall of blood glucose, (2) it is easily administered by nursing personnel, and (3) it can be stopped abruptly in the event of hypoglycemia.

Padilla and Loeb (1977) declared that attempting to manage the patient with the lowest possible dose of insulin is pointless and potentially hazardous in the presence of ketoacidosis. On the basis of a survey of the literature, they concluded that dose and mode of insulin administration are relatively unimportant as long as adequate concentrations of insulin are present in responsive tissues. They suggest that if continuous low-dose infusion is to be used, an initial loading dose of 10–20 U should be given, followed by constant infusion at the rate of 10–15 U/hr. They judged that 50–100 U by bolus injection hourly is equally effective and is simpler than the intravenous method. Protracted deliberations at bedside to plan a "tailor-made" insulin dose early in the course of therapy is probably naïve and time-wasting.

Sherwin (1977) also concluded that the quantity and mode of insulin administration are of little consequence with regard to the rate at which abnormalities in glucose and ketone metabolism are reversed in diabetic ketoacidosis. He stated that there was no evident reduction in requirements for potassium, in risk of hypoglycemia, or in incidence of cerebral edema with the low-dose infusion treatment mode. He feared that physicians will not monitor the patient intensively and may leave the bedside if the low-dose infusion technique is used.

An Editorial (1977c) in the *British Medical Journal* claims simplicity and reliability of low-dose intravenous and low-dose intramuscular therapy of ketoacidosis. At 0.1 or 1 U/ml saline, loss of insulin on the containers is minimal and obviates the need for adding albumin or the patient's own blood to prevent absorption of insulin to glassware.

Piters *et al.* (1977) compared three treatment protocols in three groups with ketoacidosis: (1) 50 U insulin i.v. initially, and at intervals of 2 hr; (2) continuous infusion of 10 U/hr; and (3) loading intravenous dose of 3 U followed by 2 U/hr by infusion. The authors concluded that 10 U/hr infusion of insulin is as effective in normalizing plasma glucose, bicarbonate, ketone bodies, and blood pH as 50 U administered intravenously as a bolus every 2 hr, but that the lowest-dose protocol was ineffective as compared to the other two. In fact, two patients in the third group had worsening of these parameters during the first 6 hr; they did respond to boluses of 50 U insulin and administered intravenously every 2 hr. These authors felt that intravenous infusion of insulin produced constant serum levels of insulin, enabled a prompt cessation of action to be accomplished, provided for absorption of the full dose, and assured predictable linear changes in most biochemical variables. They suggested that if infusion is to be given, 10 U/hr is effective, but the dose should be reduced to 5 U/hr when plasma glucose has fallen to 300 mg/dl.

7.6.2. Lactic Acidosis

Alberti and Nattrass (1977), in reviewing lactic acidosis, noted that decreased activity of pyruvate dehydrogenase associated with diabetes makes more likely the occurrence of increased circulating lactate or lactic acidosis or both. Clinical signs of acidosis, blood lactate concentration consistently above 5 mmol/liter, and arterial pH of 7.25 or less describe the majority of patients who can be said to have lactic acidosis. Unlike type A lactic acidosis, in type B (associated with diabetes) there is no evidence of tissue anoxia. The first phase of therapy, the authors state, is alkalinization with massive amounts of bicarbonate (up to 2500 mmol bicarbonate). Hemodialysis should be considered and probably should be performed whenever pH is less than 7. In the authors' opinion, insulin therapy does not improve lactic acidosis *per se*.

7.7. Long-Term Complications

7.7.1. Diabetic Neuropathy

7.7.1.1. Evidence of Genetic Heterogeneity

Further evidence of the heterogeneous nature of diabetes, with particular respect to the presence of neuropathy, was demonstrated by McLaren *et al.* (1977) in a study of acetylator phenotypes. A group of 64 diabetic patients who had clinical signs of peripheral neuropathy were compared to 66 patients who had no evidence of peripheral neuropathy. The incidence of patients who acetylated sulfadimidine rapidly was significantly greater in the diabetics without neuropathy than in those with neuropathy, and in a group of 57 normal patients. The authors interpreted these findings as evidence that genetic factors, apart from the diabetic diathesis *per se,* may determine the development of neuropathy in any particular diabetic.

7.7.1.2. Radiculopathy

Longstreth and Newcomer (1977) described a syndrome of pain as a beltlike constriction, pressure with needlelike characteristics, and deep burning and stabbing sensations. These symptoms were located principally in the central and upper abdomen, and occasionally in the lower thorax, and were accompanied by electromyographic signs of involvement of many thoracic and/or lumbar nerve roots. Paresthesias were sometimes experienced. Additional diabetic complications such as peripheral neuropathy, gastric atony, impotence, and anhydrosis of the feet were also noticed. The value of electromyographic examination in identifying the cause of such pain was emphasized.

7.7.1.3. Peripheral Neuropathy

In a study of 56 patients having adult-onset type diabetes (64% treated with insulin), 71% were judged to have peripheral neuropathy (Braddom *et al.,* 1977). For this diagnosis, two or more indices of abnormal nerve function [(1) sural nerve latency, (2) median nerve sensory or motor latency, and (3) ulnar nerve sensory latency] were required because of the prevalence of confounding conditions in diabetes, e.g., coolness of the lower extremity, carpal tunnel syndrome, and selective trauma to ulnar nerve. The longer the duration of diabetes, the greater were the number of abnormal nerve conduction parameters per patient. The mean age of the patients, however, did not increase with increase in number of nerve condition abnormalities. Thus, the authors concluded that diabetic neuropathy was more related to the duration of diabetes than to the age of the patient. Abnormality in nerve conduction studies was associated with other clinical findings. Fifty-five percent of men said they were impotent, Achilles reflex was absent in 56%, and vibratory sense was decreased or absent in the toes in 50% of patients. The interpretation of these three clinical findings was made difficult, however, by their known association with increasing age.

7.7.1.4. Diabetic Amyotrophy

Chokroverty *et al.* (1977) concluded from a study of 12 patients that diabetic amyotrophy is a proximal intramuscular crural neuropathy, a special manifestation of diabetic neuropathy. The characteristic clinical picture is moderate to marked weakness and wasting of pelvifemoral muscles (quadriceps femoris, gluteal, hamstring, adductor, and iliopsoas muscles), characteristically without sensory impairment. Its insidious and slowly progressive onset differentiates it from the onset of ischemic mononeuropathy multiplex, which is relatively sudden. It is usually recognized in middle-aged or older patients shortly after, or simultaneous with, onset of manifest diabetes. Distal leg muscles are normal, or in some patients mildly weakened. Manifestations may be unilateral. Patellar reflexes are usually diminished or absent, but ankle reflexes may be normal or diminished. The syndrome is accompanied by diffuse aching or sharp pain in thighs or lumbosacral region. Most, but not all, fail to show diabetic retinopathy or nephropathy, and prognosis is generally good if there is adequate control of hyperglycemia. The onset of diabetic amyotrophy simultaneous with or early in the course of manifest diabetes mellitus and the improvement of the patients with good control of hyperglycemia were thought to support the concept of a metabolic cause of diabetic amyotrophy.

7.7.1.5. Autonomic Neuropathy

Hollis *et al.* (1977) concluded that the esophageal muscle *per se* was intact in diabetes, but found significantly lower velocity of contraction waves and abnormality of esophageal motility in 24 of 30 patients with peripheral neuropathy, but in only 4 of 20 who had no peripheral neuropathy. No patient had esophageal symptoms.

Gastroparesis is considered to be a neurological complication of diabetes and one whose treatment is often unsatisfactory. Longstreth *et al.* (1977) administered 15 mg metoclopramide orally, four times daily with meals, to a 19-year-old woman who had vomiting, epigastric pain, and decreased gastric peristalsis and retention of food particles. The frequency of type II gastric contractions markedly increased, gastric emptying rate strikingly increased, and the patient experienced marked improvement including a 9-kg weight gain. Brady and Richardson (1977) found that intravenous metoclopramide was associated with shortening of gastric half-time of emptying in a patient with gastric phytobezoar, postural hypotension, impotence, and peripheral neuropathy. These observations promise help for patients with gastric motility disturbance secondary to diabetes, but need to be confirmed.

Aberrations in cardiac rhythmicity are a consequence of abnormality of the autonomic nerves regulating heart rate and rhythm. Gundersen and Neubauer (1977) measured three types of pulse rate variations: (1) standard deviation of differences between R–R intervals (a measure of the variation in heart rate from one beat to the next), (2) the standard deviation of R–R intervals (this is more sensitive to long-term than short-term fluctuations in heart rate), and (3) the number of runs-up and runs-down. An increased number of runs would be indicative of loss of cyclic influence of respiration. All three types of measurements were reduced in parallel in long-term diabetics. The standard deviation of differences between R–R intervals, easily measured with an ordinary ECG apparatus, was affected earliest, correlated negatively with duration of diabetes, and therefore seems to be good for the early detection of autonomic nervous system abnormalities of the heart in diabetes. Maher *et al.* (1977) found plasma levels of glucagon in response to similar degrees of insulin-induced hypoglycemia to be 308 pg/ml for normal subjects and 209 and 115 pg/ml for nonneuropathic and neuropathic diabetic patients. The diminished to absent glucagon response in the patients with neuropathy was thought to be indicative of loss of neuromechanisms of glucagon secretion, in addition to a glucose receptor defect (neuropathics had normal increases of glucagon in response to arginine). A lack of a glucagon response to hypoglycemia was thought to contribute to metabolic instability in diabetes. A similar conclusion was reached by Reynolds *et al.* (1977).

Another clinical correlate of autonomic neuropathy in diabetes was proposed by Faerman *et al.* (1977). In their study of the sympathetic and parasympathetic nerve fibers in the heart muscles, they found in five patients who died of painless myocardial infarction what they considered typical lesions of diabetic neuropathy: beaded thickenings, spindle-shaped thickenings, fragmentation of fibers, and diminution of the number of nerve fibers. No such lesions were noted in five diabetics who had painful infarctions, five diabetics without infarction, five nondiabetics with painful infarction, and five nondiabetics without infarction. The authors concluded that the absence of pain in some diabetic patients with myocardial infarction was due to abnormality of the afferent nerves that conduct pain.

Gunderson and Christensen (1977) studied diabetic patients without neuropathy by tilting them from the supine to the near-upright position before and 45 min after intravenous injection of insulin. After insulin, supine and tilt pulse rates and plasma norepinephrine concentrations were increased significantly, whereas intravascular mass of albumin and plasma volume decreased significantly; supine, the relative decrease in plasma volume correlated with a relative increase in plasma norepinephrine. It was suggested that patients with abnormal cardiovascular reflexes might not be able to maintain arterial blood pressure after intravenous insulin. The authors suggested that insulin, either directly or secondarily to its metabolic effects, may alter the function or the volume of the endothelial cells and thereby increase the transfer of fluid and albumin out of the vascular system.

Alexander and Oake (1977) found significant attenuation of vascular reactivity to norepinephrine in the tails of male rats when insulin was infused into the isolated perfused tail at physiological and pharmacological concentrations; this was found less consistently in the female rats. The authors concluded that the hypotension cometimes observed with insulin therapy can be produced, at least in part, by an attenuation of the normal vasoconstrictor response of peripheral blood vessels to norepinephrine. A decrease in plasma volume and intravascular pool of albumin (Gundersen and Christensen, 1977) could also be a factor contributing to the development of hypotension in insulin-treated diabetic subjects.

7.7.1.6. Myoinositol Metabolism

Since nerve myoinositol is decreased in rats made diabetic with streptozotocin and since supplementation of their diet with myoinositol improved nerve conduction in these rats (Greene *et al.*, 1975), Clements and Reynertson (1977) studied the metabolism of myoinositol in diabetic patients. They found that whereas dietary intake of myoinositol and fecal excretion were similar in diabetic and nondiabetic subjects, urinary myoinositol in the untreated diabetic patients was ten times that of the healthy subjects. Further, when diabetic patients ingested a standard myoinositol load or ate regular meals, plasma myoinositol levels became significantly higher than in normal subjects, although the basal levels were not significantly different. After six diabetic patients were treated with insulin, increments in plasma myoinositol levels after a myoinositol load returned to normal, urinary excretion returned toward normal, and the myoinositol pool size increased to nearly normal. The authors speculated that the improvement of myoinositol tolerance was due to an influence of insulin treatment to increase intracellular disposition of myoinositol and possibly to decrease absorption of myoinositol from the gastrointestinal tract. Recently, Clements *et al.* (1978) obtained some evidence that a diet high in myoinositol improves conduction in peripheral nerves in human diabetes.

7.7.1.7. Experimental Diabetes and Diabetic Neuropathy

Sharma *et al.* (1977) produced diabetes in rats with streptozotocin. Measurements on tibial nerve were made before and 5 weeks after induction of diabetes. They found no effect of diabetes on maximum and average myelinated fiber diameter. There was also no change in the relationship between the myelin sheath thickness and the axon circumference. These findings suggested that reduced nerve conduction velocity, which is known to occur in such animals made diabetic, is likely to depend on metabolic alterations rather than structural changes.

7.7.2. Diabetic Microangiopathy

7.7.2.1. Muscle Capillary Basement Membrane Thickening

Williamson and Kilo (1977) published a review article, the main purposes of which were to (1) summarize and reconcile discordant reports of the influence of methods of fixation and morphometric techniques on capillary basement membrane thickening (CBMT) prevalence data reported by different investigators and (2) refocus attention on the pathophysiological significance of CBMT. They review recent contradictory points of view. Siperstein *et al.* (1968) found that CBMT was present in 98% of 51 diabetic subjects with fasting blood glucose values greater than 140 mg/dl (degree of CBMT was not correlated with duration of diabetes) and was present in over 50% of 30 prediabetic subjects (subjects had normal oral glucose tolerance tests, but both their parents were diabetic). On the basis of these findings, these authors proposed that diabetic microangiopathy is not the consequence of insulin deficiency, but is instead an independent expression of "genetic diabetes" that generally precedes onset of insulin deficiency. The clinical implication of this interpretation is that reversal of metabolic perturbations associated with the insulin-deficient state to normal (if possible) will neither prevent the onset nor alter the progression of diabetic vascular disease. However, even Siperstein and his co-investigators found CBMT with a prevalence of only 30%, rather than 100%, in diabetics under 20 years of age (Raskin *et al.*, 1975). The reports of Williamson *et al.* (1973), Østerby-Hansen and Lundbaek (1970), and Pardo *et al.* (1972) indicate that CBMT is virtually nonexistent in newly diagnosed juvenile-onset-type diabetics and is a consequence of insulin deficiency and hyperglycemia. Williamson and Kilo (1977) state that there are no substantive intrinsic differences in sensitivity for detection of CBMT attributable to fixation procedures or morphometric techniques employed by Williamson and Siperstein, as shown by various investigators. They also state that the high prevalence of CBMT in diabetics and prediabetics observed by Siperstein *et al.* (1968) may be an artifact attributable to abnormally low CBMW values for control subjects. These authors summarize various observations and conclude that thickening of capillary basement membrane associated with diabetes mellitus follows rather than precedes the onset of metabolic perturbations associated with insulin deficiency. They also stress the multifactorial pathogenesis of CBMT and the number of pathophysiological variables substantially influencing CBMT in nondiabetics as well as in diabetics, such as sex-related hormonal factors. In view of the association between the manifestation of insulin deficiency and diabetic vascular disease, the relationship between the two, if not linear, might be a continuum extending from fasting hyperglycemia to the upper limits of normal on the standard glucose tolerance test. Although JOD and MOD appear to be different diseases, CBMT does develop in both types. The fact that clinical manifestations of vascular disease and CBMT are present in a much higher percentage of newly diagnosed MOD (approximately 50%) than in newly diagnosed JOD (less than 10%) can be attributed to a much longer duration of undetected carbohydrate intolerance prior to diagnosis of diabetes in the former. The authors conclude that (1) CBMT associated with diabetes mellitus appears to be a complication of the insulin-deficient state, (2) the pathogenesis of diabetic CBMT is multifactorial, and (3) CBMT is most likely a nonspecific reaction to a manifestation of abnormal vascular function or injury. As such, it provides a useful index, perhaps the best available, for monitoring deleterious effects of the diabetic state on the vascular system. The cellular mechanism by which these effects are mediated remain to be identified.

Significant experimental studies were published in 1977 that provide important evidence that diabetic control can effect CBMT and microvascular disease. Fox *et al.* (1977) studied the effect of diabetic control on basement membrane thickening in rats. Glomerular capillary basement membrane thickness (BMT) was measured in 23 rats that had had streptozotocin-induced diabetes for 14 months and in age-matched controls. The diabetic rats were randomly allocated to four different groups, receiving either no treatment, or treatment with low-carbohydrate diet or insulin, or treatment with both. The diabetic rats treated with low-carbohydrate diet and insulin had lower plasma glucose and BMT values than those treated with insulin and a normal diet. A highly significant positive relationship was found between BMT and plasma glucose concentrations. The strong relationship between BMT and hyperglycemia found in this study suggests strongly that hyperglycemia is a main determinant in the development of BMT. Thus, blood glucose control rather than insulin administration determines BMT. These findings should offer encouragement to those who treat diabetic patients with the aim of maintaining good blood glucose control and also to those who search for improved methods of achieving such control (Fox *et al.*, 1977).

The interpretation that CBMT is in some way a consequence of the metabolic disturbance associated with insulin deficiency rather than a genetic factor independent of insulin deficiency is also the conclusion of Ganda *et al.* (1977). The propositus of monozygotic triplets developed JOD at the age of 13 years. One developed JOD at 21 years, and the third triplet is still normal at age 24 years. Muscle capillary basement membrane width of the nondiabetic triplet was normal, whereas both diabetic triplets manifested evidence of CBMT. These findings are in agreement with those in a set of discordant diabetic twins reviewed in last year's chapter (Karam *et al.*, 1976) that showed that CBMT was present in the diabetic and absent in the nondiabetic twin of a pair of monozygotic twins. These observations are consistent with the concept that CBMT follows rather than precedes the onset of carbohydrate intolerance associated with insulin deficiency.

7.7.2.2. Diabetic Microangiopathy and Intravascular Factors

Intravascular factors, in addition to changes in microvascular permeability (see Fajans, 1978) and in thickening of the capillary basement membrane, may play a role in the pathogenesis of microangiopathy. Abnormalities in platelet aggregation may be involved in capillary closure, which is one of the earliest manifestations of diabetic angiopathy. Platelet aggregation and release play a part in the development of atherosclerosis and its thromboembolic complications in addition to its possible role in the pathogenesis of microangiopathy.

Colwell *et al.* (1977) demonstrated that platelets from diabetics have an abnormal sensitivity to aggregating agents, and that this sensitivity may be related to plasma factors present in diabetics. This was found in overt diabetics and in latent diabetics, but not in prediabetic patients. Only a prospective study can show whether abnormal platelet aggregation has a role in the development of vascular disease, is a consequence of it, or is simply a characteristic of the diabetic state regardless of whether vascular disease is present or not.

Halushka *et al.* (1977) investigated factors that may be associated with and related to the increased sensitivity to platelet aggregation. The platelets synthesize significantly greater amounts of immunoreactive PgE-like material (iPGE) when they are exposed to ADP, epinephrine, and collagen than do platelets from normal subjects. Arachidonic acid, a precursor of prostaglandins, had the same effect. The increased iPGE synthesis seen in platelet-rich plasma obtained from diabetic subjects may reflect increased activity of the prostaglandin synthetase system at one or more sites. Marked changes in glucose concentration may enhance the formation of labile aggregating substances.

Waitzman *et al.* (1977) present a review of the sites at which abnormal metabolism of prostaglandins and thromboxanes may contribute to abnormal vascular and blood cell dysfunction in diabetes mellitus.

β-Thromboglobulin is a recently isolated platelet-specific protein that is released during platelet aggregation. Campbell *et al.* (1977) measured the content of plasma β-thromboglobulin in 56 patients with known complications of the disease. Although two patients were found to have elevated levels beyond the normal range, there was no significant difference between the diabetic group as a whole and a group of 35 controls. Von Willebrand factor (VWF) activity is required for vascular integrity and for normal platelet function. Sarji *et al.* (1977) performed studies that show that there is a relationship between growth hormone levels implicated in the pathogenesis of microangiopathy and VWF activity. The heightened platelet aggregation in diabetes mellitus parallels the increase in the VWF activity. The relationship appears to be complex, however, and needs further elucidation.

There is good evidence that blood viscosity in the microcirculation is determined predominantly by plasma viscosity and erythrocyte flexibility. Barnes *et al.* (1977b) designed a study to determine whether blood viscosity is increased in diabetic patients and to examine the possible relationship between changes in blood viscosity and the presence of diabetic complications. Blood viscosity at low shear rates was significantly higher in 64 patients with diabetes of more than 20 years' duration than in 61 matched nondiabetic controls. The increase was most striking in patients with either proliferative retinopathy or nephropathy, although it was present to a lesser extent in diabetic patients with evidence of myocardial or peripheral ischemia. Erythrocyte deformability was lower in the 14 diabetic patients with the most extensive microangiopathy than in 22 patients with slight or no complications or in controls. Hyperviscosity and reduced erythrocyte deformability may well be important potentially treatable factors in the etiology or progression of microvascular disease in diabetes. The increase in blood viscosity at low shear rates was principally related to changes in fibrinogen and other plasma proteins. Rigid cells and increased viscosity are likely to promote stasis in the capillaries and postcapillary venules, where the very early vasculitis in diabetes occurs. Such alterations in blood flow may lead to hypoxia, a factor previously implicated in the etiology of diabetic microangiopathy.

7.7.2.3. Diabetic Retinopathy

Engerman *et al.* (1977) studied the relationship of experimental diabetic retinopathy to metabolic control in dogs. Dogs were made alloxan-diabetic and randomly distributed into either of two prospective treatment groups. One group was poorly controlled. Commercial insulin was administered in doses inadequate to prevent chronic severe hyperglycemia and glycosuria. In the other group, it was intended that metabolic control be good, and the animals received food and commercial insulin twice daily so that their hyperglycemia and glycosuria became mild. After

5 years of diabetes, retinal capillary aneurysm, pericyte ghosts, obliterated vessels, and microvascular abnormalities typical of diabetes were apparent in each animal in the poorly controlled group. Better control was found to reduce significantly the incidence and severity of microvascular lesions. The data suggested that the mechanism responsible for diabetic retinopathy is initiated as a result of deficient insulin activity and that the development of microvascular complications of diabetes are preventable and may be inhibited by careful control of the metabolic disorder.

Although metabolic factors are undoubtedly of great importance in the pathogenesis of diabetic microangiopathy, this does not eliminate genetic factors in the predisposition of patients to diabetic microangiopathy. Evidence for heterogeneity in the occurrence of vascular disease was pointed out in the chapter on diabetes mellitus in *The Year in Metabolism 1975–1976* (Fajans, 1976). Additional evidence that genetic factors may be at play in the pathogenesis of diabetic microangiopathy come from the findings of Pyke and Tattersall (1973) that proliferative retinopathy was more frequent in concordant pairs of twins than in discordant pairs.

Barbosa *et al.* (1976) attempted to gain further insight into the genetic determinants of diabetic small-vessel disease by studying 22 HLA antigens in 110 juvenile-onset, insulin-dependent diabetics with terminal glomerular sclerosis and retinopathy, who were being prepared for kidney transplantation. The frequency of antigens A1 and B8 was significantly higher in diabetics than in controls. From this, the authors concluded that JOD with microangiopathy is one of the HLA-B8-associated disorders. Since HLA-B8 occurs in JODs, and since the authors studied a highly selected population of JODs with advanced microangiopathy and compared them with nondiabetic kidney transplant recipients and with healthy controls rather than with JODs of similar duration of disease without microangiopathy, the authors' studies do not specifically relate the finding of HLA positivity to the occurrence of microangiopathy.

In a study of histocompatibility antigens in patients with diabetic retinopathy, Becker *et al.* (1977) came to different conclusions. In 90 patients with onset of diabetes before age 30 years, the authors confirmed the reported significant increase in HLA-B8 and a decrease in HLA-B7, but there was no difference in the distribution of these antigens between those with and without retinopathy. Of 160 patients with onset of diabetes at or after 30 years of age, the 84 with no evidence of diabetic retinopathy were found to have significantly increased prevalence of HLA-A1 and B8, when compared with 76 with retinal complications or with the 282 healthy blood donors. The authors believe that HLA-A1 is the primary factor, and the increase in B8 may be due in part to linkage disequilibrium. The authors postulate heterogeneity of microangiopathy in diabetes with onset at or after age 30 years. One group with increased prevalence of HLA-A1 and B8 had a lesser predilection to retinopathy, while the other group with no significant increase of A1 or B8 had a greater chance of developing retinopathy. This hypothesis should be confirmed by prospective studies.

The retinal vasculature was evaluated by fluorescein angiography in 154 children age 5–18 years who had had symptomatic diabetes for 1 year or less (Malone *et al.*, 1977). Of these children, 25% showed no vascular abnormalities. The severity of vascular abnormalities increased with the duration of diabetes, as reported in all previous studies. The vascular abnormalities did not appear to be related to diabetic management or control when evaluated by growth failure as an index of poor control. The authors point out that a meaningful method to evaluate control in this population was not available. Growth failure is an index of such extremely poor control that it does not provide a way to correlate the presence of microangiopathy with control of the disease. The authors suggest that there may be two types of clinical diabetes mellitus, one with and one without associated vascular abnormalities, a concept supporting heterogeneity of vascular disease in JOD as previously proposed by this reviewer (Fajans *et al.*, 1976).

Paetkau *et al.* (1977) investigated the effect of smoking as an additional factor in the evolution of proliferative retinopathy. They studied 181 patients, 97 with nonproliferative and 84 with proliferative retinopathy. The number of patients with proliferative retinopathy rose with increasing tobacco consumption. In nonsmokers, no association existed between diabetes duration and proliferative retinopathy, but in smokers, the number with proliferative retinopathy rose with increasing diabetes duration. In the longer-duration group, proliferative retinopathy was significantly associated with smoking, while in the shorter-duration group, there was no relationship. This suggests that deterioration from nonproliferative to proliferative retinopathy is a function of the combination of duration of disease and exposure to tobacco. There was no association between age and degree of retinopathy. In the discussion of the findings, the authors mention that an association between proliferative retinopathy and hypoxia has been suggested. Heavy smokers were found to have carboxyhemoglobin levels as high as 15%. Chronic exposure to low levels of carbon monoxide may further embarrass oxygen supply in disease states in which oxygen delivery to tissues is already marginal. It has been suggested from both animal and human studies that carbon monoxide causes separation of arterial endothelial cells and causes edema. Such an effect could aggravate retinopathy. Also, patients with retinopathy were found to have an increased tendency to platelet aggregation. This could be due to nicotine, which is known to cause an increase in platelet stickiness. The authors state that if their findings are confirmed, the practical clinical recommendation is that diabetics be strongly urged to avoid tobacco. An Editorial (1977a) in *The Lancet* reviews the contribution of Paetkau and co-workers and notes that there were insufficient control data in several respects.

Another report attempts to investigate the possible role of levels of plasma growth hormone in the pathogenesis of diabetic retinopathy. Passa *et al.* (1977) found retinopathy in 8 of 23 patients with idiopathic hemochromatosis and diabetes, between 30 and 60 years of age at onset of diabetes and with the same duration of the disease. Retinopathy was of mild degree in these 8 patients. The plasma growth hormone response to arginine and to insulin-induced hypoglycemia was significantly lower compared with the response in uncomplicated diabetes and in nondiabetic subjects. The authors suggest that the blunted growth hormone secretion in idiopathic hemochromatosis acts as a protective factor and could explain the mild degree of retinopathy. This would support the hypothesis of a possible role of growth hormone in the development of diabetic microangiopathy. Other factors for the decreased growth hormone responses in these particular subjects have not been excluded.

A group of 100 patients with symmetrical proliferative diabetic retinopathy had one eye randomly chosen to have xenon-arc photocoagulation (British Multicenter Trial, 1977). This cooperative study showed that vision of the untreated eye deteriorated more than that of the treated eye in patients with new vessels on the optic discs. The difference in deterioration was significant after 1 year, 2 years, and 3 years. There was no difference in patients with new vessels only in the periphery of the retina. The study confirms similar results of the United States Diabetic Retinopathy Study Research Group reported in 1976 and reviewed in last year's chapter (Fajans, 1978).

7.7.2.4. Renal Changes and Nephropathy

Large kidneys are found in diabetic patients shortly after the clinical appearance of the disease (Morgensen and Andersen, 1975). Seyer-Hansen (1977) showed that streptozotocin-diabetic rats have larger kidneys than nondiabetic rats and that the rate of kidney growth during the first 7 days of diabetes was correlated with the blood glucose concentration. Over a wide range of blood glucose concentrations (116–340 mg/dl), the kidney weight, protein content, and protein/DNA ratio were closely correlated with the glucose values. Butcher *et al.* (1977) demonstrated that human diabetic glomeruli are significantly larger and heavier than nondiabetic glomeruli. The mean diameter of human diabetic glomeruli is 45% greater than that of nondiabetic glomeruli, and the mass of the diabetic glomeruli is 2.5 times greater than the mean nondiabetic glomerular mass.

Gunderson and Østerby (1977) studied autopsy kidney material from long-term diabetics and controls. Duration of diabetes was from 16 to 31 years, but the patients died from causes other than renal insufficiency. Diabetic microangiopathy progresses steadily from measurable thickening of the peripheral capillary basement membrane after 2 years of the disease, leading eventually to large accumulation of basement membrane material within the glomerular tuft, thereby reducing the capillary lumen and the capillary blood flow. The authors' studies show that the destruction of glomeruli due to diabetic microangiopathy is compensated for some years by hypertrophy of the least-affected glomeruli. This compensatory hypertrophy of the glomeruli might well account for the preservation of renal function in long-term diabetics for a number of years despite the progressive basement membrane lesions of diabetic microangiopathy. Studies of kidney function have shown that glomerular filtration rate remains high and unchanged for many years of diabetes until finally renal insufficiency sets in.

Doud *et al.* (1977) described the unique development of a lesion strongly resembling diffuse diabetic nephropathy in the renal homograft of a patient receiving a transplant because of obstructive neuropathy. The patient demonstrated clinical and morphological evidence of diabetic nephropathy in his transplanted kidney 2 years following steroid-induced diabetes mellitus (not steroid diabetes). The patient had a family history of diabetes, but the donor of the kidney did not. Diabetic nephropathy was evident by light-microscopic changes and by immunological studies.

Diabetic nephropathy occurs 10–15 years after the onset of insulin-dependent diabetes, but frequently occurs in less time after the recognition of maturity-onset diabetes. It is usually manifested by the development of the nephrotic syndrome. The sudden onset of massive proteinuria with a rapid deterioration of renal function in the stable diabetic should suggest that an additional pathological condition is affecting the kidney. Olivero and Suki (1977) reported three cases of diabetic nephropathy complicated by other superimposed renal diseases. Some of these diseases may be reversible, and the authors suggest that whenever the course of a diabetic patient's nephropathy deviates from that which is customary, a vigorous diagnostic program be instituted. Two patients had acute postinfectious and proliferative glomerulonephritis, and both patients recovered and returned to what was presumably their premorbid renal function.

As described previously, Zincke *et al.* (1977) reported that renal transplantation in the juvenile diabetic patient is superior to hemodialysis. A total of 40 patients including 37 juvenile diabetic patients with insulin-dependent diabetes mellitus and end-stage renal failure received 42 renal allografts. Of the 30 patients who are alive, 19 have been fully rehabilitated. Gangrene of peripheral extremities occurred in 30% of the survivors. The use of cadaveric kidneys in the diabetic patient may become an attractive alternative to grafts from living related donors.

In another publication from the same institution, the author provides a more comprehensive and realistic view of attempts to prolong the useful life of the juvenile diabetic with end-stage renal disease (Mitchell, 1977). In a group of 43 juvenile diabetic patients accepted for renal transplantation, and followed for as long as 5 years, the cumulative survival of the group was 66% in 1 year and 58% at 5 years. In those who had living related donor transplantation, 88% survived as compared to 65% receiving cadaveric renal allografts and 55% for those on dialysis alone. Of patients who survived transplantation 1 year or more, 50% required amputation of one or more extremities. Only 25% of the patients who had survived 1 year after transplantation were without blindness or severe peripheral vascular problems or both.

Kamdar *et al.* (1977) observed acute renal failure following intravenous administration of roentgenologic contrast media in seven diabetic patients. The renal failure occurred within 48 hr of the procedure, and oliguria occurred in six patients. Renal function returned toward prestudy levels within 4 weeks. None of the patients required dialysis. Analysis of the data obtained in these patients and those of 30 cases reported in the literature suggests that certain factors make diabetic patients prone to dye-induced acute renal failure. These include old age, long duration of diabetes, preexisting impaired renal function, the presence of retinopathy, neuropathy, and cardiovascular disease, and dehydration. The authors recommend that all diabetic patients be monitored closely after radiocontrast study to detect the development of acute renal failure so that appropriate management can be instituted early in the course of the disease.

Patients with chronic diabetes mellitus, with and without renal insufficiency, may manifest an impairment of potassium homeostasis and may be particularly at risk of hyperkalemia (Perez *et al.*, 1977a,b; DeFronzo *et al.*, 1977). This syndrome has been referred to as "hyporeninemic hypoaldosteronism." Mechanisms that may contribute to nonuremic hyperkalemia are decreased sympathetic activity, defective renin production, decreased aldosterone production as measured by decreased levels of plasma aldosterone, a renal tubular secretory defect, as well as insulinopenia leading to failure of cellular potassium uptake. Extracellular fluid volume expansion may also be a factor in the suppression of the renin–aldosterone system. Such patients may exhibit impairment not only of renin but also of aldosterone responsiveness to appropriate stimuli. These abnormalities enhance the risk of hyperkalemia in patients with decreased renal function. However, these defects were present not only in diabetics of long duration with associated renal and neurological complications, but also in patients with diabetes of more recent onset. The recognition of hyporeninemic hypoaldosteronism in the diabetic population may have important therapeutic implications. Hyperkalemia has been noted to be a surprisingly common complication of oral potassium supplementation. The use of potassium-retaining diuretics may be particularly hazardous in diabetic patients with this syndrome.

Impairment of potassium homeostasis is probably related to combined aldosterone and insulin deficiency (DeFronzo et al., 1977). These abnormalities may predispose to unexpected and occasionally life-threatening hyperkalemia, particularly in the setting of acidosis, diminished renal function, and severe hyperglycemia, or with the administration of potassium salts or potassium-sparing diuretics. Low renin and low aldosterone levels also occur in groups of diabetic patients without hyperkalemia.

7.7.3. Bone Mass in Diabetes Mellitus

In last year's chapter (Fajans, 1978), studies describing a decrease in bone mass in diabetic patients were reviewed. Further studies have appeared in which bone mass and bone density were determined in diabetic patients. Some of the results and conclusions are at variance with those reported previously. Rosenbloom et al. (1977b) confirmed the high frequency of bone density loss in insulin-dependent diabetes mellitus in a large and younger population than previously reported. A total of 196 insulin-dependent diabetic patients, age 6–26 years, were compared with 124 control subjects. White females averaged 8.2% bone loss compared with white males, whose loss averaged 4.7%. Bone loss was seen in 29% of white males and 48% of white females. This defect was seen particularly in white female children with diabetes of less than 5 years' duration. The authors postulate that osteopenia is not due to a basic cellular defect, as previously proposed by Levin et al. (1976), but that bone density loss of the diabetic state is a result of insulin deficiency. They suggest that this is expressed particularly in the population most susceptible to osteopenia, and that bone collagen synthesis and calcium transport have been shown to be influenced by insulin. In this regard, the study by Silberberg et al. (1977) may be relevant. In diabetic animals, enzyme activities of articular cartilage engaged in the synthesis and degradation of mucopolysaccharides were increased, those of the degrading enzymes more than those of the others. Implantation of pancreatic islets reversed the changes produced by diabetes, enzyme activities returning to near-normal levels.

The findings of Santiago *et al.* (1977) were somewhat different. In 107 diabetic children, 25% had bone cortical thickness values below the 5% limit for normal children. However, this was more common in boys than in girls, and was unrelated to the duration of diabetes. It was not due to delayed skeletal maturation. The authors had no explanation for the cause of the osteopenia of diabetic children.

DeLeeuw and Abs (1977) also determined bone mass and bone density with a photon-absorption technique in a Belgian group of maturity-onset-type diabetics. Mean values of bone mass and bone density were higher in the diabetic population, differing from previously reported studies. A detailed individual study revealed the existence of two diabetic populations. A smaller group had more than 10% bone gain and was characterized by higher body weight. This was true particularly in those treated with oral antidiabetic agents, differing from the findings of Levin *et al.* (1976).

7.8. Treatment of Diabetes Mellitus

7.8.1. General Considerations

In an editorial in the *New England Journal of Medicine,* Siperstein *et al.* (1977) commented on an editorial by Cahill *et al.* (1976) that suggested that the goals of appropriate therapy should include a serious effort to achieve levels of blood glucose as close to those in the nondiabetic state as feasible. Siperstein and co-authors questioned the interpretation of several recent publications on animal studies and human studies as supporting the view that tight glucose regulation may have a beneficial effect on diabetic vascular disease.

Although the authors of these two editorials differ in their interpretation of studies relating "control" to vascular disease, both groups recommend that the physician try to achieve the best control of blood glucose possible (in the absence of harmful side effects). In another editorial in the same journal, Ingelfinger (1977) points out that both editorials appeared to be very close to each other when it comes to practical application of therapeutic goals to the treatment of diabetes mellitus (also see Section 7.7.2).

7.8.2. Glycosylated Hemoglobin and Diabetic Control

Further reports appeared in 1977 that indicate that determination of glycosylated hemoglobin is a useful indicator of the degree of hyperglycemia that exists over prolonged periods of time. Gabbay *et al.* (1977)

showed that the glycosylated minor hemoglobin components Hb_{A1a+b} as well as Hb_{A1c} are elevated in insulin-dependent juvenile diabetic patients, Hb_{A1c} more than the former. Total glycosylated hemoglobin components, $Hb_{A1a+b+c}$, correlated with the degree of blood glucose regulation as measured by antecedent 24-hr glucose excretion determined in 220 diabetic patients. The highest correlation coefficient was observed between the glycosylated hemoglobin levels and the urinary glucose excretion measured 2 months previously. Hemoglobin A_{1a+b+c} levels correlated with plasma cholesterol levels, suggesting that long-term hyperglycemia is associated with hypercholesterolemia. The authors suggested that measurements of glycosylated hemoglobin levels every 2 months may allow an accurate estimate of the degree of hyperglycemia in the diabetic patient over a long time period. Serial measurements of glycosylated hemoglobin levels allow long-term studies on the effects of good control of hyperglycemia in the prevention of the various diabetic complications. At present, the determination of total glycosylated hemoglobin components is simpler than measurement of Hb_{A1c}.

Gonen *et al.* (1977) also tried to define the relationship between diabetic control, assessed by various methods, and the levels of glycosylated hemoglobin. The levels of hemoglobin A_{1c} correlated closely with the physicians' ratings of the degree of control, fasting plasma glucose (single measurement or mean of single daily values), mean daily plasma glucose levels, and highest daily plasma glucose levels. The authors concluded that the hemoglobin A_{1c} measurement is a simple, rapid, and objective procedure to assess diabetic control over long periods and may serve as a screening test for uncontrolled diabetes. They also suggested that it may be an indicator of the efficacy of various therapeutic regimens, although determination of hemoglobin A_{1c} is not helpful in deciding how diabetic control can be improved.

In 11 insulin-dependent diabetic outpatients, Lanoe *et al.* (1977) studied the correlation between hemoglobin A_{1c} concentration and diabetic control as judged by a thrice-daily semiquantitated estimation of urinary sugar excretion (Clinitest), during the 8 weeks before hemoglobin A_{1c} determination. Also determined were 24-hr glycosuria and fasting and postprandial blood glucose levels from one to five times during this period. Hemoglobin A_{1c} concentration determined by the electrofocusing technique varied inversely with the quality of control (urinary glucose indices), but not with fasting or postprandial blood glucose levels or with 24-hr glycosuria. The authors concluded that hemoglobin A_{1c} determination appears to be a far better method for measuring diabetic control than the usual criteria of determination of fasting and postprandial blood sugar and 24-hr excretion of glucose, and was as effective as and more precise than semiquantitated urinary sugar estimation three times a day.

Peterson *et al.* (1977b) showed in 10 nonketotic diabetic subjects, studied before and after control of carbohydrate metabolism, that there was a high degree of correlation between hemoglobin A_{1c} concentrations and serum triglyceride levels. The latter correlated more closely with hemoglobin A_{1c} than did serum cholesterol, and was thus indicative of a more direct relationship to carbohydrate metabolism. In another report, Peterson *et al.* (1977a) showed that there was an inverse correlation of the concentration of hemoglobin A_{1c} and specific abnormalities of leukocyte, platelet, and erythrocyte function. Erythrocyte half-life, leukocyte adherence, and the length of the secondary lag phase of platelet aggregation after stimulation with epinephrine, all deranged in diabetic patients, are increased after strict control of diabetes.

7.8.3. Diet

Crapo *et al.* (1977) studied the acute effects of different types of carbohydrates on postprandial plasma glucose and insulin responses in 60 healthy subjects. All carbohydrate loads were calculated to contain 50 g glucose. Dextrose and potato elicited similar plasma glucose responses, whereas rice, corn, and bread elicited lower responses. Similarly, dextrose and potato elicited similar and greater plasma insulin responses than did rice and corn, with the response to bread being intermediate. These differences were accentuated in patients with reduced glucose tolerance. Although these experiments have not been extended to diabetic patients, it appears that if it is a therapeutic aim to lower postprandial plasma glucose or insulin responses, or both, then specifying the type of complex carbohydrate to use in the diet may be an important adjunct in achieving these goals.

Jenkins *et al.* (1977b) showed that in healthy subjects, the presence of unabsorbable carbohydrates in various test meals reduced the rise in blood glucose and plasma insulin that otherwise follows ingestion of such meals that contain absorbable carbohydrate. This was shown after a liquid test meal to which guar gum flour was added, after a breakfast test meal in which pectin was added to the marmalade, and after a similar meal in which guar was added to the bread and pectin to the marmalade. Guar and pectin are gel-forming carbohydrates of vegetable origin. Guar gum is a storage polysaccharide obtained from the cluster bean; pectin is a partially methoxylated polymer of galacuronic acid, a constituent of plant cell walls (dietary fiber) obtained commercially from apples and citrus fruits. Both are classed as unavailable carbohydrates and may prove useful in the dietary control of diabetes by reducing insulin requirement.

In another study, Jenkins *et al.* (1977a) studied the effect of dietary fiber on glucose excretion of diabetics whose insulin dosage ranged from

38 to 92 U/day. Nine diabetic patients supplemented either their normal home diets (four patients) or metabolic ward diets (five patients) with 25 g guar gum daily for 5–7 days. The mean urinary glucose excretion fell by 46 and 54%, respectively. Gel-forming type of dietary fiber of leguminous origin may have an advantage over cereal fiber used in earlier studies as a useful adjunct to antidiabetic therapy, irrespective of the type of treatment or insulin dosage used.

In an editorial, Mendeloff (1977) reviewed the definition of dietary fiber, the physical properties of dietary fiber, and what is known about the function of dietary fiber, particularly in the large intestine of man. He offered the opinion that health could be improved by replacing some of the calories of the present American diet by increased amounts of whole grain cereals, bread, potatoes, vegetables, and fruits. That functions among the various types of dietary fiber may differ qualitatively and quantitatively was pointed out; e.g., postulated effects of plant gums on glucose metabolism may be totally inapplicable to insoluble hemicelluloses. Diabetes, like obesity, is thought to be rare in populations eating most of their carbohydrates in the form of starches containing large amounts of fiber. Farinaro *et al.* (1977) studied 150 middle-aged men prone to coronary disease. In this study, which spanned 4 years, men began to consume a diet in which total fat was reduced from the usual 40% to about 32% of calories and carbohydrate was increased from the usual 38% to about 44%. In addition, the diet was low in cholesterol and saturated fat, and moderate in unsaturated and polyunsaturated fat, and the carbohydrate contained an increased proportion of calories from simple sugar of about 15% to 18%. Cholesterol levels were significantly reduced throughout the 4 years of the diet program in all groups. For the group that sustained weight loss, at both 2 and 4 years, fasting plasma glucose was modestly but significantly reduced, as were postglucose levels; at 4 years, fasting glycemia still remained slightly below baseline. In five men with suspect fasting hyperglycemia at baseline (mean plasma glucose 120 mg/dl), sustained fall in weight and serum cholesterol was associated with sizable reductions in fasting glycemia (mean fasting plasma glucose at 2 and 4 years, 103 and 105 mg/dl) and an improvement of glucose tolerance. A moderate increase in percentage of calories from total carbohydrate and simple sugars in a fat-modified diet appears actually beneficial for glucose tolerance when calories are controlled so as to effect weight reduction in middle-aged obese men. The authors commented that control of glycemia can be years-long in duration in both normal glycemic and mildly hyperglycemic middle-aged persons when a diet of this type is used and reasonable control of obesity is obtained. Further, it can be accompanied by sustained reduction of serum lipid levels.

7.8.4. Insulin

7.8.4.1. Chronic Insulin Therapy

Yue and Turtle (1977) state that preparations of single component (SC) insulin manufactured by Eli Lilly and Company and monocomponent (MC) insulin manufactured by the Novo Company are antigenic in man; both preparations are of purity greater than 99%. Patients treated only with MC insulin were said to have significantly lower concentrations of insulin antibody in plasma than patients treated with conventional insulin, but to require a similar dose of insulin. In patients switched to MC porcine insulin, the requirement for insulin did not change; further, patients with insulin resistance treated with MC insulin experienced no decrease in insulin requirement or in plasma antibody level. The authors concluded that purified (MC and SC) insulins do not alter the "stability" of diabetes, but apparently do reduce the incidence of local pain and swelling at the site of insulin injection. In systemic insulin allergy, the response to purified insulins is variable. The authors believe that if completely nonimmunogenic insulin could be produced, it is unlikely that dramatic therapeutic benefits would result, and in addition, losses of insulin during preparation of such highly purified materials would be prohibitive commercially.

Logie and Stowers (1976) believe they have observed a decrease in requirement of insulin in a 15-year-old boy, diabetic for 3 years, who was switched from less pure insulins to MC porcine insulin. The patient initially took soluble insulin, then Lente insulin. An episode of ketoacidosis was followed by increasing insulin requirements over the next year to the level of 280 U beef soluble insulin daily. On neutral soluble pork insulin, the requirement decreased over months and stabilized at 188 U daily. After a transfer to MC porcine insulin, insulin requirement dropped by 35% over 3 days. The authors concluded that the fall in insulin requirement was related to the institution of MC insulin treatment, and that serious consequences could have occurred had it been done outside the hospital. They suggest that when patients are changed from less pure preparations of beef insulins to MC insulins, the dosage initially be cut 20%, and when changed from less pure preparations of pork insulins to MC insulins, the dosage be cut 15%. In an editorial (1977b) in *The Lancet*, a survey of daily insulin doses in Denmark over 30 years was cited. During that time, the quality of insulin preparations steadily improved and the percentage of patients receiving more than 40 U/day steadily decreased. The reduction in dose was thought to be related to the use of more highly purified insulins; this advantage must be set against production losses, higher prices, and the possible hazards of changing to the more highly purified insulins. In the opinion of the editorial writer, no convincing change in the quality of diabetic control has been reported when patients have switched to high-purity MC insulins, which are therefore probably of little importance to most diabetics; those who might be controlled with lower dosages of high-purity insulins may be identified by refinement of methods to measure plasma insulin-binding capacity (see below). However, in diabetics receiving insulin for the first time, it is reasonable to suggest that they be treated with a highly purified insulin (Mustaffa *et al.*, 1977).

Mustaffa *et al.* (1977) found that when the insulin-binding capacity of plasma was greater than 40 μU/ml, changing to a highly purified insulin is likely to be associated with a reduction of insulin requirement. In about 75% of patients treated with highly purified insulin, insulin-binding capacity and insulin requirement decreased. In most patients, the maximal reductions of insulin requirement were seen at 3–4 months. In about 25% of cases, insulin-binding capacity increased, and in most of these, more insulin was needed. The authors concluded that measurement of the insulin-binding capacity is simple and indicates those patients who are likely to be as well controlled on a smaller dose of highly purified insulin as they are on a larger dose of less purified insulin.

Of 101 patients, aged 2–21 years, seen by Rosenbloom and Giordano (1977) in several clinics in northern Florida, overtreatment occurred in 70%, and in those referred to them because of instability, overtreatment occurred in 90%. The mean overdose was 38% of the readjusted dose. Among the most common indicators of overtreatment were frank hypoglycemic episodes and excessive appetite.

7.8.4.2. Insulin Antibodies

Kurtz *et al.* (1977) studied 96 diabetic patients who had been taking insulin for at least 3 months. Free insulin, total insulin, and insulin-binding capacity were determined. Binding capacity ranged from 6 to 940 mU/liter; total insulin, from 20 to 5240 mU/liter; and free insulin, from 0 to 64 mU/liter. As total insulin and insulin-binding capacity increased, concentration of free insulin, but not glucose, fell. It was possible to maintain diabetic control, or even to produce hypoglycemia, with unmeasurable or very low plasma free concentrations of insulin. The authors speculated that high-affinity plasma binding of insulin does not necessarily limit the shift of insulin from plasma to cell receptors and suggested that as insulin dissociates from antibodies circulating in plasma, it might be actively taken up by cells. This "vacuum" effect, they thought, might be analagous to that invoked to explain the rapid uptake by tissue of some drugs that circulate bound to plasma proteins.

Little *et al.* (1977) compared the effects of sulfated insulin treatment with that of treatment with Lente insulin. A group of 74 patients were treated with Lente insulin or sulfated insulin for an average of 66 months. With sulfated insulin, antibody indices remained low throughout the 5 years of observation, and mean dose of insulin tended to decrease. In the Lente-insulin-treated group, antibody levels were significantly higher throughout the 5 years, though they did tend to decrease toward the end of the fifth year. Mean insulin dose did not decrease in the Lente group. The incidence of local skin reactions at injection sites was lower throughout the study in the group treated with sulfated insulin. In no case did diabetes become resistant or brittle. The authors thought that long-term effects of sulfated insulin on the development of insulin antibody could have benefits not obtainable with unmodified insulin. However, sulfation of beef insulin results in about a 50% loss of biological potency and about a 400% increase in cost.

Witters *et al.* (1977) presented a case report suggesting that desensitization therapy for insulin allergy can lead to insulin resistance of the immune type. This had also been observed by others (Kumar, 1977).

7.8.4.3. Lipoatrophy

Kumar *et al.* (1977) found that six of nine patients with insulin lipoatrophy of the thighs noted significant filling in of atrophic areas during the first 4 months of treatment with NPH insulin that contained 4 μg dexamethasone per insulin dose. The use of 4 μg dexamethasone in each dose of injected insulin did not change the total insulin dose for these patients.

7.8.4.4. Insulin Delivery Systems

Marliss *et al.* (1977) employed as an artificial pancreas an extracorporeal, "closed-loop" system that provided complete normalization of blood glucose concentration in nine diabetic patients during and between meals. The artificial pancreas consisted of a device for measuring plasma glucose concentration, and a control unit that received the signal corresponding to the level and rate of change of glycemia and, in turn, gave a control signal to pumps, which infused insulin and glucagon. The need for glucagon to prevent hypoglycemia could almost always be obviated by careful adjustment of insulin delivery. In only a few individual cases did blood glucose fall below 70 mg/dl. The system is considered to be applicable to clinical investigation. In studies by the same group, Albisser *et al.* (1977) employed this artificial pancreas without glucagon infusion. Mean maximal rises in glycemia after breakfast, lunch, and dinner were, respectively, 20, 25, and 25 mg/dl. The mean amounts of insulin required for these responses were 13, 18, and 9 units. When subjects ingested 50 g glucose, the average glycemic excursion was 130 mg/dl without vs. 30 mg/dl with the artificial pancreas, and in the latter circumstance the plasma glucose area was reduced by 50%. The time to return to fasting value was 4.2 and 1.3 hr, respectively. These improvements with the artificial pancreas occurred without any alterations in the patterns of plasma glucagon concentrations observed without the artificial pancreas. In depancreatized dogs, these same authors showed that during steady state and during glucose loading, there was no statistical difference between the effects of portal and peripheral intravenous infusions of insulin in terms of glycemic response, peripheral levels of insulin, patterns of infusion of insulin, and total insulin required. From these observations, it appears that the peripheral route would probably be satisfactory for studies using the artificial endocrine pancreas and possibly for future studies with implantable prostheses.

Mirouze *et al.* (1977) used an artificial pancreas that included a continuous blood glucose recording, and a noncomputerized analogue system that informed a pump system infusing insulin; neither glucose nor glucagon was infused. The doses of insulin needed for control of postprandial glycemia were 0.53 U/hr per g carbohydrate for breakfast and 0.15 U for dinner; it appeared that exogenous insulin exhibits a circadian rhythm of efficacy. The authors thought that the technique was of considerable value in the evaluation of exogenous insulin homeostasis in insulin-dependent diabetic patients.

Kerner *et al.* (1977) employed a glucose-controlled system for the infusion of insulin (Biostator) to treat 11 patients in diabetic coma or precoma. In 7 patients, insulin infusion was regulated manually or with an adjustable pump. In all patients, controlled reduction of blood glucose to the range of 150 mg/dl was achieved in 2.3–18 hr, during which time 17–320 U (in one instance 1950 U) insulin was infused; there was no hypoglycemia or hypokalemia. Provided that blood glucose was measured frequently, the results of automated vs. manual methods of giving insulin did not seem to be significantly different.

Genuth and Martin (1977) treated nine adult diabetic subjects for 2 weeks with an intravenous insulin delivery system that provided preprogrammed 5-hr pulses of insulin with each meal. They produced a normal diurnal pattern of plasma insulin. Plasma insulin peaked at 800% of basal level at 45 min after the onset of each pulse. On treatment day 14, mean plasma glucose (22 hourly samples) was 94 mg/dl with a range of 66–125 mg/dl. Of values of all treatment days, 88% were between 50 and 159 mg/dl. The authors concluded that insulin replacement coordinated with meals in a physiological manner can virtually normalize plasma glucose even without a feedback control of delivery rates. The success of this treatment depends to a considerable degree on a rather fixed character of the biological response to the pulsed delivery of insulin. The selection of the patients was favorable in this respect; i.e., none had circulating antibodies to insulin that could have altered the time course of availability of administered insulin, and seven of the nine were obese, making likely the presence of some degree of insulin resistance that may have mitigated the effects of inadvertent administration of too much insulin. The authors found that a similar program met with far less satisfactory initial results when the patients were long-standing brittle juvenile-diabetic patients.

7.8.5. Transplantation

Gates and Lazarus (1977) reported on reversal of streptozotocin-induced diabetes in rats by means of intraperitoneal implantation of chambers of nucleopore membrane filled with diced rabbit pancreas. In rats receiving two chambers, blood glucose returned to normal and glucose tolerance was identical with that in normal rats. At 6 weeks, the implanted pancreas secreted insulin, glucagon, and pancreatic polypeptide *in vivo*. Rats made diabetic, but that had received no implants, died within 5 weeks. The authors thought that rabbit neonatal pancreatic implants may be feasible therapy in insulin-requiring diabetic patients. They concluded that several dangers might be associated with this treatment, but felt that it ought to be tried.

Kretschmer *et al.* (1977) obtained evidence that diabetes in depancreatized dogs could be ameliorated by autotransplanting collagenase-digested pancreas fragments into the spleen. Dogs that received undigested pancreas fragments or fragments digested in collagenase for 10 min remained hyperglycemic following pancreatectomy and died within 28 days. Pancreas fragments that had been digested for 20 min prior to implantation produced the most normal pattern of plasma glucose in surviving dogs; in them, splenectomy at 10 weeks after implantation was followed immediately by hyperglycemia and thereafter by death. Such extirpated spleens showed islet and exocrine tissues and no apparent destruction of splenic parenchyma. In the authors' opinion, the ultimate application of this technique to clinical diabetes appears promising, although they recognized that the response of spleen to allogeneic pancreas might be quite different from the response of the spleen in dogs to autogenous tissue.

Sun *et al.* (1977) demonstrated the efficacy of artificial capillary units containing cultured islets of Langerhans in ameliorating experimental diabetes. Islets of Langerhans from normal rats were implanted into spaces surrounding Emicon hollow fibers. These fiber units were attached to the vascular system of rats made diabetic by streptozotocin and monkeys made diabetic by subtotal pancreatectomy and streptozotocin. The effects were similar in both; in the former, mean basal blood glucose concentration of 448 mg/dl was lowered to 132 mg/dl within 1 hr.

Georgakakis (1977) implanted islets into the pancreas tissue or into the submandibular gland of rats made diabetic with streptozotocin. Provided no infection occurred, diabetes was only relatively improved. The author thought this was because current isolation techniques for islets (modified collagenase method) are not at all satisfactory, and that islets are implanted in small numbers and mixed with some acinar debris.

Najarian *et al.* (1977) reported concerning transplantation of human islets in seven patients with insulin-dependent diabetes mellitus who had received renal allografts 10 to 36 months previously. All were on standard immunosuppressive therapy and had normal renal function. Pancreas donors were two 1-year-old infants and four adults. Islet tissue was obtained by collagenase digestion and implanted intraperitoneally in five instances or into a muscle pocket in the groin in one instance, and infused into the portal vein in four instances. No patient was cured of diabetes, but: (1) chemical or bacterial peritonitis did not occur, (2) portal vein pressure did not rise, (3) transplantation in the portal vein did not cause measurable hepatic dysfunction, and (4) no rejection of previously transplanted kidney developed. The only complication was a superficial wound infection after one intramuscular transplant. The authors state that if new techniques of experimental pancreatic islet preparation should become clinically applicable to human pancreas, the prospects for human islet transplantation are excellent. Intervals of 2–9 weeks of reduced insulin requirement occurred in three of the four receiving transplantation via portal vein and in three of the five receiving intraperitoneal transplantation. In the fourth subject receiving transplant via portal vein, reduction of insulin dose was by two thirds of the pretransplant requirement, and this reduction had been maintained for more than 18 months.

7.8.6. Oral Hypoglycemic Agents

The mechanisms by which oral hypoglycemic agents exert their blood-glucose-lowering effect have been the subject of further investigations. Potentially harmful side effects have been reported further.

Lebovitz *et al.* (1977) assessed insulin action by measuring insulin-mediated glucose disposal in nonketotic diabetic patients before and after normalization of fasting plasma glucose by diet (109 mg/dl) or diet plus glipizide (106 mg/dl). The slope of the glucose disappearance curve was significantly increased in the diet plus glipizide group. The authors thought that this potentiation of insulin action by glipizide therapy might account for the antidiabetic effect of this drug.

Tan *et al.* (1977) observed the effects of long-term therapy with several oral hypoglycemic agents on oral glucose tolerance tests with each subsequent test for each therapeutic group (chlorpropamide, tolbutamide, phenformin, acetohexamide, placebo groups). There was improvement in glucose tolerance but not in insulin secretion in the chlorpropamide group, but only at the end of year 1. This suggested an extra beta cell effect of chlorpropamide. Possible suppression of plasma glucagon by chlorpropamide was discussed as a possible mechanism of such an effect.

Tsalikian *et al.* (1977) state that the beneficial effect of sulfonylureas on hyperglycemia may in part be explained by the stimulation of endogenous insulin secretion postprandially and by partial suppression of postprandial and basal secretion of plasma glucagon. When 19 subjects with MOD discontinued sulfonylurea: (1) grams of urinary glucose per 24 hours increased significantly; (2) plasma glucose rose both in the basal state and after meals; and (3) postprandial plasma insulin decreased, and basal and postprandial plasma glucagon levels rose significantly (20 and 30 pg/ml increase, respectively).

Nattrass *et al.* (1977) studied the comparative effects of glibenclamide, phenformin, and metformin on metabolic rhythms in MOD. Studies were performed at the end of a month of phenformin spansules, a month of metformin, and a final month of glibenclamide. Significant increases in plasma concentrations of ketone bodies, in lactate/pyruvate ratio, and in gluconeogenic precursors were noted during phenformin and metformin but not during glibenclamide therapy. Glibenclamide therapy was associated with normalization of plasma glucose, gluconeogenic precursors, and ketone bodies.

Turkington (1977) encountered three patients who while being treated with chlorpropamide or phenformin, or both, developed hypoglycemia and encephalopathy. They were found to have abnormal EEGs and cerebral cortical atrophy. Only one was able to return to work and regain a high performance level without recurrence of symptoms.

Johnson *et al.* (1977) found that whereas glucose therapy alone was not sufficient to control hypoglycemia induced by massive ingestion of chlorpropamide by a 16-year-old boy, the infusion of 300 mg diazoxide over 30 min every 4 hr, added to the glucose treatment, was sufficient.

References

Alberti, K. G. M. M., 1977, Low-dose insulin in the treatment of diabetic ketoacidosis, *Arch. Intern. Med.* **137**:1367–1376.

Alberti, K. G. M. M., and Nattrass, M., 1977, Lactic acidosis, *Lancet* **2**:25–29.

Albisser, A. M., Leibel, B. S., Zinman, B., Murray, F. T., Zingg, W., Botz, C. K., Denoga, A., and Marliss, E. B., 1977, Studies with an artificial endocrine pancreas, *Arch. Intern. Med.* **137**:639–649.

Alexander, W. D., and Oake, R. J., 1977, Effect of insulin on vascular reactivity to norepinephrine, *Diabetes* **26**:611–614.

Aronoff, S. L., Bennett, P. H., Gorden, P., Rushforth, N., and Miller, M., 1977, Unexplained hyperinsulinemia in normal and "prediabetic" Pima Indians compared with normal Caucasians, *Diabetes* **26**:827–840.

Asplin, C. M., and Hartog, M., 1977, Serum free insulin concentrations during the treatment of diabetic coma and precoma with low dose intramuscular insulin, *Diabetologia* **13**:475–480.

Ayromlooi, J., Mann, L. J., Weiss, R. R., Tejani, N. A., and Paydar, M., 1977, Modern management of the diabetic pregnancy, *Obstet. Gynecol.* **49**:137–143.

Bar, R. S., and Roth, J., 1977, Insulin receptor status in disease states of man, *Arch. Intern. Med.* **137**:474–481.

Barbosa, J., King, R., Noreen, H., and Yunis, E. J., 1977, The histocompatibility system in juvenile, insulin-dependent diabetic multiplex kindreds, *J. Clin. Invest.* **60**:989–998.

Barbosa, J., Noreen, H., Emme, L., Goetz, F., Simmons, R., deLeiva, A., Najarian, J., and Yunis, E. J., 1976, Histocompatibility (HLA) antigens and diabetic microangiopathy, *Tissue Antigens* **7**:233.

Barbosa, J., Noreen, H., King, R., and Yunis, E. J., 1978, Genetics of juvenile diabetes (letter to the editor), *N. Engl. J. Med.* **298**:462.

Barnes, A. J., Bloom, S. R., Alberti, K. G. M. M., Smythe, P., Alford, F. P., and Chisholm, D. J., 1977a, Ketoacidosis in pancreatectomized man, *N. Engl. J. Med.* **296**:1250–1253.

Barnes, A. J., Locke, P., Scudder, P. R., Dormandy, T. L., Dormandy, J. A., and Slack, J., 1977b, Is hyperviscosity a treatable component of diabetic microcirculatory disease?, *Lancet* **2**:789–791.

Barta, L., and Simon, S., 1977, Role of HLA-B8 and BW15 antigens in diabetic children, *N. Engl. J. Med.* **296**:397.

Becker, B., Shin, D. H., Burgess, D., Kilo, C., and Miller, W. V., 1977, Histocompatibility antigens and diabetic retinopathy, *Diabetes* **26**:997–999.

Beck-Nielsen, H., Pedersen, O., Kragballe, K., and Schwartz-Sorensen, N., 1977, The monocyte as a model for the study of insulin receptors in man, *Diabetologia* **13**:563–569.

Berger, M., Berchtold, P., Cüppers, H. J., Drost, H., Kley, H. K., Müller, W. A., Wiegelmann, W., Zimmermann-Telschow, H., Gries, F. A., Krüskemper, H. L., and Zimmermann, H., 1977, Metabolic and hormonal effects of muscular exercise in juvenile type diabetics, *Diabetologia* **13**:355–365.

Blackard, W. G., Anderson, J. H., and Mullinax, F., 1977, Anti-insulin receptor antibodies and diabetes, *Ann. Intern. Med.* **86**:584–585.

Bodmer, J. G., Mann, J., Hill, A., Hill, H., Young, D., and Winearls, B., 1977, The association of Ia antigens with juvenile onset diabetes and rheumatoid arthritis, *Tissue Antigens* **10**:197.

Braddom, R. L., Hollis, J. B., and Castell, D. O., 1977, Diabetic peripheral neuropathy: A correlation of nerve conduction studies and clinical findings, *Arch. Phys. Med. Rehabil.* **58**:308–313.

Brady, P. G., and Richardson, R., 1977, Gastric bezoar formation secondary to gastroparesis diabeticorum, *Arch. Intern. Med.* **137**:1729.

British Multicenter Trial (H. Cheng), 1977, Proliferative diabetic retinopathy: Treatment with xenon-arc photocoagulation—Interim report of multicenter randomized, controlled trial, *Br. Med. J.* **1**:739–741.

Butcher, D., Kikkawa, R., Klein, L., and Miller, M., 1977, Size and weight of glomeruli isolated from human diabetic and nondiabetic kidneys, *J. Lab. Clin. Med.* **89**:544–553.

Cahill, G. F., Jr., Etzwiler, D. D., and Freinkel, N., 1976, "Control" and diabetes (editorial), *N. Engl. J. Med.* **294**:1004–1005.

Campbell, I. W., Dawes, J., Fraser, D. M., Pepper, D. S., Clarke, B. F., Duncan, L. J. P., and Cash, J. D., 1977, Plasma β-thromboglobulin in diabetes mellitus, *Diabetes* **26**:1175–1177.

Chokroverty, S., Reyes, M. G., Rubino, F. A., and Tonaki, B. S., 1977, The syndrome of diabetic amyotrophy, *Ann. Neurol.* **2**:181–194.

Clements, R. S., Jr., and Reynertson, R., 1977, Myoinositol metabolism in diabetes mellitus: Effect of insulin treatment, *Diabetes* **26**:215–221.

Clements, R., Vourganti, B., Darnell, B., and Oh, S., 1978, Effect of low and high dietary myoinositol (MI) content upon nerve conduction velocities (NCVs) in neuropathic diabetics, *Diabetes* **27**:436 (abstract).

Colwell, J. A., Sagel, J., Crook, L., Chambers, A., and Laimins, M., 1977, Correlation of platelet aggregation, plasma factor activity, and megathrombocytes in diabetic subjects with and without vascular disease, *Metabolism* **26**:279–285.

Crapo, P. A., Reaven, G., and Olefsky, J., 1977, Postprandial plasma-glucose and -insulin responses to different complex carbohydrates, *Diabetes* **26**:1178–1183.

Cudworth, A. G., and Woodrow, J. C., 1975, HL–A system and diabetes mellitus, *Diabetes* **24**:345–349.

Cudworth, A. G., Gamble, D. R., White, G. B. B., Lendrum, R., Woodrow, J. C., and Bloom, A., 1977, Etiology of juvenile-onset diabetes, *Lancet* **1**:385–388.

Davidson, M. B., and Kaplan, S. A., 1977, Increased insulin binding by hepatic plasma membranes from diabetic rats, *J. Clin. Invest.* **59**:22–30.

DeFronzo, R. A., Sherwin, R. S., Felig, P., and Bia, M., 1977, Nonuremic diabetic hyperkalemia, *Arch. Intern. Med.* **137**:842–843.

DeJong, A., Strubbe, J. H., and Steffens, A. B., 1977, Hypothalamic influence on insulin and glucagon release in the rat, *Am. J. Physiol.* **233**:E380.

De Leeuw, I., and Abs, R., 1977, Bone mass and bone density in maturity-type diabetics measured by the ^{125}I photon-absorption technique, *Diabetes* **26**:1130–1135.

Del Prete, G. F., Betterle, C., Padovan, D., Erle, G., Toffolo, A., and Bersahi, G.,

1977, Incidence and significance of islet-cell autoantibodies in different types of diabetes mellitus, *Diabetes* **26**:909–915.

DeNobel, E., van't Laar, A., and Benraad, T. J., 1977, Is a lag-storage curve an early sign of diabetes? Early insulin responses to i.v. glucose in normal subjects, mild maturity-onset diabetes and patients with lag-storage curves, *Diabetologia* **13**:35–41.

Doud, R., Lee, D. B. N., Waisman, J., and Bergstein, J. M., 1977, Development of a lesion resembling diabetic nephropathy in a renal homograft, *Arch. Intern. Med.* **137**:945–947.

Drury, M. I., Greene, A. T., and Stronge, J., 1977, Pregnancy complicated by clinical diabetes mellitus, *Obstet. Gynecol.* **49**:519–522.

Editorial, 1977a, Cigarette smoking and diabetic retinopathy, *Lancet* **1**:841.

Editorial, 1977b, High-purity insulins, *Lancet* **1**:128.

Editorial, 1977c, Insulin regime for diabetic ketoacidosis, *Br. Med. J.* **1**:405–406.

Engerman, R., Bloodworth, J. M. B., Jr., and Nelson, S., 1977, Relationship of microvascular disease in diabetes to metabolic control, *Diabetes* **26**:760–769.

Faber, O. K., and Binder, C., 1977, β-Cell function and blood glucose control in insulin dependent diabetics within the first month of insulin treatment, *Diabetologia* **13**:263–268.

Faerman, I., Faccio, E., Milei, J., Nunez, R., Jadzinsky, M., Fox, D., and Rapaport, M., 1977, Autonomic neuropathy and painless myocardial infarction in diabetic patients: Histologic evidence of their relationships, *Diabetes* **26**:1147–1158.

Fajans, S. S., 1976, Diabetes mellitus, in: *The Year in Metabolism 1975–1976* (N. Freinkel, ed.), pp. 45–71, Plenum Medical Book Company, New York.

Fajans, S. S., 1978, Diabetes mellitus, in: *The Year in Metabolism 1977* (N. Freinkel, ed.), pp. 33–99, Plenum Medical Book Company, New York.

Fajans, S. S., Floyd, J. C., Jr., Tattersall, R. B., Williamson, J. R., Pek, S., and Taylor, C. I., 1976, The various faces of diabetes in the young, *Arch. Intern. Med.* **136**:194–202.

Farinaro, E., Stamler, J., Upton, M., Mohonnier, L., Hall, Y., Moss, D., and Berkson, D., 1977, Plasma glucose levels: Long-term effect of diet in the Chicago Coronary Prevention Evaluation Program, *Ann. Intern. Med.* **86**:147–154.

Fisher, J. N., Shahshahani, M. D., and Kitabchi, A. E., 1977, Diabetic ketoacidosis: Low-dose insulin therapy by various routes, *N. Engl. J. Med.* **297**:238–241.

Flier, J. S., Kahn, C. R., Jarrett, D. B., and Roth, J., 1977, Autoantibodies to the insulin receptor: Effect on the insulin-receptor interaction in IM-9 lymphocytes, *J. Clin. Invest.* **60**:784–794.

Fox, C. J., Darby, S. C., Ireland, J. T., and Sonksen, P. H., 1977, Blood glucose control and glomerular capillary basement membrane thickening in experimental diabetes, *Br. Med. J.* **2**:605–607.

Gabbay, K. H., Hasty, N., Breslow, J. L., Ellison, R. C., Bunn, H. F., and Gallop, P. M., 1977, Glycosylated hemoglobins and long-term blood glucose control in diabetes mellitus, *J. Clin. Endocrinol. Metab.* **44**:859–864.

Gabbe, S. G., Lowensohn, R. I., Mestman, J. H., Freeman, R. K., and Goebelsmann, U., 1977, Lecithin/sphingomyelin ratio in pregnancies complicated by diabetes mellitus, *Am. J. Obstet. Gynecol.* **128**:757–760.

Ganda, O. P., Soeldner, J. S., Gleason, R. E., Smith, T. M., Kilo, C., and Williamson, J. R., 1977, Monozygotic triplets with discordance for diabetes mellitus and diabetic microangiopathy, *Diabetes* **26**:469–479.

Gates, R. J., and Lazarus, N. R., 1977, Reversal of streptozotocin-induced diabetes in rats by intraperitoneal implantation of encapsulated neonatal rabbit pancreatic tissue, *Lancet* **2**:1257–1259.

Gedik, O., and Zileli, M. S., 1977, Effects of hypocalcemia and theophylline on glucose tolerance and insulin release in human beings, *Diabetes* **26**:813–819.

Genuth, S. M., 1977, Insulin secretion in obesity and diabetes: An illustrative case, *Ann. Intern. Med.* **87**:714–716.

Genuth, S., and Martin, P., 1977, Control of hyperglycemia in adult diabetics by pulsed insulin delivery, *Diabetes* **26**:571–581.

Georgakakis, A., 1977, Experimental pancreatic islet transplantation, *Annu. Rev. Coll. Surg. Engl.* **59**:231–235.

Ginsberg, H. N., 1977a, Investigation of insulin sensitivity in treated subjects with ketosis-prone diabetes mellitus, *Diabetes* **26**:278–283.

Ginsberg, H. N., 1977b, Investigation of insulin resistance during diabetic ketoacidosis: Role of counterregulatory substances and effect of insulin therapy, *Metabolism* **26**:1135–1146.

Gonen, B., Rubenstein, A. H., Rochman, H., Tanega, S. P., and Horwitz, D. L., 1977, Hemoglobin A1: An indicator of the metabolic control of diabetic patients, *Lancet* **2**:734–736.

Greene, D. A., DeJesus, P. V., Jr., and Winegrad, A. I., 1975, Effects of insulin and dietary myoinositol on impaired peripheral motor nerve conduction velocity in acute streptozotocin diabetes, *J. Clin. Invest.* **55**:1326–1336.

Gundersen, H. J. G., and Christensen, N. J., 1977, Intravenous insulin causing loss of intravascular water and albumin and increased adrenergic nervous activity in diabetes, *Diabetes* **26**:551–557.

Gundersen, H. J. G., and Neubauer, B., 1977, A long-term diabetic autonomic nervous abnormality: Reduced variations in resting heart rate measured by a simple and sensitive method, *Diabetologia* **13**:137–140.

Gundersen, H. J. G., and Østerby, R., 1977, Glomerular size and structure in diabetes mellitus. II. Late abnormalities, *Diabetologia* **13**:43–48.

Halushka, P. V., Lurie, D., and Colwell, J. A., 1977, Increased synthesis of prostaglandin-E-like material by platelets from patients with diabetes mellitus, *N. Engl. J. Med.* **297**:1306–1310.

Harano, Y., Ohgaku, S., Kidaka, K., Haneda, K., Kikkawa, R., Shigeta, Y., and Abe, H., 1977, Glucose, insulin and somatostatin infusion for the determination of insulin sensitivity, *J. Clin. Endocrinol. Metab.* **45**:1124–1127.

Hare, J. W., and White, P., 1977, Pregnancy in diabetes complicated by vascular disease, *Diabetes* **26**:953–955.

Heber, D., Molitch, M. E., and Sperling, M. A., 1977, Low-dose continuous insulin therapy for diabetic ketoacidosis, *Arch. Intern. Med.* **137**:1377–1380.

Hendriksen, C., Faber, O. K., Drejer, J., and Binder, C., 1977, Prevalence of residual B-cell function in insulin-treated diabetics evaluated by the plasma C-peptide response to intravenous glucagon, *Diabetologia* **13**:615–620.

Hill, D. E., Mayes, S., DiBattista, D., Lockhart-Ewart, R., and Martin, J. M., 1977. Hypothalamic regulation of insulin release in rhesus monkeys, *Diabetes* **26**:726–731.

Hollis, J. B., Castell, D. O., and Braddom, R. L., 1977, Esophageal function in diabetes mellitus and its relation to peripheral neuropathy, *Gastroenterology* **73**:1098–1102.

Holst, J. J., Guldberg Madsen, O., Knop, J., and Schmidt, A., 1977, The effect of intraportal and peripheral infusions of glucagon on insulin and glucose concentrations and glucose tolerance in normal man, *Diabetologia* **13**:487–490.

Hommel, H. H., and Fischer, U., 1977, The mechanism of insulin secretion after oral glucose administration. V. Portal venous IRI concentration in dogs after ingestion of glucose, *Diabetologia* **13**:269–272.

Horowitz, S. D., Borcherding, W., and Bargman, G. J., 1977, Suppressor T cell function in diabetes mellitus, *Lancet* **2**:1291.

Horwitz, D. L., Rubenstein, A. H., and Katz, A. I., 1977, Quantitation of human pancreatic beta-cell function by immunoassay of C-peptide in urine, *Diabetes* **26**:30–35.

Hsu, T. H., Hsu, S. H., Chase, G. A., and Bias, W. B., 1977, Further data on HLA recombination in juvenile-onset diabetes, *Transplant Proc.* **9**:1855–1858.

Illeni, M. T., Pellegris, G., Del Guercio, M. J., Tarantino, A., Busetto, F., DiPietro, C., Clerici, E., Garotta, G., and Chiumello, G., 1977, HLA antigens in diabetic children, *Diabetes* **26**:870–873.

Ingelfinger, F. J., 1977, Debates on diabetes (editorial), *N. Engl. J. Med.* **296**:1228–1229.

Irvine, W. J., 1977, Classification of idiopathic diabetes, *Lancet* **1**:638–641.

Irvine, W. J., McCallum, C. J., Gray, R. S., Campbell, C. J., Duncan, L. J. P., Farquhar, J. W., Vaughan, H., and Morris, P. M., 1977a, Pancreatic islet-cell antibodies in diabetes mellitus correlated with the duration and type of diabetes, coexistent autoimmune disease, and HLA type, *Diabetes* **36**:138–147.

Irvine, W. J., McCallum, C. J., Gray, R. S., and Duncan, L. J. P., 1977b, Clinical and pathogenic significance of pancreatic-islet-cell antibodies in diabetics treated with oral hypoglycaemic agents, *Lancet* **1**:1025–1027.

Irvine, W. J., Toft, A. D., Holton, D. E., Prescott, R. J., Clarke, B. F., and Duncan, L. J. P., 1977c, Familial studies of Type-I and Type-II idiopathic diabetes mellitus, *Lancet* **2**:325–328.

Jansen, F. K., Müntefering, H., and Schmidt, W. A. K., 1977, Virus induced diabetes and the immune system, *Diabetologia* **13**:545–549.

Jaspan, J. B., Mako, M. E., Kuzuya, H., Blix, P. M., Horwitz, D. L., and Rubenstein, A. H., 1977, Abnormalities in circulating beta cell peptides in chronic renal failure: Comparison of C-peptide, proinsulin and insulin, *J. Clin. Endocrinol. Metab.* **45**:441–446.

Jaworski, M., Colle, E., Guttman, R., Belmonte, M. M., Poirier, R., and Wilkins, J.,

1977, HLA typing in families with multiple diabetic offspring, *Clin. Res.* **25**:701A.

Jenkins, D. J. A., Hockaday, T. D. R., Howarth, R., Apling, E. C., Wolever, T. M. S., Leeds, A. R., Bacon, S., and Dilawari, J., 1977a, Treatment of diabetes with guar gum: Reduction of urinary glucose loss in diabetics, *Lancet* **2**:779–780.

Jenkins, D. J. A., Leeds, A. R., Gassull, M. A., Cochet, B., and Alberti, K. G. M. M., 1977b, Decrease in postprandial insulin and glucose concentrations by guar and pectin, *Ann. Intern. Med.* **86**:20–23.

Johnson, S. F., Schade, D. S., and Peake, G. T., 1977, Chlorpropamide-induced hypoglycemia: Successful treatment with diazoxide, *Am. J. Med.* **63**:799–804.

Kahn, C. R., Baird- K., Flier, J. S., and Jarrett, D. B., 1977, Effects of autoantibodies to the insulin receptor on isolated adipocytes: Studies of insulin binding and insulin action, *J. Clin. Invest.* **60**:1094–1106.

Kalhan, S. C., Savin, S. M., and Adam, P. A. J., 1977, Attenuated glucose production rate in newborn infants of insulin-dependent diabetic mothers, *N. Engl. J. Med.* **296**:375–376.

Kamdar, A., Weidmann, P., Makoff, D. L., and Massry, S. G., 1977, Acute renal failure following intravenous use of radiography contrast dyes in patients with diabetes mellitus, *Diabetes* **26**:643–649.

Kanter, Y., Gerson, J. R., and Bessman, A. N., 1977, 2,3-Diphosphoglycerate, nucleotide phosphate, and organic and inorganic phosphate levels during the early phases of diabetic ketoacidosis, *Diabetes* **26**:429–433.

Karam, J. H., Rosenthal, M., O'Donnell, J. J., Tsalikian, E., Lorenzi, M., Gerich, J. E., Siperstein, M. D., and Forsham, P. H., 1976, Discordance of diabetic microangiopathy in identical twins, *Diabetes* **25**:24–28.

Kawamori, R., and Vranic, M., 1977, Mechanism of exercise-induced hypoglycemia in depancreatized dogs maintained on long-acting insulin, *J. Clin. Invest.* **59**:331–337.

Kerner, W., Beischer, W., Tamas, G. Y., Jr., Raptis, S., and Pfeiffer, E. F., 1977, Insulin treatment of decompensated diabetes mellitus with a new artificial endocrine pancreas, *Dtsch. Med. Wochenschr.* **102**:1500–1505.

Kitabchi, A. E., 1977, Proinsulin and C-peptide: A review, *Metabolism* **26**:547–587.

Koncz, L., Soeldner, J. S., Otto, H., Smith, T. M., and Gleason, R. E., 1977, Deranged insulin-secretory dynamics in offspring of two diabetic parents after double stimulation with intravenous glucose, *Diabetes* **26**:1184.

Kosaka, K., Hagura, R., and Kuzuya, T., 1977, Insulin responses in equivocal and definite diabetes, with special reference to subjects who had mild glucose intolerance but later developed definite diabetes, *Diabetes* **26**:944–952.

Kretschmer, G. J., Sutherland, D. E. R., Matas, A. J., Steffes, M. W., and Najarian, J. S., 1977, The dispersed pancreas: Transplantation without islet purification in totally pancreatectomized dogs, *Diabetologia* **13**:495–502.

Kumar, D., 1977, Anti-insulin IgE in diabetics, *J. Clin. Endocrinol. Metab.* **45**:1159.

Kumar, D., Miller, L. V., and Mehtalia, S. D., 1977, Use of dexamethasone in treatment of insulin lipoatrophy, *Diabetes* **26**:296–299.

Kurtz, A. B., Daggett, P. R., Mustaffa, B. E., and Nabarro, J. D. N., 1977, Effect of insulin antibodies on free and total plasma-insulin, *Lancet* **2**:56–58.

Kuzuya, H., Blix, P. M., Horwitz, D. L., Steiner, D. F., and Rubenstein, A. H., 1977a, Determination of free and total insulin and C-peptide in insulin-treated diabetics, *Diabetes* **26**:22–29.

Kuzuya, H., Blix, P. M., Horwitz, D. L., Rubenstein, A. H., Steiner, D. F., Binder, C., and Faber, O. K., 1977b, Heterogeneity of circulating C-peptide, *J. Clin. Endocrinol. Metab.* **44**:952–962.

Lanoe, R., Soria, J., Thibult, N., Soria, C., Eschwege, E., and Tchobroutsky, G., 1977, Glycosylated hemoglobin concentrations and Clinitest results in insulin-dependent diabetes, *Lancet* **2**:1156–1157.

Lebovitz, H. E., Feinglos, M. N., Bucholtz, H. K., and Lebovitz, F. L., 1977, Potentiation of insulin action: A probable mechanism for the antidiabetic action of sulfonylurea drugs, *J. Clin. Endocrinol. Metab.* **45**:601–604.

Lerner, R. L., 1977, The augmentation effect of secretin on the insulin responses to known stimuli: Specificity for glucose, *J. Clin. Endocrinol. Metab.* **45**:1–9.

Levin, M. E., Boisseau, V. C., and Avioli, L. V., 1976, Effects of diabetes mellitus on bone mass in juvenile and adult-onset diabetes, *N. Engl. J. Med.* **294**:241.

Lev-Ran, A., and Goldman, J. A., 1977, Brittle diabetes in pregnancy, *Diabetes* **26**:926–930.

Like, A. A., and Rossini, A. A., 1976, Streptozotocin-induced pancreatic insulitis: New model of diabetes mellitus, *Science* **193**:415–417.

Little, J. A., Lee, R., Sebriakova, M., and Csima, A., 1977, Insulin antibodies and clinical complications in diabetics treated for five years with lente or sulfated insulin, *Diabetes* **26**:980–988.

Logie, A. W., and Stowers, J. M., 1976, Hazards of monocomponent insulins, *Br. Med. J.* **1**:879–880.

Longstreth, G. F., and Newcomer, A. D., 1977, Abdominal pain caused by diabetic radiculopathy, *Ann. Intern. Med.* **86**:166–168.

Longstreth, G. F., Malagelada, J. R., and Kelly, K. A., 1977, Metoclopramide stimulation of gastric motility and emptying in diabetic gastroparesis, *Ann. Intern. Med.* **86**:195–196.

Ludvigsson, J., Säfwenberg, J., and Heding, L. G., 1977, HLA-types, C-peptide and insulin antibodies in juvenile diabetes, *Diabetologia* **13**:13–17.

Ludwig, H., Schernthaner, G., and Mayr, W. R., 1977, The importance of HLA genes to susceptibility in the development of juvenile diabetes mellitus. A study of 93 patients and 68 first degree blood relations, *Diabetes Metab.* **3**:43–48.

Lufkin, E. G., Reagen, T. J., Doan, D. H., and Yanagihara, T., 1977, Acute cerebral dysfunction in diabetic ketoacidosis: Survival followed by panhypopituitarism, *Metabolism* **26**:363–370.

MacMillan, D. R., Kotoyan, M., Zeidner, D., and Hafezi, B., 1977, Seasonal variation in the onset of diabetes in children, *Pediatrics* **59**:113–115.

Maher, T. D., Tanenberg, R. J., Greenberg, B. Z., Hoffman, J. E., Doe, R. P., and Goetz, F. C., 1977, Lack of glucagon response to hypoglycemia in diabetic autonomic neuropathy, *Diabetes* **26**:196–200.

Mako, M. E., Starr, J. I., and Rubenstein, A. H., 1977, Circulating proinsulin in patients with maturity onset diabetes, *Am. J. Med.* **63**:865–869.

Malone, J. I., VanCader, T. C., and Edwards, W. C., 1977, Diabetic vascular changes in children, *Diabetes* **26**:673–679.

Marliss, E. B., Murray, F. T., Stokes, E. F., Zinman, B., Nakhooda, A. F., Denoga, A., Leibel, B. S., and Albisser, A. M., 1977, Normalization of glycemia in diabetics during meals with insulin and glucagon delivery by the artificial pancreas, *Diabetes* **26**:663–672.

McCarthy, S. T., Harris, E., and Turner, R. C., 1977, Glucose control of basal insulin secretion in diabetes, *Diabetologia* **13**:93–97.

McLaren, E. H., Burden, A. C., and Moorhead, P. J., 1977, Acetylator phenotype in diabetic neuropathy, *Br. Med. J.* **2**:291–293.

Mendeloff, A. I., 1977, Dietary fiber and human health (editorial), *N. Engl. J. Med.* **297**:811–814.

Mirouze, J., Selam, J. L., Pham, T. C., and Cavadore, D., 1977, Evaluation of exogenous insulin homeostasis by the artificial pancreas in insulin-dependent diabetics, *Diabetologia* **13**:273–278.

Mitchell, J. C., 1977, End-stage renal failure in juvenile diabetes mellitus, *Mayo Clin. Proc.* **52**:281–288.

Mogensen, C. E., and Andersen, M. J. F., 1975, Increased kidney size and glomerular filtration rate in untreated juvenile diabetes: Normalization by insulin treatment, *Diabetologia* **11**:221–224.

Muggeo, M., Bar, R. S., and Roth, J., 1977, Change in affinity of insulin receptors following oral glucose in normal adults, *J. Clin. Endocrinol. Metab.* **44**:1206–1209.

Murray, F. T., Zinman, B., McClean, P. A., Denoga, A., Albisser, A. M., Leibel, B. S., Nakhooda, A. F., Stokes, E. F., and Marliss, E. B., 1977, The metabolic response to moderate exercise in diabetic man receiving intravenous and subcutaneous insulin, *J. Clin. Endocrinol. Metab.* **44**:708–720.

Mustaffa, B. E., Daggett, P. R., and Nabarro, J. D. N., 1977, Insulin binding capacity in patients changed from conventional to highly purified insulins, *Diabetologia* **13**:311–315.

Najarian, J. S., Sutherland, D. E. R., Matas, A. J., Steffes, M. W., Simmons, R. L., and Goetz, F. C., 1977, Human islet transplantation: A preliminary report, *Transplant Proc.* **9**:233–236.

Nakao, Y., Fukunishi, T., Koide, M., Akasawa, K., Ikeda, M., Yahata, M., and Imura, H., 1977, HLA antigens in Japanese patients with diabetes mellitus, *Diabetes* **26**:736–739.

Nattrass, M., Todd, P. G., Hinks, L., Lloyd, B., and Alberti, K. G. M. M., 1977, Comparative effects of phenformin, metformin and glibenclamide on metabolic rhythms in maturity-onset diabetes, *Diabetologia* **13**:145–152.

Neel, J. V., 1977, The genetics of juvenile-onset-type diabetes mellitus (editorial), *N. Engl. J. Med.* **297**:1062–1063.

Nerup, J., Andersen, O. O., Buschard, K., Christau, B., Christy, M., Kronmannm, H., Platz, P., Ryder, L., Svejgaard, A., and Thomsen, M., 1977, HLA-D typing in insulin-dependent diabetes mellitus (IDDM), *Acta Endocrinol. (Copenhagen)* **85**:48 (Suppl. 209) (abstract).

Notkins, A. L., 1977, Virus-induced diabetes mellitus: Brief review, *Arch. Virol.* **54**:1–17.

Olefsky, J. M., and Reaven, G. M., 1977, Insulin binding in diabetes: Relationships with plasma insulin levels and insulin sensitivity, *Diabetes* **26**:680–688.

Olefsky, J. M., Sperling, M. A., and Reaven, G. M., 1977, Does glucagon play a role in the insulin resistance of patients with adult non-ketotic diabetes?, *Diabetologia* **13**:327–330.

Olivero, J., and Suki, W. N., 1977, Acute glomerulonephritis complicating diabetic nephropathy, *Arch. Intern. Med.* **137**:732–734.

Oseid, S., Beck-Nielsen, H., Pedersen, O., and Sovik, O., 1977, Decreased binding of insulin to its receptor in patients with congenital generalized lipodiptrophy, *N. Engl. J. Med.* **296**:245–248.

Osterby-Hansen, R., and Lundbaek, K., 1970, The basement membrane morphology in diabetes mellitus, in: *Diabetes Mellitus: Theory and Practice* (M. Ellenberg and H. Rifkin, eds.), pp. 178–209, McGraw-Hill, New York.

Padilla, A. J., and Loeb, J. N., 1977, "Low-dose" versus "high-dose" insulin regimens in the management of uncontrolled diabetes, *Am. J. Med.* **63**:843–848.

Paetkau, M. E., Boyd, T. A. S., Winship, B., and Grace, M., 1977, Cigarette smoking and diabetic retinopathy, *Diabetes* **26**:46–49.

Pardo, V., Perez-Stable, E., Alzamora, D. B., and Cleveland, W. W., 1972, Incidence and significance of muscle capillary basal lamina thickness in juvenile diabetes, *Am. J. Pathol.* **68**:67–78.

Passa, P., Rousselie, F., Gauville, C., and Canviet, J., 1977, Retinopathy and plasma growth hormone levels in idiopathic hemochromatosis with diabetes, *Diabetes* **26**:113–120.

Patel, R., Ansuri, A., and Covarrubias, C. L.-P., 1977, Leukocyte antigens and disease. III. Association of HLA-B8 and HLA-BW15 with insulin-dependent diabetes in three different population groups, *Metabolism* **26**:487–492.

Perez, G. O., Lespier, L., Jacobi, J., Oster, J. R., Katz, F. H., Vaamonde, C. A., and Fishman, L. M., 1977a, Hyporeninemia and hypoaldosteronism in diabetes mellitus, *Arch. Intern. Med.* **137**:852–855.

Perez, G. O., Lespier, L., Knowles, R., Oster, J. R., and Vaamonde, C. A., 1977b, Potassium homeostasis in chronic diabetes mellitus, *Arch. Intern. Med.* **137**:1018–1022.

Peterson, C. M., Jones, R. L., Koenig, R. J., Melvin, E. T., and Lehrman, M. L., 1977a, Reversible hematologic sequelae of diabetes mellitus, *Ann. Intern. Med.* **86**:425–429.

Peterson, C. M., Koenig, R. J., Jones, R. L., Saudek, C. D., and Cerami, A., 1977b, Correlation of serum triglyceride levels and hemoglobin A_{1c} concentrations in diabetes mellitus, *Diabetes* **26**:507–509.

Piters, K. M., Kumar, D., Pei, E., and Bessman, A. N., 1977, Comparison of continuous and intermittent intravenous insulin therapies for diabetic ketoacidosis, *Diabetologia* **13**:317–321.

Pyke, D. A., and Tattersall, R. B., 1973, Diabetic retinopathy in identical twins, *Diabetes* **22**:613–618.

Raskin, P., Marks, J. F., Burns, H., Jr., Plumer, M. E., and Siperstein, M. D., 1975, Capillary basement membrane width in diabetic children, *Am. J. Med.* **58**:365–372.

Reaven, G. M., and Olefsky, J. M., 1977, Relationship between heterogeneity of insulin responses and insulin resistance in normal subjects and patients with chemical diabetes, *Diabetologia* **13**:201–206.

Reaven, G. M., Sageman, W. S., and Swenson, R. S., 1977, Development of insulin resistance in normal dogs following alloxan-induced insulin deficiency, *Diabetologia* **13**:459–462.

Reynolds, C., Molnar, G. D., Horwitz, D. L., Rubenstein, A. H., Taylor, W. F., and Jiang, N.-S., 1977, Abnormalities of endogenous glucagon and insulin in unstable diabetes, *Diabetes* **26**:36–45.

Robertson, R. P., and Chen, M., 1977, A role for prostaglandin E in defective insulin secretion and carbohydrate intolerance in diabetes mellitus, *J. Clin. Invest.* **60**:747–753.

Rosenbloom, A. L., and Giordano, B. P., 1977, Chronic overtreatment with insulin in children and adolescents, *Am. J. Dis. Child.* **131**:881–885.

Rosenbloom, A. L., Goldstein, S., and Yip, C. C., 1977a, Normal insulin binding to cultured fibroblasts from patients with lipoatrophic diabetes, *J. Clin. Endocrinol. Metab.* **44**:803–806.

Rosenbloom, A. L., Lezotte, D. C., Weber, F. T., Gudat, J., Heller, D. R., Weber, M. L., Klein, S., and Kennedy, B. B., 1977b, Diminution of bone mass in childhood diabetes, *Diabetes* **26**:1052–1055.

Ross, S. A., Brown, J. C., and Dupre, J., 1977, Hypersecretion of gastric inhibitory polypeptide following oral glucose in diabetes mellitus, *Diabetes* **26**:525–529.

Rossini, A. A., Appel, M. C., Williams, R. M., and Like, A. A., 1977a, Genetic influence of the streptozotocin-induced insulitis and hyperglycemia, *Diabetes* **26**:916–920.

Rossini, A. A., Like, A. A., Appel, M. C., Chick, W. L., and Cahill, G. F., Jr., 1977b, Studies of streptozotocin-induced insulitis and diabetes, *Proc. Natl. Acad. Sci. U.S.A.* **74**:2485–2489.

Roth, J., Neville, D. M., Kahn, C. R., and Gorden, P., 1977, Hormone resistance and hormone sensitivity, *N. Engl. J. Med.* **296**:277–278.

Rubinstein, P., Suciu-Foca, N., and Nicholson, J. F., 1977, Genetics of juvenile diabetes mellitus: A recessive gene closely linked to HLA D and with 50 per cent penetrance, *N. Engl. J. Med.* **297**:1036–1040.

Santiago, J. V., McAlister, W. H., Ratzan, S. K., Bussman, Y., Haymond, M. W., Shackelford, G., and Weldon, V. V., 1977, Decreased cortical thickness and osteopenia in children with diabetes mellitus, *J. Clin. Endocrinol. Metab.* **45**:845–848.

Sarji, K. E., Levine, J. H., Nair, R. M. G., Sagel, J., and Colwell, J. A., 1977, Relation between growth hormone levels and von Willebrand factor activity, *J. Clin. Endocrinol. Metab.* **45**:853–856.

Schade, D. S., and Eaton, R. P., 1977, The controversy concerning counterregulatory hormone secretion: A hypothesis for the prevention of diabetic ketoacidosis?, *Diabetes* **26**:596–601.

Schernthaner, G., Ludwig, H., and Mayr, W. R., 1977, B-lymphocyte alloantigens and insulin-dependent diabetes mellitus, *Lancet* **2**:1128.

Schultz, T. A., Lewis, S. B., Westbie, D. K., Wallin, J. D., and Gerich, J. E., 1977, Glucose delivery: A modulator of glucose uptake in contracting skeletal muscle, *Am. J. Physiol.* **233**:E514–518.

Seyer-Hansen, K., 1977, Renal hypertrophy in experimental diabetes: Relation to severity of diabetes, *Diabetologia* **13**:141–143.

Sharma, A. K., Thomas, P. K., and DeMolina, A. F., 1977, Peripheral nerve fiber size in experimental diabetes, *Diabetes* **26**:689–692.

Sherwin, R. S., 1977, Low-dose insulin therapy in diabetic ketoacidosis: Valid physiological approach, not a panacea (editorial), *Arch. Intern. Med.* **137**:1361–1362.

Sherwin, R. S., Fisher, M., Hendler, R., and Felig, P., 1976, Hyperglucagonemia and blood glucose regulation in normal obese and diabetic subjects, *N. Engl. J. Med.* **294**:455–461.

Shima, K., Tanaka, R., Morishita, S., Tarui, S., Kumahara, Y., and Nishikawa, M., 1977, Studies on the etiology of "brittle diabetes": Relationship between diabetic instability and insulinogenic reserve, *Diabetes* **26**:717–775.

Silberberg, R., Hirshberg, G. E., and Lesker, P., 1977, Enzyme studies in the articular cartilage of diabetic rats and of rats bearing transplanted pancreatic islets, *Diabetes* **26**:732–735.

Siperstein, M. D., Unger, R. H., and Madison, L. L., 1968, Studies of muscle capillary basement membranes in normal subjects, diabetic and prediabetic patients, *J. Clin. Invest.* **47**:1973–1999.

Siperstein, M. D., Foster, D. W., Knowles, H. C., Levine, R., Madison, L. L., and Roth, J., 1977, Control of blood glucose and diabetic vascular disease (editorial), *N. Engl. J. Med.* **296**:1060–1063.

Sun, A. M., Parisius, W., Healy, G. M., Vacek, I., and Macmorine, H. G., 1977, The use, in diabetic rats and monkeys, of artificial capillary units containing cultured islets of Langerhans (artificial endocrine pancreas), *Diabetes* **26**:1136–1139.

Sutton, C., 1977, Practical approach to problems of the paturient diabetic in developing countries, *Br. Med. J.* **2**:1069–1072.

Tan, M. H., Graham, C. A., Bradley, R. F., Gleason, R. E., and Soeldner, J. S., 1977, The effects of long-term therapy with oral hypoglycemic agents on the oral glucose tolerance test dynamics in male chemical diabetics, *Diabetes* **26**:561–570.

Tiengo, A., Del Prete, G. F., Nosadini, R., Betterle, C., Garotti, C., and Bersani, G., 1977, Insulin and glucagon secretion in diabetic and non-diabetic patients with circulating islet cell antibodies, *Diabetologia* **13**:451–458.

Tsalikian, E., Dunphy, T. W., Bohannon, N. V., Lorenzi, M., Gerich, J. E., Forsham, P. H., Kane, J. P., and Karam, J. H., 1977, The effect of chronic oral antidiabetic therapy on insulin and glucagon responses to a meal, *Diabetes* **26**:314–321.

Turkington, R. W., 1977, Encephalopathy induced by oral hypoglycemic drugs, *Arch. Intern. Med.* **137**:1082–1083.

Turner, R. C., Harris, E., Bloom, S. R., and Uren, C., 1977, Relation of fasting plasma glucose concentration to plasma insulin and glucagon concentrations: Studies in latent diabetics and women who have produced large-for-date babies, *Diabetes* **26**:166–171.

Van Thiel, D. H., Smith, W. I., Jr., Rabin, B. S., Fisher, S. E., and Lester, R., 1977, A syndrome of immunoglobulin A deficiency, diabetes mellitus, malabsorption, and a common HLA haplotype, *Ann. Intern. Med.* **86**:10–19.

Volpé, R., 1977, The role of autoimmunity in hypoendocrine and hyperendocrine function—with special emphasis on autoimmune thyroid disease, *Ann. Intern. Med.* **87**:86–99.

Waitzman, M. D., Colley, A. M., and Nardelli-Olkowska, K., 1977, Metabolic approaches to studies on diabetic microangiopathy, *Diabetes* **26**:510–519.

Warth, M. R., and Knopp, R. H., 1977, Lipid metabolism in pregnancy. V. Interactions of diabetes, body weight, age, and high carbohydrate diet, *Diabetes* **26**:1056–1062.

Webb, S. R., Loria, R. M., Madge, G. E., and Kibrick, S., 1976, Susceptibility of mice to Group B Coxsackie virus is influenced by the diabetic gene, *J. Exp. Med.* **143**:1239–1248.

Whitelaw, A., 1977, Subcutaneous fat in newborn infants of diabetic mothers: An indication of quality of diabetic control, *Lancet* **1**:15–18.

Williamson, J. R., and Kilo, C., 1977, Current status of capillary basement-membrane disease in diabetes mellitus, *Diabetes* **26**:65–73.

Williamson, J. R., Vogler, N., and Kilo, C., 1973, The natural history of basement membrane disease in diabetes mellitus, in: *Proceedings of the Eighth Congress of the International Diabetes Federation, Brussels, July, 1973* (W. J. Malaisse and J. Pirart, eds.), pp. 424–428, Excerpta Medica, Amsterdam.

Wilson, C., Connolly, J. H., and Thomson, D., 1977, Coxsackie B2 virus infection and acute-onset diabetes in a child, *Br. Med. J.* **1**:1008.

Witters, L. A., Ohman, J. L., Weir, G. C., Raymond, L. W., and Lowell, F. C., 1977, Insulin antibodies in the pathogenesis of insulin allergy and resistance, *Am. J. Med.* **63**:703–709.

Yoon, J. W., Huang, S. W., MacLaren, N. K., Wheeler, C. J., Selvaggio, S. S., and Notkins, A. L., 1977, Antibody to encephalomyocarditis virus in juvenile diabetes, *N. Engl. J. Med.* **297**:1235–1236.

Yue, D. K., and Turtle, J. R., 1977, New forms of insulin and their use in the treatment of diabetes, *Diabetes* **26**:341–345.

Zincke, H., Woods, J. E., Palumbo, P. J., Leary, F. J., and Johnson, W. J., 1977, Renal transplantation in patients with insulin-dependent diabetes mellitus, *J. Am. Med. Assoc.* **237**:1101–1103.

Zinman, B., Murray, F. T., Vranic, M., Albisser, A. M., Leibel, B. S., McClean, P. A., and Marliss, E. G., 1977, Glucoregulation during moderate exercise in insulin treated diabetics, *J. Clin. Endocrinol. Metab.* **45**:641–652.

Glucagon and Somatostatin

Richard E. Dobbs and Roger H. Unger

8.1. Anatomy of the Islets of Langerhans

8.1.1. Topographical Relationships of the Islet Cells

The islets of Langerhans contain at least four major cell types—the A, A_2, or α cell; the B or β cell; the D or A_1 cell; and the F cell— containing, respectively, glucagon, insulin, somatostatin, and pancreatic polypeptide. In every species thus far examined, these four cell types bear a constant topographical relationship to one another, although the particular cellular arrangements may differ from species to species. In man and in the rat, the A cells are situated in the outer rim of the islet and make up approximately 25% of the total islet cell population (Fujita *et al.*, 1976; Orci *et al.*, 1976b). The D cells are situated immediately under this outer A-cell rim and make up approximately 10% of the endocrine cells of the endocrine pancreas. The B cells form the central mass of the islets, accounting for at least 65% in the rat. F cells replace A cells in islets

Abbreviations used in this chapter: (BPG) big plasma glucagon; (cAMP) cyclic AMP; (FFA) free fatty acid(s); (GH) growth hormone; (GIP) gastric inhibitory polypeptide; (GLI) glucagonlike immunoreactivity; (IRG) immunoreactive glucagon; (VIP) vasoactive intestinal polypeptide.

RICHARD E. DOBBS • Veterans Administration Hospital, Dallas, Texas 75216; Department of Physiology, University of Texas Southwestern Medical School, Dallas, Texas 75235. ROGER H. UNGER • Veterans Administration Hospital, Dallas, Texas 75216; Department of Internal Medicine, University of Texas Southwestern Medical School, Dallas, Texas 75235.

situated close to the duodenum (Orci, 1976a); these islets are particularly rich in polypeptide-containing cells and poor in glucagon-containing cells.

8.1.2. Vascular and Neural Relationships

Afferent nerves and blood vessels enter the islets in the heterocellular cortical region (Fujita *et al.*, 1976), the area in which local contacts between heterologous cells are maximal.

8.1.3. "Paracrine" Relationships

A second unique function of the heterocellular region may involve local interactions of the various secretory products of neighboring islet cells on one another—so-called "paracrine" functions (Feyrter, 1963); insulin suppresses glucagon (Samols *et al.*, 1972), glucagon stimulates both insulin (Samols *et al.*, 1965) and somatostatin (Patton *et al.*, 1976b), and somatostatin inhibits both insulin and glucagon secretion (Koerker *et al.*, 1974; Mortimer *et al.*, 1974). A paracrine system of interlocking local hormonal influences has therefore been postulated (Unger and Orci, 1977a).

8.1.4. Subcellular Specializations

8.1.4.1. Tight Junctions

At the subcellular level, the islets of Langerhans have certain specializations with probable functional significance. Tight junctions, linear sites of fusion between the outer leaflets of the plasma membranes of adjacent cells (Orci *et al.*, 1973, 1975b,c), may create constantly changing compartments in the space between islet cells. Such compartmentalization could control access of secretory products to potential receptors on surrounding cells, perhaps guiding secreted polypeptides toward the perivascular spaces, thereby permitting them to enter the circulation to serve an endocrine function without exciting local receptors, or, alternatively, guiding secreted products to local receptors for paracrine action without changing plasma concentrations.

8.1.4.2. Gap Junctions

Gap junctions have also been identified in islet cells. These low-resistance pathways make possible electrotonic and metabolic coupling of adjacent cells (Staehelin, 1974), permitting molecules of less than 800 daltons to pass from the cytosol of one cell to that of another cell without entering the intercellular space. The recent demonstration by T. S. Lawrence *et al.* (1978) that cyclic nucleotides may pass via such channels from one cell type to another may have important implications for islet cell function. Their presence between all islet cells, irrespective of type (Orci *et al.*, 1973, 1975b,c), suggests the possibility that each islet constitutes a functional syncytium, perhaps to provide a means of coordinated secretion of its principal hormones. These intercellular communications could be involved in the reciprocal high-frequency oscillation of insulin and glucagon secretion observed by Goodner *et al.* (1976).

8.2. Structure–Function Relationships of Glucagon

The primary structure of glucagon, a 29-amino-acid polypeptide with a molecular weight of 3485 (Bromer *et al.*, 1957), is identical in all the mammalian species thus far studied with the exception of the guinea pig (Sundby, 1976). (For a more complete review, see *The Year in Metabolism 1977*, Chapter 3.)

8.2.1. Biological Structure–Function Relationships

It is not clear whether the binding of glucagon to its membrane receptor involves the entire glucagon molecule (Epand *et al.*, 1976) or only specific hydrophobic regions at positions 6–14 and 22–27 (Blundell *et al.*, 1976), but the tyrosine residues at positions 10 and 13 appear to be of key importance (Linn *et al.*, 1976). The N-terminal and central portions of glucagon are important for both binding and adenylate cyclase activation (Hruby *et al.*, 1976). Fragments containing residues 18–29 and 19–29 have a conformation similar to that of glucagon 1–29 (Ross *et al.*, 1977).

8.2.2. Immunologic Structure–Function Relationships

Assan and Slusher (1972) and Heding *et al.* (1976) proposed that so-called "specific" antiglucagon antibodies that react primarily with pancreatic-type glucagon are directed toward the 24–29 residue C-terminal section of the molecule, while "nonspecific" antisera that cross-react with "glucagonlike immunoreactivities" ("enteroglucagons") are directed toward the N-terminal 2–23 amino acid segment. Fragments of glucagon that are incapable of binding to receptors and are therefore devoid of biological activity may retain their immunoreactivity (Hruby *et al.*, 1976; Heding *et al.*, 1976; Srikant *et al.*, 1977b).

8.3. Pancreatic and Extrapancreatic Immunoreactive Glucagons

8.3.1. Immunoreactive Glucagon Fractions in Tissue Extracts

8.3.1.1. Pancreas

Extracts of mammalian, fish, and bird pancreas contain several immunoreactive glucagon (IRG) moieties (Table I). The most abundant immunoreactive fraction corresponds to 3500-molecular-weight glucagon. It is identical to crystalline beef–pork glucagon in glycogenolytic activity (Rigopoulou et al., 1970) and in its ability to activate adenylate cyclase and displace [^{125}I]glucagon from isolated liver membranes (Srikant et al., 1977b). A smaller IRG of about 2000 may be a degradation product, whereas other larger fractions have been considered to be possible glucagon precursor molecules (see below). IRGs of molecular weight 50,000 (Tager and Markese, 1976) and 65,000 (Srikant, unpublished

Table I. Characteristics of Pancreatic and Extrapancreatic Immunoreactive Glucagons

Origin	Molecular size of IRG	pI	Glycogenolytic activity	Displacement of [^{125}I]glucagon	Activation of adenylate cyclase
			Percentage response to immunoequivalent concentration of glucagon		
Pancreas	2000	—	—	—	—
	3500	6.25	100	104	100
	4900	—	—	—	—
	9000	4.65	0	10	0
	12,000	—	—	—	—
	20,000	—	—	—	—
	50,000	—	—	—	—
	65,000	—	—	—	—
Stomach (fundus)	2000	—	—	—	—
	3500	6.15	120	107	180
	9000	4.50	0	10	0
	65,000	6.40	110	97.5	82.5
Salivary gland	29,000	—	100	—	—
	70,000	—	100	—	—

observations) have been recovered from rat islets; however, their role as possible precursors of glucagon is unknown.

8.3.1.2. Stomach

The fundus of the canine stomach contains three major IRG fractions (Srikant *et al.*, 1977a) in addition to a 3500-molecular-weight biologically active "true glucagon": (1) an IRG of about 2000 daltons; (2) an IRG of about 9000 daltons, which corresponds to the biologically inactive 9000-molecular-weight proglucagon of islets (Noe and Bauer, 1971); and (3) an IRG fraction of 65,000 that binds to hepatic membranes and has approximately the same glycogenolytic activity in the isolated perfused rat liver as 3500-molecular-weight glucagon (Table I).

8.3.1.3. Intestine

Pancreatic type IRG is also present in the extracts of small bowel and colon of pigs (Holst, 1977), a species resembling primates with respect to "true glucagon" distribution, and in baboons (Bloom *et al.*, 1975b).

8.3.1.4. Salivary Gland

An IRG estimated to have a molecular weight of approximately 70,000 was noted in saline extracts of rodent and human submaxillary salivary glands (Lawrence, A. M., *et al.*, 1976); its hyperglycemic activity is similar to that of porcine glucagon. Bhathena *et al.* (1976) identified a 29,000-molecular-weight IRG in rodent and human salivary glands that has glycogenolytic activity and competes with pancreatic glucagon for binding to specific glucagon receptors of rat liver membranes; however, on incubation in urea, it dissociates into several smaller molecular weight fragments, including a 3500-molecular-weight moiety.

8.3.2. Biosynthesis of Pancreatic Glucagon

The pathway of pancreatic glucagon biosynthesis remains undetermined. Experiments in anglerfish islets suggest that a 12,000-molecular-weight IRG is cleaved to a 9000-dalton moiety (Noe, 1976) [previously referred to as "proglucagon" (Noe and Bauer, 1971) and "large glucagon immunoreactivity" (Rigopoulou *et al.*, 1970)]. This is converted to a 4900-molecular-weight polypeptide, perhaps a glucagon molecule with additional amino acid residues at the C terminus (Tager and Steiner, 1973). This, in turn, is presumably converted to 3500-molecule-weight glucagon. Hellerstrom *et al.* (1972, 1974) identified a 9000-molecular-weight "proglucagon" fraction that was slowly converted to a 3500-molecular-weight glucagon fraction before secretion. However, in pigeon islets, O'Connor and Lazarus (1976) were unable to detect a precursor–product relationship between a 20,000- and a 3500-molecular-weight IRG. The various IRG moieties thus far described and certain of their properties are listed in Table I.

8.3.3. Extrapancreatic A Cells and Glucagon Secretion

8.3.3.1. A Cells

IRG-containing A cells indistinguishable from those of A cells in the pancreas are present in the canine gastric fundus (Larsson *et al.*, 1975; Baetens *et al.*, 1976b). In the human gastic fundus, however, glucagon-containing A cells were detected in only one of eight specimens obtained at autopsy Muñoz-Barragan *et al.*, 1977). A cells were demonstrated by electron microscopy in the duodenum and colon of humans (Sasagawa *et al.*, 1973).

8.3.3.2. Glucagon

In normal dogs, the gastric contribution of glucagon to total circulating immunoreactive glucagon appears to be modest (Muñoz-Barragan *et al.*, 1976), but in insulin-deprived, totally depancreatized dogs (Vranic *et al.*, 1974; Matsuyama and Foà, 1975; Mashiter *et al.*, 1975), substantial hyperglucagonemia is present, derived largely from the gastric fundus (Blazquez *et al.*, 1976). Release of fundus glucagon is also increased in insulin-deprived alloxan-diabetic dogs (Blazquez *et al.*, 1977). Hypersecretion of gastric glucagon in insulin-deficient dogs is abolished promptly by insulin in small doses (Dobbs *et al.*, 1975; Blazquez *et al.*, 1976; Lefebvre and Luyckx, 1977) and by somatostatin (Valverde *et al.*, 1975). In the absence of insulin, the fundic A cell seems to contribute substantially to the hyperglucagonemia of diabetes mellitus (Dobbs *et al.*, 1975). The IRG present in the canine gastric fundus has glycogenolytic and cyclic-AMP (cAMP)-stimulating activity indistinguishable from that of pancreatic glucagon (Srikant *et al.*, 1976), suggesting that at least in dogs, fundic glucagon may participate in the hyperglycemia of insulin deficiency.

According to most investigators, IRG is present in the plasma of totally depancreatized humans (Müller *et al.*, 1974; Palmer *et al.*, 1976; Miyata *et al.*, 1976; Villanueva *et al.*, 1976). Palmer *et al.* (1976) reported basal IRG levels in the normal range in three totally depancreatized patients, and in two of the three, IRG levels increased following the infusion of arginine. The arginine-stimulated rise in IRG in these two patients was associated with an increase in hyperglycemia, suggesting that the circulating glucagon was biologically active (Palmer *et al.*, 1976). In contrast, Barnes and Bloom (1976) reported the complete absence of plasma glucagon in totally depancreatized patients, both during arginine stimulation (Barnes and Bloom, 1976) and after insulin withdrawal (Barnes *et al.*, 1977) (cf. Section 8.9.1.5.).

8.3.4. Immunoreactive Glucagon in Plasma

Plasma contains at least four IRG components. In addition to IRG^{3500} (Valverde *et al.*, 1976), which presumably is true glucagon, there is an IRG^{9000} and an IRG^{2000}; these three fractions correspond in molecular size to the fractions identified in glucagon-secreting tissues (Table I). A fourth fraction not yet identified in tissues is "big plasma glucagon" (BPG), a globulin-sized immunoreactive substance (Valverde *et al.*, 1974), previously referred to as "interfering factor" (Weir *et al.*, 1973) and "macro-IRG" (Valverde *et al.*, 1975), and reported by Kuku *et al.* (1976) to comprise most of the basal plasma IRG in normal subjects. It remains to be characterized chemically and biologically.

8.4. Glucagon Metabolism, Clearance, and Degradation

It is estimated that the liver removes 64% of true glucagon, i.e., the 3500-molecular-weight IRG, as quantitated by gel filtration (Jaspan and Rubenstein, 1977), whereas hepatic extraction of the larger-molecular-weight IRG components is far less. Only 30% of the total unfractionated plasma IRG is removed by the liver (Felig *et al.*, 1974). The importance of the kidney in glucagon clearance is indicated by the fact that bilateral kidney exclusion in dogs is followed by an immediate increase in total plasma IRG, even when further glucagon secretion is inhibited by somatostatin (Lefebvre and Luyckx, 1976). The hyperglucagonemia of renal failure (Bilbrey *et al.*, 1974) is in large part the result of a decrease in the removal of true glucagon by the kidney (Lefebvre and Luyckx, 1976).

8.5. Actions of Glucagon

8.5.1. Mechanisms

8.5.1.1. Receptor Binding

Glucagon action is initiated by its binding to a specific receptor on the plasma membrane of its target cell. This activates adenylate cyclase and begins the cascade of biochemical events. Even a small change in the molecular structure of mammalian glucagon, such as the substitution of a single amino acid as in avian glucagon (Sundby, 1976), reduces its binding affinity to the glucagon receptor of rat liver plasma membranes (Tung *et al.*, 1977). The glucagon receptor has been separated from hepatocyte membranes (Bregman and Levy, 1977; Welton *et al.*, 1977); the former workers obtained a membrane protein with a molecular weight of approximately 23,000–25,000, which they suggest may be a component of the glucagon receptor and which behaves like a membrane receptor with respect to its glucagon-binding properties.

There is evidence that changes in plasma glucagon concentration may influence the sensitivity of its target tissues through changes in the binding and action of the hormone, as has been proposed for other hormones (Gavin *et al.*, 1972). Glucagon binding was reduced in rats made chronically hyperglucagonemic by starvation (Fouchereau-Peron *et al.*, 1976; Srikant *et al.*, 1977b), insulin deficiency, or repeated glucagon injections (Srikant *et al.*, 1977b). Yet, despite this "down-regulation" of glucagon receptors, the ability of glucagon to activate adenylate cyclase in their liver membranes was undiminished through an increased efficiency of the reduced number of occupied glucagon receptors (Srikant *et al.*, 1977b). However, increased binding of glucagon and an associated increase in glucagon-stimulated adenylate cyclase activity was reported in the liver plasma membranes of partially nephrectomized uremic rats (Soman and Felig, 1977) and in untreated insulin-deficient rats with hyperglucagonemia (Soman and Felig, 1978).

8.5.1.2. Adenylate Cyclase Activation

Hammes and Rodbell (1976) suggest that the adenylate cyclase system exists in an A and a B state. Activating ligands bind preferentially to the B state, and only the B state is active. Rodbell and Londos (1976) propose that the adenylate cyclase system in rat liver membranes contains four effector sites, three of which (sites for glucagon, GTP, and divalent cations) enhance activity, while occupation of the fourth, the adenosine site, results in inhibition of enzyme activity. All the sites are allosterically linked to give a finely controlled regulatory system; control is exerted by a shift in equilibrium between inactive (A) and active (B) states of the enzyme, and preferential binding of the effectors to the B state.

8.5.1.3. Glycogenolysis

Binding of glucagon to its specific receptor on the hepatocyte plasma membrane activates adenylate cyclase on the cytosol surface of the cell membrane and increases the conversion of ATP to cAMP, thereby initiating a cascade of reactions. The first of these is the activation of the cAMP-dependent protein kinase, which in turn activates phosphorylase kinase. Activated phosphorylase kinase converts inactive glycogen phosphorylase to the active form, and glycogenolysis is accelerated. The protein kinase concomitantly inactivates glycogen synthetase, thereby reducing glycogen synthesis. This system appears to be separate from epinephrine-stimulated glycogenolysis, which occurs via α receptors that activate phosphorylase and inactivate glycogen synthase without accumulation of cAMP or activation of cAMP-dependent protein kinase (Hutson *et al.*, 1976; Cherrington *et al.*, 1976).

8.5.1.4. Gluconeogenesis

Rapid increases in the activity of hepatic phosphoenolpyruvate (PEP) carboxykinase, the rate-limiting enzyme of gluconeogenesis, occur in response to gluconeogenic hormones such as glucagon (Exton and Park, 1969; Blair *et al.*, 1973; Pilkis *et al.*, 1975). PEP carboxykinase activity is also increased during starvation and experimental diabetes (Ballard and Hopgod, 1973; Murphy and Anderson, 1974), conditions in which glucagon levels are elevated. PEP carboxykinase requires a "ferroactivator," an iron-containing liver cytosol protein (Bentle and Lardy, 1977). This protein, which has a molecular weight of approximately 100,000, is elevated in alloxan diabetes and returns to normal in parallel with PEP carboxykinase following insulin treatment (MacDonald *et al.*, 1977).

8.5.1.5. Ketogenesis

Ketogenesis requires that the insulin/glucagon ratio be low (McGarry *et al.*, 1977). The low insulin level contributes to ketogenesis primarily at the adipocyte level through enhanced lipolysis, which augments the delivery to the liver of free fatty acids (FFA), the substrates for ketogenesis. At the same time, the relatively high glucagon level converts the liver to a ketogenic organ capable of oxidizing long-chain fatty acids to ketones. A high ketogenic capacity of the liver requires both the presence of carnitine for the transport of fatty acids into the mitochondria by carnitine acyltransferase, and the presence of glucagon, which halts the flow of glucose-derived carbon into pathways of fatty acid synthesis and/or blocks fatty acid synthesis at the acetyl-CoA carboxylase level (Cook *et al.*, 1977). This reduces the levels of malonyl-CoA, the first committed step in fatty acid synthesis, and the inhibitor of fatty acid oxidation and ketone formation (McGarry *et al.*, 1976, 1977; McGarry and Foster, 1977). A glucagon-induced decline in malonyl-CoA (Cook *et al.*, 1977) permits enhanced fatty acid oxidation and ketogenesis (McGarry *et al.*, 1977). Normally, during carbohydrate feeding, when glucagon is low, fatty acid synthesis increases and the resulting high levels of malonyl-CoA repress fatty acid oxidation; in contrast, in hyperglucagonemic states, such as starvation and diabetes, low malonyl-CoA levels permit accelerated fatty acid oxidation and ketogenesis.

8.5.1.6. Effects on Lipids

In concert with its ketogenic action, glucagon inhibits fatty acid synthesis (Geelen et al., 1977; Cook et al., 1977), and in physiologic concentrations stimulates lipolysis (Schade and Eaton, 1977) by activating adipocyte adenylate cyclase, which increases the cAMP production and activates cAMP-dependent protein kinase. The active protein kinase phosphorylates hormone-sensitive triglyceride lipase, producing the active form of the enzyme, which acts to break down triglycerides to FFA and glycerol (for a review, see Lefebvre, 1972).

8.5.2. Physiology

8.5.2.1. Glycogenolysis

Glucagon has long been known to be a potent glycogenolytic agent (Sutherland and DeDuve, 1948). It plays an important role in maintaining hepatic glucose production and preventing hypoglycemia under basal conditions (Liljenquist et al., 1977; Cherrington et al., 1978), after a protein meal (Müller et al., 1970; Wahren et al., 1976), and during strenuous exercise (Vranic et al., 1976). Insulin levels decline and glucagon increases during exercise (Böttger et al., 1972a; Harvey et al., 1974), the reduced insulin/glucagon ratio promoting a rate of hepatic glucose production sufficient to replace the glucose utilized by the exercising muscle and thereby to prevent hypoglycemia (Vranic et al., 1976; Galbo et al., 1977). Increased adrenergic activity and elevated epinephrine levels are probably partially responsible for the increase in glucagon and decrease in insulin observed during very strenuous exercise (Galbo et al., 1976). When epinephrine-induced glucagon secretion is blocked by concomitant infusion of somatostatin, there is a delay in the glucose rise, indicating that glucagon mediates, in part, epinephrine-induced glycogenolysis (Chideckel et al., 1977).

8.5.2.2. Gluconeogenesis

The gluconeogenic effects of glucagon have been demonstrated both in vitro (Mallette et al., 1969) and in vivo (Chiasson et al., 1975). Glucagon promotes the hepatic uptake of gluconeogenic precursors (Brockman *et al.*, 1975; Sestoft *et al.*, 1977) and the intrahepatic shunting of alanine into gluconeogenic pathways (Chiasson *et al.*, 1975). In the postabsorptive state, glucagon-mediated gluconeogenesis (Jennings *et al.*, 1977) accounts for approximately one third of the basal glucose production (Cherrington *et al.*, 1976). The gluconeogenic potential of glucagon is markedly enhanced by insulin deficiency and reduced by insulin, evidence of the importance of the relative concentrations of insulin and glucagon in the regulation of basal hepatic gluconeogenesis. An elevation of glucagon levels without a concomitant change in insulin stimulates gluconeogenesis (Bomboy *et al.*, 1977; Liljenquist *et al.*, 1977). The high glucagon and low insulin levels in the plasma of suckling lambs, humans, and rats (Beaudry *et al.*, 1977) (probably a result of the high-protein, high-fat, low-carbohydrate milk diet) are associated with increased gluconeogenesis, which prevents hypoglycemia in the early neonatal period.

8.6. Control of Glucagon Secretion

8.6.1. Control by Nutrients

8.6.1.1. Glucose

Hyperglycemia reduces glucagon secretion and abolishes or reduces the glucagon responses to various stimuli such as protein (Müller *et al.*, 1970) and exercise (Böttger *et al.*, 1972a). The mechanism by which glucose blocks glucagon secretion is unknown. It has been proposed that the A cell contains a stereospecific glucoreceptor responsible for the inhibition of glucagon secretion by glucose (Matschinsky *et al.*, 1975; Grodsky *et al.*, 1975). Others have proposed that glucose suppresses glucagon secretion through enhanced glucose entry, which is believed to be an insulin-requiring process (Unger and Lefebvre, 1972). Leclercq-Meyer *et al.* (1977) observed that metabolic intermediates, including fumarate, glutamate, and pyruvate, stimulated glucagon release at low glucose concentrations; this argues against the view that glucose-induced suppression of A-cell secretion is due to an increase in an energy-providing substrate, as do the observations of comparable ATP content of islets from diabetics rats with and without insulin treatment (Matschinsky *et al.*, 1976).

The possible role of a glucose-stimulated increase in insulin in the mediation of the A-cell response to hyperglycemia was first suggested by Samols *et al.* (1972), who demonstrated its ability to suppress glucagon. Insulin suppresses glucagon release from the isolated islets of streptozotocin-diabetic rats (Buchanan and Mawhinney, 1973), and in humans a quantitative relationship between the glucose-stimulated insulin response and glucagon suppression was demonstrated (Hatfield *et al.*, 1977). However, Pagliara *et al.* (1975) were unable to suppress aminogenic glucagon secretion with insulin in perfused pancreases of streptozotocin-diabetic rats, and proposed that glucose-induced changes in glucagon secretion are independent of insulin.

The relative hyperglucagonemia seen during insulin deprivation in juvenile diabetics can be restored to normal by insulin (Braaten *et al.*, 1973; Gerich *et al.*, 1975a; Raskin *et al.*, 1975, 1976; Sperling *et al.*, 1977; Seino *et al.*, 1977). In addition to a loss of hyperglycemia-induced suppression of glucagon, juvenile-type diabetics may fail to respond to hypoglycemia, a potent stimulus for glucagon secretion in nondiabetics (Gerich *et al.*, 1973; Maher *et al.*, 1977; Benson *et al.*, 1977).

8.6.1.2. Amino Acids

The release of glucagon in response to ingested protein (Müller *et al.*, 1971) and infused amino acids (Assan *et al.*, 1967; Ohneda *et al.*, 1968; Rocha *et al.*, 1972) serves to prevent hypoglycemia secondary to aminogenic insulin secretion (Unger *et al.*, 1969; Cherrington and Vranic, 1971; Wahren *et al.*, 1976). The mechanism of this stimulatory effect is not clear, but it appears to occur with nonmetabolizable amino acids (Assan *et al.*, 1977), suggesting a receptor mechanism.

8.6.1.3. Free Fatty Acids

Elevated plasma FFA suppress plasma IRG levels (Madison *et al.*, 1968; Luyckx and Lefebvre, 1970; Gerich *et al.*, 1976a). When plasma FFA are reduced by nicotinic acid, plasma IRG levels rise (Lefebvre, 1972), a response that is markedly inhibited by exogenous replacement of the FFA (Luyckx and Lefebvre, 1976) or glucose (Quabbe *et al.*, 1977). Inasmuch as glucagon can stimulate lipolysis *in vivo* at physiologic doses (Schade and Eaton, 1977), the feedback relationships between glucagon and FFA levels may be physiologically relevant (Lefebvre, 1972).

8.6.2. Influence of Hormones

8.6.2.1. Gastrointestinal Hormones

Gastrin (Unger *et al.*, 1967), pancreozymin-cholecystokinin (Unger *et al.*, 1967; Frame *et al.*, 1975), gastric inhibitory polypeptide (GIP) (Rabinovitch and Dupre, 1974), and vasoactive intestinal polypeptide (VIP) (Schebalin *et al.*, 1977; Kaneto *et al.*, 1977; Ohneda *et al.*, 1977) have been identified as glucagon secretagogues, and secretin is a weak inhibitor (Santeusanio *et al.*, 1972; Ipp *et al.*, 1977b). Those hormones released during the absorption of nutrients from the gut may serve to prime islet cell secretion for an incoming nutrient load (Unger and Eisentraut, 1967).

8.6.2.2. Neurotensin and Substance P

The hyperglycemic effect of neurotensin (Carraway *et al.*, 1976; Brown and Vale, 1976; Ukai *et al.*, 1977) is associated with low insulin and high glucagon levels (Carraway *et al.*, 1976; Ishida *et al.*, 1976), and is believed to be glucagon-dependent (Ukai *et al.*, 1977). Similar changes in glucagon secretion were observed in the isolated canine pancreas during perfusion of neurotensin and substance P, indicating a direct effect on the pancreas (Patton *et al.*, 1976a).

8.6.2.3. Bombesin

Bombesin, a tetradecapeptide originally isolated from frog skin (Anastasi *et al.*, 1971) and found in mammalian intestine (Erspamer and Melchiorri, 1975) and brain (Brown *et al.*, 1977), produces hyperglycemia (Brown *et al.*, 1977) and an increase in glucagon secretion (Fallucca *et al.*, 1977; Brown *et al.*, 1977; Gambardella *et al.*, 1977). It is more effective in producing hyperglycemia when administered intracisternally than intravenously (Brown *et al.*, 1977), suggesting that its actions are mediated via the central nervous system, possibly through catecholamine-induced changes of glucagon secretion.

8.6.2.4. Other Factors

Finally, the recent discovery in the islets of other peptides such as GIP (Smith *et al.*, 1977), gastrin (Erlandsen *et al.*, 1976), VIP (Said and Rosenberg, 1976; Buffa *et al.*, 1977), thyrotropin-releasing hormone (Morley *et al.*, 1978), and glucagonlike immunoreactivity (GLI) (Moody *et al.*, 1976) in nerve endings of the pancreas within certain islet cells may prove to be of functional significance. Ipp *et al.* (1978) reported that endogenous opioids may alter the secretion of islet cell hormones, including glucagon.

8.6.3. Neural Control

8.6.3.1. Hypothalamic Influences

Electrical stimulation of the ventromedial hypothalamus enhances glucagon secretion and inhibits insulin secretion (Frohman and Bernardis, 1971), changes that may be mediated via the autonomic nervous system (Woods and Porte, 1974). Stimulation of the sympathetic nerves (Marliss *et al.*, 1973) and infusion of catecholamines similarly affect A-cell (Iversen, 1973) and B-cell function (Porte *et al.*, 1975). The hypothalamus contains other substances capable of influencing insulin and glucagon release from isolated islets (Moltz *et al.*, 1977) and *in vivo* (Brown and Vale, 1976; Alberti *et al.*, 1973; Koerker *et al.*, 1974). Whether these substances are released into the circulation or serve as neurotransmitters is not clear.

8.6.3.2. Adrenergic Stimulation—Stress and Exercise

Glucose homeostasis during stress and exercise appears, in large part, to be the consequence of a simultaneous rise in glucagon and decline in insulin. β-Adrenergic blockade does not diminish the glucagon response in prolonged exercise (Galbo *et al.*, 1977).

8.6.3.3. Dopaminergic Influence

The administration of a catecholamine precursor, L-dopa, increases plasma glucose, insulin, and glucagon levels in normal man (Rayfield *et al.*, 1975; Leblanc *et al.*, 1977; Lorenzi *et al.*, 1977), perhaps through conversion of L-dopa to dopamine and the stimulation of dopaminergic receptors in the hypothalamus or in the A and B cells of the pancreas. However, apomorphine, a reported stimulator of postsynaptic dopamine receptors, fails to affect glucagon secretion in normal subjects and in insulin-deprived diabetics (Lorenzi *et al.*, 1977).

8.6.3.4. Serotonin

Serotonin was reported to have an inhibitory action on A-cell secretion in humans (Marco *et al.*, 1976), and the serotonin precursor 5-hydroxytryptophan decreases arginine-stimulated glucagon release in isolated islets (Marco *et al.*, 1977a). These observations provide support for possible serotonergic control of basal and stimulated glucagon release.

8.7. Glucagonlike Immunoreactivity (Enteroglucagon)

"Glucagonlike immunoreactivity" (GLI) or "enteroglucagon" are terms used to refer to a group of polypeptides present throughout the postduodenal small intestine (Unger *et al.*, 1961, 1966, 1968; Samols *et al.*,

1965; Valverde *et al.*, 1968), stomach, and colon (Frame, 1976, 1977) that cross-react with antiglucagon sera directed against the N-terminus of the hormone but not with C-terminally directed antisera (Heding *et al.*, 1976). GLI was identified by immunocytochemical technics in "EG" (for entero-glucagon) cells of the gut (Pelletier *et al.*, 1975), the "A-like" cells first described by Orci *et al.* (1968). GLI levels in plasma rise during the absorption of glucose (Samols *et al.*, 1965; Unger *et al.*, 1968) and other monosaccharides (Marco *et al.*, 1971), fat and protein (Böttger *et al.*, 1973), and various cations (Böttger *et al.*, 1972b), but its physiologic role is unknown.

The GLIs of crude gut extracts constitute a heterogeneous family of polypeptides ranging from 2900 to 12,000 in molecular weight. The only GLI thus far purified and partially characterized is a 12,000-molecular-weight moiety called "GLI-1" or "glicentin" (Sundby *et al.*, 1976; Jacobsen *et al.*, 1977). GLI-1 contains an immunodeterminant similar to that of the glucagon N-terminal 2–23 amino acid residue plus a C-terminal sequence that may be identical to the 8-amino-acid residue fragment of progluca-gon described by Tager and Steiner (1973). It was proposed (Jacobsen *et al.*, 1977) that GLI-1 may contain the full sequence of glucagon but that it does not react with C-terminally directed antiglucagon sera because of structural masking of the C-terminal immunodeterminant by the proglu-cagon sequence. Using antibodies against "GLI-1," specific immunofluo-rescence for GLI-1 was observed in glucagon-containing pancreatic A_2 cells of the pancreas (Moody *et al.*, 1976), raising the possibility that the GLI-1 molecule may be a precursor of both glucagon and smaller GLI moieties (Moody *et al.*, 1976). GLI was also reported to be present in pancreatic extracts and commercial preparations of glucagon (Srikant and Unger, 1976). If, in fact, glucagon and the smaller GLI moieties are both derived from a common precursor containing both the N-terminal and C-terminal sequences of glucagon, perhaps the A_2 cells of the pancreas and the EG cells of the small intestine differ only with respect to the enzymes required to produce their respective secretory products.

The biological activities of GLI-containing extracts are qualitatively similar to those of glucagon (Table II). There is a "true," or "pancreatic type," glucagon in the gut, as well as the small molecular form of GLI (Valverde *et al.*, 1968), and they both bind to liver cell membranes and activate cyclase (Sasaki *et al.*, 1975a; Srikant *et al.*, 1976; Holst *et al.*, 1977), and both exhibit glycogenolytic activity, although the activity of GLI is less than that of glucagon. It has been suggested that GLI, like glucagon, inhibits gastrointestinal motility (Rehfeld *et al.*, 1973), in which case the postprandial hypersecretion of GLI observed in gastrectomized patients (Marco *et al.*, 1977b; D'sa and Buchanan, 1977), in patients with dumping syndrome (Bloom *et al.*, 1972), and in patients with jejunoileal bypass

Table II. Comparison of Pancreatic Glucagon, Gastrointestinal
Glucagon, and Glucagonlike Immunoreactivity

Property	Pancreatic glucagon	GI glucagon	GLI
Molecular weight	3485	≈ 3500	≈ 2900
Isoelectric point	6.2	6.2	10
Immunoreactive ratio of 78J/30K[a]	1.0	0.9	61
Glycogenolytic activity (% of 10 ng glucagon)	100	100	50
70% of maximum adenylate cyclase stimulation	10^{-8} M	10^{-8} M	10^{-7} M
Affinity for rat liver membranes	4×10^{-9}	3×10^{-9}	5×10^{-8}

[a]Ratio of values obtained by measuring with antiserum 78J, which reacts with the 3–23 residues of glucagon thought to be contained in the GLI molecule, and 30K, which reacts with 24–29 residues of glucagon, which are presumed to be absent or inaccessible in the GLI molecule.

surgery (Barry *et al.*, 1977) might represent a compensatory attempt to slow gastrointestinal activity.

8.8. Somatostatin

8.8.1. Distribution in Tissues

8.8.1.1. Central Nervous System

Somatostatin, a 14-amino-acid polypeptide first identified by its ability to inhibit growth hormone (GH) release (Krulich *et al.*, 1968) and later isolated from ovine (Brazeau *et al.*, 1973) and porcine (Schally *et al.*, 1976) hypothalamic extracts, is distributed in the central nervous system, gastrointestinal tract, and pancreas (Vale *et al.*, 1976; Kronheim *et al.*, 1977; Arimura *et al.*, 1975; Patel and Reichlin, 1978).

Somatostatin has been localized immunocytochemically in cells (Elde and Parsons, 1975) and nerve fibers (Pelletier *et al.*, 1977) of the hypothalamus, suggesting a neurosecretory mechanism via the hypothalmo–hypophyseal portal system to the adenohypophysis. The distribution of somatostatin in synaptosomes from medial basal hypothalamus, preoptic areas, and amygdala suggests a possible neurotransmitter role for the peptide (Epelbaum *et al.*, 1977). Studies of brain lesions and hypothalamic deafferentation suggest that most hypothalamic somatostatin originates from neurons in the periventricular region (Epelbaum *et al.*, 1977). The localization of immunoreactive somatostatin in peripheral noradrenergic neurons and nerve fibers of the myenteric (Auerbach's) plexus in the colon (Hökfelt *et al.*, 1977) appears to conflict with Dale's "one neuron, one transmitter" principle (for a review, see Burnstock, 1976).

Numerous reports have confirmed the inhibitory action of somatostatin on GH secretion under a variety of conditions both *in vivo* and *in vitro* (for a review, see Vale *et al.*, 1977). That the administration of antisomatostatin antibodies to rats increases basal GH levels and prevents stress-induced GH suppression is evidence of somatostatin's physiologic importance in regulation of GH secretion (Arimura *et al.*, 1976; Ferland *et al.*, 1976; Terry *et al.*, 1976). Antisomatostatin serum enhances cold-induced thyrotropin (TSH) release (Arimura *et al.*, 1976; Ferland *et al.*, 1976) and inhibits stress-induced suppression of TSH secretion, suggesting a possible role in regulation of TSH secretion (Arimura *et al.*, 1976).

8.8.1.2. Gastrointestinal Tract

Gastrointestinal D cells are found in highest concentration in the gastric antrum closely associated with gastrin-producing cells, and in lesser concentration in fundic mucosa with a pattern of distribution resembling that of glucagon-producing A cells (Helmsteadter *et al.*, 1977; Fritsch *et al.*, 1978). This pattern of D-cell distribution may make it possible for somatostatin to exert local effects on certain gastrointestinal functions.

8.8.1.3. Pancreas

Hellman and Lernmark (1969) suggested that the pancreatic D-cell contained a substance that could inhibit insulin release. Several years later, it was reported that pancreatic D cells contained somatostatin (Luft *et al.*, 1974; Dubois, 1975; Orci *et al.*, 1975a). The location of the D cells between A and B cells of the islets, together with demonstrations by Koerker *et al.* (1974) and by Mortimer *et al.* (1974) that somatostatin lowers plasma insulin and glucagon levels in baboons and humans, and that antisomatostatin serum increases secretion of glucagon (Barden *et al.*, 1977) and insulin (Taniguchi *et al.*, 1977) from isolated islets, raised the possibility that somatostatin may exert direct local control of insulin and glucagon secretion (Orci and Unger, 1975; Unger and Orci, 1977a).

8.8.2. Pancreatic Somatostatin Release

Pancreatic somatostatin release is stimulated by arginine (Patton *et al.*, 1976c), glucose (Schauder *et al.*, 1976; Ipp *et al.*, 1977a; Weir *et al.*,

1977a), leucine, amino acid mixtures, pancreozymin-cholecystokinin, gastrin, GIP, secretin (Ipp *et al.*, 1977b), and cAMP (Barden *et al.*, 1976). Epinephrine (Schauder *et al.*, 1976) and diazoxide (Samols *et al.*, 1977) inhibit somatostatin release. The parallelism between the responses of pancreatic insulin and somatostatin to various secretagogues introduces the possibility that the two islet hormones may have a common function, one perhaps relating to nutrient homeostasis (Unger *et al.*, 1977). Somatostatin in pharmacologic doses inhibits the following gastrointestinal functions: gastrin release (Bloom *et al.*, 1974), gallbladder contraction (Creutzfeldt *et al.*, 1975), gastrin-stimulated HCl secretion (Bloom *et al.*, 1975a), splanchnic blood flow and xylose absorption (Wahren and Felig, 1976), pancreatic exocrine function (Wilson *et al.*, 1977), and cholecystokinin-pancreozymin release (Schmitt *et al.*, 1978). Intraportal infusion of somatostatin at a physiologic rate also reduces the rate of xylose absorption after a xylose meal (Schusdziarra *et al.*, 1977a,b), raising the possibility that it may have a role in regulating the rate at which ingested nutrients enter the circulation. That gastrointestinal hormones stimulate secretion of somatostatin, which, even in physiologic concentrations, may inhibit gastrointestinal functions, raises the possibility of a feedback circuit, a gut–islet–gut axis. This would permit the islets to regulate the entry rate of exogenous nutrients into the circulation and coordinate their influx with insulin-mediated nutrient disposal (Unger *et al.*, 1977), thereby minimizing changes in nutrient concentration during meals.

8.8.3. Mechanism of Action

Specific receptors for somatostatin have been isolated from anterior pituitary gland homogenates (Ogawa *et al.*, 1976), from a clonal strain of rat pituitary tumor cells (Schonbrunn and Tashjian, 1977), and from isolated anterior pituitary secretory granules (Dular and LaBella, 1977). There is present in the cytosol fractions of rat, human, and bovine tissue extracts a soluble somatostatin-binding protein that has a molecular weight of approximately 80,000 (Ogawa *et al.*, 1977), but its function has not been identified.

Somatostatin's effects on the anterior pituitary (Borgeat *et al.*, 1974) and pancreatic islets (Efendic *et al.*, 1975; Claro *et al.*, 1977) may be partially mediated by inhibition of cAMP accumulation. However, somatostatin can also inhibit exogenous cAMP-induced insulin release, indicating an effect of somatostatin at a more distal point (Basabe *et al.*, 1977; Claro *et al.*, 1977). High concentrations of somatostatin inhibit *in vitro* glucagon stimulation of hepatic adenylate cyclase activity (Vinicor *et al.*, 1977), and cAMP-induced hepatic glucose production (Sacks *et al.*, 1977), as well as cAMP-induced cell-free protein synthesis in hepatic ribosomes (Tragl and Kinast, 1977).

Somatostatin's inhibition of glucose-induced insulin secretion can be overcome by increasing the calcium concentration (Curry and Bennett, 1974; Taminato *et al.*, 1975), and by high concentrations of the calcium ionophore A23187 (Fujimoto and Ensinck, 1976; Wollheim *et al.*, 1977a; Basabe *et al.*, 1977), suggesting that somatostatin may act by changing calcium transport. Currently, there are conflicting results on somatostatin's effect on calcium uptake in islets (Wollheim *et al.*, 1977b; Bhathena *et al.*, 1976).

Somatostatin inhibition of both basal and glucose-stimulated insulin secretion (Smith *et al.*, 1976) is prevented by infusion of phentolamine, whereas phentolamine-stimulated glucagon secretion is not blocked by somatostatin (Smith *et al.*, 1977). These results imply that the effects of somatostatin may be regulated by the level of sympathetic nervous system activity.

8.8.4. Abnormalities of Somatostatin

Diminished content of somatostatin (Patel *et al.*, 1976, 1977) and D cells has been observed in obese hyperglycemic mice. Volume density of D cells is increased in juvenile diabetics (Orci *et al.*, 1976b) and in rats following streptozotocin destruction of B cells (Baetens *et al.*, 1976a). A striking decrease in somatostatin concentration and a relative decrease in somatostatin-containing cells are observed in spontaneously diabetic mice (Patel *et al.*, 1977).

Somatostatin-containing D-cell tumors of the endocrine pancreas were first described by Larsson *et al.* (1977) and Ganda *et al.* (1977). In the plasma of both patients, insulin and glucagon levels were low; the patients exhibited mild diabetes with an abnormal glucose tolerance, but without severe endogenous hyperglycemia or ketosis (Unger, 1977).

Achlorhydria and steatorrhea were noted in Larsson's patient, perhaps the result of inhibitory effects of somatostatin on gastric acid (Bloom *et al.*, 1974) and pancreatic enzyme secretion (Creutzfeldt *et al.*, 1975). Both patients had gallbladder disease, conceivably the result of increased stasis caused by somatostatin's inhibitory actions on gallbladder contraction (Creutzfeldt *et al.*, 1975).

Somatostatinoma is difficult to diagnose; however, a combination of steatorrhea, achlorhydria, gallbladder disease, and impaired glucose tolerance may be clues for the presence of a D-cell tumor.

8.8.5. Somatostatin Degradation

The biological half-life of somatostatin as gauged by suppression of GH secretion is 2–4 min (Redding and Coy, 1974). Brain and serum contain peptidases that rapidly inactivate somatostatin (Marks and Stern,

1975; Marks *et al.*, 1976). Marks *et al.* (1976) proposed that the less rapidly degraded D-Trp[8]-somatostatin analogue is more stable in plasma, but that once it reaches its tissue binding site, it can be inactivated by enzymes attacking secondary positions on the moleucle.

8.8.6. Somatostatin Analogues

The short biological half-life and relative broad specificity of somatostatin have limited its usefulness as a therapeutic agent. In an effort to produce a substance that would have a longer duration of activity, a greater biological potency, and differing specificities, numerous analogues of somatostatin have been synthesized. Current interest in the use of somatostatin to inhibit glucagon secretion in diabetes mellitus initiated a search for an analogue with selective A-cell inhibitory specificity. The cyclic configuration of somatostatin is necessary for full biological activity (Rivier *et al.*, 1975). Somatostatin analogues that do not contain cysteine but contain carbon–carbon bonds between residues 3 and 14, thereby forming a cyclic peptide, suppress GH, but not insulin and glucagon (Grant *et al.*, 1976; Garsky *et al.*, 1976; Sarantakis *et al.*, 1976). The substitution of L-tryptophan in position 8 with D-tryptophan yields a molecule 8 times more potent than somatostatin in suppressing insulin, glucagon, and GH secretion (Rivier *et al.*, 1975; Vale *et al.*, 1976; Brown *et al.*, 1976). The analogue des-Asn[5]-D-Trp[8]-somatostatin inhibits insulin but not glucagon secretion (Sarantakis *et al.*, 1976). D-Cys[14]-somatostatin is more effective in suppressing glucagon than insulin secretion (Brown *et al.*, 1976). The double-substituted D-Trp[8]-D-Cys[14]-somatostatin and D-Trp[8]-somatostatin analogues enhance the effectiveness of insulin therapy in the treatment of hyperglycemia in alloxan-diabetic dogs (Schusdziarra *et al.*, 1977a).

8.9. Glucagon in Clinical Medicine

8.9.1. Diabetes Mellitus

8.9.1.1. A-Cell Function in Diabetes

A-cell function is abnormal in diabetes mellitus (Aguilar-Parada *et al.*, 1969; Unger *et al.*, 1970; Müller *et al.*, 1970; Buchanan and McCarroll, 1972). In insulin-deficient patients, relative or absolute hyperglucagonemia is invariably present; striking absolute hyperglucagonemia may be present in ketoacidosis (Assan *et al.*, 1969; Unger *et al.*, 1970; Müller *et al.*, 1973) and in nonketotic, hyperosmolar, hyperglycemic coma (Lindsey *et al.*, 1974). It is presumed to be the consequence not only of increased glucagon secretion, but also of decreased glucagon removal resulting from dehydration with diminished glomerular filtration and renal removal of glucagon (Lefebvre and Luyckx, 1975; Bilbrey *et al.*, 1974). On rehydration and insulin treatment, glucagon levels return to normal (Assan *et al.*, 1969; Müller *et al.*, 1973; Lindsey *et al.*, 1974).

Relatively well controlled diabetic patients, i.e., juvenile-type diabetics receiving maintenance doses of insulin, and adult-onset type diabetics irrespective of therapy, also exhibit abnormalities in A-cell function. These may be separated into two categories: (1) impairment of the A-cell response to steady-state hyperglycemia and to acute change in glucose concentration and (2) an exaggerated A-cell response to stimuli, such as a protein meal or an arginine infusion. The loss of the normal glucose–glucagon relationship is manifested by a relative increase in glucagon levels in patients with fasting hyperglycemia (Unger *et al.*, 1970), and by a failure of glucagon levels to suppress in response to orally or intravenously induced hyperglycemia (Müller *et al.*, 1970; Buchanan and McCarroll, 1972; Heding and Rasmussen, 1972; Gossain *et al.*, 1974; Kurahachi *et al.*, 1977). In the latter study, the glucagon responses of 80 insulin-independent diabetics to an intravenous and oral glucose load were compared with those of 22 normal controls. Whereas nondiabetics suppressed normally following an oral glucose meal, in mild diabetics (mean fasting glucose 110 mg%), suppression was minimal; in moderate diabetics (mean fasting glucose 166 mg%), it was absent; and in severe diabetics (fasting plasma glucose averaging 275 mg%), a paradoxical rise was observed. The index of glucagon suppression per rise of blood glucose ($-\Sigma\Delta IRG/\Sigma\Delta BS$) was approximately 2 in normal subjects and only 0.11 or less in the diabetics. It is accurate to state that in all forms of overt diabetes, the A cell is autonomous of glycemic control, either because of a defect in glucose sensing or in the glucagon response, or both.

The second abnormality in A-cell function, hyperresponsiveness to stimulation, is manifested by an exaggerated rise in plasma glucagon levels in response to arginine (Aguilar-Parada *et al.*, 1969; Unger *et al.*, 1970), alanine (Wise *et al.*, 1973), and protein meals (Müller *et al.*, 1970). In nondiabetics, hyperglycemia completely abolishes the protein-induced rise in glucagon (Müller *et al.*, 1970), whereas in diabetics, the ambient glucose concentration does not influence the magnitude of the glucagon response to a protein meal (Raskin *et al.*, 1978). Thus, in hyperglycemic or normoglycemic diabetics, a carbohydrate-free protein meal may result in a glucagon-mediated increase in glycemia.

8.9.1.2. Effect of Insulin on A-Cell Function in Juvenile-Type Diabetes Mellitus

In juvenile-type diabetics, the infusion of insulin reduces fasting glucagon levels to normal (Raskin *et al.*, 1975; Warne *et al.*, 1977) and corrects the exaggerated response to arginine (Gerich *et al.*, 1975a; Raskin *et al.*, 1976). However, a constant infusion of insulin does not restore the glucose–glucagon relationship to normal; in contrast to nondiabetics, when hyperglycemia is induced in juvenile diabetics receiving a constant infusion of insulin, the protein-induced rise in glucagon is not abolished (Raskin *et al.*, 1978). But if the glucose load is accompanied by the constant insulin infusion, plus a supplementary bolus of insulin plus an additional insulin superinfusion, the protein-induced glucagon response is reduced toward normal (Raskin *et al.*, 1978). Similarly, although the abnormal response to orally and intravenously administered glucose is improved by a constant insulin infusion, a sudden rise in insulin levels produced by a bolus of insulin may be required to simulate the normal suppression of glucagon during the hyperglycemia (Sperling *et al.*, 1977; Aydin *et al.*, 1977; Yamamoto *et al.*, 1979).

On the basis of these findings, it has been concluded that in juvenile diabetics, the abnormal IRG response to protein is the simple consequence of insulin lack. However, the loss of the normal glucose–glucagon relationships may be a consequence of the loss of a normal glucose–insulin relationship; i.e., the normal IRG response to glucose may require a relatively normal glucose-induced insulin response (Unger and Orci, 1977b). The possibility that a rise in insulin is the signal, or one of several signals, that determines its response to hyperglycemia is based on the concepts of Samols *et al.* (1972) and supported by the studies of Weir *et al.* (1976), Laurent and Mialhe (1976), and Hatfield *et al.* (1977); the latter group observed a significant relationship between glucagon suppression by glucose and the pancreatic B-cell response to glucose in normal and in mild diabetics with varying degrees of B-cell function. However, in a sense, the *in vitro* studies of Pagliara *et al.* (1975) and Matschinsky *et al.* (1976) suggest otherwise.

8.9.1.3. Effect of Insulin in Adult-Onset Diabetics

Adult-onset diabetics exhibit the same abnormalities in A-cell function as juvenile-type diabetics, i.e., loss of the normal glucose–glucagon relationship and hyperresponsiveness of glucagon to arginine and protein meals (Unger *et al.*, 1970; Müller *et al.*, 1970). As in juvenile-type diabetics, fasting glucagon levels of adult-onset diabetics are reduced by a constant infusion of insulin (Raskin *et al.*, 1975). However, in contrast to juvenile-type diabetics, neither their exaggerated response of glucagon to aminogenic stimulation nor the loss of the glucose–glucagon relationship can be restored by exogenous insulin, even when constant-dose insulin infusion is supplemented by a bolus and superinfusion at a rate that produces superphysiologic increments in plasma insulin (Aydin *et al.*, 1977; Raskin *et al.*, 1976; Yamamoto *et al.*, 1979; Unger *et al.*, 1978). The ineffectiveness of insulin in restoring A-cell function to normal in this form of diabetes may reflect the fact that insulin *is* present in the islets of such patients (Unger and Orci, 1977c). If the islets of human adult-onset diabetics resemble those of ob/ob mice, with which they share such abnormalities as hyperglycemia, obesity, and relative hyperinsulinemia, one might predict a deficiency of somatostatin-containing D cells (Patel *et al.*, 1976). Glucose (Ipp *et al.*, 1977c; Schauder *et al.*, 1976; Weir *et al.*, 1977a), amino acids (Patton *et al.*, 1977; Ipp *et al.*, 1977c), and gastrointestinal hormones (Ipp *et al.*, 1977b) stimulate the secretion of pancreatic somatostatin, a powerful inhibitor of glucagon secretion by the adjacent A cells, raising the possibility, as yet unproved, that an inadequate somatostatin response during glucose loading contributes to the abnormal glucagon responses; i.e., in the normal islet, both somatostatin and insulin are involved in restraining glucagon release (Unger and Orci, 1977a).

8.9.1.4. Pathophysiologic Importance of Glucagon in Insulin Deficiency

It was recently proposed (Unger and Orci, 1975; Dobbs *et al.*, 1975) that complete expression of the metabolic syndrome of diabetes mellitus requires, in addition to diminished insulin secretion or effectiveness or both, the presence of a relative or absolute excess of glucagon. According to this concept, deficiency of insulin or of its action is the *sine qua non* of diabetes, without which few of the metabolic aberrations of the diabetic state can occur, but in the absence of glucagon, it was proposed, the insulin abnormality leads only to decreased utilization of glucose, increased lipolysis, and increased mobilization of amino acids from muscle, with little, if any, hepatic overproduction of glucose or ketones. The evidence in support of this concept has been extensively reviewed (Unger and Orci, 1977b,c; Unger *et al.*, 1978) and is based on the work of many groups (Gerich *et al.*, 1975a; 1976b; Sakurai *et al.*, 1975; Sherwin *et al.*, 1977a) demonstrating that when glucagon levels are suppressed by somatostatin, insulin deficiency generates neither the marked endogenous hyperglycemia nor the ketoacidosis that would otherwise occur. More recently, elegant studies by Cherrington *et al.* (1978) and Keller *et al.* (1977) provided evidence of glucagon's role in hepatic glucose and ketone production in insulin deficiency and of the fact that when both glucagon and insulin are deficient, overproduction of these fuels does not occur. The studies of McGarry et al. (1975a,b, 1977) elucidated the mechanism of ketogenesis and delineated glucagon's essential role in this process (see Section 8.5.1.5.).

The two recently described patients with chronic hypersomatostatinemia resulting from somatostatin-producing tumors of pancreatic D cells (Larsson et al., 1977; Ganda et al., 1977) may represent a model of chronic hypoinsulinemia and hypoglucagonemia (Unger, 1977). Despite their hypoinsulinemia, neither of these patients had clinical evidence of marked overproduction of glucose and neither developed ketoacidosis. A similarly benign diabetic syndrome occurs in the Houssay preparation, another example of combined insulin and glucagon deficiency (Nakabayashi et al., 1978).

8.9.1.5. Controversy Concerning the Importance of Glucagon in Diabetes Mellitus

It was reported that late hyperglycemia appeared during the infusion of somatostatin for 5 hr in nondiabetic subjects (Sherwin et al., 1977b), and that in maturity-onset diabetics (Tamborlane et al., 1977) both hyperglycemia and hyperketonemia occurred despite ongoing suppression of glucagon. However, the "hyperglycemia" and "hyperketonemia" in these studies was trivial; in the maturity-onset diabetics, for example, glucose rose only 10 mg% and $\beta\text{-}OH$-butyrate less than 0.3 mmol. The studies can therefore be employed as evidence that hypoinsulinemia does *not* give rise either to severe hyperglycemia or to severe hyperketonemia when glucagon is suppressed.

Additionally, it was reported that glucagon replacement in normal subjects during suppression of both insulin and glucagon by means of somatostatin infusion did not substantially increase glycemia, glucose production, or ketone levels (Sherwin et al., 1977b). Yet in similar studies, others (Cherrington et al., 1976, 1978; Keller et al., 1977) demonstrated that glucagon causes a sustained increase in hyperglycemia and ketone production. The apparent conflict in results may be the consequence of important differences in experimental design. The study of Sherwin and co-workers was carried out in humans, and glucagon was necessarily infused via a peripheral vein, thereby depriving the liver, its major target organ, of full access to the infused glucagon and reducing the magnitude of its hepatic effects relative to the rise in the concentration of glucagon in the peripheral circulation (Holst et al., 1977). In the important studies of Cherrington et al. (1976, 1978), glucagon was infused at a similar rate but via the physiologic portal venous route, thereby exposing the liver to 100% of the administered hormone; hepatic glucose production increased and hyperglycemia in excess of 250 mg% was observed without a rise in plasma glucagon levels above their preexperimental basal values. And when neither insulin nor glucagon were replaced, i.e., when a bihormonal deficiency was produced, hepatic glucose production did not rise, suggesting that the presence of glucagon is required to mediate the increase in hepatic glucose production that occurs in the insulin-deficient state. Another extremely important observation in the Cherrington study was that although the glucagon-mediated increase in hepatic glucose production returned toward preexperimental basal levels after the first hour, its hyperglycemic actions persisted considerably longer, obviously because of diminished glucose utilization resulting from the insulin deficiency. This observation demonstrates that relatively short-lived increments of hepatic glucose production may result in a persistent endogenous hyperglycemia. These issues were reviewed in greater detail by Unger *et al.* (1978).

The most powerful evidence against glucagon's essentiality in mediating the severe endogenous hyperglycemia and enhanced ketogenesis of the insulin-deficient state is based on the studies of Barnes and co-workers in totally depancreatized patients (Barnes and Bloom, 1976; Barnes *et al.*, 1977). Using a specific immunoabsorbent to "strip" glucagon from the serum of their patients, they added "glucagon-free" plasma to the glucagon standards used to make up the standard curves of their radioimmunoassay; this maneuver was designed to exclude materials other than true pancreatic glucagon from measurement (Alford *et al.*, 1977). By this technique, glucagon levels in totally depancreatized human subjects were found to be zero (Barnes and Bloom, 1976; Barnes *et al.*, 1977). They compared the effects of insulin withdrawal in four totally depancreatized patients with those in six juvenile-type diabetics (Barnes *et al.*, 1977). In the latter group, plasma glucagon rose promptly, and within 12 hr after insulin withdrawal, β-hydroxybutyrate and glucose had increased by more than 3.0 mmol/liter and 200 mg%, respectively, whereas in the totally depancreatized patients, glucagon levels remained at unmeasurable levels throughout and yet β-hydroxybutyrate rose by almost 1.0 mmol/liter and glucose by 124 mg%. In the "aglucagonemic" depancreatized group, the increase in glucose and ketones was considerably less than in the hyperglucagonemic juvenile diabetics, evidence that glucagon *did* play a role in the differences; yet ketones and glucose *did* rise following insulin withdrawal despite the total absence of assayable glucagon. It was therefore concluded that glucagon is *not* essential for these metabolic changes, which could have been the direct consequence of insulin lack.

While this conclusion is certainly tenable, alternative interpretations may also be considered. First, in all other studies of totally depancreatized patients, in which glucagon was assayed by conventional techniques, circulating immunoreactivity was detected (Müller *et al.*, 1974; Palmer *et al.*, 1976; Miyata *et al.*, 1976), and the assumption that all this residual IRG (see Section 8.2.2) is biologically inactive is not necessarily warranted; other glycogenolytic substances, such as GLI (enteroglucagon) cross-react with the glucagon receptor and increase hepatic adenylate cyclase activity (Sasaki et al., 1975b), and withdrawal of insulin would be expected to enhance their biological activity, perhaps by increasing glucagon-binding sites (Soman and Felig, 1977). The failure of hepatic glucose production to rise in combined insulin–glucagon deficiency (Cherrington et al., 1978) (cf. Section 8.5.2.2) raises the possibility that the increase of glycogenolysis in depancreatized humans with a deficiency of "true glucagon" was not the result of insulin lack by itself, but rather was caused by other glycogenolytic factors unopposed by insulin action.

8.9.1.6. Controversy Concerning the Role of Glucagon in the Presence of Insulin

Of far more practical importance than the role of glucagon in the absence of insulin is its role in the presence of insulin, i.e., in insulin-secreting maturity-onset diabetics and insulin-treated juvenile-onset diabetics. The studies of Sherwin et al. (1976, 1977b) have been interpreted as demonstrating that while glucagon may be biologically active in the complete absence of insulin, it is devoid of hyperglycemic activity in insulin-treated juvenile-type diabetics and in maturity-onset diabetics in whom endogenous insulin is present. Their conclusions were supported by more recent studies of Holst et al. (1977) and Clarke et al. (1978). Yet, a more recent study showed that in juvenile-type diabetics and in an adult-type diabetic, the infusion of glucagon for 24 hr at a rate identical to that employed by Sherwin et al. (1976) increases hyperglycemia and induces massive glycosuria (Fig. 1) and ketonuria and a significant increase in urea nitrogen excretion (Table III) despite the continued intravenous infusion of insulin at a rate that, without the glucagon infusion, had maintained normal fasting plasma glucose levels (Raskin and Unger, 1977). A rise in endogenous glucagon has a similar effect; in juvenile-type and adult-onset type diabetics rendered normoglycemic by a constant overnight infusion of insulin, the ingestion of a carbohydrate-free protein meal elicited a 50 mg% increase in plasma glucose levels in concert with the protein-induced increase in endogenous glucagon levels (Raskin et al., 1978), findings that may have therapeutic implications with respect to the clinical management of hyperglycemia.

8.9.1.7. Mechanism of Somatostatin-Induced Amelioration of Diabetic Hyperglycemia

Originally, the amelioration of diabetic hyperglycemia by constant intravenous infusion of somatostatin (Gerich et al., 1975b) was attributed

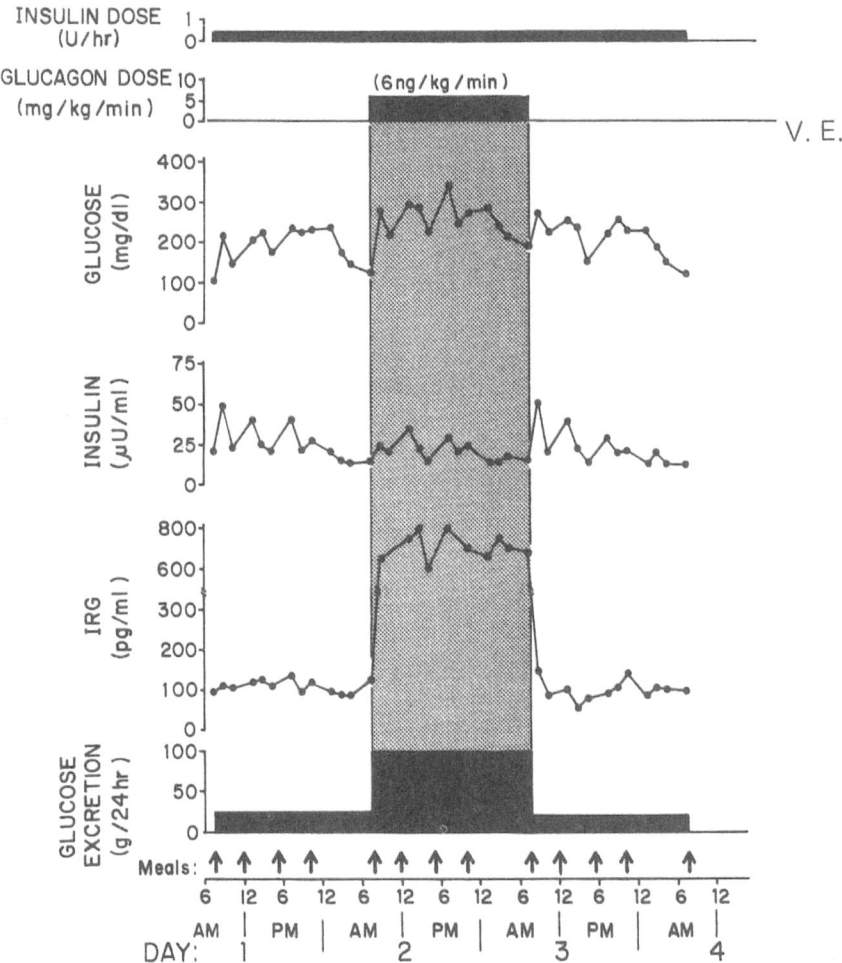

Fig. 1. Effect of intravenous administration of glucagon in a dose of 6 ng/kg per min on the plasma glucose, insulin, and IRG concentration and on 24-hr glucose excretion in a 50-year-old adult-onset diabetic woman. A total dose of 6 U/day of insulin was administered intravenously at a rate of 0.25 U/hr. Reprinted from Raskin and Unger (1977) with the permission of *Diabetes.*

solely to its glucagon-lowering actions. However, Wahren and Felig (1976) demonstrated that somatostatin can reduce the absorption of glucose and xylose, and proposed that much of the amelioration of diabetic hypertriglyceridemia is the consequence of reduced influx from the gut, rather than of inhibition of glucagon-mediated hepatic glucose production. While the gastrointestinal effects of somatostatin are probably important, more recent evidence suggests that the glucose-lowering effects of soma-

Table III. 24-Hour Urinary Glucose, Urea Nitrogen, and Ketone Excretion before, during, and after Intravenous Administration of Glucagon to Diabetics at a Rate of 6 ng/kg per min (Study A) or 3 ng/kg per min (Study B)

Patient	Before Glucose (g/24 hr)	Before Control day urea nitrogen (g/24 hr)	Before Ketones (μmol/24 hr)	During Glucose (g/24 hr)	During Glucagon day urea nitrogen (g/24 hr)	During Ketones (μmol/24 hr)	After Glucose (g/24 hr)	After Control day urea nitrogen (g/24 hr)	After Ketones (μmol/24 hr)
				Study A					
C.P.	44	5.4	340	158	9.2	690	33	5.7	320
D.B.	5	9.6	553	188	15.4	2445	21	10.7	1286
P.T.	69	4.3	296	163	7.6	3265	51	4.7	753
V.E.	26	8.9	738	99	14.7	1331	19	12.2	609
MEAN	36 ± 14	7.0 ± 1	482 ± 102	152 ± 19^a	11.7 ± 2^a	1933 ± 573^a	31 ± 7^a	8.3 ± 2^a	742 ± 202^a
				Study B					
C.P.	5	5.6	307	18	9.1	708	6	5.5	346
D.B.	3	10.2	936	59	13.7	1308	16	9.8	867
P.T.	44	10.2	506	168	12.6	3248	36	5.7	616
MEAN	17 ± 13	8.7 ± 1.5	583 ± 186	82 ± 45	11.8 ± 1.4	1755 ± 766	19 ± 9	7.0 ± 1.4	550 ± 104

[a] $p < 0.05$ vs. preceding day.

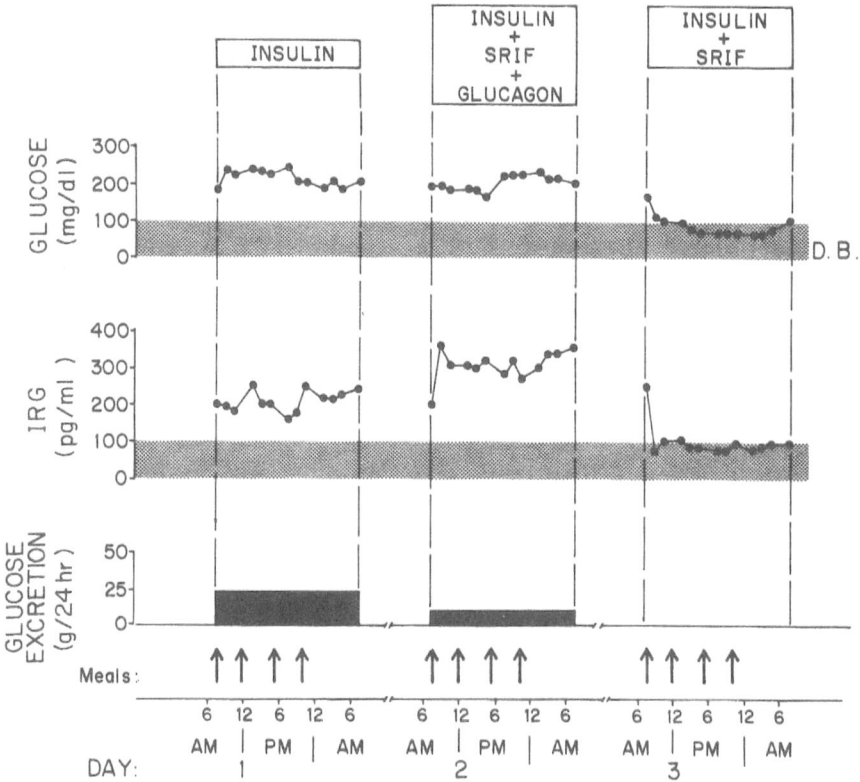

Fig. 2. Comparison of plasma glucose and glucagon profiles in a juvenile-type diabetic during constant insulin infusion, constant infusion of somatostatin (SRIF) and glucagon, and insulin plus somatostatin without glucagon. Hyperglycemia and glycosuria are absent when hyperglucagonemia is reduced.

tostatin in juvenile-type diabetics also occur on diets that are virtually free of carbohydrate, and thereby eliminate glucose absorption as a significant variable; moreover, in these studies, superinfusion of glucagon during somatostatin-induced suppression of endogenous glucagon was accompanied by sustained hyperglycemia, glycosuria, and ketonuria, despite continuing somatostatin infusion (Fig. 2) (Unger and Raskin, 1978). At present, it would seem that somatostatin improves diabetic hyperglycemia by reducing the entry into the circulation of both ingested glucose and endogenously produced glucose.

8.9.2. Glucagonoma

Becker *et al.* (1942) reported what was probably the first described case of glucagonoma syndrome in a patient with pancreatic neoplasm containing islet cell features. The patient exhibited an abnormal glucose tolerance test, anemia, and necrolytic dermatitis. The characteristics of glucagonoma syndrome are currently recognized to include elevated plasma glucagon (McGavran *et al.*, 1966), a dermatitis described as "migratory necrolytic erythemia" (Church and Crane, 1967; Binnick, 1977), frank diabetes or an abnormal glucose tolerance test, weight loss, anemia, and occasionally hypocholesterolemia (Mallinson *et al.*, 1974). These symptoms usually improve or disappear following chemotherapy or tumor removal (Boden and Owen, 1977; Danforth *et al.*, 1976).

Glucagon secretion from A-cell tumors in response to secretagogues such as arginine is greater than normal (Boden and Owen, 1977; Weir *et al.*, 1977b) and may respond paradoxically to agents such as tolbutamide and oral glucose (Boden and Owen, 1977).

The glucagonoma syndrome has been well characterized clinically (McGavran *et al.*, 1966; Mallinson *et al.*, 1974; Recant *et al.*, 1976), and it is now well established that in addition to an increase in 3500-molecular-weight IRG, 9000-molecular-weight IRG may also be increased (Valverde *et al.*, 1976; Danforth *et al.*, 1976; Recant *et al.*, 1976; Weir *et al.*, 1977b; Boden and Owen, 1977; for a review of various immunoreactive glucagon fractions see Jaspan and Rubenstein, 1977). Studies of the kinship of a patient with glucagonoma (Boden and Owen, 1977) revealed high levels of whole plasma IRG in some of the members; the increased levels were due not only to increased IRG[9000] but also to increased BPG in some instances, although in the glucagonoma patient, BPG levels were normal.

8.9.3. Nondiabetic Hyperglucagonemia

BPG appeared to be the main IRG component in a family with apparent hyperglucagonemia transmitted as an autosomal dominant characteristic (Ensinck and Palmer, 1976; Palmer *et al.*, 1978). None of the family members had diabetes mellitus or any disorders that might be related to this abnormality. Boden and Owen (1977) described a hereditary form of hyperglucagonemia in the family of a patient with glucagonoma syndrome in which over 85% of the plasma IRG of four unaffected relatives had a molecular weight of at least 30,000 daltons. A patient with agammaglobulinemia was found to have no measurable IRG of molecular size close to IgG, indicating that some immunoglobulins may be a component of BPG or may bind in a competitive manner to glucagon antisera (Von Schenck, 1977).

In renal insufficiency (Kuku *et al.*, 1976; Emmanouel *et al.*, 1976; Valverde *et al.*, 1976), both IRG[9000] and true glucagon levels are high (for a review, see Jaspan and Rubenstein, 1977). In portocaval shunts (Bilheimer *et al.*, 1975) and cirrhotics, high plasma IRG levels are present.

8.9.4. Glucagon Deficiency

The first fully described case of glucagon deficiency was reported by Vidnes and Oyasaeter (1977). The patient was a 3-month-old Pakistani infant with closely related parents both of whom exhibited subnormal aminogenic glucagon responses; moreover, two siblings were thought to have died from hypoglycemia, suggesting an autosomal recessive disorder. Severe persistent hypoglycemia without hyperinsulinemia but with a high insulin/glucagon ratio was present. Treatment with glucagon resulted in striking improvement and a return of glucose levels to normal.

ACKNOWLEDGMENTS

This work was supported by Veterans Administration Institutional Research Support Grant 549-8000-01; National Institutes of Health Grants AM 02700-16, 1-RO1-AM 18179, and 1-MO1-RR 00633; National Institutes of Health Contract NO1-AM-62219; Pfizer Laboratories, New York; Bristol Myers Company, New York; Dr. Karl Thomae GmbH, Germany; Merck, Sharpe and Dohme, Rahway, New Jersey; CIBA-Geigy Corporation, Summit, New Jersey; The Upjohn Company, Kalamazoo, Michigan; Eli Lilly, Indianapolis, Indiana; and the Salk Institute–Texas Research Foundation.

References

Aguilar-Parada, E., Eisentraut, A. M., and Unger, R. H., 1969, Pancreatic glucagon secretion in normal and diabetic subjects, *Am. J. Med. Sci.* **257**:415–419.

Alberti, K. G. M. M., Christensen, N. J., Christensen, S. E., Hansen, A. P., Iversen, J., Lundbaek, K., Seyer-Hansen, K., and Orskov, H., 1973, Inhibition of insulin secretion by somatostatin, *Lancet* **2**:1299–1301.

Alford, F. P., Bloom, S. R., and Nabarro, J. D. N., 1977, Glucagon levels in normal and diabetic subjects: Use of a specific immunoabsorbent for glucagon radioimmunoassay, *Diabetologia* **13**:1–6.

Anastasi, A., Erspamer, V., and Bucci, M., 1971, Isolation and structure of bombesin and alytesin, two analogous actine peptides from the skin of the European amphibians, *Bombina* and *Alytes, Experientia* **27**:166–167.

Arimura, A., Sato, H., Dupont, A., Nishi, N., and Schally, A. V., 1975, Somatostatin: Abundance of immunoreactive hormone in rat stomach and pancreas, *Science* **189**:1007–1009.

Arimura, A., Smith, W. D., and Schally, A. V., 1976, Blockade of the stress-induced decrease in blood GH by antisomatostatin serum in rats, *Endocrinology* **98**:540–543.

Assan, R., and Slusher, N., 1972, Structure/function and structure/immunoreactivity relationships of the glucagon molecule and related synthetic peptides, *Diabetes* **21**:843–855.

Assan, R., Roselin, G., and Dollias, J., 1967, Effets sur la glucagonemia des perfusions et ingestions d'acides amines, in: *Journ. Annu. Diabetol. Hotel*, Vol. 7, pp. 25–41, Medicales Falmmarion, Paris.

Assan, R., Hautecouverture, G., Guillemant, S., Douchy, F., Protin, P., and Derot, M., 1969, Evolution de parametres hormonaux (glucagon, cortisol, hormone somatotrope) et energetiques (glucose, acides gras libre glycerol) dans dix acido-cetoses diabetiques graves traitees, *Pathol. Biol.* **17**:1095–1105.

Assan, R., Attali, J. R., Ballerio, G., Boillot, J., and Girard, J. R., 1977, Glucagon secretion induced by natural and artificial amino acids in the perfused rat pancreas, *Diabetes* **26**:300–307.

Aydin, I., Raskin, P., and Unger, R. H., 1977, The effect of short-term intravenous insulin on the glucagon response to a carbohydrate meal in adult onset and juvenile-type diabetics, *Diabetologia* **13**:629–636.

Baetens, D., Coleman, D. L., and Orci, L., 1976a, Islet cell population in ob/ob and db/db mice, *Diabetes* **25** (Suppl.):344.

Baetens, D., Rufener, C., Srikant, C. B., Dobbs, R., Unger, R., and Orci, L., 1976, Identification of glucagon-producing cells (A-cells) in dog gastric mucosa, *J. Cell Biol.* **69**:455–464.

Ballard, F. J., and Hopgood, M. F., 1973, Phosphopyruvate: Carboxylase induction by L-tryptophan—Effects on synthesis and degradation of the enzyme, *Biochem. J.* **136**:259–264.

Barden, N., Alvarado-Urbina, G., Cote, J., and Dupont, A., 1976, Cyclic AMP-dependent stimulation of somatostatin secretion by isolated rat islets of Langerhans, *Biochem, Biophys, Res. Commun.* **3**:840.

Barden, N., Lavoie, M., Dupont, A., Cote, J., and Cote, J. P., 1977, Stimulation of glucagon release by addition of antisomatostatin serum to islets of Langerhans *in vitro*, *Endocrinology* **101**:635–638.

Barnes, A. J., and Bloom, S. R., 1976, Pancreatectomized man: A model for diabetes without glucagon, *Lancet* **1**:219–221.

Barnes, A. J., Bloom, S. R., Alberti, K. G. M. M., Smythe, P., Alford, F. P., and Chisholm, D. J., 1977, Ketoacidosis in pancreatectomized man, *N. Engl. J. Med.* **296**:1250–1253.

Barry, R. E., Barisch, J., Bray, G. A., Sperling, M. A., Morin, R. J., and Benfield, J., 1977, Intestinal adaptation after jejunoileal bypass in man, *Am. J. Clin. Nutr.* **30**:32–42.

Basabe, J. C., Cresto, J. C., and Aparicio, N., 1977, Studies on the mode of action of somatostatin on insulin secretion, *Endocrinology* **101**:1436–43.

Beaudry, M. A., Chiasson, J. L., and Exton, J. H., 1977, Gluconeogenesis in the suckling rat, *Am. J. Physiol.* **233**(3):E175–180.

Becker, S. W., Kahn, D., and Rothman, S., 1942, Cutaneous manifestation of internal malignant tumors, *Arch. Dermatol. Syphilol.* **45**:1069–1080.

Benson, J. W., Jr., Johnson, D. G., Palmer, J. P., Werner, P. L., and Ensinck, J. W., 1977, Glucagon and catecholamine secretion during hypoglycemia in normal and diabetic man, *J. Clin. Endocrinol. Metab.* **44**:459–464.

Bentle, L. A., and Lardy, H. A., 1977, P-enolpyruvate carboxykinase ferroactivator: Purification and some properties, *J. Biol. Chem.* **252**:1431–1440.

Bhathena, S. J., Perrino, P. V. , Voyles, N. R., Smith, S. S., Wilkins, S. D., Coy, D. H., Schally, A. V., and Recant, L., 1976, Reversal of somatostatin inhibition of insulin and glucagon secretion, *Diabetes* **25**:1031–1040.

Bilbrey, G. L., Faloona, G. R., White, M. C., and Knochel, J. P., 1974, Hyperglucagonemia of renal failure, *J. Clin. Invest.* **53**:841–847.

Bilheimer, D. W., Goldstein, J. L., Grundy, S. M., and Brown, M. S., 1975, Reduction in cholesterol and low density lipoprotein synthesis after portacaval shunt surgery in a patient with homozygous familial hypercholesterolemia, *J. Clin. Invest.* **56**:1420–1430.

Binnick, A. N., 1977, Glucagonoma syndrome: Report of two cases and literature review, *Arch. Dermatol.* **113**(6):749–754.

Blair, J. B., Cook, D. E., and Lardy, H. A., 1973, Influence of glucagon on the metabolism of xylitol and dihydroxyacetone in the isolated perfused rat liver, *J. Biol. Chem.* **248**:3601–3607.

Blazquez, E., Muñoz-Barragan, L., Patton, G. S., Orci, L., Dobbs, R. E., and Unger, R. H., 1976, Gastric A-cell function in insulin-deprived depancreatized dogs, *Endocrinology* **99**:1182–1188.

Blazquez, E., Muñoz-Barragan, L., Patton, G. S., Dobbs, R. E., and Unger, R. H., 1977, Demonstration of gastric glucagon hypersecretion in insulin-deprived alloxan diabetic dogs, *J. Lab. Clin. Med.* **89**:971–977.

Bloom, S. R., Royston, C. M. S., and Thomson, J. P. S., 1972, Plasma enteroglucagon levels in the dumping syndrome, *Clin. Sci.* **43**:18P.

Bloom, S. R., Mortimer, C. H., Thorner, M. O., Besser, G. M., Hall, R., Gomez-Pan, A., Roy, V. M., Russell, R. C. G., Coy, D. H., Kastin, A. J., and Schally, A. V., 1974, Inhibition of gastrin and gastric acid secretion by growth-hormone release-inhibiting hormone, *Lancet* **2**:1106–1109.

Bloom, S. R., Ralphs, D. N., Besser, G. M., Hall, R., Coy, D. H., Kastin, A. J., and Schally, A. V., 1975a, Effect of somatostatin on motilin levels and gastric emptying, *Gut* **16**:834.

Bloom, S. R., Bryant, M. G., and Polak, J. M., 1975b, Distribution of gut hormones, *Gut* **16**:821.

Blundell, T. L., Dockerill, S., Sasaki, K., Tickle, I. J., and Wood, S. P., 1976, The relation of structure to storage and receptor binding of glucagon, *Metabolism* **25**(Suppl.):1331–1338.

Boden, G., and Owen, O. E., 1977, Familial hyperglucagonemia—an autosomal dominant disorder, *N. Engl. J. Med.* **296**:534–538.

Bomboy, J. D., Jr., Lewis, S. B., Lacy, W. W., Sinclair-Smith, B. C., and Liljenquist, J. E., 1977, Transient stimulatory effect of sustained hyperglucagonemia on splanchnic glucose production in normal and diabetic man, *Diabetes* **26**:177–184.

Borgeat, T., Labrie, F., Drouin, J., Belanger, H., Immer, H., Sestanj, K., Nielson, V., Gotz, M., Schally, A. V., Coy, D. H., and Coy, E. J., 1974, Inhibition of cyclic 3'-5' monophosphate stimulation in anterior pituitary gland *in vitro* by growth hormone release inhibiting hormones, *Biochem. Biophys. Res. Commun.* **56**:1052–1059.

Böttger, I., Schlein, E., Faloona, G. R., Knochel, J. P., and Unger, R. H., 1972a, The effect of exercise on glucagon secretion, *J. Clin. Endocrinol. Metab.* **35**:117–125.

Böttger, I., Faloona, G. R., and Unger, R. H., 1972b, The effect of calcium and other salts upon the release of glucagon-like immunoreactivity from the gut, *J. Clin. Invest.* **51**:831–836.

Böttger, I., Dobbs, R., Faloona, G. R., and Unger, R. H., 1973, The effects of triglyceride absorption upon glucagon, insulin and gut glucagon-like immunoreactivity, *J. Clin. Invest.* **52**:2532–2541.

Braaten, J. T., Faloona, G. R., and Unger, R. H., 1973, Comparison of alpha-cell dysfunction in acquired and inherited diabetes mellitus, *Diabetes* **22**(Suppl.):302.

Brazeau, P., Vale, W., Burgus, R., Ling, N., Butcher, M., Rivier, J., and Guillemin, R., 1973, Hypothalamic polypeptide that inhibits the secretion of immunoreactive pituitary growth hormone, *Science* **179**:77–79.

Bregman, M. D., and Levy, D., 1977, Labeling of glucagon binding components in hepatocyte plasma membranes, *Biochem. Biophys. Res. Commun.* **78**:584–590.

Brockman, R. P., Bergman, E. N., Joo, P. K., and Manns, J. G., 1975, Effects of glucagon and insulin on net hepatic metabolism of glucose precursors in sheep, *Am. J. Physiol.* **229**:1344–1349.

Bromer, W. W., Sinn, L. G., and Behrens, O. K., 1957, The amino acid sequence of glucagon. V. Location of amide groups, acid degradation studies and summary of sequential evidence, *J. Am. Chem. Soc.* **79**:2807–2810.

Brown, M., and Vale, W., 1976, Effects of neurotensin and substance P on plasma insulin, glucagon and glucose levels, *Endocrinology* **98**:819–822.

Brown, M., Rivier, J., and Vale, W., 1976, Somatostatin analogs with selected biologic activities, *Metabolism* **25**(Suppl.):1501–1503.

Brown, M. R., Rivier, J., and Vale, W. W., 1977, Bombesin affects the central nervous system to produce hyperglycemia in rats, *Life Sci.* **21**:1729–1734.

Buchanan, K. D., and Mawhinney, W. A. A., 1973, Insulin control of glucagon release from insulin deficient rat islets, *Diabetes* **22**:801–803.

Buchanan, K. D., and McCarroll, A. M., 1972, Abnormalities of glucagon metabolism in untreated diabetes mellitus, *Lancet* **2**:1394–1395.

Buffa, R., Capella, C., Solcia, E., Frigerio, B., and Said, S. I., 1977, Vasoactive intestinal peptide (VIP) cells in the pancreas and gastrointestinal mucosa. An immunohistochemical and ultrastructural study, *Histochemistry* **50**:217–227.

Burnstock, G., 1976, Do some nerve cells release more than one neurotransmitter? *Neurosci.* **1**:239–248.

Carraway, R. E., Demers, L. M., and Leeman, S. E., 1976, Hyperglycemic effect of neurotensin; a hypothalamic peptide, *Endocrinology* **99**:1452–1462.

Cherrington, A., and Vranic, M., 1971, Role of glucagon and insulin in control of glucose turnover, *Metabolism* **20**:625–628.

Cherrington, A. D., Chiasson, J. L., Liljenquist, J. E., Jennings, A. S., Keller, U., and Lacy, W. W., 1976, The role of insulin and glucagon in the regulation of basal glucose production in the postabsorptive dog, *J. Clin. Invest.* **58**:1407–1418.

Cherrington, A. D., Lacy, W. W., and Chiasson, J. L., 1978, Effect of glucagon on glucose production during insulin deficiency in the dog, *J. Clin. Invest.* **62:**664–677.

Chiasson, J. L., Liljenquist, J. E., Sinclair-Smith, B. C., and Lacy, W. W., 1975, Gluconeogenesis from alanine in normal postabsorptive man: Intrahepatic stimulatory effect of glucagon, *Diabetes* **24:**571 584.

Chideckel, E. W., Goodner, C. J., Koerker, D. J., Johnson, D. G., and Ensinck, J. W., 1977, Role of glucagon in mediating metabolic effects of epinephrine, *Am. J. Physiol.* **232**(5):PE464–470.

Church, R. E., and Crane, W. A. J., 1967, A cutaneous syndrome associated with islet-cell carcinoma of the pancreas, *Br. J. Dermatol.* **79:**284–286.

Clarke, W. L., Santiago, J. V., Thomas, L., and Kipnis, D. M., 1978, The effect of hyperglucagonemia on blood glucose concentrations and insulin require-ments in insulin-requiring diabetes mellitus, *Diabetes,* **27:**649–652

Claro, A., Grill, V., Efendic, S., and Luft, R., 1977, Studies on the mechanisms of somatostatin action on insulin release, *Acta Endocrinol.* **85:**379–388.

Cook, G. A., Nielsen, R. C., Hawkins, R. A., Mehlman, M. A., Lakshamanan, M. R., and Veech, R. L., 1977, Effect of glucagon on hepatic malonyl coenzyme A concentration and on lipid synthesis, *J. Biol. Chem.* **252:**4421–4424.

Creutzfeldt, W., Lankisch, P. G., and Folsch, U. R., 1975, Hemmung der Sekretin-und Cholezystokinin-pankreozymin induzierten Saft- und Enzymsekretin des Pankreas undder fallenblase Kontraktion beim Menschen durch Somato-statin, *Dtsch. Med. Wochenschr.* **100:**1135–1138.

Curry, D. L., and Bennett, L. L., 1974, Reversal of somatostatin inhibition of insulin secretion by calcium, *Biochem. Biophys. Res. Commun.* **60:**1015–1019.

Danforth, D. N., Jr., Triche, T., Doppman, J. L., Beazley, R. M., Perrino, P. V., and Recant, L., 1976, Elevated plasma proglucagon-like component with a glucagon-secreting tumor: Effect of streptozotocin, *N. Engl. J. Med.* **295:**242–245.

Dobbs, R., Sakurai, H., Sasaki, H., Faloona, G. R., Valverde, I., Baetens, D., Orci, L., and Unger, R. H., 1975, Glucagon: Role in the hyperglycemia of diabetes mellitus, *Science* **187:**544–547.

D'sa, A. B. B., and Buchanan, K. D., 1977, Role of gastrointestinal hormones in the response to massive resection of the small bowels, *Gut* **18:**877–881.

Dubois, M. P., 1975, Immunoreactive somatostatin is present in discrete cells of the endocrine pancreas, *Proc. Natl. Acad. Sci. U.S.A.* **72:**1340–1343.

Dular, R., and LaBella, F., 1977, Actions of releasing factors on isolated secretory granules mediated by calcium, *Life Sci.* **21:**1527–1534.

Efendic, S., Grill, V., and Luft, R., 1975, Inhibition by somatostatin of glucose induced 3′:5′-monophosphate (cyclic AMP) accumulation and insulin release in the isolated pancreatic islets of the rat, *FEBS Lett.* **55:**131–133.

Elde, R. P., and Parsons, J. A., 1975, Immunocytochemical localization of somato-statin in cell bodies of the rat hypothalamus, *Am. J. Anat.* **144:**541–548.

Emmanouel, D. S., Jaspan, J. B., Kuku, S. F., Rubenstein, A. H., and Katz, A. I., 1976, Pathogenesis and characterization of hyperglucagonemia in the uremic rat, *J. Clin. Invest.* **58:**1266–1272.

Ensinck, J. W., and Palmer, J. P., 1976, Dominant inheritance of large molecular weight species of glucagon, *Metabolism* **25**(Suppl.):1409–1414.

Epand, R. M., Cote, T. E., Hui Bon Hoa, D., Rosselin, G., and Schreier, S., 1976, Biologic activity and conformational properties of glucagon and glucagon analogs, *Metabolism* **25**(Suppl.):1317–1318.

Epelbaum, J., Willoughby, J. O., Brazeau, P., and Martin, J. B., 1977, Effects of brain lesions and hypothalamic deafferentation on somatostatin distribution in the rat brain, *Endocrinology* **101**:1495–1502.

Erlandsen, S. L., Hegre, O. D., Parsons, J. A., McEvoy, R. C., and Elde, R. P., 1976, Pancreatic islet cell hormones: Distributions of all types in the islet and evidence for the presence of somatostatin and gastrin within the D-cell, *J. Histochem. Cytochem.* **24**:883–897.

Erspamer, V., and Melchiorri, P., 1975, Actions of bombesin on secretions and motility on the gastrointestinal tract, in: *Gastrointestinal Hormones* (J. C. Thompson, ed.), pp. 575–589, University of Texas Press, Austin.

Exton, J. H., and Park, C. R., 1969, Control of gluconeogenesis in liver. III. Effects of L-lactate, pyruvate, fructose, epinephrine and adenosine 3′-5′-monophosphate on gluconeogenic intermediates in the perfused rat liver, *J. Biol. Chem.* **244**:1424–1433.

Fallucca, F., Delle Fave, G. F., Gambardella, S., Mirabella, C., De Magistris, L., and Carratu, R., 1977, Glucagon secretion induced by bombesin in man, *Lancet* **2**:609–610.

Felig, P., Gusberg, R., Hendler, R., Gump, F. E., and Kinney, J. M., 1974, Concentrations of glucagon and the insulin : glucagon ratio in the portal and peripheral circulation (38286), *Proc. Soc. Exp. Biol. Med.* **147**:88–90.

Ferland, L., Labrie, F., Jobin, M., Arimura, A., and Schally, A. V., 1976, Physiological role of somatostatin in the control of growth hormone and thyrotropin secretion, *Biochem. Biophys. Res. Commun.* **68**:149–156.

Feyrter, F., 1963, *Über die peripheren endokrinen (parakrinen) Drusen des Menchen*, p. 2, Maudrich, Vienna and Dusseldorf.

Fouchereau-Peron, M., Rancon, F., Freychet, P., and Rosselin, G., 1976, Effect of feeding and fasting on the early steps of glucagon action in isolated rat liver cells, *Endocrinology* **98**:755–760.

Frame, C. M., 1976, The contribution of the distal gastrointestinal tract to glucagon-like immunoreactivity secretion in the rat (39464), *Proc. Soc. Exp. Biol. Med.* **152**:667–670.

Frame, C. M., 1977, Regional release of glucagon-like immunoreactivity from the intestine of the cat, *Horm. Metab. Res.* **9**:117–120.

Frame, C. M., Davidson, M. B., and Sturdevant, R. A. L., 1975, Effects of the octapeptide of cholecystokinin on insulin and glucagon secretion in the dog, *Endocrinology* **97**:549–553.

Fritsch, H. A. R., Van Noorden, S. N., and Pearse, A. G. E., 1978, Localisation of somatostatin- and gastrin-like immunoreactivity in the gastrointestinal tract of *Ciona intestinalis* L., *Cell Tissue Res.* **186**:181–185.

Frohman, L. A., and Bernardis, L. L., 1971, Effect of hypothalamic stimulation on plasma glucose, insulin and glucagon levels, *Am. J. Physiol.* **221**:1596–1603.

Fujimoto, W. Y., and Ensinck, J. W., 1976, Somatostatin inhibition of insulin and glucagon secretion in rat islet culture: Reversal by ionophore A23187, *Endocrinology* **98**:259–262.

Fujita, T., Yanatori, Y., and Murakami, T., 1976, Insulo-acinar axis, its vascular basis and its functional and morphological changes caused by CCK-PZ and caerulein, in: *Endocrine, Gut and Pancreas* (T. Fujita, ed.), pp. 347–357, Elsevier, Amsterdam.

Galbo, H., Holst, J. J., Christensen, N. J., and Hilsted, J., 1976, Glucagon and plasma catecholamines during beta-receptor blockade in exercising man, *J. Appl. Physiol.* **40**:855–863.

Galbo, H., Richter, E. A., Holst, J. J., and Christensen, N. J., 1977, Diminished hormonal responses to exercise in trained rats, *J. Appl. Physiol.* **43**:953–958.

Gambardella, S., Delle Fave, G., Mirabella, C., Caccamo, C., De Magistris, L., and Caratu, R., 1977, Glucagon secretion induced by bombesin in man, *Diabetologia* **13**:395.

Ganda, O. P., Weir, G. C., Soeldner, J. S., Legg, M. A., Chick, W. L., Patel, Y. C., Ebeid, A. M., Gabbay, K. H., and Reichlin, S., 1977, Somatostatinoma: A somatostatin containing tumor of the endocrine pancreas, *N. Engl. J. Med.* **296**:963–967.

Garsky, V. M., Clark, D. E., and Grant, N. H., 1976, Synthesis of a nonreducible cyclic analog of somatostatin having only growth hormone release inhibiting activity, *Biochem. Biophys. Res. Commun.* **73**:911–916.

Gavin, J. R., III, Roth, J., Jen, P., and Freychet, P., 1972, Insulin receptors in human circulating cells and fibroblasts (lymphocytes/monoiodoinsulin/glucose oxidation), *Proc. Natl. Acad. Sci. U.S.A.* **69**:747–751.

Geelen, M. J. H., Vaartjes, W. J., and Gibson, D. M., 1977, Levels of cyclic 3'-5'-adenosine monophosphate (cAMP) in maintenance cultures of rat hepatocytes in response to insulin and glucagon, *Lipids* **12**:577–580.

Gerich, J. E., Langlois, M., Noacco, C., Karam, J. H., and Forsham, P. H., 1973, Lack of glucagon response to hypoglycemia in diabetes: Evidence for an intrinsic pancreatic alpha cell defect, *Science* **182**:171–173.

Gerich, J. E., Tsalikian, E., Lorenzi, M., Karam, J. H., Schneider, V., Gustafson, G., and Bohannon, N. V., 1975a, Normalization of fasting hyperglucagonemia and excessive glucagon responses to intravenous arginine in human diabetes mellitus by prolonged perfusion of insulin, *J. Clin. Endocrinol. Metab.* **41**:1178–1180.

Gerich, J. E., Lorenzi, M., Schneider, V., Tsalikian, E., Karam, J. H., and Forsham, P. H., 1975b, Prevention of human diabetic ketoacidosis by somatostatin. Evidence for an essential role of glucagon, *N. Engl. J. Med.* **292**:985–989.

Gerich, J. E., Langlois, M., Noacco, C., Lorenzi, M., Karam, J. H., and Forsham, P. H., 1976a, Comparison of the suppressive effects of elevated plasma glucose and free fatty acid levels on glucagon secretion in normal and insulin-dependent diabetic subjects: Evidence for selective alpha-cell insensitivity to glucose in diabetes mellitus, *J. Clin. Invest.* **58**:320–325.

Gerich, J. E., Lorenzi, M., Bier, D. M., Tsalikian, E., Schneider, V., Karam, J. H., and Forsham, P. H., 1976b, Effects of physiologic levels of glucagon and growth hormone on human carbohydrate and lipid metabolism: Studies involving administration of exogenous hormone during suppression of endogenous hormone secretion with somatostatin, *J. Clin. Invest.* **57**:875–884.

Goodner, C. J., Walike, B. C., Koerker, D. J., Brown, A. C., Ensinck, J. W., Chideckel, E. W., Palmer, J., and Kalnasy, L. W., 1976, Insulin, glucagon and glucose: Synchronous, stable oscillations in the rhesus monkey, *Diabetes* **25**(Suppl.):340.

Gossain, V. V., Matute, M. L., and Kalkhoff, R. K., 1974, Relative influence of obesity and diabetes on plasma alpha-cell glucagon, *J. Clin. Endocrinol. Metab.* **38**:238–243.

Grant, N., Clark, D., Garsky, V., Jaunakais, I., McGregor, W., and Sarantakis, D., 1976, Dissociation of somatostatin effects: Peptides inhibiting the release of growth hormone but not glucagon or insulin in rats, *Life Sci.* **19**:629–632.

Grodsky, G. M., Fanska, R., and Lundquist, I., 1975, Interrelationship between alpha and beta anomer of glucose effecting insulin and glucagon secretion in the perfused rat pancreas, *Endocrinology* **97**:573–580.

Hammes, G. G., and Rodbell, M., 1976, Simple model for hormone-activated adenylate cyclase systems, *Proc. Natl. Acad. Sci. U.S.A.* **73**:1189–1192.

Harvey, W. D., Faloona, G. R., and Unger, R. H., 1974, The effect of adrenergic blockade on exercise-induced hyperglucagonemia, *Endocrinology* **94**:1254–1258.

Hatfield, H. H., Banasiak, M. F., Driscoll, T., Kim, H. J., and Kalkhoff, R. K., 1977, Glucose suppression of glucagon: Relationship to pancreatic beta cell function, *J. Clin. Endocrinol. Metab.* **44**:1080–1087.

Heding, L. G., and Rasmussen, S. M., 1972, Determination of pancreatic and gut glucagon-like immunoreactivity (GLI) in normal and diabetic subjects, *Diabetologia* **8**:408–411.

Heding, L. G., Frandsen, E. K., and Jacobsen, H., 1976, Structure–function relationship: Immunologic, *Metabolism* **25**(Suppl.):1327–1329.

Hellerstrom, C., Howell, S. L., Edwards, J. C., and Anderson, A., 1972, An investigation of glucagon biosynthesis in isolated pancreatic islets of guinea pigs, *FEBS Lett.* **27**:97–101.

Hellerstrom, C., Howell, S. L., Edwards, J. C., Andersson, A., and Ostenson, C. G., 1974, Biosynthesis of glucagon in isolated pancreatic islets of guinea pigs, *Biochem. J.* **140**:13–23.

Hellman, B., and Lernmark, A., 1969, Inhibition of the *in vitro* secretion of insulin by an extract of pancreatic A_1 cells, *Endocrinology* **84**:1484–1488.

Helmstedter, V., Feurle, G. E., and Forssmann, W. G., 1977, Relationship of glucagon-somatostatin and gastrin-somatostatin cells in the stomach of the monkey, *Cell Tissue Res.* **177**:29–46.

Hökfelt, T., Elfnin, L. G., Elde, R. P., Schultzberg, M., Goldstein, M., and Luft, R., 1977, Occurrence of somatostatin-like immunoreactivity in some peripheral sympathetic noradrenergic neurons, *Proc. Natl. Acad. Sci.* **74**:3587.

Holst, J. J., 1977, Extraction, gel filtration pattern, and receptor binding of porcine gastrointestinal glucagon-like immunoreactivity, *Diabetologia* **13**:159–169.

Holst, J. J., Guldberg Madsen, O., Knop, J., and Schmidt, A., 1977, The effect of intraportal and peripheral infusions of glucagon on insulin and glucose concentrations and glucose tolerance in normal man, *Diabetologia* **13**:487–490.

Hruby, V. J., Wright, D. E., Lin, M. C., and Rodbell, M., 1976, Semisynthetic glucagon derivatives for structure–function studies, *Metabolism* **25**(Suppl.):1323–1326.

Hutson, N. J., Brumley, F. T., Assimacopoulos, F. D., Harper, S. C., and Exton, J. H., 1976, Studies on the alpha-adrenergic activation of hepatic glucose output. I. Studies on the alpha-adrenergic activation of phosphorylase and gluconeogenesis and inactivation of glycogen synthase in isolated rat liver parenchymal cells, *J. Biol. Chem.* **251**:5200–5208.

Ipp, E., Patton, G., Dobbs, R., Harris, V., Vale, W., and Unger, R. H., 1977a, Endogenous immunoreactive somatostatin (IRS) secretion by the pancreas, *Diabetes* **26**:359.

Ipp, E., Dobbs, R. E., Harris, V., Arimura, A., Vale, W., and Unger, R. H., 1977b, The effects of gastrin, GIP, secretin, and the octapeptide of cholecystokinin upon immunoreactive somatostatin release by the perfused canine pancreas, *J. Clin. Invest.* **60**:1216–1219.

Ipp, E., Dobbs, R. E., Arimura, A., Vale, W., Harris, V., and Unger, R. H., 1977c, Release of immunoreactive somatostatin from the pancreas in response to glucose, amino acids, pancreozymin-cholecystokinin, and tolbutamide, *J. Clin. Invest.* **60**:760–765.

Ipp, E., Dobbs, R. E., Guillemin, R., and Unger, R. H., 1978, Responses of the endocrine pancreas to morphine and β-endorphin, *Clin. Res.* **26**:418A.

Ishida, T., Kawamura, K., Goto, A., Nishina, Y., Takahara, J., Yamamoto, S., Kawanishi, K., and Ofuji, T., 1976, Comparison studies of neurotensin and xenopsin upon pancreatic secretion in dog, *Metabolism* **25**(Suppl.):1467–1468.

Iversen, J., 1973, Adrenergic receptors in the secretion of glucagon and insulin from the isolated perfused canine pancreas, *J. Clin. Invest.* **42**:2102–2116.

Jacobsen, H., Demandt, A., Moody, A. J., and Sundby, F., 1977, Sequence analysis of porcine gut GLI-1, *Biochim. Biophys. Acta* **493**:452–459.

Jaspan, J. B., and Rubenstein, A. H., 1977, Circulating glucagon plasma profiles and metabolism in health and disease, *Diabetes* **26**:887.

Jennings, A. S., Cherrington, A. D., Liljenquist, J. E., Keller, U., Lacy, W. W., and Chiasson, J. L., 1977, The roles of insulin and glucagon in the regulation of gluconeogenesis in the postabsorptive dog, *Diabetes* **26**:847–856.

Kaneto, A., Kaneko, T., Kajinuma, H., and Kosaka, K., 1977, Effect of vasoactive intestinal polypeptide infused intrapancreatically on glucagon and insulin secretion, *Metabolism* **26**:781–786.

Keller, U., Chiasson, J., Liljenquist, J. E., Cherrington, A. D., Jennings, A. S., and Crofford, O. B., 1977, The roles of insulin, glucagon, and free fatty acids in the regulation of ketogenesis in dogs, *Diabetes* **26**:1040–1051.

Koerker, D. J., Ruch, W., Chideckel, E., Palmer, J., Goodner, C. J., Ensinck, J., and Gale, C. C., 1974, Somatostatin: Hypothalamic inhibitor of the endocrine pancreas, *Science* **184**:482–484.

Kronheim, S., Berelowitz, M., and Pimstone, B. L., 1977, The characterization of growth hormone release inhibiting hormone-like immunoreactivity in normal urine, *Clin. Endocrinol.* **7**:343–347.

Krulich, L., Dhariwal, A. P. S., and McCann, S. M., 1968, Stimulatory and inhibitory effects of purified hypophalamic extracts on growth hormone release from the rat pituitary *in vitro*, *Endocrinology* **83**:783–790.

Kuku, S. F., Jaspan, J. B., Emmanouel, D. S., Zeidler, A., Katz, A. I., and Rubenstein, A. H., 1976, Heterogeneity of plasma glucagon, circulating components in normal subjects and patients with chronic renal failure, *J. Clin. Invest.* **58**:742–750.

Kurahachi, H., Seino, Y., Ikeda, M., Sakurai, H., Yoshimi, T., and Imura, H., 1977, Insuppressibility of plasma glucagon by orally or intravenously administered glucose in diabetes mellitus, *Endocrinol. Jpn.* **24**(5):413–419.

Larsson, L. I., Holst, J., Hakanson, R., and Sundler, F., 1975, Distribution and properties of glucagon immunoreactivity in the digestive tract of various mammals: An immunohistochemical and immunochemical study, *Histochemistry* **44**:281–290.

Larsson, L. I., Hirsch, M. A., Holst, J. J., Ingemansson, S., Kuhl, C., Lindkaer, J. S., Lundqvist, G., Rehfeld, J. F., and Schwartz, T. W., 1977, Pancreatic somatostatinoma: Clinical features and physiological implications, *Lancet* **1**:666–668.

Laurent, F., and Mialhe, P., 1976, Insulin and the glucose–glucagon feedback mechanism in the duck, *Diabetologia* **12**:23–33.

Lawrence, A. M., Tan, S., Hojvat, S., Kirsteins, L., and Mitton, J., 1976, Salivary gland glucagon in man and animals, *Metabolism* **25**(Suppl.):1405–1408.

Lawrence, T. S., Beers, W. H., and Gilula, N. B., 1978, Transmission of hormonal stimulation by cell-to-cell communication, *Nature (London)* **272**:501–506.

Leblanc, H., Lachelin, G. C. L., Abu-Fadil, S., and Yen, S. S. C., 1977, The effect of dopamine infusion on insulin and glucagon secretion in man, *J. Clin. Endocrinol. Metal.* **44**:196–198.

Leclercq-Meyer, V., Marchand, J., and Malaisse, J., 1977, The arginine-like effect of "fumerate + glutamate + pyruvate" mixture on glucagon release, *Life Sci.* **20**:1193–1198.

Lefebvre, P. J., 1972, Glucagon and lipid metabolism, in: *Glucagon: Molecular Physiology, Clinical and Therapeutic Implications* (P. J. Lefebvre and R. H. Unger, eds.), pp. 175–180, Pergamon Press, Oxford.

Lefebvre, P. J., and Luyckx, A. S., 1975, Effect of acute kidney exclusion of renal arteries on peripheral plasma glucagon levels and pancreatic glucagon production in the anesthetized dog, *Metabolism* **24**:1169–1176.

Lefebvre, P. J., and Luyckx, A. S., 1976, Plasma glucagon after kidney exclusion: Experiments in somatostatin-infused and in eviscerated dogs, *Metabolism* **25**:761–768.

Lefebvre, P. J., and Luyckx, A. S., 1977, Factors controlling gastric-glucagon release, *J. Clin. Invest.* **59**:716–722.

Liljenquist, J. E., Mueller, G. L., Cherrington, A. D., Keller, U., Chiasson, J. L., Perry, J. M., Lacy, W. W., and Rabinowitz, D., 1977, Evidence for an important role of glucagon in the regulation of hepatic glucose production in normal man, *J. Clin. Invest.* **59**:369–374.

Linn, M. C., Nicosia, S., and Rodbell, M., 1976, Effects of iodination of tyrosyl residues on the binding and action of glucagon and its receptor, *Biochemistry* **15**:4537–4540.

Lindsey, C. A., Faloona, G. R., and Unger, R. H., 1974, Plasma glucagon in nonketotic hyperosmolar coma, *J. Am. Med. Assoc.* **229**:1771–1773.

Lorenzi, M., Tsalikian, E., Bohannon, N. V., Gerich, J. E., Karam, J. H., and Forsham, P. H., 1977, Differential effects of L-dopa and apomorphine on glucagon secretion in man: Evidence against central dopaminergic stimulation of glucagon, *J. Clin. Endocrinol. Metab.* **45**:1154–1158.

Luft, R., Efendic, S., Hokfelt, T., Johansson, O., and Arimura, A., 1974, Immunohistochemical evidence for the localization of somatostatin-like immunoreactivity in a cell population of the pancreatic islets, *Med. Biol.* **52**:428.

Luyckx, A. S., and Lefebvre, P. J., 1970, Arguments for a regulation of pancreatic glucagon secretion by circulating free fatty acids (34511), *Proc. Soc. Exp. Biol. Med.* **133**:524–528.

Luyckx, A. S., and Lefebvre, P. J., 1976, Effect of somatostatin on metabolic and hormonal changes induced by nicotinic acid in insulin-dependent diabetics, *Diabetologia* **12**:447–453.

MacDonald, M. J., Huang, M. T., and Lardy, H. A., 1977, 3-aminopicolinate: A metal complexing activation of P-enolpyruvate carboxykinase, *Fed. Proc. Fed. Am. Soc. Exp. Biol.* **36**:932.

Madison, L. L., Seyffert, W. A., Jr., Unger, R. H., and Baker, B., 1968, Effect of plasma free fatty acids on plasma glucagon and serum insulin concentrations, *Metabolism* **17**:301–304.

Maher, T. D., Tanenberg, R. J., Greenberg, B. Z., Hoffman, J. E., Doe, R. P., and Goetz, F. C., 1977, Lack of glucagon response to hypoglycemia in diabetic autonomic neuropathy, *Diabetes* **26**:196–200.

Mallette, L. E., Exton, J. H., and Park, C. R., 1969, Control of gluconeogenesis from amino acids in the perfused rat liver, *J. Biol. Chem.* **244**:5713–5723.

Mallinson, C. N., Bloom, S. R., Warin, A. P., Salmon, P. R., and Cox, B., 1974, A glucagonoma syndrome, *Lancet* **2**:1–5.

Marco, J., Faloona, G. R., and Unger, R. H., 1971, Effect of endogenous intestinal glucagon-like immunoreactivity (GLI) on insulin secretion and glucose concentration in dogs, *J. Clin. Endocrinol. Metab.* **33**:318–325.

Marco, J., Hedo, J. A., Martinell, J., Calle, C., and Villanueva, M. L., 1976, Potentiation of glucagon secretion by serotonin antagonists in man, *J. Clin. Endocrinol. Metab.* **42**:215–221.

Marco, J., Hedo, J. A., and Villanueva, M. L., 1977a, Inhibition of glucagon release by serotonin in mouse pancreatic islets, *Diabetologia* **13**:585–588.

Marco, J., Hedo, J. A., Villanueva, M. L., Calle, C., Corujedo, A., and Segovia, J. M., 1977b, Effect of food ingestion on intestinal glucagon-like immunoreactivity (GLI) secretion in normal and gastrectomized subjects, *Diabetologia* **13**:131–135.

Marks, N., and Stern, F., 1975, Inactivation of somatostatin (GH-RIH) and its analogs by crude and partially purified rat brain extracts, *FEBS Lett.* **55**:220–224.

Marks, N., Stern, F., and Benuck, M., 1976, Correlation between biological potency and biodegradation of a somatostatin analogue, *Nature (London)* **261**:511–512.

Marliss, E. B., Girardier, L., Seydoux, J., Wollheim, C. B., Kanazawa, Y., Orci, L., Renold, A. E., and Porte, D., Jr., 1973, Glucagon release induced by pancreatic nerve stimulation in the dog, *J. Clin. Invest.* **52**:1246–1259.

Mashiter, K., Harding, P. E., Chou, M., Mashiter, G. D., Stout, J., Diamond, D., and Field, J. B., 1975, Persistent pancreatic glucagon but not insulin response to arginine in pancreatectomized dogs, *Endocrinology* **96**:678–693.

Matschinsky, F. M., Pagliara, A. S., Hover, B. A., Haymond, M. W., and Stillings, S. N., 1975, Differential effects of α- and β-D-glucose on insulin and glucagon secretion from the isolated perfused rat pancreas, *Diabetes* **24**:369–372.

Matschinsky, F. M., Pagliara, A. S., Stillings, S. N., and Hover, B. A., 1976, Glucose and ATP levels in pancreatic islet tissue of normal and diabetic rats, *J. Clin. Invest.* **58**:1193–1200.

Matsuyama, I., and Fòa, P. P., 1975, Plasma glucose, insulin, pancreatic and enteroglucagon levels in normal and depancreatized dogs (38288), *Proc. Soc. Exp. Biol. Med.* **147**:97–102.

McGarry, J. D., and Foster, D. W., 1977, Hormonal control of ketogenesis, *Arch. Intern. Med.* **137**:495–501.

McGarry, J. D., Wright, P. H., and Foster, D. W., 1975a, Hormonal control of ketogenesis: Rapid activation of hepatic ketogenic capacity in fed rats by anti-insulin serum and glucagon, *J. Clin. Invest.* **55**:1202–1209.

McGarry, J. D., Robles-Valdes, C., and Foster, D. W., 1975b, Role of carnitine in hepatic ketogenesis, *Proc. Natl. Acad. Sci. U.S.A.* **72**:4385–4388.

McGarry, J. D., Robles-Valdes, C., and Foster, D. W., 1976, Glucagon and ketogenesis, *Metabolism* **25**(Suppl.):1387–1391.

McGarry, J. D., Mannaerts, G. P., and Foster, D. W., 1977, A possible role for malonyl-CoA in the regulation of hepatic fatty acid oxidation and ketogenesis, *J. Clin. Invest.* **60**:265–270.

McGavran, M. H., Unger, R. H., Recant, L., Pol, H. C., Kilo, C., and Levin, M. E., 1966, A glucagon-secreting alpha cell carcinoma of the pancreas, *N. Engl. J. Med.* **274**:1408–1413.

Miyata, J., Yamamoyo, T., Yamaguchi, M., Nakao, K., and Yoshida, T., 1976, Plasma glucagon after total resection of the pancreas in man, *Proc. Soc. Exp. Biol. Med.* **152**:540–543.

Moltz, J. H., Dobbs, R. E., McCann, S. M., and Fawcett, C. P., 1977, Effects of hypophalamic factors on insulin and glucagon release from the islets of Langerhans, *Endocrinology* **101**:196–202.

Moody, A. J., Frandsen, E. K., Jacobsen, H., Sundby, F., and Orci, L., 1976, Discussion: The structural and immunologic relationship between gut GLIs and glucagon, *Metabolism* **25**(Suppl.):1336–1338.

Morley, J. E., Levin, S. R., Pehlevanian, M., Adachi, R., Garvin, T. J., Pekary, A. E., and Hersham, J. M., 1978, Thyrotropin releasing hormone (TRH) and the pancreas, *Clin. Res.* **26**:160A.

Mortimer, C. H., Turnbridge, W. J. G., Carr, D., Yeomans, L., Lind, T., Coy, D. H., Bloom, S. R., Kastin, A., Mallinson, C. N., Besser, G. M., Schally, A. V., and Hall, R., 1974, Effects of growth hormone release–inhibiting hormone on circulating glucagon, insulin and growth hormone in normal, diabetic, acromegalic and hypopituitary patients, *Lancet* **1**:697–701.

Muller, W. A., Faloona, G. R., Unger, R. H., and Aguilar-Parada, E., 1970, Abnormal alpha cell function in diabetes: Response to carbohydrate and protein ingestion, *N. Engl. J. Med.* **283**:109–115.

Müller, W. A., Faloona, G. R. , and Unger, R. H., 1971, The influence of the antecedent diet upon glucagon and insulin secretion, *N. Engl. J. Med.* **285**:1450–1454.

Müller, W. A., Faloona, G. R., and Unger, R. H., 1973, Hyperglucagonemia in diabetic ketoacidosis: Its prevalence and significance, *Am. J. Med.* **54**:52–57.

Müller, W. A., Brennan, M. F., Tan, M. H., and Aoki, T. T., 1974, Studies of glucagon secretion in pancreatectomized patients, *Diabetes* **23**:512–516.

Muñoz-Barragan, L., Blazquez, E., Patton, G. S., Dobbs, R. E., and Unger, R. H., 1976, Gastric A-cell function in normal dogs, *Am. J. Physiol.* **231**:1057–1061.

Muñoz-Barragan, L., Rufener, C., Srikant, C. B., Dobbs, R. E., Shannon, W. A., Baetens, D., and Unger, R. H., 1977, Immunocytochemical evidence for glucagon-containing cells in the human stomach, *Horm. Metab. Res.* **9**:37–39.

Murphy, E. D., and Anderson, J. W., 1974, Tissue glycolytic and gluconeogenic enzyme activities in mildly and moderately diabetic rats: Influence of tolbutamide administration, *Endocrinology* **94**:27–34.

Nakabayashi, H., Dobbs, R. E., and Unger, R. H., 1978, The role of glucagon deficiency in the Houssay phenomenon of dogs, *J. Clin. Invest.* **61**:1355–1362.

Noe, B. D., 1976, Biosynthesis of glucagon, *Metabolism* **25**(Suppl.):1339–1341.

Noe, B. D., and Bauer, G. E., 1971, Evidence for glucagon biosynthesis involving a protein intermediate in islets of the anglerfish *(Lophius amencauus)*, *Endocrinology* **89**:642–651.

O'Connor, K. J., and Lazarus, N. R., 1976, Studies on the biosynthesis of pancreatic glucagon in the pigeon *(Columba livia)*, *Biochem. J.* **156**:279–288.

Ogawa, N., Friesen, H. G., Martin, J. B., and Brazeau, P., 1976, Radioreceptor assay for somatostatin, *Endocrinology (Suppl.)* **98**:154.

Ogawa, N., Thompson, T., Friesen, H. G., Martin, J. B., and Brazeau, P., 1977, Properties of soluble somatostatin-binding protein, *Biochem. J.* **165**:269–277.

Ohneda, A., Parada, E., Eisentraut, A., and Unger, R. H., 1968, Characterization of response of circulating glucagon to intraduodenal and intravenous administration of amino acids, *J. Clin. Invest.* **47**:2305–2322.

Ohneda, A., Ishii, S., Horigome, K., Chiba, M., Sakai, T., Kai, Y., Watanabe, K., and Yamagata, S., 1977, Effect of intrapancreatic administration of vasoactive intestinal peptide upon the release of insulin and glucagon in dogs, *Horm. Metab. Res.* **9**(6):447–452.

Orci, L., 1977, Discussion, in: *Recent Progress in Hormone Research* (R. O. Greep, ed.), p. 511, Academic Press, New York.

Orci, L., and Unger, R. H., 1975, Functional subdivision of islets of Langerhans and possible role of D-cells, *Lancet* **2**:1243–1244.

Orci, L., Pictet, R., Forssmann, W. G., Renold, A. E., and Rouiller, C., 1968, Structural evidence for glucagon producing cells in the intestinal mucosa of the rat, *Diabetologia* **4**:56–67.

Orci, L., Unger, R. H., and Renold, A. E., 1973, Structural coupling between pancreatic islet cells, *Experientia* **29**:1015–1018.

Orci, L., Baetens, D., Dubois, M. P., and Rufener, C., 1975a, Evidence for the D-cell of the pancreas secreting somatostatin, *Horm. Metab. Res.* **7**:400–402.

Orci, L., Malaisse-Lagae, F., Amherdt, M., Ravazzola, M., Weisswange, A., Dobbs, R., Perrelet, A., and Unger, R., 1975b, Cell contacts in human islets of Langerhans, *J. Clin. Endocrinol. Metab.* **41**:841–844.

Orci, L., Malaisse-Lagae, F., Ravazzola, M., Rouiller, D., Renold, A. E., Perrelet, A., and Unger, R., 1975c, A morphological basis for intercellular communication between A- and B-cells in the endocrine pancreas, *J. Clin. Invest.* **56**:1066–1070.

Orci, L., Baetens, D., Ravazzola, M., Stefan, Y., and Malaisse-Lagae, F., 1976a, Pancreatic polypeptides and glucagon: Non-random distribution in pancreatic islets, *Life Sci.* **19**:1811–1816.

Orci, L., Baetens, D., Rufener, C., Amherdt, M., Ravazzola, M., Studer, P., Malaisse-Lagae, F., and Unger, R. H., 1976b, Hypertrophy and hyperplasia of somatostatin-containing D-cells in diabetes, *Proc. Natl. Acad. Sci. U.S.A.* **73**:1338–1342.

Pagliara, A. S., Stillings, S. N., Haymond, M. W., Hover, B. A., and Matschinsky, F. M., 1975, Insulin and glucose as modulators of the amino acid–induced glucagon release in the isolated pancreas of alloxan and streptozotocin diabetic rats, *J. Clin. Invest.* **55**:244–255.

Palmer, J. P., Werner, P. L., Benson, J. W., and Ensinck, J. W., 1976, Immunoreactive glucagon responses to arginine in three pancreatectomized humans, *Metabolism* **25**(Suppl.):1483–1485.

Palmer, J. P., Werner, P. L., Benson, J. W., and Ensinck, J. W., 1978, Dominant inheritance of large molecular weight immunoreactive glucagon, *J. Clin. Invest.* **61**:763–769.

Patel, Y. C., and Reichlin, S., 1978, Somatostatin in hypothalamus, extrahypothalamic brain, and peripheral tissues of the rat, *Endocrinology* **102**:523–530.

Patel, Y. C., Orci, L., Bankier, A., and Cameron, D. P., 1976, Decreased pancreatic somatostatin (SRIF) concentration in spontaneously diabetic mice, *Endocrinology* **99**:1415–1418.

Patel, Y. C., Cameron, D. P., Stefan, Y., Malaisse-Lagae, F., and Orci, L., 1977, Somatostatin: Widespread abnormality in tissues of spontaneously diabetic mice, *Science* **198**:930–931.

Patton, G., Brown, M., Dobbs, R., Vale, W., and Unger, R. H., 1976a, Effects of neurotensin and substance P on insulin and glucagon release by the perfused dog pancreas, *Metabolism* **25**(Suppl.):1465.

Patton, G. S., Dobbs, R., Orci, L., Vale, W., and Unger, R. H., 1976b, Stimulation of pancreatic immunoreactive somatostatin (IRS) release by glucagon, *Metabolism* **25**(Suppl.):1499.

Patton, G. S., Ipp, E., Dobbs, R. E., Vale, W., Orci, L., and Unger, R. H., 1976c, Response of pancreatic immunoreactive somatostatin to arginine, *Life Sci.* **19**:1957–1960.

Patton, G. S., Ipp, E., Dobbs, R. E., Orci, L., Vale, W., and Unger, R. H., 1977, Pancreatic immunoreactive somatostatin release, *Proc. Natl. Acad. Sci. U.S.A.* **74**:2140–2143.

Pelletier, G., Leclerc, R., Arimura, A., and Schally, A. V., 1975, Immunohistochemical localization of somatostatin in the rat pancreas, *J. Histochem. Cytochem.* **23**:699–701.

Pelletier, G., Dube, D., and Puviani, R., 1977, Somatostatin: Electron microscope immunohistochemical localization in secretory neurons of rat hypothalamus, *Science* **196**:1469–1470.

Pilkis, S. J., Claus, T. H., Johnson, R. A., and Park, C. R., 1975, Hormonal control of cyclic 3':5'-AMP levels and gluconeogenesis in isolated hepatocytes from fed rats, *J. Biol. Chem.* **250**:6328–6336.

Porte, D., Jr., Woods, S. C., Chen, M., Smith, P. H., and Ensinck, J. W., 1975, Central factors in the control of insulin and glucagon secretion, *Pharmacol. Biochem. Behav.* **3**:127–133.

Quabbe, H. J., Ramek, W., and Luyckx, A. S., 1977, Growth hormone, glucagon, and insulin response to depression of plasma free fatty acids and the effect of glucose infusion, *J. Clin. Endocrinol. Metab.* **44**:383–391.

Rabinovitch, A., and Dupre, J., 1974, Effects of gastric inhibitory polypeptide present in impure pancreozymin-cholecystokinin on plasma insulin and glucagon in the rat, *Endocrinology* **94**:1139–1144.

Raskin, P., and Unger, R. H., 1977, Effects of exogenous hyperglucagonemia in insulin-treated diabetics, *Diabetes* **26**:1034–1039.

Raskin, P., Fujita, Y., and Unger, R. H., 1975, Effect of insulin–glucose infusions on plasma glucagon levels in fasting diabetics and nondiabetics, *J. Clin. Invest.* **56**:1132–1138.

Raskin, P., Aydin, I., and Unger, R. H., 1976, The effect of insulin on the exaggerated glucagon response to arginine stimulation in diabetes mellitus, *Diabetes* **25**:227–229.

Raskin, P., Aydin, I., Yamamoto, T., and Unger, R. H., 1978, Abnormal alpha cell function in human diabetes, *Am. J. Med.* **64**:988–997.

Rayfield, E. J., George, D. T., Eichner, H. L., and Hsu, T. H., 1975, L-Dopa stimulation of glucagon secretion in man, *N. Engl. J. Med.* **293**:589–591.

Recant, L., Perrino, P. V., Bhathena, S. J., Danforth, D. N., Jr., and Lavine, R. L., 1976, Plasma immunoreactive glucagon fractions in four cases of glucagonoma: Increased "large glucagon immunoreactivity," *Diabetologia* **12**:319–326.

Redding, T. W., and Coy, D. H., 1974, The disappearance, distribution and excretion of ^{125}I-tyrosine[1]-growth hormone release inhibiting hormone in mice, rats, and man, 56th Meeting of the American Endocrine Society, Atlanta, Georgia, Abstract 198.

Rehfeld, J. F., Heding, L. G., and Holst, J. J., 1973, Increased gut glucagon release as pathogenetic factor in reactive hypoglycemia, *Lancet* **1**:116–118.

Rigopoulou, D., Valverde, I., Marco, J., Faloona, G., and Unger, R. H., 1970, Large glucagon immunoreactivity in extracts of pancreas, *J. Biol. Chem.* **245**:496–501.

Rivier, J., Brown, M., and Vale, W., 1975, [D-Trp^8]-somatostatin: An analog of somatostatin more potent than the native molecule, *Biochem. Biophys. Res. Commun.* **65**:746–751.

Rocha, D. M., Faloona, G. R., and Unger, R. H., 1972, Glucagon stimulating activity of twenty amino acids in dogs, *J. Clin. Invest.* **51**:2346–2351.

Rodbell, M., and Londos, C., 1976, Regulation of hepatic adenylate cyclase by glucagon, GTP, divalent cations, and adenosine, *Metabolism* **25**(Suppl.):1347–1349.

Ross, J. B. A., Rousslang, K. W., Deranleau, D. A., and Kwiram, A. L., 1977, Glucagon conformation: Use of optically detected magnetic resonance and phosphorescence of tryptophan to evaluate critical requirements for folding of the polypeptide chain, *Biochemistry* **16**(24):5398–5402.

Sacks, H., Waligora, K., Matthews, J., and Pimstone, B., 1977, Inhibition by somatostatin of glucagon-induced glucose release from the isolated perfused rat liver, *Endocrinology* **101**:1751–1759.

Said, S. I., and Rosenburg, R. N., 1976, Vasoactive intestinal polypeptide: Abundant immunoreactivity in neural cell lines and normal tissues, *Science* **192**:907–908.

Sakurai, H., Dobbs, R. E., and Unger, R. H., 1975, The role of glucagon in the pathogenesis of the endogenous hyperglycemia of diabetes mellitus, *Metabolism* **24**:1287–1297.

Samols, E., Marri, G., and Marks, V., 1965, Promotion of insulin secretion by glucagon, *Lancet* **2**:415–416.

Samols, E., Tyler, J., and Marks, V., 1972, Glucagon–insulin interrelationships, in: *Glucagon: Molecular Physiology, Clinical and Therapeutic Implications* (P. J. Lefebvre and R. H. Unger, eds.), pp. 151–174, Pergamon Press, Oxford, England.

Samols, E., Weir, G. C., Patel, Y. C., Fernandez-Durango, R., Arimura, A., and Loo, S. W., 1977, Suppression of canine pancreatic A, B, D, and PP cell secretion by diazoxide, *Diabetes* **26**(Suppl.):375.

Santeusanio, F., Faloona, G. R., and Unger, R. H., 1972, Suppressive effect of secretin upon pancreatic alpha cell function, *J. Clin. Invest.* **51**:1743–1749.

Sarantakis, D., Teichman, J., Lien, E. L., and Fenichel, R. L., 1976, A novel cyclic tetradecapeptide, WY-40, 770, with prolonged growth hormone release inhibiting activity, *Biochem. Biophys. Res. Commun.* **73**:336–342.

Sasagawa, T., Kobayashi, S., and Fujita, T., 1973, Electron microscopy of GEP endocrine cells, in: *Symposium on the GEP Endocrine System* (T. Fujita, ed.), p. 31, Igaku Shoin, Tokyo.

Sasaki, H., Rubalcava, B., Baetens, D., Blazquez, E., Srikant, C. B., Orci, L., and Unger, R. H., 1975a, Identification of glucagon in the gastrointestinal tract, *J. Clin. Invest.* **56**:135–145.

Sasaki, H., Rubalcava, B., Srikant, C. B., Baetens, D., Orci, L., and Unger, R. H., 1975b, Gut glucagonoid (GLI) and gastrointestinal glucagon, in: *Gastrointestinal Hormones* (J. C. Thompson, ed.), pp. 519–528, University of Texas Press, Austin.

Schade, D. S., and Eaton, R. P., 1977, The effect of short term physiological elevations of plasma glucagon concentration on plasma triglyceride concentration in normal and diabetic man, *Horm. Metab. Res.* **9**(4):253–257.

Schally, A. V., Dupont, A., Arimura, A., Reding, T. W., Nishi, N., Linthicum, G., and Schlesinger, D. H., 1976, Isolation and structure of somatostatin from porcine hypothalamus, *Biochemistry* **15**:509–514.

Schauder, P., McIntosh, C., Arends, J., Arnold, R., Frerichs, H., and Creutzfeldt, W., 1976, Somatostatin and insulin release from isolated rat pancreatic islets stimulated by glucose, *FEBS Lett.* **68**:225–227.

Schebalin, M., Said, S. I., and Makhlouf, G. M., 1977, Stimulation of insulin and glucagon secretion by vasoactive intestinal peptide, *Am. J. Physiol.* **232**:E197–E200.

Schmitt, J., Lorenzi, M., Gerich, J., Bohannon, N., Karam, J. H., and Forsham, P. H., 1978, Effect of phentolamine on somatostatin's action in man, *Clin. Res.* **26**:131A.

Schonbrunn, A., and Tashjian, A. H., Jr., 1977, Characterization of specific functional receptors for somatostatin in pituitary tumor cells in culture, Program and Abstracts, 59th Annual Meeting, Endocrine Society, Chicago, abstract 242.

Schusdziarra, V., Ipp, E., and Unger, R. H., 1977a, Somatostatin, a physiologic regulator of nutrient influx, *Diabetes* **26**(Suppl.):359.

Schusdziarra, V., Dobbs, R. E., Harris, V., and Unger, R. H., 1977b, Immunoreactive somatostatin levels in plasma of normal and alloxan diabetic dogs, *FEBS Lett.* **81**:69–72.

Seino, Y., Ikeda, M., Nakan, K., Nakahara, H., Seino, S., and Imura, H., 1977, Amino acid modulation of glucose-induced insulin and glucagon release in diabetic patients, *Metabolism* **26**:911–919.

Sestoft, L., Bartels, P. D., Fleron, P., Folke, M., Gammeltaff, S., and Kristensen, L. Ø., 1977, Influence of thyroid state on the effects of glycerol on gluconeogenesis and energy metabolism in perfused rat liver, *Biochim. Biophys. Acta* **499**:119–130.

Sherwin, R. S., Fisher, M., Hendler, R., and Felig, P., 1976, Hyperglucagonemia and blood glucose regulation in normal, obese, and diabetic subjects, *N. Engl. J. Med.* **294**:455–461.

Sherwin, R. S., Hendler, R., DeFronzo, R., Wahren, J., and Felig, P., 1977a, Glucose homeostasis during prolonged suppression of glucagon and insulin secretion by somatostatin, *Proc. Natl. Acad. Sci. U.S.A.* **74**:348–352.

Sherwin, R. S., Tamborlane, W., Hendler, H., Sacca, L., DeFronzo, R. A., and Felig, P., 1977b, Influence of glucagon replacement on the hyperglycemic and hyperketonemic response to prolonged somatostatin infusion in normal man, *J. Clin. Endocrinol. Metab.* **45**:1104–1107.

Smith, P. H., Woods, S. C., and Porte, D., Jr., 1976, Phentolamine blocks the somatostatin-mediated inhibition of insulin secretion, *Endocrinology* **98**:1073–1076.

Smith, P. H., Woods, S. C., Ensinck, J. W., and Porte, D., Jr., 1977, Phentolamine prevents the somatostatin-mediated inhibition of pancreatic glucagon secretion, *Metabolism* **26**:841–846.

Soman, V., and Felig, P., 1977, Glucagon and insulin binding to liver membranes in partially nephrectomized uremic rat model, *J. Clin. Invest.* **60**:224–232.

Soman, V., and Felig, P., 1978, Glucagon binding and adenylate cyclase activity in liver membranes from untreated and insulin-treated diabetic rats, *J. Clin. Invest.* **61**:552–560.

Sperling, M. A., Aleck, K., and Voina, S., 1977, Suppressibility of glucagon secretion by glucose in juvenile diabetes, *J. Pediatr.* **90**:543–547.

Srikant, C. B., and Unger, R. H., 1976, Evidence for the presence of glucagon-like immunoreactivity (GLI) in the pancreas, *Endocrinology* **99**:1655–1658.

Srikant, C. B., McCorkle, K., and Unger, R. H., 1976, Characteristics of tissue IRGs in the dog, *Metabolism* **25**(Suppl. 1):1403–1404.

Srikant, C. B., McCorkle, K., and Unger, R. H., 1977a, Properties of immunoreactive glucagon (IRG) fractions of canine stomach and pancreas, *J. Biol. Chem.* **251**:1847–1851.

Srikant, C. B., Freeman, D., McCorkle, K., and Unger, R. H., 1977b, Binding and biologic activity of glucagon in liver cell membranes of chronically hyperglucagonemic rats, *J. Biol. Chem.* **252**:7434–7438.

Staehelin, L. A., 1974, Structure and function of intercellular junctions, *Int. Rev. Cytol.* **39**:191–283.

Sundby, F., 1976, Species variations in the primary structure of glucagon, *Metabolism* **25**(Suppl.):1319–1321.

Sundby, F., Jacobsen, H., and Moody, A. J., 1976, Purification and characterization of a protein from porcine gut with glucagon-like immunoreactivity, *Horm. Metab. Res.* **8**:366–371.

Sutherland, E. W., and DeDuve, C., 1948, Origin and distribution of the hyperglycemic–glycogenolytic factor of the pancreas, *J. Biol. Chem.* **175**:663–674.

Tager, H. S., and Markese, J., 1976, Immunoreactive "glucagons" in pancreatic islets, *Metabolism* **25**(Suppl.):1343–1346.

Tager, H. S., and Steiner, D. F., 1973, Isolation of a glucagon-containing peptide: Primary structure of a possible fragment of proglucagon, *Proc. Natl. Acad. Sci. U.S.A.* **70**:2321–2325.

Tamborlane, W. V., Sherwin, R. S., Hendler, R., and Felig, P., 1977, Metabolic effects of somatostatin in maturity-onset diabetes, *N. Engl. J. Med.* **297**:181–183.

Taminato, T., Seino, Y., Goto, Y., and Imura, H., 1975, Interaction of somatostatin and calcium in regulating insulin release from isolated pancreatic islets of rats, *Biochem. Biophys. Res. Commun.* **66**:928–934.

Taniguchi, H., Utsumi, M., Hasegawa, M., Kobayashi, T., Watanabe, Y., Murakami, K., Seki, M., Tsutou, A., Makimura, H., Sakoda, M., and Baba, S., 1977, Physiologic role of somatostatin: Insulin release from rat islets treated by somatostatin antiserum, *Diabetes* **26**:700–702.

Terry, L. C., Martin, J. B., Willoughby, J. O., Brazeau, P., and Patel, Y., 1976, Antiserum to somatostatin prevents stress induced inhibition of growth hormone secretion in the rat, *Science* **192**:565–567.

Tragl, K. H., and Kinast, H., 1977, Inhibition by somatostatin of adenosine-3′,5′-monophosphate stimulated hepatic ribosomal protein synthesis, *Klin. Wochenschr.* **55**:707–709.

Tung, A. K., Rosenzweig, S. A., and Foa, P. P., 1977, Glucagon from avian pancreatic islets: Radioreceptor studies, *Can. J. Biochem.* **55**:915–918.

Ukai, M., Inoue, I., and Itatsu, T., 1977, Effect of somatostatin on neurotensin-induced glucagon release and hyperglycemia, *Endocrinology* **100**:1284–1286.

Unger, R. H., 1977, Somatostatinoma, *N. Engl. J. Med.* **296**:998–1000.

Unger, R. H., and Eisentraut, A. M., 1967, Glucagon, in: *Hormones in Blood* (C. H. Gray and A. L. Bacharach, eds.), pp. 83–128, Academic Press, New York and London.

Unger, R. H., and Lefebvre, P. J., 1972, Glucagon physiology, in: *Glucagon: Molecular Physiology, Clinical and Therapeutic Implications* (P. J. Lefebvre and R. H. Unger, eds.), pp. 213, Pergamon Press, Oxford.

Unger, R. H., and Orci, L., 1975, The essential role of glucagon in the pathogenesis of diabetes mellitus, *Lancet* 1:14–16.

Unger, R. H., and Orci, L., 1977a, Hypothesis: The possible role of the pancreatic D-cell in the normal and diabetic states, *Diabetes* 26:241–244.

Unger, R. H., and Orci, L., 1977b, Role of glucagon in diabetes, *Arch. Intern. Med.* 137:482–491.

Unger, R. H., and Orci, L., 1977c, The role of glucagon in the endogenous hyperglycemia of diabetes mellitus, *Annu. Rev. Med.* 28:119–130.

Unger, R. H., and Raskin, P., 1978, The effect of glucagon and of its suppression upon diabetic hyperglycemia, *Diabetes* 27(Suppl. 2):99.

Unger, R. H., Eisentraut, A., Sims, K., McCall, M. S., and Madison, L. L., 1961, Site of origin of glucagon in dogs and humans, *Clin. Res.* 9:53.

Unger, R. H., Ketterer, H., and Eisentraut, A. M., 1966, Distribution of immunoassayable glucagon in gastrointestinal tissues, *Metabolism* 15:865–867.

Unger, R. H., Ketterer, H., Dupre, J., and Eisentraut, A. M., 1967, The effects of secretin, pancreozymin, and gastrin on insulin and glucagon secretion in anesthetized dogs, *J. Clin. Invest.* 46:630–645.

Unger, R. H., Ohneda, A., Valverde, I., Eisentraut, A. M., and Exton, J., 1968, Characterization of the responses of circulating glucagon-like immunoreactivity to intraduodenal and intravenous administration of glucose, *J. Clin. Invest.* 47:48–65.

Unger, R. H., Ohneda, A., Aguilar-Parada, E., and Eisentraut, A. M., 1969, The role of aminogenic glucagon secretion in blood glucose homeostasis, *J. Clin. Invest.* 48:810–822.

Unger, R. H., Aguilar-Parada, E., Muller, W. A., and Eisentraut, A. M., 1970, Studies of pancreatic alpha cell function in normal and diabetic subjects, *J. Clin. Invest.* 49:837–848.

Unger, R. H., Ipp, E., Schusdziarra, V., and Orci, L., 1977, Hypothesis: Physiologic role of pancreatic somatostatin and the contribution of D-cell disorders to diabetes mellitus, *Life Sci.* 20:2081–2085.

Unger, R. H., Dobbs, R. E., and Orci, L., 1978, Insulin, glucagon, and somatostatin secretion in the regulation of metabolism, *Annu. Rev. Physiol.* 40:307–343.

Vale, W., Ling, N., Rivier, J., Villarreal, J., Rivier, C., Brown, M., and Douglas, C., 1976, Anatomic and phylogenetic distribution of somatostatin, *Metabolism* 25(Suppl.):1491–1494.

Vale, W., Rivier, C., and Brown, M., 1977, Regulatory peptides of the hypothalamus, *Annu. Rev. Physiol.* 39:473–527.

Valverde, I., Rigopoulou, D., Exton, J., Ohneda, A., Eisentraut, A., and Unger, R. H., 1968, Demonstration and characterization of a second fraction of glucagon-like immunoreactivity in jejunal extracts, *Am. J. Med. Sci.* 255:415–420.

Valverde, I., Villanueva, M. L., Lozano, I., and Marco, J., 1974, Presence of glucagon immunoreactivity in the globulin fraction of human plasma ("big plasma glucagon"), *J. Clin. Endocrinol. Metab.* 39:1090–1098.

Valverde, I., Dobbs, R., and Unger, R. H., 1975, Heterogeneity of plasma glucagon immunoreactivity in normal, depancreatized, and alloxan diabetic dogs, *Metabolism* **24**:1021–1028.

Valverde, I., Lemon, H. M., Kessinger, A., and Unger, R. H., 1976, Distribution of plasma glucagon immunoreactivity in a patient with a suspected glucagonoma, *J. Clin. Endocrinol. Metab.* **42**:804–808.

Vidnes, J., and Oyasaeter, S., 1977, Glucagon deficiency causing severe neonatal hypoglycemià in a patient with normal insulin secretion, *Pediatr. Res.* **11**:943–949.

Villanueva, M. L., Hedo, J. A., and Marco, J., 1976, Plasma glucagon immunoreactivity in a totally pancreatectomized patient, *Diabetologia* **12**:613–616.

Vinicor, F., Higdon, G., and Clark, C. M., Jr., 1977, Effects of somatostatin on the hepatic adenylate cyclase system in the rat, *Endocrinology* **101**:1071–1077.

Von Schenck, H., 1977, Production and characterization of an antiserum against pancreatic glucagon, *Clin. Chim. Acta* **80**(3):455–463.

Vranic, M., Pek, S., and Kawamori, R., 1974, Increased "glucagon immunoreactivity" (IRG) in plasma of totally depancreatized dogs, *Diabetes* **23**:905–912.

Vranic, M., Kawamori, R., Pek, S., Koracevic, N., and Wrenshall, G. A., 1976, The essentiality of insulin and the role of glucagon in regulating glucose utilization and production during strenuous exercise in dogs, *J. Clin. Invest.* **57**:245–255.

Wahren, J., and Felig, P., 1976, Influence of somatostatin on carbohydrate disposal and absorption in diabetes mellitus, *Lancet* **2**:1213–1216.

Wahren, J., Felig, P., and Hagenfeldt, L., 1976, Effect of protein ingestion on splanchnic and leg metabolism in normal man and in patients with diabetes mellitus, *J. Clin. Invest.* **57**:987–999.

Warne, G. L., Alford, F. P., Chisholm, D. J., and Court, J., 1977, Glucagon and diabetes: Complete suppression of glucagon by insulin in human diabetes, *Clin. Endocrinol.* **6**:277–284.

Weir, G. C., Turner, R. C., and Martin, D. B., 1973, Glucagon radioimmunoassay using antiserum 30K: Interference by plasma, *Horm. Metab. Res.* **5**:241–244.

Weir, G. C., Knowlton, S. D., Atkins, R. F., McKennan, K. X., and Martin, D. B., 1976, Glucagon secretion from the perfused pancreas of streptozotocin-treated rats, *Diabetes* **25**:275–282.

Weir, G. C., Samols, E., Ramseur, R., Day, J. A., Jr., and Patel, Y. C., 1977a, Influence of glucose and glucagon upon somatostatin secretion from the isolated perfused canine pancreas, *Clin. Res.* **25**:403A.

Weir, G. C., Horton, E. S., Aoki, T. T., Slovik, D., Jaspan, J., and Rubenstein, A. H., 1977b, Secretion by glucagonomas of a possible glucagon precursor, *J. Clin. Invest.* **59**:325–330.

Welton, A. F., Lad, P. M., Newby, A. C., Yamamura, H., Nicosia, S., and Rodbell, M., 1977, Solubilization and separation of the glucagon receptor and adenylate cyclase in guanine nucleotide–sensitive states, *J. Biol. Chem.* **252**(17):5947–5950.

Wilson, R. M., Boden, G., Shore, L. S., and Essa-Koumar, N., 1977, Effect of somatostatin on meal-stimulated pancreatic exocrine secretions in dogs, *Diabetes* **26**:7–10.

Wise, J. K., Hendler, R., and Felig, P., 1973, Evidence of alpha cell function by infusion of alanine in normal, diabetic, and obese subjects, *N. Engl. J. Med.* **288**:487–490.

Wollheim, C. B., Blondel, B., Renold, A. E., and Sharp. G. W. G., 1977a, Somatostatin inhibition of pancreatic glucagon release from monolayer cultures and interactions with calcium, *Endocrinology* **101**:911–919.

Wollheim, C. B., Kikuchi, M., Renold, A. E., and Sharp, G. W. G., 1977b, Somatostatin- and epinephrine-induced modifications of $^{45}Ca^{++}$ fluxes and insulin release in rat pancreatic islets maintained in tissue culture, *J. Clin. Invest.* **60**:1165–1173.

Woods, S. C., and Porte, D., Jr., 1974, Neural control of the endocrine pancreas, *Physiol. Rev.* **54**:596–619.

Yamamoto, T., Raskin, P., Aydin, I., and Unger, R. H., 1979, The effects of insulin on the response of immunoreactive glucagon to an intravenous glucose load in human diabetes (submitted for publication).

Recent Advances in Body Fuel Metabolism

Philip Felig and Veikko Koivisto

9.1. Introduction

The major fuels involved in body metabolism are carbohydrate, fat (including ketones), and amino acids. In this review, we focus on recent studies that deal with the regulation of fuel production and utilization. Hormonal interactions, particularly as they relate to diabetes mellitus, are discussed. In addition, the effects of exercise on fuel homeostasis and insulin metabolism are reviewed.

9.2. Glucose Metabolism

9.2.1. Is Glucagon Essential in Diabetes?

The relative importance of glucagon excess and insulin deficiency in the pathogenesis of diabetes has been the subject of considerable investigative interest and debate in recent years (Felig *et al.*, 1976b; Unger, 1976). The discovery of somatostatin, a polypeptide that inhibits secretion

PHILIP FELIG and VEIKKO KOIVISTO • Section of Endocrinology, Department of Internal Medicine, Yale University School of Medicine, New Haven, Connecticut 06510.

of glucagon (Koerker *et al.*, 1974) as well as insulin (Siler *et al.*, 1973), has provided a powerful tool for investigating the roles of these glucoregulatory hormones. In addition, recent studies in pancreatectomized humans have provided additional insights.

9.2.1.1. Somatostatin-Induced Hypoglucagonemia

In *The Year in Metabolism 1977*, the effects of prolonged suppression (6–7 hr) of glucagon and insulin secretion were reviewed (Felig and Koivisto, 1978). In normal subjects, ongoing infusion of somatostatin results in an initial fall in glucose production and plasma glucose. However, after 2 hr, glucose production rises to values in excess of basal preinfusion levels while plasma glucose levels reach fasting concentrations of 150–160 mg/100 ml, despite continued suppression of glucagon secretion (Sherwin *et al.*, 1977a). Those data were interpreted as indicating that insulin lack rather than glucagon excess is the primary determinant of the diabetic state.

The failure to observe more severe hyperglycemia with prolonged infusion of somatostatin could be interpreted as indicating the need for basal or increased glucagon secretion to achieve full expression of the diabetic syndrome (i.e., severe hyperglycemia). To test this hypothesis, Sherwin *et al.* (1977b) infused somatostatin along with replacement doses of glucagon to normal subjects for 6 hr. The addition of glucagon caused a 2-fold increase in glucose production during the initial 1–2 hr of infusion. However, by 3 hr glucose production fell to slightly below preinfusion levels despite ongoing infusion of glucagon. Thus, after 3 hr, glucagon replacement had no stimulatory effect on glucose production. Furthermore, after 6 hr of infusion, the blood glucose level was identical regardless of the presence or absence of glucagon in the infusate. These data indicate that the failure to observe more severe hyperglycemia with prolonged infusion of somatostatin cannot be ascribed to glucagon lack. The more likely explanation is that some insulin secretion persists in the face of somatostatin infusion.

Further evidence that changes in insulin rather than glucagon secretion govern the overall response to somatostatin is derived from studies with maturity-onset diabetics and patients with somatostatin-producing tumors.

Tamborlane *et al.* (1977) infused somatostatin for 5 hr to maturity-onset diabetics. The infusion resulted in a sustained 45–55% fall in plasma insulin and glucagon concentration. Plasma glucose, which before infusion ranged from 120 to 295 mg/100 ml, initially fell by 20–25 mg/100 ml but returned to baseline by 2–3 hr and thereafter rose to levels 45–50 mg/100 ml higher than in saline-infused controls. The rise in plasma glucose was inversely proportional to the fall in insulin. Plasma branched-chain amino acids (leucine, isoleucine, and valine), which are known to rise in circumstances of insulin deficiency (Felig *et al.*, 1970a), increased by 40–45%. In addition, a 5-fold increase in betahydroxybutyrate was observed during somatostatin infusion (Tamborlane *et al.*, 1977). These findings thus indicate that fasting hyperglycemia in maturity-onset diabetes is not reduced to normal by suppression of glucagon secretion with somatostatin. In contrast, during hypoinsulinemia caused by somatostatin, an intensification of hyperglycemia, hyperketonemia, and hyperaminoacidemia occurs, thus arguing against the use of somatostatin in diabetics with residual insulin secretion (Tamborlane *et al.*, 1977).

During the past year, two patients with a somatostatin-producing tumor were reported (Ganda *et al.*, 1977; Larsson *et al.*, 1977). High somatostatin secretion resulted in a low level of plasma glucagon and insulin (Ganda *et al.*, 1977). Despite the lack of glucagon, both patients had diabetes. These findings thus underscore the primary role of insulin lack rather than glucagon excess in the development of the diabetic syndrome (Felig *et al.*, 1976b). In addition, the patient of Larsson *et al.* (1977) had steatorrhea, which is in keeping with the earlier observations of Wahren and Felig (1976) that somatostatin may interfere with nutrient absorption.

9.2.1.2. Pancreatectomized Man

Recent studies in pancreatectomized subjects have further clarified the effect of hypoglucagonemia on glucose homeostasis (Barnes and Bloom, 1976; Barnes *et al.*, 1977a,b). In pancreatectomized subjects, no basal glucagon was detectable in the plasma and no glucagon response to arginine infusion occurred (Barnes and Bloom, 1976). Nevertheless, these patients demonstrated marked fasting hyperglycemia (251 ± 46 mg/100 ml), and hyperketonemia. The elevations in glucose and ketones were, however, less than those observed in similarly insulin-deprived diabetics in whom glucagon was available (Barnes *et al.*, 1977a,b).

Taken together, the data involving infusion of exogenous somatostatin, endogenous production of somatostatin by islet cell tumors, and observations in pancreatectomized man all fail to support an essential role for glucagon in diabetes. Fasting hyperglycemia and hyperketonemia of moderate to marked degree occur in the face of suppression or total absence of glucagon secretion. The failure to observe more severe hyperglycemia with somatostatin infusions is not due to the lack of glucagon but reflects ongoing availability of some insulin (Sherwin *et al.*, 1977b). Nevertheless, in circumstances of absolute insulin deficiency, glucagon secretion can result in further deterioration of the diabetic state.

9.2.2. Effects of Hyperglucagonemia

9.2.2.1. Normal Man

A physiologic role for glucagon in the stimulation of glucose production is recognized in three circumstances: (1) starvation (Wahren *et al.*, 1977); (2) protein feeding (Unger *et al.*, 1969; Wahren *et al.*, 1976); and (3) exercise (Felig *et al.*, 1972b). The stimulatory effect of physiologic hyperglucagonemia on hepatic glucose production was demonstrated by Felig *et al.* (1976a) to be evanescent, lasting less than 30–45 min. In a subsequent report, Bomboy *et al.* (1977) noted a similar transient effect of glucagon on splanchnic glucose production in normal as well as diabetic subjects. The loss of responsiveness to hyperglucagonemia could not be ascribed to glycogen depletion, since pharmacologic doses of glucagon continued to elicit an increase in splanchnic glucose output (Bomboy *et al.*, 1977).

As reviewed previously, Sherwin *et al.* (1976a) reported that persistent hyperglucagonemia (approximately 300 pg/ml) fails to elicit a deterioration in glucose tolerance in normal subjects. Some questions were raised regarding those observations because (1) glucagon was infused via a peripheral rather than portal vein; (2) whole blood was added to the infusate (to prevent adsorption to tubing) and may have inactivated the biological action of glucagon; and (3) a 3-hr period of hyperglucagonemia antedated the administration of glucose, during which time the diabetogenic effects of glucagon may have been dissipated (Unger, 1976). To answer these objections, Holst *et al.* (1977), studying normal subjects, infused glucagon via a portal as well as peripheral vein for 60 min prior to and 120 min following a 25 g i.v. glucose load. Human albumin rather than whole blood was added to the glucagon infusate to prevent adsorption to tubing. The findings indicated that during the glucagon infusion, glucose tolerance remained within normal limits and was uninfluenced by the route (portal vs. peripheral) of glucagon administration (Holst *et al.*, 1977). These data thus confirm the earlier observations of Sherwin *et al.* (1976b) that physiologic hyperglucagonemia does not of itself bring about a diabetic state in previously normal subjects.

9.2.2.2. Diabetes

The effect of hyperglucagonemia on glucose homeostasis in insulin-dependent diabetics was studied by Raskin and Unger (1977). In a previous report, Sherwin *et al.* (1976b) observed no change in plasma glucose levels in insulin-dependent diabetics infused with glucagon so long as insulin was administered in its usual dosage. The infusion rate employed by Raskin and Unger was similar to that used by Sherwin *et al.* (1976b), resulting in a 3- to 5-fold rise in the plasma glucagon level. Before and during the glucagon infusion, the patients received an infusion of insulin at a rate of 1–2 U/hr. During the glucagon infusion, mean plasma glucose levels, measured at 2-hr intervals, increased by 25–45%. Close inspection of the data reveals, however, that increments in plasma glucose occurred almost exclusively during the first 6–12 hr of the infusion, and in only one subject was the increment greater than 100 mg/100 ml above pre- or postinfusion values. The data thus indicate that if glucagon has an effect in the diabetic on plasma glucose in the face of insulin, it is transient and of small magnitude. A more substantial increase, however, was observed in urinary glucose output during glucagon infusion (82–152 g) as compared with that during control day (11–36 g). This 4- to 5-fold increase in urinary glucose output in contrast to the slight rise in hyperglycemia suggests that glucagon may induce changes in the renal handling of glucose. Interestingly, recent studies in normal man demonstrated that a 2-hr glucagon infusion (10 ng/kg per min) significantly increases glomerular filtration rate, filtration fraction, and urinary β_2-microglobulin excretion rate (Parving *et al.*, 1977). Glucagon-induced changes in kidney function (Parving *et al.*, 1977) may thus explain the marked rise in urinary glucose excretion observed in the face of transient, modest elevations in plasma glucose (Raskin and Unger, 1977).

9.2.2.3. Uremia

In addition to the necessity for insulin deficiency, under certain circumstances, altered tissue responsiveness to glucagon may contribute to the diabetogenic effect of this hormone. The importance of augmented tissue sensitivity to glucagon in the pathogenesis of glucose intolerance is suggested by observations in uremic man (Sherwin *et al.*, 1976a). Chronic renal failure is characterized by an increased incidence of glucose intolerance, insulin resistance, and a 3- to 4-fold increase in circulating glucagon. Following chronic dialysis, glucose tolerance and insulin sensitivity return to normal in the absence of changes in plasma glucagon. On the basis of these observations, hyperglucagonemia did not appear to contribute to uremia-induced glucose intolerance. However, the role of glucagon in uremia is evident when responsiveness to this hormone is examined. When glucagon is infused to uremic subjects (nondialyzed) in physiologic doses, the glycemic effect is increased 3- to 4-fold in comparison with healthy controls (Sherwin *et al.*, 1976a). Furthermore, a direct linear correlation is observed between performance on glucose tolerance testing and the glycemic response to glucagon infusion. This augmented glycemic response to glucagon returns to normal following dialysis, thereby accounting for improved glucose tolerance despite persistence of the hyperglucagonemia (Sherwin *et al.*, 1976a). Recent studies with the use of the uremic rat model provide a cellular mechanism for these changes in responsiveness to glucagon (Soman and Felig, 1977). In 70 and 90% nephrectomized rats, glucagon binding to liver membranes is increased 2- to 3-fold. Furthermore, the increase in glucagon binding was accompanied by a proportionate increase in glucagon-stimulated adenylate cyclase activity. In fact, the curves describing glucagon-binding and glucagon-stimulated adenylate cyclase activity at varying concentrations of glucagon were superimposable (Soman and Felig, 1977). Thus, changes in glucagon responsiveness in uremia may result from augmented binding of this hormone to target cells. These findings provide the first evidence of an important role for glucagon receptors in a syndrome of carbohydrate intolerance.

9.2.3. Glucose Production: Gluconeogenesis from Alanine

In the postabsorptive, overnight-fasted state, approximately 75% of hepatic glucose output is due to glycogenolysis and the rest is derived from gluconeogenesis (Felig, 1973). In contrast, in circumstances in which liver glycogen stores are depleted, such as after prolonged fasting (Felig *et al.*, 1969) or during pregnancy (Felig *et al.*, 1972a), ketotic hypoglycemia (Pagliara *et al.*, 1972), or long-term exercise (Ahlborg *et al.*, 1974), hepatic glucose output is dependent on gluconeogenesis rather than glycogenolysis. In those conditions, the availability of alanine, which accounts for more than half the total amino acid utilization for hepatic gluconeogenesis, becomes important in the regulation of blood glucose concentration (Felig, 1975).

Recent studies have provided new information regarding the effect of altered availability of alanine, glucagon, and insulin on hepatic gluconeogenesis and on the intracellular mechanisms regulating gluconeogenesis from alanine. Saccá *et al.* (1977b) studied the effect of hyperalaninemia on hepatic glucose production in the dog. Alanine was infused for 60 min at a constant rate (2 mg/kg per min). Hepatic glucose production and glucose utilization were determined using a primed constant infusion of [2-^{3}H]glucose. Alanine infusion resulted in a 2-fold rise in plasma alanine concentration, a 30% rise in insulin, and a 77% increase in plasma glucagon. During the infusion, both the glucose production and disappearance rate rose. However, the production rate, which was proportional to the increase in plasma glucagon, rose more than the disappearance rate, resulting in hyperglycemia. Interestingly, at the end of the alanine infusion, the glucose production returned to baseline despite ongoing hyperglucagonemia and a fall in plasma insulin. These findings thus indicate that the effect of endogenous hyperglucagonemia on hepatic glucose production is transient even in the presence of hyperalaninemia (Saccá et al., 1977b).

Jennings et al. (1977) infused somatostatin along with insulin to induce isolated glucagon deficiency with normal insulin levels. During hypoglucagonemia, the conversion rate of [^{14}C]glucose was reduced by 44 ± 9%. In contrast, when isolated insulin deficiency with normal glucagon levels was produced, the rate of alanine conversion to glucose was enhanced by 74 ± 7%. Somatostatin together with insulin and glucagon replacement had no effect on alanine conversion to glucose.

Recently, there has been interest in the intracellular mechanism by which glucagon stimulates gluconeogenesis from alanine. Glucagon is known to stimulate hepatic uptake of some amino acids, which led to the suggestion that it might stimulate gluconeogenesis by increasing the availability of alanine in the liver cell (Mallette et al., 1969; Chiasson et al., 1975). By using a perfused rat liver, Ayuso-Parrilla et al. (1977) demonstrated that addition of alanine alone to the perfusion medium resulted in a significant rise in the intracellular concentrations of alanine, pyruvate, and oxaloacetate with a subsequent 5-fold rise in the rate of hepatic glucose production. When glucagon was added to the perfusion medium along with alanine, there was a further rise in intracellular alanine levels and a 50% increase in glucose production above that observed with alanine alone. However, the intracellular concentration of the intermediates pyruvate and oxaloacetate was decreased by glucagon. In other studies, intraperitoneal administration of glucagon to starved rats resulted in a marked rise in blood glucose despite a decrease in hepatic alanine and pyruvate concentrations. These findings thus suggest that glucagon-induced stimulation of gluconeogenesis cannot be explained primarily on the basis of acceleration of transport of alanine into the hepatocyte.

Singh and Snyder (1978) reported in rats that 1-thyroxine (T$_4$) increases gluconeogenesis from alanine. By using a perfused rat liver, they demonstrated that hepatic conversion of alanine to glucose was markedly enhanced in thyrotoxic rats as compared with normals. T$_4$ treatment increased the transport of alanine from the extracellular to the intracellular space in the liver. Intracellular pyruvate concentration was decreased, whereas intermediates in gluconeogenesis between phosphoenolpyrutate and 1,3-diphosphoglycerate were significantly increased. Thus, the control site (crossover point) for the effect of T$_4$ on gluconeogenesis seems to lie between pyruvate and phosphoenolpyruvate. The data thus suggest that T$_4$ stimulates hepatic gluconeogenesis from alanine via a mechanism that involves increased intracellular transport of alanine and accelerated conversion of pyruvate to phosphoenolpyruvate. These changes are similar to those reported with glucagon.

9.2.4. The Counterregulatory Response to Hypoglycemia

The counterregulatory response to hypoglycemia involves several hormonal factors. Garber et al. (1976a) demonstrated that after insulin injection, a hormonal response was initiated when the blood glucose level was 40–45 mg/100 ml. An increase in plasma catecholamines was observed first; a rise in plasma glucagon, cortisol, or growth hormone occurred 10–30 min later. These findings suggested that catecholamines, rather than glucagon or other hormones, play a major role in initiating the rebound in glucose production after insulin injection (Garber et al., 1976a).

The role of glucagon in the response to hypoglycemia was further studied in the rat by Saccá et al. (1977a). Rats received a somatostatin infusion, during which no glucagon response to insulin-induced hypoglycemia was observed. Control rats without a somatostatin infusion showed an 8- to 9-fold rise in glucagon during hypoglycemia. In response to the insulin injection, blood glucose fell to a nadir by 20–30 min, which was virtually identical in the two groups. The early part (20–30 min) of the recovery phase was also similar in the two groups. However, during the late recovery (at 50–60 min after insulin injection), blood glucose was significantly lower in glucagon-deficient rats.

These findings thus support the view that a rise in plasma glucagon may augment the glycemic rebound to insulin-induced hypoglycemia but does not initiate it (Garber et al., 1976a; Saccá et al., 1977a).

Hypoglycemia after ethanol comsumption in glycogen-depleted subjects is a common clinical finding. Joffe et al. (1977) recently measured plasma insulin and glucagon levels in subjects with ethanol-induced hypoglycemia. The patients had a history of excessive alcohol intake with binge drinking and no food consumption for several hours before their admission to the hospital in a stuporous state. Their plasma insulin levels were low (7 ± 1 μU/ml), as expected. Plasma glucagon concentration was increased 2- to 3-fold above normal. These findings indicate that hyperglucagonemia, even in the presence of hypoinsulinemia, cannot overcome the inhibitory effect of ethanol on hepatic glucose production (Joffe et al., 1977).

There is anecdotal clincial evidence in diabetics that hypoglycemic symptoms may occur in response to a falling blood glucose concentration before absolute hypoglycemia is achieved. As noted above, when the blood glucose falls to hypoglycemic levels after insulin injection, counterregulatory hormonal responses occur. Whether this hormonal response occurs when glucose falls from hyperglycemic levels to normoglycemic levels was recently studied in normal man by DeFronzo *et al.* (1977). By using a primed continuous infusion of glucose (glucose-clamp technique), blood glucose was raised to 250–300 mg/100 ml and maintained at that concentration for 1 hr. Thereafter, the glucose infusion was stopped and the blood glucose concentration was allowed to drop spontaneously. Despite a rapidly falling blood glucose concentration, no increase in plasma catecholamines, glucagon, cortisol, or growth hormone was observed as long as the blood glucose remained above a normal fasting level. Thus, in normal man, a fall in blood glucose from hyperglycemic levels does not trigger a counterregulatroy hormonal response before absolute hypoglycemia has been achieved (DeFronzo *et al.*, 1977). It should, however, be emphasized that this conclusion may not apply to chronically hyperglycemic diabetic patients.

In view of the importance of catecholamines in the response to hypoglycemia, treatment with antiadrenergic drugs might be expected to accentuate the likelihood of insulin-induced hypoglycemia in diabetic patients. Deacon *et al.* (1977) examined the effect of three β-adrenergic blocking drugs on insulin hypoglycemia in diabetics. The agents were propranolol (a nonselective β-blocker); acebutolol, an agent that primarily blocks β_1-receptors (heart) but has some effect on β_2-receptors (liver and muscle); and atenolol, an agent that is specific for β_2-receptors. The results showed that propranolol delayed recovery from hypoglycemia, acebutolol potentiated the magnitude of hypoglycemia, while atenolol (the highly specific β_1-blocker), did not differ from a placebo, Thus, β_1-specific adrenergic blocking drugs may be safer than nonselective drugs when used in insulin-treated diabetics (Deacon *et al.*, 1977).

9.3. Ketone and Fatty Acid Metabolism

9.3.1. Hormonal Control of Ketogenesis

Both lipid mobilization and hepatic conversion of free fatty acids (FFA) to ketone bodies are under hormonal control involving insulin, glucagon, catecholamines, corticosteroids, and growth hormone. Previous studies employing physiologic hyperglucagonemia or growth hormone excess demonstrated that these hormones cause hyperketonemia only during insulin deficiency, but are not ketogenic as long as physiologic amounts of insulin are available (Schade and Eaton, 1976; Gerich *et al.*, 1976).

More recently, studies employing somatostatin infusions have further clarified the role of insulin deficiency and glucagon in the regulation of ketogenesis in the dog (Keller *et al.*, 1977). When somatostatin was infused

along with basal amounts of glucagon to cause a selective insulin deficiency, a 2-fold increase in hepatic ketone body production was observed.
To increase substrate supply for ketogenesis, intralipid plus heparin were
added to the infusion. As a result, an additional 2-fold rise in ketone body
production occurred during selective insulin deficiency. The data suggest
that the stimulatory effect of selective insulin deficiency on ketone production is mediated, in part, by an intrahepatic mechanism independent
of FFA availability or uptake (Keller *et al.*, 1977).

The role of insulin and glucagon in ketone body production was
further evaluated in studies involving pancreatectomized patients (Barnes
et al., 1977a,b; Barnes and Bloom, 1976). Over a 12-hr period following
insulin withdrawal, pancreatectomized subjects demonstrated an increase
of 1.8 ± 0.8 mmol/liter in plasma ketone bodies despite the absence of
detectable plasma glucagon. By contrast, in control diabetics, a 6-fold
increase in plasma glucagon was observed during insulin withdrawal,
which was accompained by an increase of 4.1 ± 0.7 mmol/liter in circulating ketone acids. These findings thus indicate that the presence of glucagon is not essential for the development of hyperketonemia. However,
during absolute insulin deficiency, hyperglucagonemia can intensify
ketone body production. These studies thus underscore the primary role
of insulin deficiency in the development of hyperketonemia (Felig *et al.*,
1976a). It should also be noted that the pancreatatomized patient may not
only have glucagon deficiency. For example, the possible role of pancreatic polypeptide in ketogenesis remains to be established.

In addition to insulin and glucagon, the role of norepinephrine and
glucocorticoids in the regulation of ketogenesis has been recently evaluated. Norepinephrine increases fatty acid mobilization and substrate availability, thus leading to enhanced ketone body production (Willms *et al.*,
1969). To determine whether norepinephrine has an effect on ketogenesis independent of its lipolytic action, Schade and Eaton (1977) infused
norepinephrine to diabetic subjects. A control group was injected with
heparin so as to raise their plasma FFA level comparable to that in subjects
with norepinephrine infusion. The norepinephrine-infused subjects demonstrated a greater rise in plasma ketone bodies than the heparin-injected
subjects. Schade and Eaton (1977) conclude that norepinephrine has a
ketogenic effect independent of substrate availability. Perusal of their data
indicates that this conclusion is open to question. Thus, the greater
ketonemic effect of norepinephrine was generally restricted to the latter
part of the infusion (30–60 min), at which time FFA levels were 2- to 3-
fold higher than in the heparin study, in which FFA fell rapidly after 30
min.

Using a similar experimental design (identical substrate supply in
experimental and control group), Schade *et al.* (1977) also demonstrated

that chronic glucocorticoid administration can increase plasma ketone body concentration. In contrast, acute glucocorticoid administration had no effect on ketone body level. These findings thus suggest that glucocorticoids can raise plasma ketone concentration independent of a lipolytic effect. Whether this hyperketonemic action is due to enhanced hepatic ketone production or decreased peripheral utilization remains to be established.

9.3.2. Role of Malonyl-Coenzyme A

Ingestion of glucose can reverse starvation ketosis. The underlying mechanism was postulated to be inhibition of lipolysis and intrahepatic oxidation of fatty acids to ketone acids (McGarry *et al.*, 1973). More recently, McGarry *et al.* (1977) provided a fascinating insight into the regulation of fatty acid oxidation in the liver. Employing a mitochondrial fraction of rat liver, the authors demonstrated that malonyl-CoA inhibited ketogenesis from oleic acid but not from octanoic acid. The site of inhibition was the carnitine acyltransferase-I reaction. This inhibitory effect of malony-CoA was specific and reversible.

Malonyl-CoA, which is a product of glucose oxidation, is also an intermediate in fatty acid synthesis from glucose. After carbohydrate feeding, the rate of fatty acid synthesis from glucose is high, resulting in a high malonyl-CoA concentration as well. In these circumstances, malonyl-CoA serves a dual role: it is a substrate for fat synthesis and a repressor of fat oxidation (McGarry *et al.*, 1977). In contrast, during starvation and in diabetes when the glucose utilization rate is low, malonyl-CoA concentration is diminished, resulting in uninhibited fatty acid oxidation and ketone body production in the liver (McGarry *et al.*, 1977; McGarry and Foster, 1977).

As noted in the preceding section, the stimulatory effect of glucagon on ketogenesis was suggested to be mediated by an intrahepatic mechanism (Keller *et al.*, 1977). Interestingly, recent studies have demonstrated that glucagon can decrease malonyl-CoA concentration in isolated hepatocytes (Cook *et al.*, 1977). Thus, the regulatory factor mediating the effect of both glucagon and glucose on ketogenesis could be malonyl-CoA.

9.3.3. Hypoketonemic Action of Alanine

In addition to glucose and insulin, alanine availability may influence plasma ketone concentration. Ozand *et al.* (1977) infused alanine to fasted rats so as to raise plasma alanine concentration to nonfasted levels. A rapid, dose-dependent fall in plasma betahydroxybutyrate concentration was observed. No significant change occurred in acetoacetate level. There was no relationship between the fall in betahydroxybutyrate and changes in plasma insulin, glucagon, fatty acids, or growth hormone. Administration of dichloracetate (which decreases ketone utilization) along with alanine did not prevent the hypoketonemic effect of alanine, suggesting that the fall in plasma ketones is due to a decrease in hepatic ketone production rather than an increase in peripheral utilization.

Because the hypoketonemic effect of alanine was specific for betahydroxybutyrate, mechanisms other than malonyl-CoA availability are likely to be involved as mediator. An intracellular redistribution of reducing equivalents, shifting the reducing capacity to cytosol and thus restricting the mitochondria from reducing acetoacetate to betahydroxybutyrate, was postulated (Ozand *et al.*, 1977).

9.4. Amino Acid Metabolism

9.4.1. Origin of Alanine Synthesized in Skeletal Muscle

A variety of *in vivo* and *in vitro* studies have established that alanine and glutamine are quantitatively the most important amino acids released by muscle (Felig, 1975). Since the output of alanine greatly exceeds its content in muscle protein, *in situ* synthesis of alanine from pyruvate by muscle tissue was proposed (Pozefsky *et al.*, 1969). Other studies demonstrating that alanine is the major gluconeogenic precursor extracted by the liver led to the formulation of the glucose–alanine cycle (Mallette *et al.*, 1969; Felig *et al.*, 1970b; Felig, 1973). In this cycle, alanine is synthesized in muscle by transamination of glucose-derived pyruvate. The alanine is then released from muscle and taken up by liver, where its carbon skeleton is reconverted to glucose. Subsequent studies have shown that the branched-chain amino acids have a special role in providing the amino groups for alanine synthesis in muscle (Buse *et al.*, 1972; Odessey *et al.*, 1974; Palaiologos and Felig, 1976).

As discussed in last year's review, a variety of studies in intact man in the resting state, in exercise, in lactic acidosis, in McArdle's syndrome, and in some types of hereditary myoglobinuria strongly support the conclusion that the carbon skeleton of the alanine synthesized in muscle is derived from glucose as predicted by the glucose–alanine cycle (Felig and Koivisto, 1978). *In vitro* studies, however, have yielded conflicting results. Odessey *et al.* (1974), using isotopically labeled glucose, demonstrated that at least 60% of alanine released by rat diaphragm is formed by transamination of glucose-derived pyruvate. In contrast, Garber *et al.* (1976b,c) and Goldstein and Newsholme (1976) suggested that the carbon skeleton of alanine is not glucose-derived but is formed from other amino acids in muscle protein, notably valine, isoleucine, and perphaps leucine. These workers challenged the concept of the glucose–alanine cycle because (1) a variety of amino acids stimulated alanine output from incubated muscle, (2) inhibitors of glycolysis such as iodoacetate (Garber *et al.*, 1976c) and flouride (Goldstein and Newsholme, 1976) fail to reduce alanine output, and (3) addition of isoleucine increased the output of lactate and pyruvate as well as alanine from muscle (Goldstein and Newsholme, 1976). It should be noted that none of these observations involved isotopic studies tracing the origin of alanine, nor did they include quantitative assessments of the potential rate of pyruvate formation from amino acids released in proteolysis as compared with glycolytic rates in muscle.

In a subsequent series of elegant studies, Chang and Goldberg (1978a–c) reexamined the observations noted above and added a variety of new data that indicate that exogenous glucose molecules rather than protein-derived amino acids are the source of the carbon skeletons for alanine synthesis as originally formulated in the glucose–alanine cycle. Using incubated diaphragm as well as extensor digitorum longus and soleus, Chang and Goldberg (1978a) demonstrated the following: (1) Stimulation of alanine synthesis by branched-chain amino acids is explicable simply by increased transamination of pyruvate. (2) A specific inhibitor or glycolysis, 2-deoxyglucose, clearly decreases muscle alanine synthesis. (3) The failure of iodoacetate and fluoride to interfere with alanine synthesis was not confirmed. Furthermore, the metabolic effect of these compounds was shown not to be limited to inhibition of glycolysis, but included stimulation of proteolysis. The failure of Garber *et al.* (1976a) and Goldstein and Newsholme (1976) to observe a fall in alanine output despite inhibition of glycolysis thus may reflect simultaneous stimulation of proteolysis. (4) Using ^{14}C-labeled amino acids, it was clearly shown by Chang and Goldberg that only valine, isoleucine, glutamate, aspartate, and asparigine can provide tricarboxylic acid cycle intermediates from which pyruvate can be formed in muscle tissue. (5) Even assuming that the carbon skeletons of these five amino acids are quantitavely converted to pyruvate, comparison of the rates of glycolysis (determined with [^{3}H]glucose) and proteolysis in muscle tissue indicated that over 97% of the carbons of the alanine, lactate, and pyruvate formed in muscle are derived from blood-borne glucose, while only 3% can be derived from amino acids generated by protein breakdown. (6) Studies of the metabolic fate of the five amino acids that are potential precursors of pyruvate in muscle indicate that their carbon skeletons are converted to glutamine (50%) or CO_2, while less than 2% appear as alanine (Chang and Goldberg, 1978b). (7) Leucine and isoleucine were shown to inhibit pyruvate (and glucose) oxidation (Chang and Goldberg, 1978c). This inhibition thus accounts for the increased release of pyruvate and lactate from muscle after addition of these amino acids (Goldstein and Newsholme, 1976), even though the carbon skeletons of isoleucine and leucine are not themselves converted to pyruvate by muscle tissue.

In summary, the work of Chang and Goldberg provides direct isotopic and quantitative evidence that the carbon skeletons of virtually all the alanine synthesized in muscle are glucose-derived. Furthermore, previous data purporting to show a dissociation between glycolysis and alanine synthesis are uninterpretable (and not confirmed), since the glycolytic inhibitors employed (fluoride and iodoacetate) also accelerate proteolysis, while a more specific glycolytic inhibitor (2-deoxyglucose) does indeed block muscle alanine synthesis. In addition, the stimulatory effect of branched-chain amino acids on pyruvate and lactate release from muscle is not due to conversion of the carbon skeletons of these amino acids to pyruvate, but is a consequence of inhibition of oxidation of glucose-derived pyruvate. Taken together, these data provide direct confirmation of the original formulation of the glucose–alanine cycle.

9.4.2. Metabolic Fate of Glutamine Utilized by Intestine

As noted above, glutamine as well as alanine account for much of the alpha amino nitrogen released by muscle. A variety of studies have shown that the kidney is the major site of glutamine uptake, particularly in starvation or acidosis or both (Felig, 1975). Net uptake of glutamine by the splanchnic bed has also been observed, raising the possibility of its being an important gluconeogenic substrate (Marliss et al., 1971). However, studies examining arterial–portal venous differences in man have shown that the gut rather than the liver is the site of virtually the entire splanchnic uptake of glutamine (Felig et al., 1973a,b).

More recently, the in vivo metabolic fate of glutamine extracted by gut tissue was examined by means of arterial–venous differences and isotopic tracer studies (Windmueller and Spaeth, 1978). In perfused segments of rat jejunum, net fractional extraction of glutamine was 30% as compared with 10–15% for ketone acids and 3% for glucose. More important, over 50% of the extracted glutamine was converted to CO_2, accounting for 35% of total CO_2 production by intestine. In contrast, only 4% of glutamine carbon was converted to alanine; over 80% of the alanine carbon released by intestine was derived from glucose. These data thus indicate that glutamine is an important oxidative fuel for intestine. The findings also demonstrate that no more than 30% of the carbon skeletons of glutamine taken up by the gut are released and made available to the liver as gluconeogenic substrate in the form of lactate, alanine, or other amino acids (Windmueller and Spaeth, 1978).

9.5. Fuel Metabolism in Exercise

The increased requirement for energy during exercise causes a variety of changes in body fuel metabolism. A number of recent reports have provided new information regarding the roles of glucose, glycogen, and FFA during exercise in normal man. In addition, new insights have been obtained on glucoregulatory mechanisms in diabetes during exercise.

9.5.1. Influence of Glucose Ingestion before Exercise

Prolonged exercise leads to a fall in blood glucose due to the failure of splanchnic glucose output to keep pace with the increased glucose consumption by the exercising muscle. Glucose feeding during prolonged exercise is followed by a rise in blood glucose level and an increase in carbohydrate utilization, resulting in improved physical work capacity (Ahlborg and Felig, 1976).

The effect of glucose ingestion prior to exercise on the response to prolonged work was recently examined by Ahlborg and Felig (1977). Normal subjects ingested 200 g glucose before 4 hr of bicycle exercise at 30% of maximal oxygen uptake. The response was compared with that in controls who did not receive any glucose before a comparable 4-hr period of exercise. In the glucose-fed subjects, during exercise, arterial glucose levels were increased by 30–40%, whereas arterial glycerol was markedly reduced. In addition, FFA levels failed to increase during the initial 2 hr in the glucose-fed group, whereas they rose in controls throughout the exercise. Plasma insulin concentration was 2- to 3-fold greater than in controls, whereas glucagon levels, which rose 4-fold in controls, were 60–70% lower in glucose-fed subjects. Glucose uptake by the exercising leg was higher in the glucose-fed subjects, accounting for 48–58% of leg oxygen consumption as compared with 27–41% in controls. The total splanchnic glucose escape after glucose ingestion was 80–140% higher than in controls, although splanchnic uptake of gluconeogenic precursors (lactate, pyruvate, and glycerol) was reduced by 60–100% in the glucose-fed group.

These data thus indicate that glucose ingestion prior to prolonged exercise results in increased glucose delivery to peripheral tissue and augmented glucose uptake by the exercising leg in association with decreased hepatic gluconeogenesis. Furthermore, the exercise-induced fall in plasma insulin and rise in glucagon concentration are prevented and lipolysis is diminished. The overall effect of glucose feeding prior to prolonged exercise is thus to promote glucose delivery and uptake by exercising muscle and to spare body fat stores and utilization of gluconeogenic substrates. A similar conclusion was reached by Pirnay *et al.* (1977) in studies using [^{13}C]glucose.

Interestingly, total splanchnic glucose output over 3 hr in the glucose-fed exercising group could account for 57% of the ingested load. In nonexercising subjects, splanchnic glucose output amounts to 40% of the ingested load. Thus, exercise has the effect of enhancing peripheral delivery of ingested glucose. Nevertheless, even in circumstances of exercise, the liver remains a major site (40–45%) of disposal of ingested glucose.

9.5.2. Influence of Ethanol Ingestion

Enhanced hepatic gluconeogenesis is an important source of fuel during prolonged exercise. Ethanol alters the redox potential in the liver and inhibits splanchnic uptake of gluconeogenic precursors (lactate, glycerol), thus resulting in decreased gluconeogenesis and hypoglycemia (Freinkel *et al.*, 1967; Krebs, 1968). Ethanol may also lower circulating levels of FFA (Jones *et al.*, 1965), which is another important fuel during exercise. The interaction of ethanol and exercise on hepatic gluconeogenesis and the turnover of FFA was recently examined. When ethanol was infused to normal subjects throughout a 3-hr exercise period, gluconeogenesis declined by 50%, and splanchnic glucose output, which remained elevated in the control group, decreased by 40% (Juhlin-Dannfelt *et al.*, 1977). Furthermore, leg uptake of glucose remained unchanged as exercise was prolonged during ethanol infusion, but rose in control subjects by 3 hr of exercise. Arterial glucose levels tended to show a greater fall in the ethanol group. However, due to the concomitant decrease in glucose production and uptake, hypoglycemic levels were reached only in individual subjects (Juhlin-Dannfelt *et al.*, 1977). Arterial FFA concentration, which was reduced by ethanol at rest, rose comparable to controls during exercise and accounted for a comparable portion of leg oxidative metabolism in both groups. Acetate and lactate released from the liver after ethanol infusion were taken up by skeletal muscle, contributing about 10% of leg oxidative metabolism during exercise (Jorfeldt and Juhlin-Dannfelt, 1977).

These data thus indicate that ethanol reduces both glucose production and utilization during exercise, but fails to interfere with lipolysis and FFA utilization.

9.5.3. Glucose-Sparing Effect of Free Fatty Acids

Several studies during the past year have extended our knowledge regarding the proposal originally made by Randle *et al.* (1963) that increased availability of FFA can decrease carbohydrate utilization in exercising muscle.

By using a perfused rat hindquarter, Rennie et al. (1976) demonstrated that increased availability of FFA has a glycogen-sparing effect in red muscle fibers. However, in white fibers, whose capacity to oxidize FFA is very low, FFA had no effect on glycogen depletion. These findings in perfused skeletal muscle were further extended by Rennie and Holloszy (1977). As compared with the absence of FFA, addition of oleate at 1.8 mM to the perfusion media resulted in a 30% fall in muscle glucose uptake and lactate production both at rest and during muscle contraction. In addition, during sciatic nerve stimulation, the presence of oleate protected against glycogen depletion in the fast-twitch red and slow-twitch red types of muscle, but not in white muscle. Contraction resulted in intracellular glucose accumulation in all three muscle types, and this effect was significantly augmented in red muscle by perfusion with oleate. Thus, the availability of FFA has an inhibitory effect on both glucose uptake and glycogen utilization in red skeletal muscle.

Hickson et al. (1977) fed rats with corn oil, after which a heparin injection was given to raise plasma FFA levels prior to exercise. As compared with controls, the fall of blood glucose during exercise occurred less rapidly in animals with raised FFA levels. Furthermore, as compared with controls, glycogen concentration decreased less rapidly in all three types of skeletal muscle and in liver in the animals with raised FFA levels. The possible physiological importance of this observation lies in the finding that the rats with raised plasma FFA levels were able to run 1 hr longer than the control animals before becoming exhausted.

Whether the glucose–fatty acid cycle is operative in humans during exercise remains controversial. Costill et al. (1977) assessed the effect of enhanced plasma FFA levels on the depletion of muscle glycogen during brief (30-min) exercise at 68% of maximal capacity. The subjects ingested a fatty meal 4–5 hr prior to exercise and were then given a heparin bolus 30 min before exercise. A control group received no heparin or fat meal.

Heparin injection resulted in a 3- to 4-fold increase in plasma FFA levels. Plasma glucose rose during exercise in both groups, but the rise was significantly higher in subjects with high FFA levels than in controls. Furthermore, subjects with enhanced plasma FFA showed less muscle depletion of glycogen during exercise than did controls. Total carbohydrate oxidation and lactate production were smaller than in controls, while lipid oxidation in the heparin-treated subjects was higher.

Ahlborg and Hagenfeldt (1977) injected heparin in normal subjects prior to exercise but without a preceding fatty meal and measured net uptake of blood glucose by muscle. During exercise, fractional FFA uptake by the exercising leg was enhanced in heparin-injected subjects as compared with controls. However, leg uptake of circulating glucose and splanchnic glucose production were similar in both groups. These findings suggest that increased FFA uptake may spare muscle glycogen but fails to interfere with uptake of blood glucose by exercising muscle.

9.5.4. Interaction of Exercise and Insulin in Diabetes

Exercise-induced hypoglycemia is a common complication in diabetics treated with insulin. Although this has long been recognized, its mechanism has remained obscure. Recent studies have provided new insights regarding insulin absorption and action during exercise in diabetic patients.

Murray et al. (1977) observed that the glucose response to exercise in diabetics is dependent in part on the route of insulin administration. They gave insulin either subcutaneously or via an intravenous infusion. Infusion was given either with an infusion pump (Murray et al., 1977; Zinman et al., 1977) or an artificial pancreas (Albisser et al., 1977). During exercise, peripheral glucose disappearance rate increased by 40–50% (i.e., from 2.5 to 3.5 mg/kg per min). When insulin was administered intravenously, the increment in glucose production by the liver matched the rise in peripheral glucose utilization so that plasma glucose concentration remained unchanged. The pattern was similar to that observed in controls (Zinman et al., 1977). In contrast, when insulin was injected subcutaneously before exercise, exercise resulted in a fall in glucose production whereas the increment in glucose disappearance was similar to that seen for normals or diabetics infused with insulin. Thus, in insulin-injected diabetics, glucose production during exercise did not meet the needs of increased peripheral utilization, thereby resulting in hypoglycemia. The development of hypoglycemia suggested the possibility of enhanced insulin availability during exercise in patients treated with subcutaneous insulin injection. Indeed, findings in pancreatectomized dogs (Kawamori and Vranic, 1977) and in three diabetic subjects (Albisser et al., 1977; Zinman et al., 1977) and more recently in normal man injected with subcutaneous insulin (Dandona et al., 1978) demonstrated a rise in plasma insulin during exercise. Because no change in plasma insulin was observed in dogs given intravenous infusions of insulin (Vranic et al., 1976), the evidence suggested that exercise increases the mobilization of injected insulin rather than reduces its catabolism.

To examine the hypothesis that exercise accelerates insulin absorption, Koivisto and Felig (1978) studied the effect of leg exercise on the disappearance rate of ^{125}I-labeled short-acting insulin from various subcutaneous injection sites in diabetic subjects. Nine units of radioactive insulin was injected subcutaneously into either the leg, arm, or abdomen, and the disappearance rate was measured externally during and after 1 hr of moderate bicycle exercise. As compared with the resting control day, insulin disappearance from the thigh was increased by 135% during the first 10 min of leg exercise and remained 50% above resting levels during and after the exercise. Leg exercise had no effect on the insulin disappearance rate from the arm. Interestingly, insulin disappearance from injection sites in the abdomen was reduced during the postexercise recovery period.

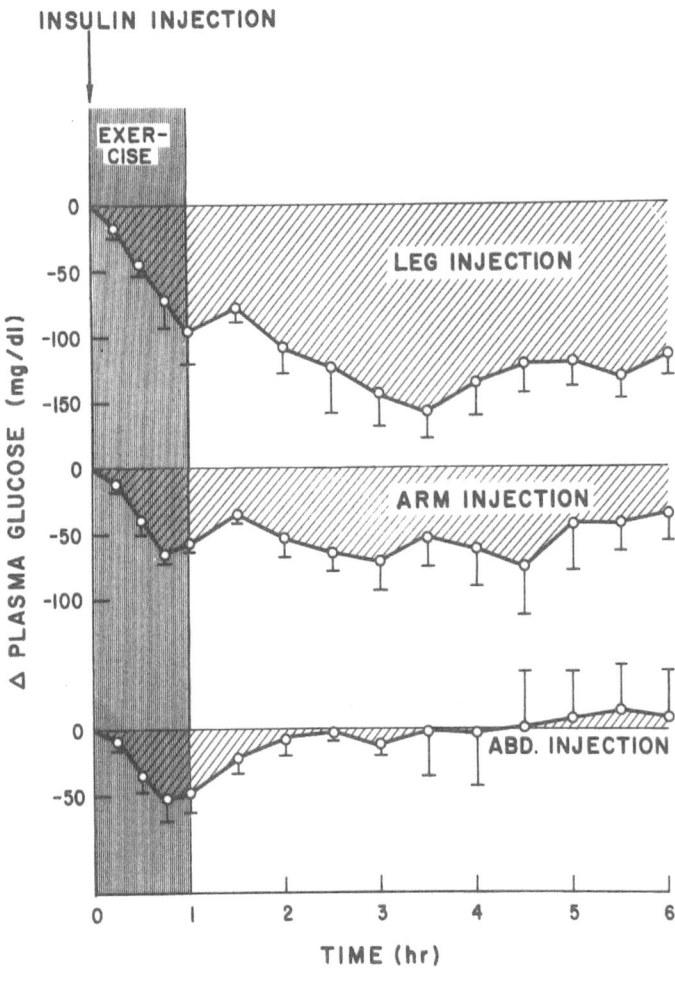

Fig. 1. Effects of varying sites of insulin injection on the blood glucose response to leg exercise in diabetic patients. From Koivisto and Felig (1978); reproduced from the *New England Journal of Medicine,* with permission.

The glycemic response to exercise was in accord with the effect of exercise on insulin absorption. As compared with insulin injection in the leg, the hypoglycemia during and after exercise was reduced by 57% when insulin was injected into the arm and by 89% when it was injected into the abdomen (Fig. 1).

Current findings thus indicate that exercise accelerates insulin absorption from the exercising limb and that the enhanced insulin delivery contributes to exercise-induced hypoglycemia. These observations have implications for the management of the insulin-dependent diabetic patient: the tendency to exercise-induced hypoglycemia may be lessened by the use of nonexercised injection sites.

Enhanced delivery of injected insulin during exercise was also observed in normal rats injected with tracer amounts of tritiated insulin (Berger *et al.*, 1978). At the very beginning of treadmill exercise, rats showed a marked rise in plasma [^{3}H]insulin levels. In addition to enhanced mobilization, exercise resulted in a redistribution of ^{3}H radioactivity in tissues, mainly increasing [^{3}H]insulin concentration in skeletal muscle and the liver.

References

Ahlborg, G., and Felig, P., 1976, Influence of glucose ingestion of fuel–hormone response during prolonged exercise, *J. Appl. Physiol.* **41**:683–688.

Ahlborg, G., and Felig, P., 1977, Substrate utilization during prolonged exercise preceded by ingestion of glucose, *Am. J. Physiol.* **233**:E188–194.

Ahlborg, G., and Hagenfeldt, L., 1977, Effect of heparin on the substrate utilization during prolonged exercise, *Scand. J. Clin. Lab. Invest.* **37**:619–624.

Ahlborg, G., Felig, P., Hagenfeldt, L., Hendler, R., and Wahren, J., 1974, Substrate turnover during prolonged exercise in man: Splanchnic and leg metabolism of glucose, free fatty acids and amino acids, *J. Clin. Invest.* **53**:1080–1090.

Albisser, A. M., Leibel, B. S., Zinman, B., Murray, F. T. P., Zingg, W., Botz, C. K., Denoga, A., and Marliss, E., 1977, Studies with an artificial endocrine pancreas, *Arch. Intern. Med.* **137**:639–649.

Ayuso-Parrilla, M. S., Martin-Requero, A., and Parrilla, R., 1977, On the mechanism of glucagon stimulation of hepatic gluconeogenesis, *Pfluegers Arch.* **370**:45–49.

Barnes, A. J., and Bloom, S. R., 1976, Pancreatectomized man: A model for diabetes without glucagon, *Lancet* **1**:219–221.

Barnes, A. J., Bloom, S. R., Albert, K. G. M. M., Smythe, P. S., Alford, F. P., and Chisholm, D. J., 1977a, Ketoacidosis in pancreatectomized man, *N. Engl. J. Med.* **296**:1250–1253.

Barnes, A. J., Bloom, S. R., Mashiter, K., Alberti, K. G. M. M., Smythe, P., and

Turnell, D., 1977b, Persistent metabolic abnormalities in diabetes in the absence of glucagon, *Diabetologia* **13**:71–75.

Berger, M., Halban, P. A., Müller, W. A., Offord, R. E., Renold, A. E., and Vranic, M., 1978, Mobilization of subcutaneously injected tritiated insulin in rats: Effects of muscular exercise, *Diabetologia* **15**:133–140.

Bomboy, J. D., Lewis, S. B., Lacy, W. W., Sinclair-Smith, B. C., and Liljenquist, J. E., 1977, Transient stimulatory effect of sustained hyperglucagonemia on splanchnic glucose production in normal and diabetic man, *Diabetes* **26**:177–184.

Buse, M. G., Biggers, J. F., Friderici, K. H., and Buse, J. F., 1972, Oxidation of branched chain amino acids by isolated hearts and diaphragms of the rat, *J. Biol. Chem.* **247**:8085–8096.

Chang, T. W., and Goldberg, A. L., 1978a, The origin of alanine produced in skeletal muscle, *J. Biol. Chem.* **253**:3677–3684.

Chang, T. W., and Goldberg, A. L., 1978b, The metabolic fates of amino acids and the formation of glutamine in skeletal muscle, *J. Biol. Chem.* **253**:3685–3695.

Chang, T. W., and Goldberg, A. L., 1978c, Leucine inhibits oxidation of glucose and pyruvate in skeletal muscles during fasting, *J. Biol. Chem.* **253**:3696–3701.

Chiasson, J. L., Liljenquist, J. E., Sinclair-Smith, B. C., and Lacy, W. W., 1975, Gluconeogenesis from alanine in normal postabsorptive man: Intrahepatic stimulatory effect of glucagon, *Diabetes* **24**:574–584.

Cook, G. A., Lakshmanan, M. R., and Veech, R. L., 1977, The effect of glucagon on hepatic malonyl-coenzyme A concentration and on lipid synthesis, *Fed. Proc. Fed. Am. Soc. Exp. Biol.* **36**:672 (abstract).

Costill, D. L., Coyle, E., Dalsky, G., Evans, W., Fink, W., and Hoopes, D., 1977, Effects of elevated plasma FFA and insulin on muscle glycogen usage during exercise, *J. Appl. Physiol.* **43**:695–699.

Dandona, P., Hooke, O., and Bell, J., 1978, Exercise and insulin absorption from subcutaneous tissue, *Br. Med. J.* **1**(611):479–480.

Deacon, S. P., Karunanayake, A., and Barnett, D., 1977, Acebutolol, atenolol, and propranolol and metabolic responses to acute hypoglycemia in diabetics, *Br. Med. J.* **2**(6097):1255–1257.

DeFronzo, R. A., Andres, R., Bledsoe, T. A., Boden, G., Faloona, G. A., and Tobin, J. D., 1977, A test of the hypothesis that the rate of fall in glucose concentration triggers counterregulatory hormonal response in man, *Diabetes* **26**:445–452.

Felig, P., 1973, The glucose alanine cycle, *Metabolism* **22**:179–207.

Felig, P., 1975, Amino acid metabolism in man, *Annu. Rev. Biochem.* **44**:933–955.

Felig, P., and Koivisto, V. A., 1978, Body fuel metabolism, in: *The Year in Metabolism 1977* (N. Freinkel, ed.), pp. 143–168, Plenum Medical Book Company, New York.

Felig, P., Owen, O. E., Wahren, J., and Cahill, G. F., Jr., 1969, Amino acid metabolism during prolonged starvation, *J. Clin. Invest.* **48**:584–594.

Felig, P., Marliss, E., and Ohman, J. L., 1970a, Plasma amino acid levels in diabetic ketoacidosis, *Diabetes* **19**:727–729.

Felig, P., Pozefsky, T., Marliss, E., and Cahill, G. F., Jr., 1970b, Alanine: Key role in gluconeogenesis, *Science* **167**:1003–1004.

Felig, P., Kim, Y. J., Lynch, V., and Hendler, R., 1972a, Amino acid metabolism during starvation in human pregnancy, *J. Clin. Invest.* **51**:1195–1202.

Felig, P., Wahren, J., Hendler, R., and Ahlborg, G., 1972b, Plasma glucagon levels in exercising man, *N. Engl. J. Med.* **287**:184–185.

Felig, P., Wahren, J., Karl, I., Cerasi, E., Luft, R., and Kipnis, D. M., 1973a, Glutamine and glutamate metabolism in normal and diabetic subjects, *Diabetes* **22**:573–576.

Felig, P., Wahren, J., and Raf, L., 1973b, Evidence of inter-organ amino acid transport by blood cells in man, *Proc. Natl. Acad. Sci. U.S.A.* **70**:1775–1779.

Felig, P., Wahren, J., and Hendler, R., 1976a, Influence of physiologic hyperglucagonemia on basal and insulin-inhibited splanchnic glucose output in normal man, *J. Clin. Invest.* **58**:761–765.

Felig, P., Wahren, J., Sherwin, R., and Hendler, R., 1976b, Insulin, glucagon and somatostatin in normal physiology and diabetes mellitus, *Diabetes* **25**:1091–1099.

Freinkel, N., Cohen, A. K., Sandler, R., and Arky, R. A., 1967, Alcohol hypoglycemia: A prototype of the hypoglycemias induced in the fasting state, in: *Proceedings of the 6th Congress of the International Diabetes Federation, Excerpta Med. Int. Congr. Ser.* **172**:873–886.

Ganda, O. P., Weir, G. C., Soeldener, J. S., Legg, M. A., Chick, W. L., Patel, Y. C., Ebeid, A. M., Gabbay, K. H., and Reichlin, S., 1977, Somatostatinoma: A somatostatin containing tumor of endocrine pancreas, *N. Engl. J. Med.* **296**:963–967.

Garber, A. J., Cryer, P. E., Santiago, J. V., Haymond, M. W., Pagliara, A. S., and Kipnis, D. M., 1976a, The role of adrenergic mechanism in the substrate and hormonal response to insulin-induced hypoglycemia in man, *J. Clin. Invest.* **58**:7–15.

Garber, A. J., Karl, I. E., and Kipnis, D. M. 1976b, Alanine and glutamine synthesis and release from skeletal muscle. I. Glycolysis and amino acid release, *J. Biol. Chem.* **251**:826–835.

Garber, A. J., Karl, I. E., and Kipnis, D. M., 1976c, Alanine and glutamine synthesis and release form skeletal muscle. II. The precursor role of amino acids in alanine and glutamine synthesis, *J. Biol. Chem.* **251**:836–843.

Gerich, J. E., Lorenzi, M., Bier, D. M., Tsalikian, E., Schneider, V., Karam, J. H., and Forsham, P. H., 1976, Effects of physiologic levels of glucagon and growth hormone on human carbohydrate and lipid metabolism: Studies involving administration of exogenous hormone during suppression of endogenous hormone secretion with somatostatin, *J. Clin. Invest.* **57**:875–884.

Goldstein, L., and Newsholme, E. A., 1976, The formation of alanine from amino acids in diaphragm muscle of the rat, *Biochem. J.* **154**:555–558.

Hickson, R. C., Rennie, M. J., Conlee, R. K., Winder, W. W., and Holloszy, J. O., 1977, Effects of increased plasma fatty acids on glycogen utilization and endurance, *J. Appl. Physiol.* **43**:829–833.

Holst, J. J., Guldberg Madsen, O., Knop, J., and Schmidt, A., 1977, The effect of intraportal and peripheral infusions of glucagon on insulin and glucose concentrations and glucose tolerance in normal man, *Diabetologia* **13**:487–490.

Jennings, A. S., Cherrington, A. D., Liljenquist, J. E., Keller, U., Lacy, W. W., and Chiasson, J. L., 1977, The roles of insulin and glucagon in the regulation of gluconeogenesis in the postabsorptive dog, *Diabetes* **26**:847–856.

Joffe, B. I., Shires, R., Seftel, H. C., and Heding, L. G., 1977, Plasma insulin, C-peptide, and glucagon levels in acute phase of ethanol-induced hypoglycaemia, *Br. Med. J.* **2**(6088):678.

Jones, D. P., Perman, E. S., and Lieber, C. S., 1965, Free fatty acid turnover and triglyceride metabolism after ethanol ingestion in man, *J. Lab. Clin. Med.* **66**:804–813.

Jorfeldt, L., and Juhlin-Dannfelt, A., 1977, The influence of ethanol on human splanchnic and skeletal muscle metabolism during exercise, *Scand. J. Clin. Lab. Invest.* **37**:609–618.

Juhlin-Dannfelt, A., Ahlborg, G., Hagenfeldt, L., Jorfeldt, L., and Felig, P., 1977, Influence of ethanol on splanchnic and skeletal muscle substrate turnover during prolonged exercise in man, *Am. J. Physiol.* **233**:PE195–202.

Kawamori, R., and Vranic, M., 1977, Mechanism of exercise-induced hypoglycemia in depancreatized dogs maintained on long-acting insulin, *J. Clin. Invest.* **59**:331–337.

Keller, U., Chiasson, J.-L., Liljenquist, J. E., Cherrington, A. D., Jennings, A. S., and Crofford, O., 1977, The roles of insulin, glucagon, and free fatty acids in the regulation of ketogenesis in dogs, *Diabetes* **26**:1040–1056.

Koerker, D. L., Ruch, W., Chideckel, E., Palmer, J., Goodner, C. J., Ensinck, J., and Gale, C. C., 1974, Somatostatin: Hypothalamic inhibitor of the endocrine pancreas, *Science* **184**:482–484.

Koivisto, V. A., and Felig, P., 1978, Effects of leg exercise on insulin absorption in diabetic patients, *N. Engl. J. Med.* **298**:79–83.

Krebs, H. A., 1968, The effects of ethanol on the metabolic activities of the liver, *Adv. Enzyme Regul.* **6**:467–480.

Larsson, L.-I., Hirsch, M. A., Holst, J. J., Ingemansson, S., Kühl, C., Lindkaer Jensen, S. L., Lundquist, G., Rehfeld, J. F., and Schwartz, T. W., 1977, Pancreatic somatostatinoma: Clinical features and physiological implications, *Lancet* **1**:666–668.

Mallette, L. E., Exton, J. H., and Park, C. R., 1969, Control of gluconeogenesis from amino acids in the perfused rat liver, *J. Biol. Chem.* **244**:5713–5723.

Marliss, E. B., Aoki, T. T., Pozefsky, T., Most, A. S., and Cahill, G. F., Jr., 1971, Muscle and splanchnic glutamine and glutamate metabolism in post absorptive and starved man, *J. Clin. Invest.* **50**:814–817.

McGarry, J. D., and Foster, D. W., 1977, Hormonal control of ketogenesis: Biochemical considerations, *Arch. Intern. Med.* **137**:495–501.

McGarry, J. D., Meier, J. M., and Foster, D. W., 1973, The effects of starvation and refeeding on carbohydrate and lipid metabolism *in vivo* and in the perfused rat liver: The relationship between fatty acid oxidation and esterification in the regulation of ketogenesis, *J. Biol. Chem.* **248**:270–278.

McGarry, J. D., Mannaerts, G. P., and Foster, D. W., 1977, A possible role for malonyl-CoA in the regulation of hepatic fatty acid oxidation and ketogenesis, *J. Clin. Invest.* **60**:265–270.

Murray, F. T., Zinman, B., McLean, P. A., Denoga, A., Albisser, A. M., Leibel, B. S., Nakhioda, A. F., Stokes, E. F., and Marliss, E. B., 1977, The metabolic response to moderate exercise in diabetic man receiving intravenous and subcutaneous insulin, *J. Clin. Endocrinol. Metab.* **44**:708–720.

Odessey, R., Khairallah, E. A., and Goldberg, A. L., 1974, Origin and possible significance of alanine production by skeletal muscle, *J. Biol. Chem.* **249**:7623–7629.

Ozand, P. T., Reed, W. D., Girard, J., Hawkins, R. L., Collins, R. M., Jr., Tildon, J. T., and Cornblath, M., 1977, Hypoketonaemic effect of L-alanine, *Biochem. J.* **164**:557–564.

Pagliara, A. S., Karl, I. E., DeVivo, D. C., Feigin, R. D., and Kipnis, D. M., 1972, Hypoalaninemia: A concomitant ketotic hypoglycemia, *J. Clin. Invest.* **51**:1440–1449.

Palaiologos, G., and Felig, P., 1976, Effects of ketone bodies on amino acid metabolism in isolated rat diaphragm, *Biochem. J.* **154**:709–716.

Parving, H.-H., Noer, I., Kehlet, H., Mogensen, C. E., Svendsen, P. A., and Heding, L., 1977, The effect of short-term glucagon and growth hormone infusion on kidney function in normal man, *Acta Endocrinol.* **85**(Suppl. 209):50.

Pirnay, F., Lacroix, M., Mosora, F., Luyckx, A., and Lefebvre, P., 1977, Glucose oxidation during prolonged exercise evaluated with naturally labeled C^{13}-glucose, *J. Appl. Physiol.* **43**:258–261.

Pozefsky, T., Felig, P., Tobin, J. D., Soeldner, J. S., and Cahill, G. F., Jr., 1969, Amino acid balance across the tissue of the forearm in postabsorptive man: Effects of insulin at two dose levels, *J. Clin. Invest.* **48**:2273–2282.

Randle, P. J., Garland, P. B., Hales, C. N., and Newsholme, E. A., 1963, The glucose fatty acid cycle: Its role in insulin sensitivity and the metabolic disturbances of diabetes mellitus, *Lancet* **1**:785–789.

Raskin, P., and Unger, R. H., 1977, Effects of exogenous hyperglucagonemia in insulin-treated diabetics, *Diabetes* **26**:1034–1039.

Rennie, M. J., and Holloszy, J. O., 1977, Inhibition of glucose uptake and glycogenolysis by availability of oleate in well-oxygenated perfused skeletal muscle, *Biochem. J.* **168**:161–170.

Rennie, M. J., Winder, W. W., and Holloszy, J. O., 1976, A sparing effect of increased plasma fatty acids on muscle and liver glycogen content in the exercising rat, *Biochem. J.* **156**:647–655.

Saccá, L., Perez, G., Carteni, G., Trimarco, B., and Rengo, F., 2977a, Role of glucagon in the glucoregulatory response to insulin-induced hypoglycemia in the rat, *Horm. Metab. Res.* **9**:209–212.

Saccá, L., Trimarco, B., Perez, G., and Rengo, F., 1977b, Studies on the mechanism underlying the influence of alanine infusion on glucose dynamics in the dog, *Diabetes* **26**:262–270.

Schade, D. S., and Eaton, R. P., 1976, Modulation of fatty acid metabolism by glucagon in man. IV. Effects of physiologic hormone infusion in normal man, *Diabetes* **25**:978–983.

Schade, D. S., and Eaton, R. P., 1977, The regulation of plasma ketone body concentration by counterregulatory hormones in man, *Diabetes* **26**:989–996.

Schade, D. S., Eaton, R. P., and Standefer, J., 1977, Glucocorticoid regulation of plasma ketone body concentration in insulin deficient man, *J. Clin. Endocrinol. Metab.* **44**:1069–1079.

Sherwin, R. S., Bastl, C., Finkelstein, F. O., Fisher, M., Black, H., Hendler, R., and Felig, P., 1976a, Influence of uremia and hemodialysis on the turnover and metabolic effects of glucagon, *J. Clin. Invest.* **57**:722–731.

Sherwin, R. S., Fisher, M., Hendler, R., and Felig, P., 1976b, Hyperglucagonemia and blood glucose regulation in normal, obese and diabetic subjects, *N. Engl. J. Med.* **294**:455–461.

Sherwin, R. S., Hendler, R., DeFronzo, R. A., Wahren, J., and Felig, P., 1977a, Glucose homeostasis during prolonged suppression of glucagon and insulin secretion by somatostatin, *Proc. Natl. Acad. Sci. U.S.A.* **74**:348–352.

Sherwin, R. S., Tamborlane, W., Hendler, R., Saccá, L., DeFronzo, R. A., and Felig, P., 1977b, Influence of glucagon replacement on the hyperglycemic and hyperketonemic response to prolonged somatostatin infusion in normal man, *J. Clin. Endocrinol. Metab.* **45**:1104–1107.

Siler, T. M., Vandenberg, G., and Yen, S. S. C., 1973, Inhibition of growth hormone release in humans by somatostatin, *J. Clin. Endocrinol. Metab.* **37**:632–634.

Singh, S. P., and Snyder, A. K., 1978, Effect of thyrotoxicosis on gluconeogenesis from alanine in the perfused rat liver, *Endocrinology* **102**:182–187.

Soman, V., and Felig, P., 1977, Glucagon and insulin binding to liver membranes in a partially nephrectomized uremic rat model, *J. Clin. Invest.* **60**:224–232.

Tamborlane, W. T., Sherwin, R. S., Hendler, R., and Felig, P., 1977, Metabolic effects of somatostatin in maturity onset diabetes, *N. Engl. J. Med.* **297**:181–183.

Unger, R. H., 1976, Glucagon and blood sugar (letter), *N. Engl. J. Med.* **294**:1239.

Unger, R. H., Ohneda, A., Aquilar-Parada, E., and Eiseutraut, A. M., 1969, The role of aminogenic glucagon secretion in blood glucose homeostasis, *J. Clin. Invest.* **48**:810–822.

Vranic, M., Kawamori, R., Pek, S., Kovacevic, N., and Wrenshall, G. A., 1976, The essentiality of insulin and the role of glucagon in regulating glucose utilization and production during strenuous exercise in dogs, *J. Clin. Invest.* **57**:245–255.

Wahren, J., and Felig, P., 1976, Influence of somatostatin on carbohydrate disposal and absorption in diabetes mellitus, *Lancet* **2**:1213–1216.

Wahren, J., Felig, P., and Hagenfeldt, J., 1976, Effect of protein ingestion on splanchnic and leg metabolism in normal man and in patients with diabetes mellitus, *J. Clin. Invest.* **57**:987–999.

Wahren, J., Efendic, S., Luft, R., Hagenfeldt, L., Björkman, O., and Felig, P., 1977, Influence of somatostatin on splanchnic glucose metabolism in postabsorptive and 60-hour fasted humans, *J. Clin. Invest.* **59**:299–307.

Willms, B., Bottcher, V., Wolters, V., Sakamoto, N., and Soling, H. D., 1969, Relationship between fat and ketone body metabolism in obese and nonobese diabetics and nondiabetics during norepinephrine infusion, *Diabetologia* 5:88–96.

Windmueller, H. G., and Spaeth, A. E., 1978, Identification of ketone bodies and glutamine as the major respiratory fuels *in vivo* for postabsorptive rat small intestine, *J. Biol. Chem.* 253:69–76.

Zinman, B., Murray, F. T., Vranic, M., Albisser, A. M., Leibel, B. S., McLean, P. A., and Marliss, E. B., 1977, Glucoregulation during moderate exercise in insulin treated diabetics, *J. Clin. Endocrinol. Metab.* 45:641–652.

What's New in Obesity: Current Understanding of Adipose Tissue Morphology

Jules Hirsch, Irving M. Faust, and Patricia R. Johnson

10.1. Introduction

Obesity is, by definition, an increase in the amount of adipose tissue. Clearly, the additional mass of fat in obesity must be stored in adipose tissue consisting of either large adipocytes or more adipocytes, or in tissue with some mixture of cellular hyperplasia and hypertrophy. This obvious fact was brought to the attention of clinicians and investigators over two decades ago by the work of Reh (1953) and Bjuiulf (1959). Yet, the meaningfulness of the cellular morphology of adipose tissue in either the pathogenesis or perpetuation of obesity remains uncertain. On the one hand, the cellular disposition of triglyceride in the unilocular adipocyte of white adipose tissue may be a totally passive event with no consequences for metabolism or energy regulation. At the other extreme, it could be that adipocyte size and number are controlling elements in a caloric–intake–storage–energy-output system and thus are of central concern to

JULES HIRSCH and IRVING M. FAUST • Department of Human Behavior and Metabolism, The Rockefeller University, New York, New York 10021. PATRICIA R. JOHNSON • Department of Human Behavior and Metabolism, The Rockefeller University, New York, New York 10021; Department of Biology, Vassar College, Poughkeepsie, New York 12601.

our understanding of obesity. The latter possibility, which might be called
the "adipocyte theory of obesity," deserves thorough investigation, since
there has been amassed a wealth of data to suggest that the adipocyte is
metabolically highly active and very sensitive to hormones. It is the
purpose of this review to consider recent findings on adipose cellularity,
chiefly from work with animals, but also with human subjects, in order to
evaluate the "adipocyte theory of obesity." In particular, several questions
will be examined:

1. What are the preferred methods for determining adipose cellu-
    larity? Are they reliable?
2. What is the cellularity of adipose tissue in man and animals?
3. How constant is adipocyte number?
4. How are new adipocytes formed?
5. Are adipocyte size and number of significance in energy
    regulation?

10.2. Techniques for Measuring Adipocyte Size and Number

The parameters that define adipose cellularity are mean cell size, the
distribution of cell sizes, and the number of cells in either a given site or
the total organism. Mean cell size can vary considerably from one site or
depot to another within the same organism. Cell diameters appear to be
normally distributed over a wide range of cell sizes. As a consequence of
the normal distribution of diameters, cell volumes (which closely reflect
cell lipid content) are found as a cubic expansion of the distribution of
diameters and are therefore markedly skewed, covering a large range of
cell volumes.

The simplest approach to the problem of measuring cellularity in
adipose tissue would at first glance appear to be the measurement of tissue
DNA and lipid. DNA would measure total cell number, and the ratio of
lipid to DNA should measure average cell lipid content. Since unilocular
adipocytes are so rich in lipid content, the measure of lipid per cell would
closely approximate cell size. However, it has been repeatedly shown that
as much as 80% of adipose tissue DNA is found outside of lipid-filled cells
in supportive tissues, wandering cells such as macrophages, and perhaps
in precursor adipocytes (Hollenberg and Vost, 1968). Thus, DNA measurement has had to be abandoned as a method for estimating adipocyte
cellularity. The methods to be described below that are currently in use
for determining the cellularity of adipose tissue are all based on the sizing
and numbering of lipid-filled cells. Yet, the issue of unfilled or precursor
adipocytes is of extreme importance and will be discussed as well.

10.2.1. Intact Tissue

Goldrick (1967) demonstrated that cell size could be determined from shreds of human or animal tissue. Photographs were made and the intact cells sized using a Zeiss Particle Size Analyzer. More recently, investigators have used slices of tissue and a similar technique of analysis. Sjostrom *et al.* (1971) suggested a method in which 100 cells are examined microscopically and diameters recorded; Lemonnier (1972) measured the surface area of cells when projected onto a ground-glass screen and then with a series of formulas arrived at average cell volume.

10.2.2. Osmium-Fixed Tissue

An alternative approach to the microscopic examination of histological sections has been to fix shreds of tissue of known lipid content in osmium tetroxide (Hirsch and Gallian, 1968). When the cells are disaggregated, the osmium-fixed suspension of cells is counted and cell size determined as a quotient: lipid content in the fixed tissue divided by total cells counted from the tissues.

10.2.3. Adipocyte Suspensions

Perhaps the most commonly used technique has been microscopic sizing and counting of cells liberated from the tissue by collagenase digestion (DiGirolamo *et al.*, 1971). Usually, suspended cells are placed in a hemocytometer chamber and cell number determined. Alternatively, cell diameters can be measured and appropriate calculations made to determine average cell volume or cell lipid content.

10.2.4. Advantages and Disadvantages of Counting Techniques

The reliability and comparative results of these various methods have been evaluated. Hirsch and Gallian (1968), Sjostrom *et al.* (1971), and Smith *et al.* (1972) found a high degree of consistency among these various methods. Nevertheless, there are advantages and disadvantages to each approach. The osmium-fixation method is expensive, since it requires the use of large amounts of osmium tetroxide and the availability of an electronic or other automatic device for determining particle number. It has the advantage of counting large numbers of cells without the tedium and potential observer bias of microscopic examination of tissue slices or intact pieces of tissue. The collagenase digestion method for liberating adipocytes almost always ruptures some cells, which creates a problem of possible selective destruction of larger cells that are more liable to disruption. This method can also lead to the creation of small lipid droplets that can be difficult to distinguish from adipocytes. In some reports (Stiles *et al.*, 1976; Ashwell and Garrow, 1973), large numbers of small "adipocytes" have been seen and counted. Unless these cells are also seen in intact tissue preparations, it is difficult to be certain that they are not artifacts created during collagenase digestion.

It must be emphasized that all these methods count only lipid-filled cells. Whether or not cells have lipid is determined visually when tissue fragments or slices are examined. The osmium-fixation method requires that osmium-fixed cells be easily separable from supportive tissue, sink readily in an aqueous suspension, and be retained by a filter usually with a pore size of 25 μm. The collagenase cell suspension method is dependent on the property of lipid-filled cells to rise quickly to the surface. The detection of "preadipocytes," or of adipocytes either depleted of lipid or not yet filled, is not possible by any of the aforementioned methods.

These methods can be used to estimate total adipocyte number of the organism by dividing average cell lipid content into the amount of total lipid stored in adipose tissue. While accurate data for this calculation are relatively easy to obtain in experimental animals in which carcass composition can be determined, the data are liable to error in human studies, since total fat storage is difficult to measure with accuracy. Furthermore, the calculation is heavily dependent on obtaining a truly average cell size from the tissue fragments that are sampled. Salans *et al.* (1973) pointed up the shortcomings of these calculations and showed the need for multiple sampling of subcutaneous tissue for accurate estimates of total cell number in man. It should be remembered that adipocyte size tends to be similar across depots both in man and animals, but is never exactly the same in all depots. When cells enlarge, the change tends to occur in all depots, although there can be systematic variations. Total lipid content is of course most accurately measured by tissue extraction in experimental animals. In human studies, independent measures of lean body mass by [40]K counting or the determination of body water have led to quite reliable estimates of total body fat. However, considerable errors, particularly in infants or in extremely obese subjects, can be encountered. Consequently, the data presented on adipose cellularity cannot at this time be considered precisely accurate, yet the directionality of the findings and the broad consistency of experimental data from many laboratories have led to the accumulation of a significant body of new information on adipose cellularity.

10.3. Cellularity of Adipose Tissue in Man and Animals

Data from many laboratories indicate that adipose tissue of nonobese adult human subjects contains $25-40 \times 10^9$ adipocytes with an average lipid content per cell of $0.3-0.7$ μg. Average cell diameters corresponding to these lipid contents are generally between 80 and 110 μm. Several investigators have examined the site-to-site variations in adipocyte size. Hirsch and Knittle (1970) found that abdominal subcutaneous cells were larger than cells from other sites. Salans *et al.* (1973) also found variations in cell size from site to site, but concluded that a satisfactory estimate of average cell size could be obtained by sampling from several subcutaneous sites.

10.3.1. Development of Adipose Cellularity in Man

Hirsch and Knittle (1970), Brook *et al.* (1972), Boulton *et al.* (1974), Dauncey and Gairdner (1975), Knittle (1976), and Hager (1977) studied the rate of appearance of lipid-filled adipocytes during infancy and childhood. The newborn, term human infant is well endowed with adipose tissue, unlike the newborn of other species. Adipose tissue accounts for 10–15% of body weight. The greater leanness of premature infants suggests that fat accumulation normally occurs during the last trimester of pregnancy. The stored lipid of the newborn has a composition that indicates the likelihood that it is made almost exclusively from carbohydrate within the fetus, rather than by placental transfer of maternal fat (Bagdade and Hirsch, 1966). At birth, the stored fat weighs roughly 400 g, as compared with 10,000 or more g to be found in the average adult adipose depot. Thus, the newborn has about $\frac{1}{25}$ the stored fat it will develop during growth and maturation. This fat is stored in about $\frac{1}{5}$ the number of adult cells and in cells that contain about $\frac{1}{5}$ as much lipid as the adipocytes of adult tissue. The adipocytes do not appear unusually small on ordinary histological study, since an 80% reduction in lipid content is accompanied by only a little more than a 40% reduction in cell diameter. Cells smaller than adult cells are seen, but extremely small cells, less than 25 μm in diameter, are generally not found in human newborn tissue.

Most data show that during the first year of life, there is a definite increase in cell size but only a slight increase in cell number. Thereafter, cell number increases gradually as does cell size, with a sharper increase of both at puberty. Adult values are attained by late adolescence. At no time is there such a sharp peak of increased appearance of cells as to be indicative of a special "critical period." If such exists, it might occur prenatally or perhaps in early adolescence when the rate of appearance of cells is most rapid. It must be remembered, however, that such cell counting is only of lipid-laden cells. What precursors exist, and when they are formed, remains completely unknown. Somewhat more information is available on the sequence of events in rodent adipose tissue.

10.3.2. Adipose Cellularity in Laboratory Rodents

A series of studies over the past decade, primarily using the osmium-fixation electronic counting method, have led to the conclusion that in the normal albino rat, adipocyte number achieves a maximum and stable value in young adulthood and does not change thereafter. After about the 14th week in the life of the normal albino rat, increases in adipose depot size occur due to adipocyte enlargement. Again, the use of this counting technique measures only the appearance of filled adipocytes. However, measurement of the incorporation of tritiated thymidine into adipocyte DNA does allow one to distinguish to some degree between proliferation and lipid-filling. The data of Greenwood and Hirsch (1974) using thymidine incorporation indicated that all cell proliferation in the epididymal fat pad of the normal Sprague–Dawley rat had ceased by about 35 days of age. Thus, the apparent increase in cell numbers from 7 to 14 weeks of age in the epididymal pad is due to lipid-filling of preexistent cells. While such thymidine incorporation studies have not been done for other depots in the rat, it seems reasonable to assume that other depots behave similarly, since cell-counting data for the retroperitoneal and subcutaneous depots in the normal rat yield data similar to those for the epididymal pad. However, species differences do occur, as the data of DiGirolamo et al. (1971) attest. They report that the epididymal fat pad in the guinea pig adds cells up to 1 year of life. Other evidence for increases in adipocyte number during the adult life of animals will be presented in more detail below.

10.3.3. Cellularity in Human Obesity

Extensive data have been accumulated on the cellular aberrations found in human obesity. It is clear that all human obesity is hypertrophic. With moderate degrees of obesity, this may be the only abnormality found, but as obesity becomes more severe, increasing disturbances of cell number are found. Indeed, all severely obese individuals have an increase in adipocyte number. The data suggest that there is a ceiling for adipocyte size. A four or fivefold enlargement of the stored fat or a 1.6- to 1.7-fold enlargement of adipocyte diameter would appear to represent an upper limit. Obesity of greater proportions is accompanied by increases in cell number that seem to have no upper limit. Most severe forms of obesity date from childhood, and thus a correlation is found between cell number and early onset of the disease. If, however, careful examinations are made of lesser degrees of obesity with lesser degrees of hypercellularity, it is hard to establish an unequivocal relationship between cell number and age of onset.

A relationship between cell number and age of onset has been carefully sought, since rats underfed in the preweaning state will have a long-standing reduction in cell number (Knittle and Hirsch, 1968). When litters are prepared so that preweaning animals are reared in either small or very large litters, the animals in the large litters will be stunted at weaning. This stunting is accompanied by a marked diminution in fat storage. Adipose tissue shows a decrease in cell number as well as cell size, which persists until at least 10 weeks of age. A comparable situation in man, with early alterations in nutrition leading to permanent changes in cellularity, has therefore seemed to be a reasonable possibility.

When obese children were examined by Knittle (1976), it was found that obesity in childhood is like that in the adult, in that an increase in cell size is always found. Furthermore, there is often an increase in cell number, when obese children are compared with nonobese children of the same age. But at no time does one find a purely hyperplastic state. If obesity were the exclusive result of a proliferative disorder of adipocytes, one might have expected that at some time during the development of obesity in childhood, an overabundance of cells of normal or even subnormal size might be found. Such a situation has not been found.

10.3.4. Cellularity in Animal Obesity

There are many experimental models of obesity in animals. These have been most thoroughly studied in rodents. In all instances, obese rodents show marked cellular enlargement, but various degrees of hyperplasia can also be found. Thus, the Zucker obese rat (fa/fa) shows striking increases in cell number along with hypertrophy when compared with lean littermates (Fa/fa or Fa/Fa) (Johnson *et al.*, 1971). In contrast, similar or even greater degrees of obesity brought about by lesion of the ventromedial portions of the hypothalamus lead only to cellular enlargement, without change in cell number (Hirsch and Han, 1969; Johnson *et al.*, 1971). The ob/ob mouse and the New Zealand obese mouse have been characterized as having hyperplastic–hypertrophic obesity, whereas the yellow mouse shows changes only in cell size (Johnson and Hirsch, 1972). It has been convenient to group these obesities as to age of onset as well as adipose tissue morphology. In general, the earlier the age of onset, the greater the change in cell number; however, as will be discussed below, under some conditions an apparent increase in cell number can be induced in rats of almost any age.

As discussed with human obesity, one might suppose that were obesity primarily a disorder of adipocyte proliferation, some situations would be found in which hyperplastic adipose tissue would be found with smaller cells. At no stage of rodent obesity has this been found to be the case.

10.4. How Constant Is Adipocyte Number?

There can be little question that adipocyte size is more mutable than cell number. The acute response of the tissue to negative or positive energy balance is a prompt decrease or increase in cell size. But increasingly it is being found that some influences over time can lead to the appearance of more fat-filled cells. Thus, evidence from several laboratories (Ashwell and Garrow, 1973; Widdowson and Shaw, 1973; Stiles *et al.*, 1976) suggests that new fat cells can appear in adult rats, well beyond the time that cellular proliferation is believed to cease. Recently completed studies of the effects of feeding highly palatable diets to adult rats show that new cells can be induced in all adipose depots (Lemonnier, 1972; Faust *et al.*, 1978). Thus, the earlier concept of a stable population of adipocytes in the adult applies to the chow-fed rat, but with either high-fat diets on sucrose-supplemented diets, more cells appear. It remains to be established whether the increased numbers of cells that appear in such diet-induced obesity are the result of proliferation or merely lipid-filling. The observation that they remain in the depots after the animals are returned to chow strongly suggests that they are indeed new cells (Faust *et al.*, 1978).

10.4.1. Stability of Cell Number

The impressive fact concerning the stability of the adipocyte population is that adipocytes formed at any stage of life remain in the tissue for exceedingly long periods of time. There is no clinical or experimental evidence that adipocyte number can ever be decreased. Even a dramatic decrement in body weight, maintained over many years, does not cause a noticeable decrease in the adipocyte population. Formerly obese patients who have maintained near-normal body weight for many years as the result of intestinal bypass operations, illness, or extraordinary willpower have just as many fat cells as they had when they were at their heaviest. Severe weight loss in adult rats is similarly ineffective in causing a reduction in adipocyte number (Hirsch and Han, 1969).

The number of adipocytes by current counting techniques may appear to decline at some point during a period of severe weight loss, but the decline is the result of cells diminishing in size through lipolytic activity and being overlooked by current methods, rather than permanent reduction in cell number. As soon as a severely reduced person begins to regain weight, adipocyte number quickly returns to the level seen prior to weight loss, a finding that supports the idea of stable cell number. Because of such persistence of fat cells, reduction of adipose cell number can be achieved only by the surgical removal of adipose tissue, not a generally accepted medical intervention.

10.4.2. Changes in Cell Number

That adipocyte number can increase in adult animals, under some conditions, is now well established. Johnson and Hirsch (1972) first showed that hypothalamic damage in mice, produced by systemic injections of goldthioglucose (GTG), causes an obesity that is primarily hypertrophic, but also significantly hyperplastic in one depot, the retroperitoneal. Shortly thereafter, Lemonnier (1972) showed that high-fat feeding produces a similar effect of increased adipocyte number in the retroperitoneal depots in both mice and rats. Such increases may have been the result of induced new adipocyte production, but it is possible that they were not. For example, it may be that during the first few weeks of life, when adipocytes are formed, a pool of incompletely differentiated adipocytes is also formed. Overeating later in life may stimulate the completion of differentiation in those cells. But whatever the mechanism, this phenomenon has been observed in several strains of rats on either high-fat or high-sucrose diets (Faust et al., 1978). In all these circumstances, there is hyperphagia and a sharp increase in the mass of adipose tissue. The cellular response is orderly and predictable. In all depots (retroperitoneal, epididymal, and subcutaneous), cells enlarge. When cells achieve a lipid content of about 1.2–1.9 μg, new cells appear. This generally occurs first in the retroperitoneal depot, but then elsewhere as well. It is as though cellular hypertrophy is the first response to a demand for increased storage capacity, but an upper limit of cell size sets in motion some process that permits further storage to occur in new cells, thereby inducing further hypertrophy, in the new cells. Indeed, cell size may actually decline at this point. Thus, Johnson et al. (1979) found that during development of the adipose tissues in the obese Zucker rat, average fat cell size increases to a maximum (around 1.9 μg lipid/cell), and then quickly decreases and plateaus at a substantially smaller size (around 1.3 μg lipid/cell), as cell number increases.

Interestingly, it has been found (Faust et al., 1978) that when cell number is increased by a high-fat diet and the animal is then restored to chow feeding, cell size declines but the new higher cell number is unchanged. Thus, this observation provides further evidence for the inability of differentiated adipocytes to dedifferentiate or disappear.

Another set of studies that demonstrate that cells can appear in the adult life of rodents is concerned with the response to lipectomy. Although it has been repeatedly shown that the removal of portions of the epididymal fat pad leads to no compensatory growth of fat at that site (Faust *et al.*, 1976), in other sites lipectomy can be followed by restorative growth (Faust *et al.*, 1977a). Thus, the removal of inguinal subcutaneous fat in the young rat is followed by a slow regeneration of lost fat cells. At 7 months after surgery, exactly the same number of cells is present in the operated sites of lipectomized and sham-operated animals (Faust *et al.*, 1977a).

Thus, the removal of fat or an imposed pressure to store more fat can lead to the appearance of new cells. It would seem reasonable to suppose, then, that some type of precursor cell must be present even in adult life. Normally, the differentiation of this cell is inhibited or inadequately stimulated and the tissue is responsive to variations in energy flux by a waxing and waning of cell size, but there are conditions that lead to the differentiation and likely the further proliferation of the hypothetical precursor cell or preadipocyte.

10.5. How Are New Adipocytes Formed?

An approach that has proved valuable for examination of the processes of both proliferation and differentiation of other tissues is *in vitro* culture of organs or cells. Several investigators have recently reported the successful culture of a non-lipid-filled cell type derived from human or rat adipose tissue. Such cells when grown in enriched medium first proliferate until they reach confluence, after which they show the capacity to accumulate substantial amounts of lipid. Poznanski *et al.* (1973) first reported the culture of cells obtained from the stromal elements of a collagenase digest of adult human subcutaneous adipose tissue. After 2 weeks in culture, these cells showed greater lipid accumulation than skin fibroblasts grown under identical conditions. They also contained more glycerol and had enhanced conversion of [^{14}C]glucose into lipid. Van *et al.* (1976) grew similar cells from human omental tissue and demonstrated that they could be subcultured for up to three passages without loss of morphological and functional characteristics. Dixon-Shanies *et al.* (1975) cultured cells derived from the supernatant (floating) fraction of a collagenase digest of human omental adipose tissue (CAT cells). CAT cells grew more slowly than did fibroblasts and converted more glucose to lipid, but insulin failed to stimulate glucose conversion to lipid as it does in true adipocytes. Thus, it is not clear what these cells are. They might be mature adipocytes in the process of losing lipid, or "dedifferentiating" in culture and regaining the capacity to divide. On the other hand, they could conceivably be a precursor cell type that was tightly associated with mature adipocytes, but once released from that association was able to proliferate in culture. Van and Roncari (1977) reported the culture and subculture of a homogeneous population of cells derived from adult rat epididymal adipose tissue. When cultured in a medium enriched with free fatty acids, these cells accumulate abundant lipid, round up, and occasionally reach the unilocular stage. Bjorntorp *et al.* (1978) also reported the culture of cells derived from the stromal–vascular fraction of young (4 to 6 week-old) rat adipose tissue. The cells that these investigators culture are derived from a population that passes through a 25 μm mesh after collagenase digestion of the tissue. They enrich the growth medium with triolein to enhance the process of lipid accumulation by the cultured cells. These studies all suggest that some type of precursor cell can be found in adult adipose tissue and that such a cell can be induced to accumulate lipid under cell culture conditions. However, it is not yet clear whether or not these cells are simply differentiated small cells containing the necessary membrane components and enzymes to function as fat cells, or whether they are a true adipocyte precursor cell that must first differentiate through new protein synthetic activity.

Unfortunately, histological examination of adult or even juvenile human or rat adipose tissue does not show large numbers of proliferating and differentiating preadipocytes or adipoblasts. The process of differentiation must be exceedingly rapid. When fat tissue is regenerating following lipectomy, mature adipocytes are found in abundance with only an occasional multilocular cell visible in histological preparations (Johnson *et al.*, 1978). Clearly, further careful histological work combined with autoradiography and tissue culture will be needed to delineate the precise cellular sequence of adipocyte formation and differentiation.

10.6. Significance of Cell Size and Number in Energy Regulation

The most crucial question facing the investigator dealing with adipose cellularity and human obesity is whether cell size or number can influence food-intake behavior. It is clear that adipocyte size can affect the metabolic behavior of adipose tissue as measured *in vitro*. For example, the rate of glycerol release and the response of cells to the effects of epinephrine and insulin are very much influenced by cell size (Bjorntorp and Sjostrom, 1972). But evidence for a connecting link between adipose tissue morphology and food intake remains more elusive. It is certainly tantalizing to believe that such a link exists. When the markedly obese individual loses weight, there are enormous forces at work to cause regain of weight. After weight loss, all known hormonal and metabolic abnormalities of obesity seem to be corrected; yet the impetus to regain weight seems stronger than can be accounted for by habit or psychological factors alone. What is impressive is the persistence of small adipocytes; yet how these can be a force for weight regain is unknown.

Recently, two types of studies have lent credence to the idea of some relationship between adipocyte size and food intake. When a group of obese individuals were observed during weight loss, it was found that difficulty in adhering to dietary restrictions became most extreme when a normal or average cell size was reached (Bjorntorp et al., 1975). Further weight reduction seemed to be resisted, as though shrinkage of cells beyond the average size generated impulses to depart from treatment and overeat. Other interpretations of the data are possible, but the findings are consonant with a cell-size–food-intake relationship.

A more telling piece of evidence comes from studies made on lipectomized animals (Faust et al., 1977b). When Osborne–Mendel rats are lipectomized, food intake appears to be the same as in sham-operated animals. As a consequence, the lipectomized animals, which continue to store increasing amounts of fat, as do the sham controls, store the fat in fewer and therefore larger cells. Since ordinary chow diets do not lead to changes in cell number, this situation persists over months, i.e., animals (sham vs. lipectomized) with the same food intake and the same total amount of stored fat, but a difference in cellularity. If the animals are then presented with a highly palatable, high-fat diet, all become hyperphagic. But the lipectomized animals, with fewer cells, quickly expand cell size to a greater degree than sham-operated animals and the lipectomized animals diminish the hyperphagic response more quickly. When the sham-operated animals fill their more numerous cells to the same degree, hyperphagia begins to abate in these animals as well. The most plausible interpretation for these data is that an upper limit of cell size acts as a brake on food intake. If the experiment were continued, eventually an increase in cell number would most likely occur, but in the early weeks of the study, cell size is clearly related to food intake. This experiment provides the clearest evidence to date linking adipose cellularity with food intake.

Thus, the "adipocyte theory of obesity," with modifications, remains a useful way of ordering data on animal and human obesity. The chemical or neural links between adipocytes and the central nervous system are subjects for active research. Without the establishment of the nature of these links, the hypothesis must remain interesting, yet arguable and tentative.

ACKNOWLEDGMENTS

This work has been supported in part by NIH grants CRC RR 00102, AM 18325, AM 20508, and AM 19382 and by NSF grant PCM 76-09324.

References

Ashwell, M., and Garrow, J. S., 1973, Full and empty fat cells, *Lancet* **2**:1036–1037.

Bagdade, J. D., and Hirsch, J., 1966, Gestational and dietary influences on the lipid content of the infant buccal fat pad, *Proc. Soc. Exp. Biol. Med.* **122**:616–619.

Bjorntorp, P., and Sjostrom, L., 1972, The composition and metabolism *in vitro* of adipose tissue fat cells of different sizes, *Eur. J. Clin. Invest.* **2**:78–84.

Bjorntorp, P., Carlgren, G., Isaksson, B., Krotkiewski, M., Larsson, B., and Sjostrom, L., 1975, The effect of an energy reducing dietary regime in relation to adipose tissue cellularity in obese women, *Am. J. Clin. Nutr.* **28**:445–452.

Bjorntorp, P., Karlsson, M., Pertoft, H., Pettersson, P., Sjostrom, L., and Smith, U., 1978, Isolation and characterization of cells from rat adipose tissue developing into adipocytes, *J. Lipid Res.* **19**:316–324.

Bjurulf, P., 1959, Atherosclerosis and body-build with special reference to size and number of subcutaneous fat cells, *Acta Med. Scand. Suppl.* **166**:349.

Boulton, T. J. C., Dunlop, M., and Court, J. M., 1974, Adipocyte growth in the first two years of life, *Aust. Paediatr. J.* **10**:301–305.

Brook, C. G. D., Lloyd, J. K., and Wolf, O. H., 1972, Relation between age of onset of obesity and size and number of adipose cells, *Brit. Med. J.* **2**:25–27.

Dauncey, M. J., and Gairdner, D., 1975, Size of adipose cells in infancy, *Arch. Dis. Child.* **50**:286–290.

DiGirolamo, M., Mendlinger, S., and Fertig, J. W., 1971, A simple method to determine fat cell size and number in four mammalian species, *Am. J. Physiol.* **221**:850–858.

Dixon-Shanies, D., Rudick, J., and Knittle, J. F., 1975, Observations on the growth and metabolic functions of cultured cells derived from human adipose tissue, *Proc. Soc. Exp. Biol. Med.* **149**:541–545.

Faust, I. M., Johnson, P. R., and Hirsch, J., 1976, Noncompensation of adipose tissue mass in partially lipectomized mice and rats, *Am. J. Physiol.* **231**:539–544.

Faust, I. M., Johnson, P. R., and Hirsch, J., 1977a, Adipose tissue regeneration following lipectomy, *Science* **197**:391–393.

Faust, I. M., Johnson, P. R., and Hirsch, J., 1977b, Surgical removal of adipose tissue alters feeding behavior and the development of obesity in the rat, *Science* **197**:393–396.

Faust, I. M., Johnson, P. R., and Hirsch, J., 1978, Diet-induced adipocyte number increase in adult rats: A new model of obesity, *Am. J. Physiol.* **4**:E279–E286.

Goldrick, R. B., 1967, Morphological changes in the adipocyte during fat deposition and mobilization, *Am. J. Physiol.* **212**:777–782.

Greenwood, M. R. C., and Hirsch, J., 1974, Postnatal development of adipocyte cellularity in the normal rat, *J. Lipid Res.* **15**:474–483.

Hager, A., 1977, Adipose cell size and number in relation to obesity, *Postgrad. Med. J.* **53**:101–110.

Hirsch, J., and Gallian, E., 1968, Methods for the determination of adipose cell size in man and animals, *J. Lipid Res.* **9**:110–119.

Hirsch, J., and Han, P. W., 1969, Cellularity of rat adipose tissue: Effects of growth, starvation and obesity, *J. Lipid Res.* **10**:77–82.

Hirsch, J., and Knittle, J., 1970, Cellularity of obese and nonobese adipose tissue, *Fed. Proc. Fed. Am. Soc. Exp. Biol.* **29**:1516–1521.

Hollenberg, C. H., and Vost, A., 1968, Regulation of DNA synthesis in fat cells and stromal elements from rat adipose tissue, *J. Clin. Invest.* **47**:2485–2498.

Johnson, P. R., and Hirsch, J., 1972, Cellularity of adipose depots in six strains of genetically obese mice, *J. Lipid Res.* **13**:2–11.

Johnson, P. R., Zucker, L. M., Cruce, J. A. F., and Hirsch, J., 1971, Cellularity of adipose depots in the genetically obese Zucker rat (*fafa*), *J. Lipid Res.* **12**:706–714.

Johnson, P. R., Roth, J., Dresner, D., and Lumb, E. S., 1978, Evidence for precursor adipocytes in regenerating tissue following lipectomy in the rat, *Fed. Proc. Fed. Am. Soc. Exp. Biol.* **37**:615.

Johnson, P. R., Stern, J. S., Greenwood, M. R. C., and Hirsch, J., 1979, Adipose tissue hyperplasia and hyperinsulinemia in Zucker obese female rats: A developmental study, *Metabolism* (in press).

Knittle, J. L., 1976, General discussion, in: *Nutrient Requirements in Adolescence* (J. I. McKigney and H. N. Munro, eds.), pp. 71–103, M.I.T. Press, Cambridge, Massachusetts.

Knittle, J. L., and Hirsch, J., 1968, Effect of early nutrition on the development of rat epididymal fat pads: Cellularity and metabolism, *J. Clin. Invest.* **47**:2091–2098.

Lemonnier, D., 1972, Effect of age, sex and site on the cellularity of the adipose tissue in mice and rats rendered obese by a high fat diet, *J. Clin. Invest.* **51**:2907–2915.

Poznanski, W. J., Waheed, I., and Van, R., 1973, Human fat cell precursors: Morphologic and metabolic differentiation in culture, *Lab. Invest.* **29**:570–576.

Reh, M., 1953, Fettzellgrosse beim Menschen und ihre Abhängigkeit vom Ernährungszustand, *Virchows Arch. Pathol. Anat. Physiol.* **324**:234–242.

Salans, L. B., Cushman, S. W., and Weismann, R. E., 1973, Studies of human adipose tissue: Adipose cell size and number in nonobese and obese patients, *J. Clin. Invest.* **52**:929–941.

Sjostrom, L., Bjorntorp, P., and Vrana, J., 1971, Microscopic fat cell size measurements on frozen–cut adipose tissue in comparison with automatic determinations of osmium-fixed fat cells, *J. Lipid Res.* **12**:521–530.

Smith, U., Sjostrom, L., and Bjorntorp, P., 1972, Comparison of two methods for determining human adipose cell size, *J. Lipid Res.* **13**:822–824.

Stiles, J. W., Francendese, A. A., and Masoro, J., 1976, Influence of age on the size and number of fat cells in the epididymal depot, *Am. J. Physiol.* **229**:1561–1568.

Van, R. L. R., and Roncari, D. A. K., 1977, Isolation of fat cell precursors from adult rat adipose tissue, *Cell Tissue Res.* **181**:197–203.

Van, R. L. R., Bayliss, C. E., and Roncari, D. A. K., 1976, Cytological and enzymological characterization of adult human adipocyte precursors in culture, *J. Clin. Invest.* **58**:699–704.

Widdowson, E. M., and Shaw, W. T., 1973, Full and empty fat cells, *Lancet* **2**:906.

Divalent Ion Metabolism

Jack W. Coburn, Kiyoshi Kurokawa, and Charles R. Kleeman

11.1. Introduction

The thrust of this review is directed to certain specific topics of divalent ion metabolism, rather than to providing a tedious, "index card" description of all topics related to divalent ion metabolism. Research and clinical studies in the field of altered vitamin D metabolism are appearing with great frequency with more investigators now involved. Thus, the focus of this review includes recent advances in the metabolism and actions of vitamin D, a discussion of clinical disorders that are believed to relate to altered vitamin D metabolism or action, the regulation of phosphate homeostasis, and a more recent update on the syndrome of phosphate depletion. Hyperparathyroidism and hypercalcemia are not included in this review; the reader may find such a review in *Contemporary Endocrinology*, Vol. 1 (Kleeman and Kleeman, 1979). Limiting the review to these few topics made possible a more cohesive text.

JACK W. COBURN and KIYOSHI KUROKAWA • Nephrology Section, Medical and Research Services, Veterans Administration Wadsworth Hospital Center and Department of Medicine, University of California at Los Angeles School of Medicine, Los Angeles, California 90073. CHARLES R. KLEEMAN • Center for Health, Enhancement, Education, and Research, Department of Medicine, University of California at Los Angeles School of Medicine, Los Angeles, California 90073.

11.2. Vitamin D

11.2.1. Introduction

Recent reports related to the metabolism and action of vitamin D, studies designed to define the role of vitamin D in the endocrine regulation of calcium metabolism, and papers on the role of vitamin D in various disease states have appeared during the past year.

In a recent review, DeLuca (1977) summarizes data on vitamin D as a member of the hormone system that regulates calcium metabolism. He provides a historical background about rickets and early work on identification and synthesis of vitamin D_2 and D_3. He summarizes his views on the functions of vitamin D, emphasizing the effect on intestinal calcium and phosphorus absorption, with his opinion that there is no definite proof that vitamin D induces bone mineralization by any mechanism other than its effect to raise calcium and phosphorus in the extracellular fluid. Moreover, most *in vitro* data suggest that 1,25-dihydroxy-vitamin D_3 [$1,25(OH)_2D_3$] acts to stimulate bone resorption. He discusses the natural sources of vitamin D, its biogenesis and metabolism, and factors that affect its absorption and transport. He reviews the regulation of the production of $1,25(OH)_2D_3$ and emphasizes the effects of either low-calcium or low-phosphorus diets as factors stimulating the bioactivation of D_3. He also briefly discusses various analogues of vitamin D that can act without the necessity of undergoing 1-hydroxylation. He briefly considers various diseases that involve altered calcium and phosphorus metabolism. The value of measuring plasma 25-hydroxy-D as an indication of vitamin D status is reviewed. This paper provides an up-to-date review; although it does reflect the personal views of the writer, he is a world authority on the subject.

Haussler and colleagues (Haussler *et al.*, 1977; Haussler and McCain, 1977) review evidence for the presence of specific receptors for $1,25(OH)_2D_3$ in both cytosol and nuclear chromatin; they summarize the evidence that hormone binding with the genome correlates with synthesis of specific new messenger RNA and protein. The proposed time course for the events following the administration of $1,25(OH)_2D_3$ in vitamin-D-deficient chicks is shown in Fig. 1. Thus, one sees, sequentially, binding of $1,25(OH)_2D_3$ to chromatin, increased RNA synthesis, and augmented template activity; enhanced intestinal calcium absorption follows these steps.

Data that show a specific receptor for $1,25(OH)_2D_3$ in the parathyroid gland are presented, and the use of the nuclear receptor for the assay of $1,25(OH)_2D$ is discussed. Data are presented indicating that patients with primary hyperparathyroidism have plasma values of $1,25(OH)_2D$ that are

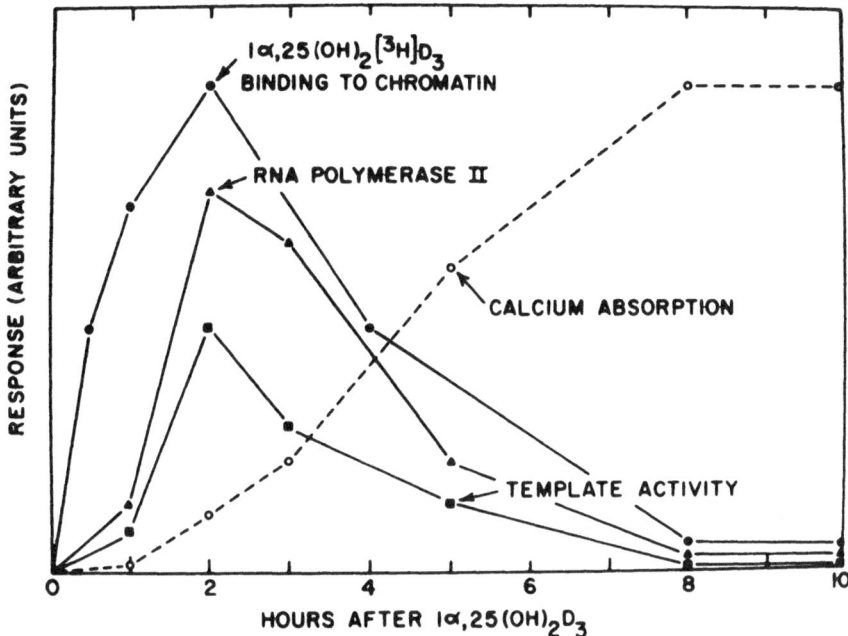

Fig. 1. Time course of 1,25(OH)$_2$D$_3$-mediated events in vitamin-D-deficient chick intestinal cells following a dose of 625 pmol 1,25(OH)$_2$D$_3$. Reproduced from Haussler *et al.* (1977) with permission of the publisher.

increased above normal. Observations in patients under treatment with anticonvulsants are of interest: Thus, levels of 25(OH)D were low in patients receiving phenobarbital, alone, and in those receiving phenytoin and phenobarbital; however, the plasma levels of 1,25(OH)$_2$D were normal or even increased in the patients receiving phenobarbital. Such observations indicate that the abnormalities of serum calcium and bone seen in association with anticonvulsant treatment cannot be explained by the subnormal levels of 1,25(OH)$_2$D; also, the data indicate that depressed circulating levels of 25(OH)D do not necessarily lead to reduced levels of 1,25(OH)$_2$D. Haussler and McCain (1977) review observations that the ingestion of certain botanical species by grazing animals can cause calcinosis and other pathological features similar to vitamin D intoxication; such observations stimulate interest in the identification of vitamin-D-like compounds in plants. A major difference between the plant product and vitamin D is that the plant material is water-soluble and has an apparent molecular weight in excess of 1000. In contrast, 1,25(OH)$_2$D$_3$ is preferentially soluble in organic solvents and has a molecular weight of 416. The structure of this compound is suggested to be that of a glycoside of

$1,25(OH)_2D_3$. The possibility that this water-soluble compound might be a therapeutic substitute for $1,25(OH)_2D_3$ is discussed in this comprehensive review of vitamin D action (Haussler *et al.*, 1977).

11.2.2. Metabolism and Transport of 25-Hydroxy-Vitamin D_3

The major circulating form of vitamin D metabolite, $25(OH)D_3$, is present in the circulation largely bound to a specific vitamin-D-binding protein (DBP). Recently developed radioimmunoassays for this binding protein for vitamin D have revealed that the majority of DBP is present in the plasma as an apoprotein not containing the bound molecule of $25(OH)D$ or of vitamin D. Indeed, only 1–2% of binding sites of DBP are occupied by $25(OH)D_3$ in circulation. While plasma levels of $25(OH)D$ may change in various disease states, plasma levels of DBP do not seem to change in such diseases as vitamin D deficiency, vitamin D excess, sarcoidosis, anticonvulsant therapy, and renal failure; significant rises in plasma levels of DBP were observed in pregnant women or those on contraceptive pills, while they were decreased in hepatic cirrhosis and in the nephrotic syndrome (Haddad and Walgate, 1976; Imawari and Goodman, 1977).

The fetus receives its $25(OH)D$ via placental transfer from maternal sources. Thus, the serum concentrations of both $25(OH)D$ and DBP were both found to be lower in serum from the cord than in maternal serum. Bouillon *et al.* (1977) calculated the free plasma levels of $25(OH)D$ based on the concentrations of both $25(OH)D$ and DBP and the measured association constants of both substances. The calculated concentration of "free $25(OH)D$" was slightly but significantly higher in cord serum than in maternal serum. A highly significant correlation was found between maternal and cord serum concentrations of DBP, total $25(OH)D$, and "free $25(OH)D$." These data indicate that the higher maternal $25(OH)D$ concentration may not indicate the favorable transfer of sterol across placenta to the fetus, and indeed, the low fetal concentration of DBP may create an unfavorable environment for the fetal storage of $25(OH)D$ during intrauterine life.

Human breast milk contains small amounts of vitamin D either as D itself or in a sulfated form. During lactation, the mother can lose a significant amount of vitamin D, a factor that could theoretically result in a relative vitamin-D-deficient state. However, studies by Fairney *et al.* (1977) demonstrated no effect of lactation for 4–6 weeks on plasma $25(OH)D$ levels in the mothers compared to observations in nonlactating mothers.

A study of children living in the upper midwestern United States (age range 0.5–6 years) revealed that levels of serum $25(OH)D$ were not different from reported values in other American children and adults

(Arnaud *et al.*, 1977). Serum 25(OH)D levels fell during the winter. This was due primarily to a decrease in 25(OH)D$_3$, while levels of 25(OH)D$_2$ remained constant throughout the year. The proportion of 25(OH)D$_3$ in total plasma 25(OH)D was 83% in summer and 67% in winter. Such observations suggest the importance of the natural biosynthesis of D$_3$ compared to sources of vitamin D$_2$ added to foodstuffs in the maintenance of the vitamin D state of children throughout the year.

In a study by Clark and Potts (1977), the metabolism of vitamin D was studied in rats deprived of vitamin D over a prolonged period. Plasma levels of 25(OH)D, measured serially, fell within 1 week, but they did not become undetectable until 9 weeks after initiation of a D-deficient diet; on the other hand, a fall in serum calcium and other signs of vitamin D deficiency were apparent by 2 weeks. When the animals were vitamin-D-deficient, they were given vitamin D$_3$ in doses ranging from 32 ng to 2.5 μg, 1 to 3 times/week. Blood samples were obtained at weekly intervals for the measurement of serum calcium and 25(OH)D. As the quantity of vitamin D$_3$ administered was increased from low to very high quantities, the plasma levels of 25(OH)D rose to 800 ng/ml. Only with the highest dose did the rats become hypercalcemic and lose weight. These data demonstrate a direct relationship between the dose of vitamin D$_3$ given and the plasma concentration of 25(OH)D$_3$. Such observations provide very little support for regulation of the 25-hydroxylase. These authors discussed the concept that a comparison of the biological actions of 1,25(OH)$_2$D$_3$ with those of 1α(OH)D$_3$ may provide a clue to the 25-hydroxylation. In normal man, they describe rapid 25-hydroxylation of radiolabeled 1α(OH)D$_3$, even in patients receiving large amounts of D$_3$, a further observation suggesting that there is little, if any, regulation of the 25-hydroxylation. They conclude that there is little to support the importance of regulation of this hydroxylase. These data do not agree with the radioisotopic studies in man of Mawer *et al.* (1971) and Lumb *et al.* (1971), nor do they fit with our preliminary observations comparing the effects of 1,25(OH)$_2$D$_3$ and 1α(OH)D$_3$ in man.

Other observations speak against the conclusion of Clark and Potts (1977). In man, it has generally been found that the larger the dose of vitamin D given, the smaller the fraction that is converted to 25(OH)D$_3$. Although it has been concluded that the conversion of D$_3$ to 25(OH)D$_3$ is modified by product inhibition of 25(OH)D$_3$ itself, Mawer and Reeve (1977) did not consider the results of the experiments carried out *in vivo* to be entirely convincing. To further explore this matter, Mawer and Reeve (1977) carried out studies of 25-hydroxylation of vitamin D using isolated perfused livers obtained from vitamin-D-deficient rats. The liver was perfused with radiolabeled vitamin D$_3$, and radiolabeled 25(OH)D$_3$ was assessed in the perfusate at hourly intervals. The various factors studied that might affect this conversion included pretreatment with cholecalciferol (D_3), 625 pmol, or 25(OH)D_3, 6250 pmol, given to the animal 12 hr before the perfusion, and pretreatment with 1,25(OH)$_2$$D_3$, 10 pmol, or 24,25(OH)$_2$$D_3$, 100 pmol, each given 6 hr before the perfusion. The results indicate no difference between the amount of [^{3}H]-25(OH)D_3 released into the perfusate in control, untreated rats compared to animals pretreated with 25(OH)D_3, 1,25(OH)$_2$$D_3$, or 24,-25(OH)$_2$$D_3$. However, pretreatment with vitamin D itself was associated with a significant reduction in the quantity of 25(OH)D_3 produced. The possibility that the nonlabeled D_3 used to pretreat had a dilutional effect was excluded by studies carried out using ^{14}C-labeled D_3. Such observations may be explained in terms of classic substrate inhibition of an enzyme, although the authors point out that it is entirely possible that D_3 and 25(OH)D_3 may compete for the same binding protein within the liver. They suggest the possibility that a transport protein may be needed to shuttle 25(OH)D_3 from the microsomes onto the surface of the cell; such a protein may have a greater affinity for D_3 than for 25(OH)D_3. Such an event could produce these results without the necessity of invoking inhibition of the 25-hydroxylase itself by D_3.

11.2.3. Regulation of 25-Hydroxy-Vitamin D$_3$-1α-Hydroxylase and Generation of 1,25-Dihydroxy-Vitamin D$_3$

1,25(OH)$_2$$D_3$ is thought to be the active form of vitamin D, and this metabolite is exclusively produced by the kidney; thus, the regulation of renal production of 1,25(OH)$_2$$D_3$ is critical for the regulation of calcium and phosphate homeostasis in the body. Many factors have been suggested as regulators of 1,25(OH)$_2$$D_3$ production, among them being serum calcium, serum inorganic phosphate concentration, parathyroid hormone, calcitonin, and the concentration of vitamin D metabolites in the serum. Indeed, 1,25(OH)$_2$$D_3$ itself is a potent inhibitor of the renal 1α-hydroxylase, and it also stimulates 24-hydroxylase to produce 24,-25(OH)$_2$$D_3$. These effects of 1,25(OH)$_2$$D_3$ are mediated by a nuclear effect, since they can be prevented by pretreatment of the animal by actinomycin D or by α-amanitin (Colston *et al.*, 1977). Thus, it seems that when a sufficient amount of 1,25(OH)$_2$$D_3$ is produced in the kidney in the vitamin-D-deficient state, the 24-hydroxylate is then activated; thus, 25(OH)D_3 delivered to the kidney may be converted to 24,25(OH)$_2$$D_3$.

Both hypocalcemia and parathyroid hormone (PTH) have been shown to stimulate renal conversion of 1,25(OH)$_2$$D_3$. Since a low calcium level may not stimulate renal 1,25(OH)$_2$$D_3$ production in the absence of parathyroid glands, the effect of hypocalcemia is believed to be mediated by increased PTH. It has been generally accepted that the renal action of

PTH is mediated by intracellular increase in cyclic AMP (cAMP). An earlier observation by Rasmussen *et al.* (1972) indicated that the *in vitro* conversion of $25(OH)D_3$ to $1,25(OH)_2D_3$ is stimulated by the addition of cAMP or dibutyryl cAMP to isolated renal tubules obtained from vitamin-D-deficient chicks. These results suggest that cAMP is an intracellular mediator for the PTH effect on renal 1-hydroxylase activity. Horiuchi *et al.* (1977) demonstrated that the *in vivo* infusion of cAMP also resulted in the accumulation of tritiated $1,25(OH)_2D_3$ in the plasma of vitamin-D-deficient, thyroparathyroidectomized (TPTX) rats, indicating that cAMP can mimic the action of PTH in stimulating the production of $1,25(OH)_2D_3$ *in vivo*.

In addition to PTH, calcium, phosphorus, and $1,25(OH)_2D_3$, which affect the synthesis of $1,25(OH)_2D_3$, strontium can also suppress the $25(OH)D_3$-1-hydroxylase and suppress PTH secretion as well. In a study designed to evaluate ionic factors affecting $1,25(OH)_2D_3$ production, Omdahl and Evan (1977) studied $25(OH)D_3$-1α-hydroxylase in isolated mitochondria obtained from kidneys of vitamin-D-deficient chicks. They found that oxidative phosphorylation and the synthesis of $1,25(OH)_2D_3$ were decreased by the addition of strontium or calcium. However, calcium and strontium both caused swelling of the mitochondria. To evaluate whether the mitochondrial swelling was related to the decreased synthesis of $1,25(OH)_2D_3$, they carried out other studies with strontium and calcium administered in the diet. Each decreased the synthesis of $1,25(OH)_2D_3$ *in vivo* and reduced the enzyme activity, as measured *in vitro;* these effects occurred in the absence of morphological changes in the mitochondria or a loss of oxidative phosphorylation activity. Thus, the *in vitro* actions of calcium and strontium do not necessarily reflect the mechanism whereby these cations can alter the renal 1-hydroxylation of $25(OH)D_3$ *in vivo*.

The concept that sex steroids may have an important effect on the bioconversion of vitamin D to its more active forms was pioneered by Kenney and associates (see Coburn *et al.*, 1978). The evaluation of the effects of estrogen, progesterone, and testosterone was extended by Tanaka *et al.* (1976) in experiments carried out in adult Japanese quail. In adult male birds, it was found that the enzyme present in the kidneys was primarily $25(OH)D_3\alpha$-24-hydroxylase, rather than the 1-hydroxylase. The single injection of estradiol, 5 mg, into a male bird completely suppressed the $25(OH)D_3\alpha$-24-hydroxylase and augmented the activity of the 1-hydroxylase. Immature male birds did not respond to estrogen alone, but responded to estradiol plus testosterone. Testosterone, given alone, had little or no effect on the hydroxylation of either vitamin D sterol. A castrated male bird showed a response to estradiol only when testosterone was given concomitantly. With optimal doses of both estradiol and testosterone, the activity of the 25(OH)D$_3$-1-hydroxylase could be increased 225-fold. Such results provide strong evidence for a major role of sex steroids in the metabolism of vitamin D. This may be particularly important in the bird, which must mobilize relatively large quantities of calcium for the production of the eggshell. To date, results are not available in other animals, although Pike *et al.* (1977) found high levels of 1,25(OH)$_2$D in both lactating rats and pregnant human females compared to levels in their normal, nonlactating and nonpregnant counterparts.

11.2.4. Measurement of Vitamin D Metabolites in Plasma

The introduction of assay of 25(OH)D and 1,25(OH)$_2$D in plasma has provided new insight into the variations in vitamin D metabolism both in disease and in health. The information obtained by the assays of 1,25(OH)$_2$D in various disease and health states was reviewed by Haussler and McCain (1977). Some of these results are indicated in Table I (Haussler *et al.*, 1977; Pike *et al.*, 1977).

Assays for serum levels of 24,25(OH)$_2$D have also been developed. Taylor *et al.* (1977) and Taylor (1977) reported values of plasma 24,-25(OH)$_2$D and concomitant levels of 25(OH)D and in a variety of clinical disorders. They found a positive correlation between serum levels of 24,25(OH)$_2$D and serum levels of 25(OH)D. Also, the plasma levels of 24,25(OH)$_2$D were found to be disproportionately elevated for any given level of plasma 25(OH)D in patients with hyperparathyroidism, while the values were low or undetectable in anephric patients. In contrast to these results, Haddad *et al.* (1977) reported normal levels of 24,25(OH)$_2$D in

Table I.   Circulating 1,25(OH)$_2$D in Disorders of Mineral Metabolism

Disease state	Number of patients	Plasma 1,25(OH)$_2$D (ng/dl ± S.D.)
Normal (>18 yr old)	58	3.4 ± 0.8
Normal (5–10 yr old)	4	6.4 ± 0.9
Chronic renal failure	50	0.4 ± 0.4
Polycystic kidneys	5	0.8 ± 0.5
Hypoparathyroidism	11	2.8 ± 0.9
Pseudohypoparathyroidism	8	2.9 ± 1.4
Primary hyperparathyroidism	26	5.4 ± 2.1
Nutritional osteomalacia	3	1.4 ± 0.5
Familial hypophosphatemic rickets	11	3.3 ± 1.4
Juvenile osteoporosis	5	3.4 ± 0.4
Sarcoidosis	4	3.6 ± 1.3
Idiopathic hypercalciuria	40	5.0 ± 1.6

the plasma of uremic patients. These contradictory results are, at the moment, somewhat confusing; unpublished observations of which we are aware from two other laboratories indicate that the plasma levels of $24,25(OH)_2D$ are reduced in patients with advanced renal insufficiency and in those who are anephric. Nonetheless, some time may be required for clarification of the true level of this sterol in plasma of various clinical disorders.

11.2.5. Actions of Vitamin D

11.2.5.1. Effects on Phosphate Homeostasis and Absorption

Vitamin D deficiency, produced in experimental animals, can lead to impaired intestinal phosphorus absorption, while the administration of $1,25(OH)_2D_3$ improves phosphate transport in animals receiving an adequate supply of vitamin D. Rizzoli *et al.* (1977) carried out a study to determine whether variations in the production of $1,25(OH)_2D_3$ in vitamin-D-replete animals can change intestinal phosphorus absorption. The endogenous production of $1,25(OH)_2D_3$ was modified by (1) high phosphate intake, (2) thyroparathyroidectomy (TPTX), or (3) treatment with the diphosphonate, disodium ethane-1-hydroxy-1,1-diphosphonate (EHDP). Intestinal phosphorus absorption was evaluated utilizing both the *in situ* duodenal loop technique and the overall net intestinal absorption as determined from metabolic balance techniques. A reduction in dietary P_i stimulated P_i absorption, and TPTX decreased P_i absorption; the latter was corrected by the administration of either PTH or $1,25(OH)_2D_3$. Also, EHDP, given at a dose known to inhibit the generation of $1,25(OH)_2D_3$, decreased duodenal absorption of P_i in both intact and TPTX animals. This effect was corrected by the administration of $1,25(OH)_2D_3$. However, the administration of PTH to TPTX, EHDP-treated animals did not restore duodenal phosphorus absorption toward normal. Such results support the hypothesis that rats with a normal supply of vitamin D can vary the endogenous production of $1,25(OH)_2D_3$ to modulate their intestinal P_i absorption. Nonetheless, these effects were relatively small compared to the effect of variations in dietary phosphorus on its dietary absorption. The authors interpret these results to indicate that the action of PTH on duodenal phosphorus transport is mediated via an effect on the production of $1,25(OH)_2D_3$. However, the probability that phosphorus deprivation induces events with a much stronger effect was also suggested. Such observations are in accord with data from our own laboratory; moreover, in preliminary studies we found that $1,25(OH)_2D_3$ stimulates a much greater increase of phosphorus transport in a rat receiving a low-phosphorus diet than occurs in animals receiving a normal phosphate intake. Thus, an increased production of $1,25(OH)_2D$ does not entirely account for the adaptation to a low-phosphorus diet.

Walling (1977) carried out careful studies of the intestinal transport of calcium and inorganic phosphate across the rat intestine *in vitro* in the absence of an electrochemical gradient. He found that $1,25(OH)_2D_3$ led to an increase in active absorption of calcium and P_i in all segments of the small intestine, with the changes occurring only in the absorptive flux, secretory fluxes being unchanged. Active calcium absorption was greatest in the duodenum, while active phosphorus absorption was highest in the jejunum. The ratio of the absorptive flux of phosphorus to the flux of calcium remained remarkably constant, even as absorption increased 80–200% with $1,25(OH)_2D_3$. From these observations, he suggested that the hormonally active metabolites of vitamin D either produced coupled calcium and phosphorus transport or coordinated the stimulation of separate absorptive processes for these two ions. He suggested that there may be differential distribution of vitamin-D-responsive cells that can account for either calcium or P_i absorption, with a predominance of calcium-absorbing cells in the duodenum, while there is a preponderance of phosphorus-absorbing cells in the jejunum.

Although data such as those cited above indicate that vitamin D augments phosphorus transport in experimental animals, less information is available in man. Early studies have shown that pharmacological doses of vitamin D can produce an increase in net absorption of both calcium and phosphorus in uremic patients. Brickman *et al.* (1977) provided a clear demonstration that $1,25(OH)_2D_3$ and $1\alpha(OH)D_3$ can each stimulate net phosphorus absorption in normal human volunteers and in patients with advanced uremia. Moreover, the data illustrate a dose-related effect with a progressively greater net absorption of phosphorus as the dose of $1,25(OH)_2D_3$ is increased. An evaluation of the relationship between the change in moles of calcium absorption and the change in moles of P_i absorption has revealed a slope of 0.46. These results, obtained during metabolic balance studies, utilize a normal calcium content in the diet; thus, they do not exclude the possibility that phosphorus absorption occurs secondarily to that of calcium. However, data in experimental animals have shown an effect of vitamin D sterols on phosphorus transport independent of calcium. These observations are of clinical significance because they indicate that net phosphorus absorption will be augmented in uremic patients by treatment with the active vitamin D sterol unless measures are taken to counteract this effect.

11.2.5.2. Actions of Vitamin D on the Kidney

The question of whether vitamin D or one of the active sterols has a direct effect on renal tubular transport of calcium and phosphorus has continued to be a subject of interest. An evaluation of these questions is complex, since an evaluation of the effects of vitamin D on the kidney must include consideration of other factors that affect the renal handling of calcium and phosphorus, in particular the blood levels of calcium and phosphorus and the status of PTH and calcitonin, which can be affected either indirectly or directly by vitamin D. Also, many studies of the renal effects of $1,25(OH)_2D_3$ or other vitamin D sterols have been evaluated within a few hours of administration of the vitamin D sterol; on the other hand, the intestinal effect of these sterols is known to be maximal only after 12–48 hr. Thus, the renal physiologist may not evaluate the renal tubular effects at the time when the effect may be optimal. In a short-term study carried out in the rat, Popovtzer *et al.* (1977) found that the administration of $25(OH)D_3$ interfered with the phosphaturic action of calcitonin. This effect on the phosphaturia was accompanied by a reduction in the augmented urinary cAMP excretion normally produced by calcitonin. These observations are analogous to previous studies by Popovtzer and Robinette (1975), which illustrated that $25(OH)D_3$ also interfered with the phosphaturic action of PTH. These observations are consistent with the previous report of Puschett *et al.* (1975), which indicated that the infusion of $1,25(OH)_2D_3$ could block the phosphaturic actions of a small quantity of PTH.

These short-term studies are in contrast to the studies of Bonjour *et al.* (1977), who reported that $1,25(OH_2D_3$, given for several days in a small dose calculated to restore intestinal calcium absorption to normal in TPTX rats, led to an *increase* in urinary phosphorus excretion. The mechanism whereby $1,25(OH)_2D_3$ produces a decrease in phosphorus excretion in one model and an increase in its excretion in another remains uncertain. The role of vitamin D in controlling the renal handling of P is reviewed in greater detail in Section 11.4. The chronically parathyroidectomized animal is hyperphosphatemic, and studies have shown that $1,25(OH)_2D_3$ causes serum phosphorus to fall in an animal with a high level of serum phosphorus, while $1,25(OH)_2D_3$ causes an increase in serum phosphorus level in an animal with hypophosphatemia. Thus, tubular mechanisms may exist whereby the phosphorus status of the animal dictates the overall net effect of a vitamin D metabolite on phosphate handling.

The effects of $1,25(OH)_2D_3$ and other vitamin D sterols on the renal handling of calcium have also been the subject of continued investigation. In a study carried out in parathyroidectomized rats, Rizzoli *et al.* (1977) found that $1,25(OH)_2D_3$, given for several days, led to an increase in the renal excretion of calcium. Previous studies carried out in dogs suggested that $25(OH)D$ may produce an early decrease in urinary calcium excretion (Puschett *et al.*, 1972). In man, the administration of $1,25(OH)_2D_3$ produces a prompt and marked increase in urinary calcium to an extent that is greater than one might expect from the increase in intestinal absorption of calcium. Thus, such results suggest that low doses of vitamin D sterols may be capable of decreasing renal tubular transport of calcium in a vitamin-D-replete animal. Such an effect may occur, in part, as a consequence of suppression of parathyroid activity; on the other hand, the acute administration of much larger quantities of $1,25(OH)_2D_3$ may enhance renal tubular calcium transport. The role of vitamin D metabolites in affecting renal handling of calcium and phosphorus under normal physiological conditions remains far from being understood at this time.

11.2.5.3. Effect of Vitamin D on the Parathyroid Glands

Several bits of evidence, some cited in *The Year in Metabolism 1977* (Coburn *et al.*, 1978), suggest that vitamin D or one of its metabolites may exert an action on the parathyroid glands and affect the secretion of PTH. Thus, it is known that $1,25(OH)_2D_3$ accumulates in the parathyroid glands, and both cytoplasmic and nuclear receptors for $1,25(OH)_2D_3$ exist in the parathyroid glands (Brumbaugh *et al.*, 1975; Cloix *et al.*, 1976). However, data on the physiological effects of $1,25(OH)_2D_3$ on PTH are somewhat conflicting. Thus, Care *et al.* (1977) reported that there may be stimulation of PTH secretion by a pulse dose of $1,25(OH)_2D_3$, an observation exactly the opposite from those previously reported by Chertow *et al.* (1975). In man, Llach *et al.* (1977) studied the acute effect of orally administered $1,25(OH)_2D_3$ on serum calcium, phosphorus, and immunoreactive PTH (iPTH) and on urinary cAMP in normal subjects. The first observable change that followed the oral administration of $1,25(OH)_2D_3$ was an increase in urinary calcium at 5–6 hr, although urinary cAMP fell shortly thereafter. Serum iPTH decreased in some of the subjects only, and these subjects generally exhibited an increase in serum calcium. There were no consistent changes in renal phosphate handling. Such observations in normal, vitamin-D-replete man provide no definite evidence for a direct effect of $1,25(OH)_2D_3$ on secretion of PTH.

In another study in which parathyroid gland weight was the parameter evaluated, Henry *et al.* (1977) reported that vitamin D_3 causes significant regression of hyperplastic parathyroid glands in association with an increase in serum calcium following its administration to vitamin-D-deficient animals. On the other hand, $1,25(OH)_2D_3$ produced the same increase in serum calcium, but caused no change in parathyroid gland size. Only when $1,25(OH)_2D_3$ was given in combination with $24,25(OH)_2D_3$ was there a decrease in the size of parathyroid glands in concert with the rise in serum calcium. These latter observations point to the possibility that $24,25(OH)_2D_3$ and $1,25(OH)_2D_3$ may somehow interact to affect proliferation of parathyroid cells. Such data point to the complex nature of interactions between vitamin D and its active forms and changes in parathyroid gland activity.

11.2.6. Biological Actions of 24,25-Dihydroxy-Vitamin D_3

Although a number of naturally occurring vitamin D sterols, including $24,25(OH)_2D_3$, have been identified in plasma and other biological samples, it has generally been assumed that $1,25(OH)_2D_3$ is responsible for most, if not all, of the effects previously attributed to vitamin D itself. In a study comparing the effects of $1,25(OH)_2D_3$, $24,25(OH)_2D_3$, and $1,24,25(OH)_3D_3$, Walling *et al.* (1977) found that $1,25(OH)_2D_3$ and $1,24,-25(OH)_3D_3$ each stimulated intestinal absorption of calcium and phosphorus in both sham-operated and nephrectomized rats. On the other hand, $24,25(OH)_2D_3$, even in a 10-fold higher dose, had no effect on intestinal absorption of calcium and phosphorus in nephrectomized rats, while it stimulated their absorption in sham-operated animals. These observations on calcium transport corroborated previous experiments from DeLuca's laboratory (Boyle *et al.*, 1973; Holick *et al.*, 1973), and the data also demonstrated that $24,25(OH)_2D_3$ and $1,24,25(OH)_3D_3$ have an effect on phosphorus transport similar to that of $1,25(OH)_2D_3$. A major point was that the effect on intestinal transport required the kidneys and, therefore, 1-hydroxylation. These observations and data obtained in chicks, which show that $24,25(OH)_2D_3$ is degraded very rapidly, led Holick *et al.* (1976) to suggest that $24,25(OH)_2D_3$ was largely an inactive degradation product of vitamin D metabolism.

A number of recent observations provide support for the view that $24,25(OH)_2D_3$ may exert biological effects different from those of its sister sterol, $1,25(OH)_2D_3$. Thus, Miravet *et al.* (1976) found that $24,25(OH)_2D_3$, given to vitamin-D-deficient rats with normal serum calcium levels as a consequence of phosphorus-restricted diet, exhibited a decrease in serum calcium rather than an increase, as occurs in animals given $1,25(OH)_2D_3$. In addition, Kanis *et al.* (1977) found that $24,25(OH)_2D_3$, when given to normal man, led to a decrease in fecal calcium but produced no increase in urinary calcium excretion. These observations stand in contrast to the effect of $1,25(OH)_2D_3$ whereby a decrease in fecal calcium is almost precisely offset by the increase in urinary calcium. Thus, little or no positive balance for calcium occurs with $1,25(OH)_2D_3$, while $24,25(OH)_2D_3$ produced a positive balance for calcium (Fig. 2). Bordier *et al.* (1977) reported that $24,25(OH)_2D_3$, when given in conjunction with $1,25(OH)_2D_3$, led to more effective mineralization of bone compared to the action of $1,25(OH)_2D_3$ alone.

Further evidence for qualitatively different effects of vitamin D metabolites, including $24,25(OH)_2D_3$, were reported by Lieberherr *et al.*

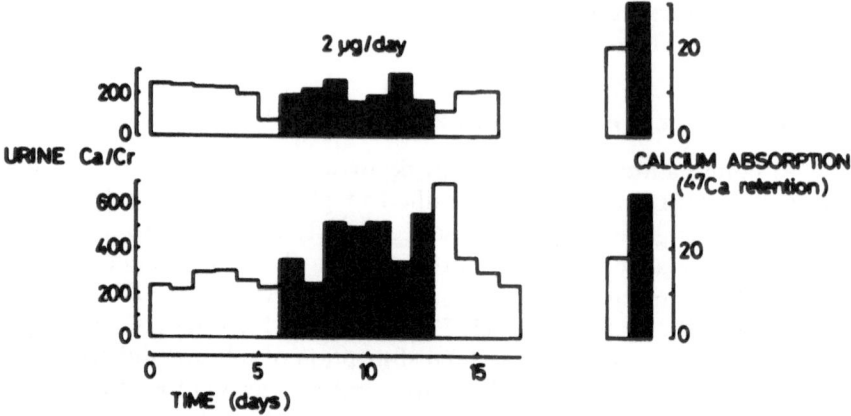

Fig. 2. Effects of 24,25(OH)$_2$D$_3$ *(top)* and of 1,25(OH)$_2$D$_3$ *(bottom)* on the intestinal absorption and urinary excretion of calcium in a normal man. Reproduced from Kanis *et al.* (1977) with permission of the publisher.

(1977). They evaluated acid and alkaline phosphatase activities in the calvaria obtained from vitamin-D-deficient rats given small doses of 25(OH)D$_3$, 24,25(OH)$_2$D$_3$, or 1,25(OH)$_2$D$_3$, *in vivo.* The 25(OH)D$_3$ caused a significant increase, while 24,25(OH)$_2$D$_3$ led to a decrease, and 1,25(OH)$_2$D$_3$ produced no change in enzyme activities. These enzyme changes did not seem to be related to alterations in the concentrations of calcium or phosphorus in the serum. Such observations provide further support for the view that various vitamin D sterols may exert qualitatively different actions. It should be noted that such studies do not, as yet, define the physiological role of these sterols; however, they do suggest that the view that 1,25(OH)$_2$D$_3$ accounts for all actions heretofore attributed to vitamin D$_3$ itself should be subjected to serious reappraisal.

11.2.7. Metabolism and Degradation of Vitamin D

Most past work has been focused on the generation of the active forms of vitamin D; recent reports have shed light on the mechanism whereby vitamin D is degraded. There is considerable evidence for side-chain cleavage and oxidation of the steroid: Thus, Kumar and associates (Kumar *et al.*, 1976; Kumar and DeLuca, 1976, 1977) measured the $^{14}CO_2$ in the expired air of vitamin-D-deficient rats and chicks given either 25(OH)[26,27-^{14}C]vitamin D$_3$, 1,25(OH)$_2$[26,27-^{14}C]vitamin D$_3$, or 24,-25(OH)$_2$[26,27-^{14}C]vitamin D$_3$ intravenously. Approximately 7% of a 650-pmol dose of labeled 25(OH)D$_3$ and 25% of a 325-pmol dose of labeled

$1,25(OH)_2D_3$ were metabolized to $^{14}CO_2$ in 48 hr by vitamin-D-deficient rats (Kumar *et al.*, 1976). Nephrectomy completely prevented the metabolism of labeled $25(OH)D_3$ to $^{14}CO_2$, but not that of $1,25(OH)_2D_3$ (Fig. 3). Less than 5% of the ^{14}C from labeled $24,25(OH)_2D_3$ was broken down to $^{14}CO_2$, but the effect of nephrectomy on the metabolism of $24,25(OH)_2D_3$ was not evaluated (Kumar *et al.*, 1976). Feeding vitamin-D-deficient rats with a diet high in calcium and supplemented with vitamin D_3 markedly suppressed the production of $^{14}CO_2$ from labeled $25(OH)D_3$ but not from labeled $1,25(OH)_2D_3$. Since the rate of the $^{14}CO_2$ evolution from labeled $1,25(OH)_2D_3$ was maximal 4–12 hr after a dose of the sterol, it is suggested that this side-chain oxidation may be of significant importance to the biological function of $1,25(OH)_2D_3$.

In other experiments designed to identify the site of side-chain oxidation of vitamin D, these investigators found that the amount of $^{14}CO_2$ formed after a 325-pmol dose of labeled $1,25(OH)_2D_3$ was reduced by 65.2% at 4 hr and by 67.1% at 8 hr in rats the jejunum, ileum, and colon of which were removed (Kumar and DeLuca, 1977). These observa-

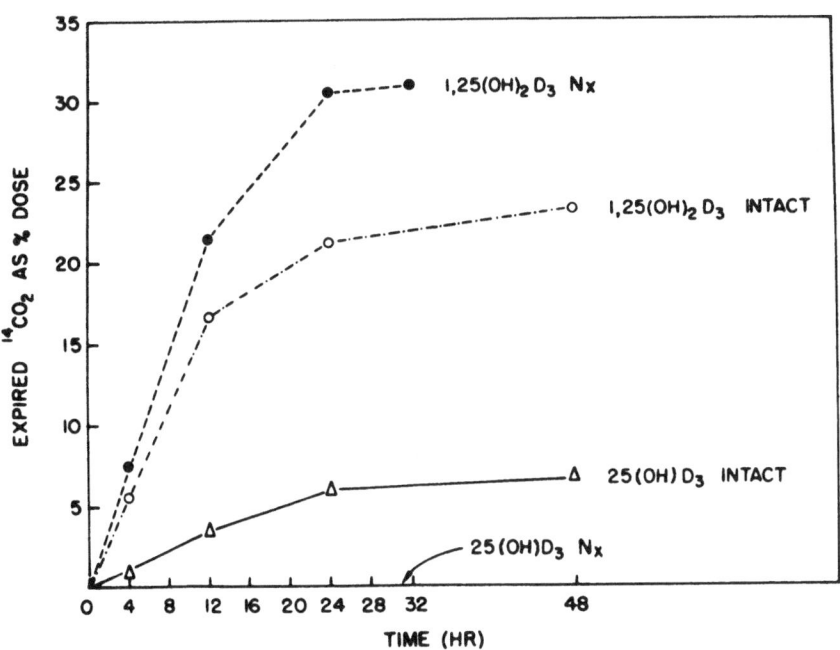

Fig. 3. Side-chain oxidation of $25(OH)D_3$ and $1,25(OH)_2D_3$ in vitamin-D-deficient rats with intact kidneys (INTACT) and with nephrectomy (Nx). Reproduced from Kumar *et al.* (1976) with permission of the publisher.

tions suggest that the intestine is one of the sites where the side-chain oxidation takes place. Intestinal bacterial flora is not likely to be of significance, since "germ-free" rats produced as much $^{14}CO_2$ from labeled $1,25(OH)_2D_3$ as was produced by animals with normal bacterial flora.

The role of the kidneys and bile in the excretion of vitamin D is being appreciated as well. In a study of normal, vitamin-D-replete, adult rats, given 200 pmol 25(OH)D [approximately 80 μg ^{3}H-labeled $25(OH)D_3$], Larsson and Lorentzon (1977) found substantial production of a vitamin D sterol that comigrated with $1,25(OH)_2D_3$ on Sephadex LH 20 column chromatography. Substantial amounts of radioactivity were found in urine of these vitamin-D-replete, normal animals. There were also sizable amounts of radioactivity in the bile, generally in the methanol-extracted rather than the chloroform phase. The physiological significance of these observations is not entirely clear because of the large dose of 25(OH)D given and because of the "pulse" administration; nonetheless, the finding of a substantial amount of vitamin D metabolites in the urine and bile suggests that further efforts should be directed to the study of the roles of the kidney and liver in the degradation and excretion of vitamin D compounds.

11.2.8. Intestinal Calcium Absorption and Mechanism of Adaptation to a Low-Calcium Diet

The mechanism by which the mammal or bird produces an adaptive increase in intestinal calcium absorption when the dietary intake of calcium is restricted has been a subject of some interest. With the newer knowledge of the steps of bioconversion of vitamin D into its active forms, it has generally been assumed that a change in the activation of $25(OH)D_3$ to $1,25(OH)_2D_3$ is a major factor that mediates this adaptation of intestinal calcium transport. In a provocative study by Michalska et al. (1976), there are data to suggest that the process of adaptation may be more complex than has previously been suspected. This group of investigators utilized the everted gut sac technique to study the effect of a low-calcium diet on active calcium transport by various segments of the small intestine of the rat at varying times following dietary calcium restriction. In young rats receiving a normal-calcium diet, they noted that active translocation of calcium was limited to the proximal 10 cm of the small intestine, i.e., the duodenum. With dietary calcium restriction, calcium transport of the duodenum was augmented maximally within 3 days; thereafter, the calcium transport gradually declined, and active calcium transport by this segment had almost disappeared after 28 days. In contrast, the calcium transport of the proximal jejunum increased only slowly after introduction of the low-calcium diet, and was highest 7–21 days after the low-calcium diet was initiated. In the distal ileum, active transport could be detected after 3 days of the low-calcium diet and increased progressively until 21 days, although it decreased after 4 weeks. In every segment, the magnitude of calcium transport returned to a normal pattern in animals returned from a low-calcium diet to a standard, normal-calcium diet. These observations suggest that there may be a rapid mechanism that accounts for the early stimulation of calcium transport by the duodenum, while a slower mechanism is responsible for the subsequent appearance of active calcium transport by the more distal portions of the intestine. All the animals were receiving vitamin D_3, and some of the adaptive responses may have been related to the bioconversion of $25(OH)D_3$ to $1,25(OH)_2D_3$; on the other hand, it seems unlikely that the different temporal responses seen in different intestinal segments can all be attributed to the same changes in vitamin D metabolism.

In another study, Pento et al. (1977) evaluated the role of the parathyroid glands in the adaptation of intestinal calcium transport in response to dietary calcium deprivation. This was evaluated utilizing both in vitro inverted duodenal sacs and the in situ ligated duodenal segment. Intact and parathyroidectomized young rats were given a low-calcium diet for either 7, 14, or 21 days before measurement of calcium transport. Parathyroidectomy was carried out 3 days prior to initiation of the low-calcium diet. Parathyroidectomy led to complete abolition of the adaptive response, measured at 7 days, but it did not prevent the response seen after 21 days. The observations at 14 days were somewhat equivocal. These data suggest that the short-term adaptation does involve PTH, while a longer-term adaptation does not require PTH, unless, of course, some hyperplasia of accessory parathyroid tissue may have occurred. These observations, as well as the study cited above, suggest that the adaptation involves more than one mechanism.

The results of these two studies are very interesting, and they may have implications in certain disease states in man. It is known that the major abnormality of intestinal calcium transport produced by uremia is a defect in active calcium transport in the proximal portion of the small intestine. The abnormality in uremia is striking, and little overlap exists between uremic patients and normal individuals. On the other hand, methods of assessing calcium absorption that measure integrated absorption in the entire intestine disclose very minor abnormalities in uremia. The implication is that more distal segments of the intestine show augmented absorption. The present experimental study may provide the clue that these processes can be separated.

11.2.8.1. Methods of Assessing Calcium Absorption

There has been a continued introduction of new methods for the assessment of calcium absorption. It is generally believed that the measurement of intestinal calcium absorption during the first 3 hr after calcium ingestion reflects the major component that involves active calcium transport. One of the most accurate, noninvasive methods for assessing this calcium absorption utilizes double isotopes, one given orally and the other intravenously, and a rather complex computation involving deconvolutional analysis. Two separate, specific activity functions of the two isotopes are involved. Roelofs and Raymakers (1976) developed a simple formula to calculate the absorption in the first 3 hr utilizing a double-isotope method. They applied this method in the analysis of 79 patients who were examined both by the abbreviated method and with the more elaborate deconvolutional method. They found very close agreement between the two; on the other hand, they emphasize that this method is capable of calculating absorption only at 3 hr and not at periods before or after the 3-hr time point after ingestion of calcium. Nonetheless, this technique may serve to simplify the procedure needed for deconvolutional analysis.

11.3. Clinical Disorders That Involve Altered Vitamin D Metabolism

Classically, the deficiency of vitamin D will produce hypocalcemia, some degree of hypophosphatemia (related to secondary hyperparathyroidism), and osteomalacia. The clarification of the steps of vitamin D metabolism has provided a better understanding of the disorders causing vitamin D deficiency. These abnormalities may occur in the steps related to formation of vitamin D_3, $25(OH)D_3$, or $1,25(OH)_2D_3$, and can be classified according to the major step of vitamin D metabolism that is affected (Coburn *et al.*, 1978). Vitamin D_3 can be reduced in individuals who have an impaired intake of vitamin D and limited exposure to sunlight. There may be decreased absorption of vitamin D on the basis of intestinal malabsorption, the short bowel syndrome, and the ingestion of drugs that can bind vitamin D, i.e., cholestyramine. The hydroxylation of vitamin D_3 to $25(OH)D_3$ can be impaired in severe liver disease. The renal production of $1,25(OH)_2D_3$ is impaired in patients with renal insufficiency. The skeletal changes found in patients with diminished vitamin D action or availability include rickets in the growing child and osteomalacia in the adult.

The symptoms of vitamin D deficiency are nonspecific, and the diagnosis of osteomalacia is frequently difficult. A great fraction of skeletal mass must be lost before routine X-ray views show the appearance of osteomalacia. Radiographic aids for making the diagnosis were proposed by Meema and Meema (1975). Using magnification techniques, they evaluated roentgenograms obtained with fine-grain film of the hands of patients with osteomalacia and osteoporosis. This method of viewing hand X rays was considered useful in separating these two skeletal disorders. Sixty percent of patients with osteomalacia but none of those with osteoporosis had increased intracortical striations, which are believed to represent enlarged Haversian canals. Subperiosteal resorption of the phalanges was present but was less frequent than were intracortical striations in patients with osteomalacia; subperiosteal resorption was absent in patients with osteoporosis. The quantitiative evaluation of cortical thickness, percentage cortical area, bone mineral mass, and bone density did not differentiate the two groups. These results, obtained by radiologists with great skill and experience in the use of skeletal X rays in metabolic bone disease, are of interest. In our experience, specific radiographic features of osteomalacia are rare in adults; if this technique and these results can be confirmed elsewhere, the technique may be of considerable value.

Nutritional rickets is rare in the United States; its incidence in underdeveloped countries is considerably greater. P. O'Connor (1977) recently reported two infants seen in the United States with nutritional rickets; they had been breast-fed and received no vitamin D supplements. Such observations point to the importance of vitamin D supplementation to breast-fed infants, since milk may provide only a limited quantity of vitamin D.

11.3.1. Abnormal Metabolism of 25-Hydroxy-Vitamin D_3

11.3.1.1. Liver Disease

Impaired production of $25(OH)D_3$ from vitamin D can occur with diffuse liver disease and in association with abnormalities of the biliary tract. Skinner *et al.* (1977) measured plasma levels of $25(OH)D$ in 39 patients with primary biliary cirrhosis. Twenty-five patients were receiving regular injections of vitamin D, and 23 of these had normal serum levels of $25(OH)D$. The serum concentrations of $25(OH)D$ increased after regular monthly injections of vitamin D to 7 patients not given vitamin D previously; such observations indicate that plasma $25(OH)D$ may increase to normal in cirrhosis if large amounts of vitamin D are provided as a substrate to the liver.

Abnormal intestinal absorption of $25(OH)D$ may be another factor leading to osteomalacia in primary biliary cirrhosis. Compston and Thompson (1977) measured intestinal absorption of $25(OH)D_3$ and evaluated bone histology in 11 patients with primary biliary cirrhosis. Following the administration of oral $25(OH)D_3$, plasma concentrations of $25(OH)D$

were lower in the patients with primary biliary cirrhosis than in normal controls. The intestinal absorption of $25(OH)D_3$ was even more depressed in 4 patients who were receiving cholestyramine therapy and who, coincidentally, had evidence of osteomalacia on bone biopsy. Thus, the appearance of osteomalacia in patients with liver disease may occur due to both impaired 25-hydroxylation of vitamin D_3 to $25(OH)D_3$ and, more important, to impaired intestinal absorption of $25(OH)D_3$; the latter may be further reduced by cholestyramine.

11.3.1.2. Anticonvulsants

The relationship between the osteomalacia or rickets associated with anticonvulsant therapy was reviewed in the preceding volume (Coburn *et al.*, 1978). Phenobarbital, phenytoin, and glutethemide are capable of inducing the activity of a hepatic microsomal P-450 enzyme, which may then hydroxylate vitamin D and other steroids in an abnormal manner and result in products that are biologically inactive. Acetazolamide, a drug commonly added in patients with refractory seizures, can also accelerate the development of anticonvulsant-associated osteomalacia.

Mosekilde *et al.* (1977) carried out quantitative morphometric analysis of bone biopsies from 20 epileptic patients receiving anticonvulsant therapy. The patients were evaluated before and after treatment with vitamin D_2, 9000 IU/day, for 4–8 months. Control biopsies revealed increased amounts of unmineralized bone, increased bone resorption, and, contrary to the findings in nutritional vitamin D deficiency, increased bone mineralization and formation, and normal cancellous bone. The skeletal abnormalities were normalized after treatment with vitamin D_2, except for a slight increase in surface area covered with osteoid in those showing osteoclastic resorption. Also, mean serum levels of $25(OH)D$ increased to a value 2.4 times the normal value during treatment. Serum iPTH levels were normal before vitamin D treatment and remained unchanged during treatment. Thus, certain features, which include an increase in both unmineralized bone and resorptive activity, are similar to those of vitamin D deficiency. However, other features, which include an increase in active mineralization, a very slight reduction in calcification rate, and increased bone turnover, differ from those seen in vitamin D deficiency. On the basis of these observations, these workers suggest that anticonvulsant osteomalacia is produced by both an abnormality of vitamin D metabolism and an alteration of the action of vitamin D sterols on target tissues.

Further uncertainties about the effect of anticonvulsants on vitamin D metabolism and osteomalacia are raised by the study of Jubiz *et al.* (1977). They reported normal or increased serum levels of $1,25(OH)_2D$ in patients treated with anticonvulsant drugs. Thus, low serum levels of

25(OH)D that are noted in anticonvulsant-treated patients are not depressed sufficiently to reduce the generation of $1,25(OH)_2D$. Such observations suggest that a lack of $1,25(OH)_2D_3$ is *not* responsible for the osteomalacia of anticonvulsant therapy, and other mechanisms must be involved in the pathogenesis of the osteomalacia. As reviewed previously (Coburn *et al.*, 1978), phenytoin may directly impair the intestinal absorption of calcium. Consistent with this notion is the report of Harrison and Harrison (1976) that phenytoin and phenobarbital given to vitamin-D-deficient rats for 5 days did not alter the response of serum calcium and phosphorus to ergocalciferol, cholecalciferol, or $25(OH)D_3$. However, these drugs significantly reduced the augmentation of intestinal calcium transport produced by the vitamin D sterols. Since the diffusibility of calcium across the mucosal barrier was not reduced, these authors suggested that the anticonvulsants may act to impair the energy-dependent extrusion of calcium at the basal–lateral surfaces of the epithelial cells of the intestine.

11.3.1.3. Nephrotic Syndrome

The hypocalcemia that is a common feature of the nephrotic syndrome is generally attributed to a reduction in the protein-bound calcium fraction due to hypoalbuminemia. Patients with nephrotic syndrome also demonstrate hypocalciuria and decreased net intestinal absorption of calcium. However, clinical evaluation of these abnormalities in calcium metabolism may be difficult in the nephrotic syndrome, since many patients with the nephrotic syndrome also exhibit impaired renal function and altered calcium metabolism due to the renal insufficiency *per se;* other patients with the nephrotic syndrome receive treatment with glucocorticoids, which can also alter calcium metabolism. Schmidt-Gayk *et al.* (1977) measured serum 25(OH)D levels in 33 patients with the nephrotic syndrome and no renal insufficiency. The values were lower in the patients with the nephrotic syndrome than were the seasonally adjusted levels of 25(OH)D in individuals without proteinuria. There was no correlation between the serum level of 25(OH)D and the amount of protein in the urine in patients whose proteinuria exceeded 3.5 g/day per 1.73 m² body surface area. Serum levels of vitamin-D-binding protein (DBP) were significantly lower in the patients with the nephrotic syndrome than in controls, and DBP was identified in the urine of the nephrotic patients. DBP migrates with α-globulin on cellulose acetate electrophoresis and has a molecular weight of approximately 59,000 daltons. In the nephrotic syndrome, the permeability of glomerular basement membrane is markedly increased for proteins with a molecular weight similar to albumin ($\approx 69,000$); thus, it is likely that the DBP is filtered in large amounts through the glomerular basement membrane and hence is lost in the urine. Haddad and Walgate (1976) also demonstrated a decrease in serum levels of DBP in patients with hypoproteinemia due to the nephrotic syndrome.

In an independent study, Barragry *et al.* (1977) found low serum levels of 25(OH)D, low plasma DBP, and the presence of DBP in urine from 10 patients with the nephrotic syndrome. The urinary excretion of DBP ranged from 20 to 170 mg with a mean of 80 mg; it was undetectable in the urine from control subjects. These workers further studied the appearance of radiolabeled vitamin D metabolites in three patients with the nephrotic syndrome and two control subjects after an oral dose of [^{3}H]cholecalciferol. In the two control subjects, nonpolar urinary radioactivity represented a negligible fraction of the dose of the labeled precursor administered. In the three patients with the nephrotic syndrome, the excretion of nonpolar radioactivity reached a maximum between 24 and 48 hr. During the first 24 hr, a significant quantity of [^{3}H]cholecalciferol appeared in the urine; however, [^{3}H]25(OH)D$_3$ constituted the major fraction of urinary radioactivity between 24 and 48 hr. The radioactivity and the urinary DBP comigrated on chromatographic separation of urine from one patient so studied. These authors also demonstrated that the plasma half-life of [^{3}H]25(OH)D$_3$ was 50% shorter than that observed in control subjects. Unfortunately, data on renal function were not given in their nephrotic patients. Nishii *et al.* (1977) demonstrated the rapid urinary excretion of intravenously administered [^{3}H]25(OH)D$_3$ in rats with experimental nephrotic syndrome from glomerulonephritis.

The pathophysiological role of low serum levels of 25(OH)D in the altered divalent ion metabolism found in the nephrotic syndrome is uncertain. Lim *et al.* (1977) reported results of calcium and phosphorus balance in 13 nephrotic patients and 8 patients during a clinical remission of the nephrotic syndrome. Mean values of creatinine clearance and the duration of the nephrotic syndrome in 13 patients were 91.6 ml/min (range 81–112 ml/min) and 14 months (range 2–48 months), respectively; creatinine clearance in the 8 patients in remission was 96.9 ml/min (range 85–126 ml/min). A marked decrease in intestinal calcium absorption was observed in the nephrotic patients, with fecal calcium equal to or exceeding dietary calcium intake in 8 of the 18 patients. The net absorption of calcium in the 8 patients in remission averaged 38.4%. The mean urinary excretion of calcium was 27 and 121 mg/day in nephrotic patients and patients in remission, respectively. The administration of calciferol, 1.25 mg/day, to 3 patients with the nephrotic syndrome had no effect on intestinal calcium absorption or renal excretion of calcium. The intestinal absorption and renal excretion of phosphorus did not differ in the two groups of patients. Bone biopsy specimens, obtained from 7 patients with the nephrotic syndrome, disclosed no evidence of osteomalacia or osteitis fibrosa. In contrast, intestinal calcium absorption, measured with a double-isotope method, was significantly reduced in patients with the nephrotic syndrome *only* when significant renal insufficiency was present; thus, 10 patients with the nephrotic syndrome and normal serum creatinine levels did not exhibit any decrease in intestinal calcium absorption (Mountokalakis *et al.*, 1977).

Goldstein *et al.* (1977) reported significantly reduced serum levels of both 25(OH)D and ionized calcium in nephrotic patients, both with and without renal insufficiency. They observed an inverse correlation between plasma 25(OH)D and urinary protein excretion and a positive correlation between plasma 25(OH)D concentration and serum albumin in the nephrotic patients. In 7 nephrotic patients with normal renal function, there was an inverse relationship between plasma ionized calcium and iPTH level. To further characterize the cause of the hypocalciuria seen in patients with the nephrotic syndrome, these authors evaluated the effect of furosemide on the renal handling of calcium and sodium. A study of the relationship between C_{Ca}/glomerular filtration rate (GFR) and C_{Na}/GFR revealed a slope lower than that previously observed in dogs with saline infusion and extracellular volume expansion or following furosemide administration. The slope was similar to that previously reported in calcium-deficient dogs receiving saline infusion, and was significantly lower than that observed in patients with advanced renal failure but without the nephrotic syndrome. Thus, the hypocalciuria cannot be explained as being due solely to alterations in the renal handling of calcium that arise secondary to changes in sodium handling.

The quantitative aspects of the urinary vitamin D losses in the nephrotic syndrome were evaluated by Barragry *et al.* (1977); they estimated the daily loss to be 2.5 μg of vitamin D and its metabolites, while Schmidt-Gayk *et al.* (1977) found 3.2 μg/day of 25(OH)D in the urine of the nephrotic patients. These quantities are equivalent to 100–120 IU vitamin D, an amount that may be equal to the daily intake of vitamin D in many parts of the world where foods are not fortified with vitamin D. However, losses of this magnitude would not be expected to lead to vitamin D deficiency in the United States. Also, it should be remembered that plasma DBP binds not only 25(OH)D$_3$ but also ergocalciferol (D$_2$), cholecalciferol (D$_3$), and 1,25(OH)$_2$D$_3$, with the highest affinity for 25(OH)D$_3$. The combined plasma content of these sterols occupies less than 5% of the available high-affinity binding sites of the DBP. Thus, it is uncertain how losses of DBP occur to an extent that there is a deficiency of 25(OH)D.

11.3.2. Defective Production of 1,25-Dihydroxy-Vitamin D$_3$

Additional data on levels of plasma 1,25(OH)$_2$D have accumulated in a variety of disorders, providing presumptive evidence of defective

Table II.   Clinical Disorders Associated with Reduced Renal Production of
1,25-Dihydroxy-Vitamin D_3

A. Conditions with reduced plasma levels of 1,25(OH)₂-vitamin D

1. Vitamin D deficiency	5. Chronic renal failure
2. Hypoparathyroidism	6. Osteomalacia associated with mesen-
3. Pseudohypoparathyroidism	chymal tumor
4. Hereditary vitamin D dependency	
rickets	

B. Conditions possibly associated with reduced production or availability of 1,25(OH)₂-vitamin D_3[a]

1. Acute renal failure	6. Strontium toxicity
2. Diabetes mellitus	7. Liver disease and biliary cirrhosis
3. Fanconi syndrome	8. Malabsorption syndromes
4. Cadmium toxicity	9. Diphosphonate treatment
5. Nephrotic syndrome	

---

[a]No clinical data are available, while observations in the experimental model may be consistent with reduced generation of 1,25(OH)₂D₃.

1,25(OH)₂D₃ production. Some of these disorders are listed in Table II, and many were reviewed in *The Year in Metabolism 1977* (Coburn *et al.*, 1978).

11.3.2.1. Renal Osteodystrophy

11.3.2.1a. Pathogenesis.   The kidney is the only organ capable of producing 1,25(OH)₂D₃, the most active form of vitamin D. In the presence of renal failure, several lines of evidence support the view that a deficiency of 1,25(OH)₂D₃ develops: There is diminished intestinal absorption of calcium that is unresponsive to vitamin D in amounts that are curative in nutritional rickets; defective skeletal mineralization (i.e., osteomalacia) is common; and there is resistance to PTH, manifested by a failure to elevate serum calcium normally following a standard infusion of parathyroid extract, a feature characteristic of vitamin D deficiency. With a deficiency of 1,25(OH)₂D₃ in renal failure, a number of consequences may be expected (Table III).

It is not known at present when during the course of progressive chronic renal failure a deficiency of 1,25(OH)₂D₃ develops. Information in a small number of patients suggests that plasma levels of 1,25(OH)₂D may not fall unless the glomerular filtration rate (GFR) is less than 30–40 ml/min (M.R. Haussler, personal communication). Van Stone *et al.* (1977) studied the conversion of [³H]-25(OH)D₃ to 1,25(OH)₂D₃ in vitamin-D-deficient rats rendered azotemic by bilateral ureteral ligation (Group A), ureteral ligation plus uninephrectomy (Group B), ureteral ligation plus 5/6 nephrectomy (Group C), or bilateral nephrectomy (Group D). The magnitude of azotemia was the same in each group at 24 hr. The percentage of ^{3}H appearing in plasma was $30.7 \pm 1.7\%$ in sham controls, $12.8 \pm 1.3\%$ in Group A, $8.2 \pm 0.5\%$ in Group B, $1.6 \pm 0.2\%$ in Group C, and 0% in Group D. These data clearly demonstrate that both the quantity of renal mass remaining and the degree of uremia *per se* can modify the production of $1,25(OH)_2D_3$ by the kidney in a model with vitamin D deficiency when renal production of $1,25(OH)_2D_3$ should be maximal. It is of interest that the intestinal content of $1,25(OH)_2D_3$ did not diminish in rats with ureteral ligation. Unilaterally nephrectomized rats had half the control rate of generation of $1,25(OH)_2D_3$ at 4 days after surgery. When such rats were studied 4 weeks later, GFR had returned to normal, but the fraction of $1,25(OH)_2D_3$ produced from $25(OH)D_3$ remained low. These data suggest that the compensatory renal hypertrophy occurring after unilateral nephrectomy was accompanied by an increase in GFR but not in the maximal capacity to produce $1,25(OH)_2D_3$. This study demonstrates that the renal mass is critical for the production of $1,25(OH)_2D_3$, and also indicates an inability of the kidney to manifest a compensatory increase in activity of 25(OH)D-1α-hydroxylase. It should be noted that the activity of the 1-hydroxylase should be maximally activated in such vitamin-D-deficient rats due to vitamin D deficiency *per se;* thus, enzyme activity might not be able to be further stimulated by other trophic factors when the enzyme is already in a maximally stimulated state. Such conditions may not hold in the state of normal vitamin D stores, as may occur in early renal insufficiency.

The relative contribution of altered vitamin D metabolism in the pathogenesis of secondary hyperparathyroidism in uremia and renal osteodystrophy remains uncertain. It is now apparent that the genesis of the reduced blood calcium and the secondary hyperparathyroidism seen in renal failure is multifactorial. Phosphate retention, reduced skeletal responsiveness to the calcemic action of PTH, as well as altered vitamin D metabolism are each major contributory factors. In addition, there may be

Table III.   Consequences of Lack of 1,25-Dihydroxy-Vitamin D_3

Intestine	Impaired suppression of PTH by an
Reduced calcium absorption	increase in serum calcium
Reduced phosphate absorption	Muscle
?Reduced magnesium absorption	Proximal myopathy
Skeleton	Plasma
Defective collagen synthesis and maturation	Hypocalcemia
Reduced PTH responsiveness of bone	Elevated iPTH
Impaired mineralization of osteoid	Hypophosphatemia (if kidneys are re-
Retarded growth	sponsive to PTH)
Parathyroid	Elevated alkaline phosphatase

altered collagen metabolism and abnormal growth and maturation of bone crystals.

Most animal models of renal osteodystrophy have been carried out over a relatively short period of time, and the information may not be relevant to human osteodystrophy. To obviate this problem, Rutherford *et al.* (1977) evaluated the effect of a reduction in dietary phosphate intake, reduced in proportion to the decrease in GFR in uremic dogs for a period of 2 years. Groups of dogs received either (1) a normal phosphate diet; (2) a diet reduced in phosphorus intake in proportion to the decrease in GFR; or (3) a reduction in phosphorus intake plus the administration of $25(OH)D_3$, 20 μg three times per week. Serum iPTH rose markedly in Group 1, rose to a lesser extent more slowly in Group 2, but remained totally normal in Group 3. Ionized blood calcium was significantly higher only in the group receiving $25(OH)D_3$; this may have occurred because the quantity of $25(OH)D_3$ given may have been pharmacological. Analysis of serial bone biopsies obtained from the rib demonstrated a linear relationship between osteoclastic resorption surface and plasma iPTH levels. In Group 1, osteoid volume and osteoid surface were increased, while the mineralization front was reduced. In Group 2, there was a mild increase in osteoid volume and an increase in osteoid surface compared to the observations in Group 1. In contrast, there were no histomorphological abnormalities of bone in Group 3. These observations support the hypothesis that phosphate retention plays an important role in the pathogenesis of secondary hyperparathyroidism, but the data indicate quite clearly that alterations in vitamin D also play an important role.

11.3.2.1b. Clinical Features of Renal Osteodystrophy. Certain symptoms present in uremia may be related to the abnormal metabolism of vitamin D. Muscle weakness, most notably of the proximal musculature, is sometimes a serious and debilitating symptom in such patients. Sometimes the afflicted patient may be confined to a wheelchair due to his muscle weakness. In many ways, this uremic myopathy resembles the muscle weakness seen in vitamin D deficiency. In both forms of myopathy, plasma activity of muscle enzymes is usually normal and electromyographic changes, if present, are nonspecific. Histological examination of muscle biopsy specimens reveals mild, nonspecific myopathic changes or severe nonspecific degenerative changes, or both, accompanied by Type II fiber atrophy by histochemistry, which is also observed in hypophosphatemic osteomalacia. Rapid improvement in muscle weakness has been observed following the administration of $1,25(OH)_2D_3$, 1–5 μg/day, or $25(OH)D_3$, 50–100 μg/day, and also after renal transplantation. In a preliminary study of three uremic patients with muscle weakness, Schoenfeld *et al.* (1977) reported electron-microscopic findings of localized areas of severe disorganization of myofibrils with dispersion of Z-band material.

These changes were normalized with clinically improved muscle strength following the administration of $25(OH)D_3$, 600–1150 μg/week, for a period of 16 weeks. Such improvement occurred without significant changes in serum calcium, phosphorus, and iPTH levels, but was associated with a significant fall in serum alkaline phosphatase, a rise in serum $25(OH)D$, and improvement in bone histology. Matthews *et al.* (1977) noted defective calcium ion transport in the fragmented sarcoplasmic reticulum of skeletal muscle of uremic rabbits. This defective calcium transport was corrected by *in vivo* administration of $1,25(OH)_2D_3$, 54 ng/ kg body weight per day or 162 ng/kg body weight per day, for 5 days. The low dose improved the capacity of the fragmented sarcoplasmic reticulum to store calcium, and the higher dose corrected the calcium-concentrating ability and the initial rate of calcium uptake in addition to augmenting the storing capacity. The addition of $1,25(OH)_2D_3$, *in vitro,* to the sarcoplasmic vesicles in a concentration comparable to circulating levels of $1,25(OH)_2D$ failed to correct the transport defect. Since calcium transport by the sarcoplasmic reticulum is believed to be important in the regulation of muscle contraction, this study may provide insight into the functional aspects of uremic myopathy and its relation to the defective production of $1,25(OH)_2D_3$.

11.3.2.1c. Management. The appropriate management of renal osteodystrophy includes: (1) reduction in serum phosphorus by decreasing its dietary intake or increasing the binding of dietary phosphate in the intestine with aluminum hydroxide or aluminum carbonate, (2) supplementation of dietary calcium to a total intake of approximately 1.5 g/day, (3) utilizing an adequate dialysate calcium concentration (6–7 mg/dl), and (4) use of an appropriate vitamin D sterol when symptomatic bone disease exists.

Vitamin D and dihydrotachysterol (DHT) are commonly effective when given in very large doses, but careful adjustment is required. In the last few years, treatment with $25(OH)D_3$, 40–100 μg/day, $1\alpha(OH)D_3$, 2–4 μg/day, or $1,25(OH)_2D_3$, 0.5–2 μg/day, has been successfully employed in the treatment of uremic bone disease and of the muscle weakness found in uremia. There is considerable risk of hypercalcemia with the highly active agents, but the serum calcium returns promptly to normal within 2– 7 days after withdrawal of the treatment.

Use of 25-Hydroxy-Vitamin D_3. Recent results of treatment with $25(OH)D_3$ have confirmed its effectiveness in treating renal osteodystrophy. Eastwood *et al.* (1977) evaluated 5 uremic patients with osteomalacia given 52–100 nmol (20–40 μg) $25(OH)D_3$/day i.v. for 4 weeks. A marked increase in plasma $25(OH)D$ levels occurred, and there was significant improvement in bone mineralization, intestinal calcium absorption, and muscle strength in 3 of the 5 patients. These results support their previous experience that a deficiency of $25(OH)D_3$ may be a factor in the development of osteomalacia in the uremic patients they encounter in the United Kingdom. The effects of $25(OH)D_3$ on bone lesions in children with renal osteodystrophy were evaluated by Witmer *et al.* (1976). X rays in 9 of the 14 children evaluated were normal or showed minimal alterations, but bone biopsies taken at the beginning of hemodialysis treatment period showed defective mineralizaton or increased bone resorption, or both, in all 4 of the 9 patients given calcium supplementation of $25(OH)D_3$, 25–50 μg/day; 5 patients received calcium supplementation alone. On rebiopsy, the bone lesions were more severe in the latter group of patients not treated with $25(OH)D_3$. On the other hand, bone biopsies in the patients treated with $25(OH)D_3$ showed improved mineralization and a disappearance of marrow fibrosis. Serum calcium levels exceeded 11 mg/dl in 4 of the 5 patients treated with $25(OH)D_3$. Five other patients with evidence of severe metabolic bone disease had either changes of osteomalacia or osteofibrosis at the outset. These patients had been treated previously with vitamin D_2, 345–685 μg/day, without effect. Four of the 5 patients were treated with $25(OH)D_3$, 25–200 μg/day, for 1–6 months. There was improvement in mineralization and a reduction in osteitis fibrosa, osteoblasts, and osteoclast surface. These results indicate the effectiveness of $25(OH)D_3$ in treating children with renal osteodystrophy, but they emphasize the need for careful monitoring for hypercalcemia. Very probably, smaller amounts of $25(OH)D_3$ would have also been effective.

Use of 1 α-Hydroxy-Vitamin D_3. There has been greater clinical experience with $1\alpha(OH)D_3$, a compound now clinically available in Europe, reported during the past year. Several reports dealing with the clinical use of this sterol were included in a supplement to Vol. 7 of *Clinical Endocrinology* edited by Peacock (1977). Pierides *et al.* (1977) described 30 patients, 23 of whom were undergoing regular hemodialysis and 7 uremic patients who were treated conservatively. Two of the 7 patients not treated with hemodialysis had X-ray evidence of osteodystrophy. Five patients had bone biopsies taken after $3\frac{1}{2}$–8 months of treatment with $1\alpha(OH)D_3$, 0.5–3 μg/day orally. Osteitis fibrosis improved in 4 of 5 biopsies, and the osteomalacia that was present in 2 of these biopsies resolved. Hypocalcemia improved steadily, and there was a fall in serum iPTH and alkaline phosphatase to within normal limits. Treatment with $1\alpha(OH)D_3$ ranged from $4\frac{1}{2}$ to 24 months in the 23 patients on regular hemodialysis, with oral doses ranging from 2 μg/week to 2 μg/day. Twelve patients improved significantly by clinical, biochemical, radiological, and histological criteria, and 11 patients failed to improve. In general, the patients who responded had raised serum iPTH levels, increased alkaline phosphatase, predominantly the bone enzyme fraction, and histological evidence of osteitis fibrosa with or without osteomalacia prior to the treatment. The nonresponding patients had almost always a pure osteomalacia with minimal if any evidence of osteitis fibrosa, and both serum alkaline phosphatase levels and iPTH values were within the normal range. The latter patients tended to have predialysis serum calcium levels in the high normal range, and $1\alpha(OH)D_3$ treatment promptly led to symptomatic hypercalciuria. Some patients in the latter group had concurrent treatment with anticonvulsant drugs, phenobarbital and phenytoin, but serum 25(OH)D levels were normal. Some of these patients showed significant hypophosphatemia, and the authors speculate on a possible role of phosphate depletion due to a poor dietary intake and the unwise use of phosphate binders in leading to the vitamin D [$1\alpha(OH)D_3$]-resistant osteomalacia. We have also encountered uremic patients with a mineralizing defect not improved by administration of vitamin D [i.e., D_2, DHT, or $1,25(OH)_2D_3$], but we have not found phosphate depletion to be an etiological factor except in rare instances (Coburn *et al.*, 1977).

A comparison of results of treatment of patients with renal osteodystrophy with either $1\alpha(OH)D_3$ or $25(OH)D_3$ was reported by Fournier *et al.* (1976). Thirteen patients were treated with either 4 μg $1\alpha(OH)D_3$ or 200 μg $25(OH)D_3$ every other day for 1–12 weeks. Bone biopsies and serial measurements of serum iPTH, serum calcium, phosphorus, and alkaline phosphate were obtained. Either agent improved the secondary hyperparathyroidism in two thirds of the cases and also improved the mineralization defect. Complete correction of histopathology was not observed, and serum iPTH levels did not revert to normal over a period of up to 12 weeks.

Use of 1,25-Dihydroxy-Vitamin D_3. Long-term experience with the use of $1,25(OH)_2D_3$ in treating patients with renal osteodystrophy has been reported by several groups. Pierides *et al.* (1976) reported results of treatment of 5 patients with $1,25(OH)_2D_3$, 1–1.5 μg/day, for 6–8 months. They demonstrated a significant improvement in intestinal calcium absorption without significant hypercalcemia. Histological evidence of secondary hyperparathyroidism improved in all patients, and serum iPTH and serum alkaline phosphatase returned to normal. Muscle strength improved both clinically and electromyographically. In a study at three centers, Coburn *et al.* (1977) reported 46 patients who were treated with either $1,25(OH)_2D_3$ (44 studies) or with $1\alpha(OH)D_3$ (6 studies) for 2–90 weeks. Thirty-eight patients presented with skeletal pain, and 27 of them noted a decrease or disappearance of pain. Muscle strength improved in 19 of 26 patients with muscular weakness prior to the treatment. Improvement of most symptoms in patients correlated with a decrease in serum alkaline phosphatase levels. Serum iPTH levels fell in many of the patients, although values rarely decreased to normal.

Two groups of patients failed to respond to $1,25(OH)_2D_3$; in some, there was marked secondary hyperparathyroidism, and treatment with $1,25(OH)_2D_3$ quickly led to hypercalcemia in these patients. A second subgroup of nonresponders had skeletal biopsy evidence of an "inactive" skeleton with abundant unmineralized osteoid, little evidence of excess parathyroid action, and low serum iPTH levels.

This last group of patients appears to have a mineralizing defect that is not corrected by the administration of vitamin D or the appropriate elevation of serum calcium and phosphorus. The pathogenesis of this disorder remains, at this time, uncertain.

11.3.2.2. Diabetes Mellitus

Experimentally produced diabetes mellitus may be associated with impaired production of $1,25(OH)_2D_3$. The restoration of the impaired intestinal calcium transport in rats made diabetic with streptozotocin following treatment with an extract of *Solanum malacoxylon,* a source of $1,25(OH)_2D_3$, supports the notion that production of $1,25(OH)_2D_3$ is impaired in this model of experimental diabetes. Schneider *et al.* (1977) extended their studies and reported data confirming the postulate. Serum levels of $25(OH)D$ and $1,25(OH)_2D$ were measured in control rats, streptozotocin-induced diabetic rats, and insulin-treated rats with streptozotocin-induced diabetes. The mean serum concentration of $1,25(OH)_2D$ was 6.7 ± 0.5 ng/dl in controls compared to 0.8 ± 0.2 ng/dl in untreated diabetic rats. There were no differences in serum levels of $25(OH)D$ in the three groups of rats. These data strongly support these investigators' previous contention that impaired calcium transport in diabetic rats arises either from failure of renal production of $1,25(OH)_2D_3$ or from increased catabolism of $1,25(OH)_2D_3$. These experiments were done after 10 days of streptozotocin treatment, making it unlikely that diabetic nephropathy could play a role in the pathogenesis.

Such alterations of vitamin D metabolism in experimental animals with diabetes may be extrapolated to the presence of bone disease in diabetic patients: Thus, Levin *et al.* (1976) measured skeletal mass of the forearm using photon absorptiometry in 35 insulin-treated, juvenile diabetic patients and 101 patients with adult-onset diabetes, who were treated with diet alone, insulin, or oral hypoglycemic agents. Bone mass was significantly decreased in both the juvenile and adult-onset diabetic patients compared to results in control subjects matched for age and sex. The decrease in bone mass could be detected within 5 years of the appearance of the diabetes. However, a demonstration of a decreased forearm bone mass in some patients with both the juvenile and adult-onset diabetes at the time of clinical onset of diabetes suggests that the basic defect may be that of decreased bone formation rather than that due to excess bone loss. These investigators suggest that the skeletal abnormality may occur as part of the basic disease rather than develop as a complication of hyperglycemia or insulin deficiency or both. The insulin-treated diabetic patients tended to have less decrease of bone mass, raising the possibility that insulin may affect bone metabolism either directly or via an indirect mechanism, e.g., altered vitamin D metabolism, and lead to secondary hyperparathyroidism.

11.3.2.3. Osteomalacia Related to Mesenchymal Tumor

Sporadic, hypophosphatemic, vitamin-D-resistant rickets occurring in association with a mesenchymal tumor of bone or soft tissue is a unique and potentially treatable form of osteomalacia. There have been at least 15 cases of this syndrome reported; it is characterized by bone lesions of osteomalacia, hypophosphatemia, normal or slightly low plasma calcium levels, elevated plasma alkaline phosphatase activity, and normal iPTH levels in plasma. In the past, it has been suggested that the tumor may release a humoral factor that causes renal wasting of phosphate. Three additional cases were reported during the last year:

Wyman *et al.* (1977) reported a 44-year-old male patient with a malignant sarcoma of the tibia. The patient was treated with oral phosphate, up to 40 g bisodium phosphate per day, and a short intensive course of vitamin D, in a dose up to 100,000 IU/day. With deterioration of his symptoms, the leg involved with the sarcoma was amputated; this was followed by immediate increases of serum phosphorus to normal and of calcium to a hypercalcemic level and a decrease in serum alkaline phosphatase. On prolonged follow-up, serum calcium returned to normal, but the serum phosphorus level fell to hypophosphatemic levels after 2 years and persisted for 1 more year until the time of the report. The cause of the hypophosphatemia is not clear, but a recurrence of the tumor was not convincingly excluded.

Aschinberg *et al.* (1977) reported a 5-year-old boy with severe rickets in association with hyperpigmented, linear, verrucous epidermal tumors, typical of the "epidermal nevus syndrome." The patient had normocalcemia, hypophosphatemia, elevated serum alkaline phosphatase levels, decreased renal tubular reabsorption of phosphorus, radiological evidence of rickets, and a lack of response to vitamin D, 50,000–100,000 IU/day. Further therapy with vitamin D, in massive doses up to 750,000 IU/day, and oral phosphate, 2 g/day, failed to induce healing of the rickets. A subtotal parathyroidectomy performed at the age of 9 was without effect. Several fibroangiomas of the face and left lower limb were excised when the patient was 12 years old; this was followed by resolution of all biochemical abnormalities within 3 months and radiological evidence of healing of rickets. The patient continuously improved and was ambulatory after corrective osteotomies. The authors further extended their study by injecting an extract of the tumor into puppies. A single injection of tumor extract produced a significant fall in tubular reabsorption of phosphorus from 78 to 46% at 60 min and to 12% at 120 min without a concomitant change in blood pressure, hematocrit, GFR, or the excretion of sodium. Control injections of saline or an extract of normal skin did not affect the tubular reabsorption of phosphorus. This case report provides evidence for the presence of a humoral factor present in the tumor, which can inhibit the renal tubular reabsorption of phosphorus; such a factor may produce the hypophosphatemia and lead to osteomalacia or rickets.

Drezner and Feinglos (1977) reported the case of a 42-year-old female, presenting with generalized bone pain, normal serum calcium, low serum phosphorus, and an elevated serum alkaline phosphatase. She was treated for many years with ergocalciferol (up to 200,000 IU/day), and oral calcium and phosphorus (up to 4 g/day), either singly or in combination; all were without beneficial effect on the hypophosphatemia. She was found to have a lytic lesion in her right iliac crest, which was shown by biopsy to be a giant cell tumor of bone. In this well-studied case, plasma iPTH, determined by radioimmunoassay using three different antibodies, was normal; maximum tubular reabsorption of phosphate/glomerular filtration rate was decreased, plasma 25(OH)D was normal, and the level of $1,25(OH)_2D$ was decreased. Under the assumption that a deficiency of $1,25(OH)_2D$ could be important in the genesis of this tumor-related osteomalacia, the authors treated this woman with $1,25(OH)_2D_3$, 3 μg/day, for 10 days (Fig. 4). The treatment resulted in a prompt increase in serum phosphorus and a small increase in calcium. The balances for calcium and phosphorus, both negative before treatment, became positive. The calcemic response to exogenous parathyroid extract became normal with improvement of bone histology judged by quantitative microradiography. Subsequent resection of the tumor was associated with a persistently normal serum level of calcium and phosphorus and positive balances for calcium and phosphorus. Aminoaciduria, present before treatment, was corrected by therapy with $1,25(OH)_2D_3$. On the basis of their data, these workers postulated the following sequence of events underlying the pathogenesis of this disorder: (1) a factor is synthesized and secreted by the tumor, (2) this factor decreases the synthesis of $1,25(OH)_2D_3$ by inhibiting the renal $25(OH)D_3$-1-hydroxylase activity, and (3) the resultant deficiency of $1,25(OH)_2D_3$ causes the osteomalacia and renal phosphate wasting.

These case studies raise an intriguing question regarding this peculiar syndrome: If the syndrome arises simply due to a lack of $1,25(OH)_2D_3$, as proposed by Drezner and Feinglos (1977), then it is difficult to explain the lack of significant hypocalcemia in this syndrome. Also, how can hypophosphatemia develop due to an isolated deficiency of

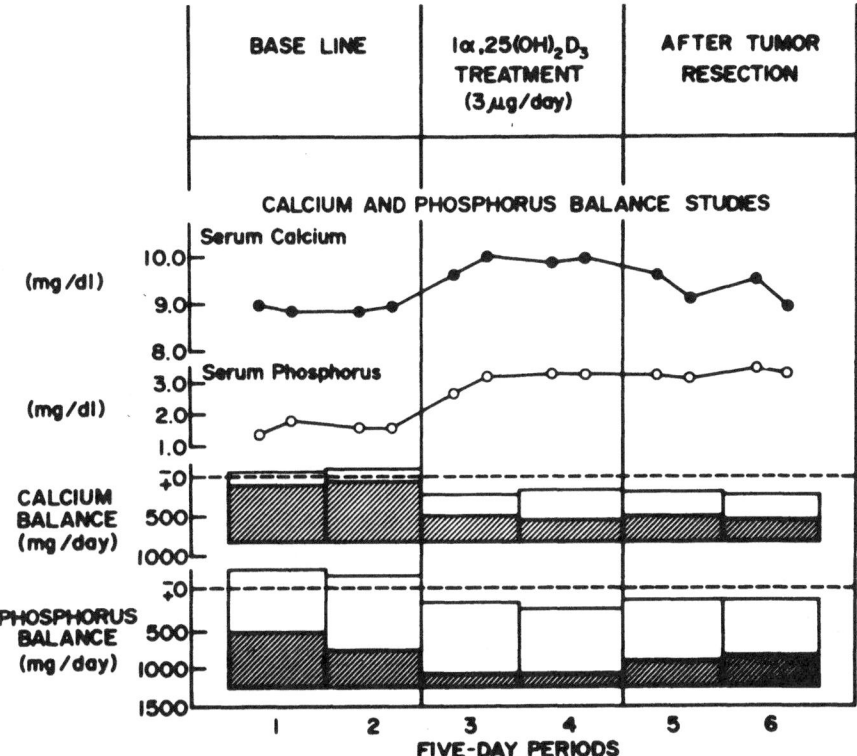

Fig. 4. Calcium and phosphorus balance in the base-line state, during treatment with 1α,25(OH)₂D₃ (3 μg/day), and after tumor resection in a patient with osteomalacia associated with a giant cell tumor of bone. The dietary calcium and phosphorus are plotted below the 0 line. Fecal excretion is represented by the shaded areas and urinary excretion by the white areas. Extension of the columns above 0 indicates negative balance and termination of the columns below 0 indicates positive balance. Reproduced from Drezner and Feinglos (1977) with permission of the publisher.

1,25(OH)₂D₃ but without concurrent secondary hyperparathyroidism? In an experimental model of vitamin D deficiency, hypophosphatemia and phosphaturia almost routinely arise, presumably from secondary hyperparathyroidism. Most reported cases do *not* have elevated levels of iPTH, and the patients remain normocalcemic. The observation of Aschinberg *et al.* (1977) that a tumor extract produced brisk phosphaturia suggests that a tumor product may have a direct effect on tubular transport of phosphate. It would seem more attractive to postulate that the tumor product may block phosphate transport and concomitantly inhibit the renal production of 1,25(OH)₂D₃.

11.3.2.4. Fanconi Syndrome

Rickets in children and osteomalacia in adults are common features of the Fanconi syndrome, which is characterized by proximal renal tubular dysfunction with impaired reabsorption of amino acids, glucose, bicarbonate, and phosphate. Hypophosphatemia often arises due to the renal loss of this ion and contributes to the genesis of the bone disease; however, the bone lesions of this syndrome often respond to pharmacological doses of vitamin D without measurable changes in plasma phosphorus levels. These clinical observations suggested a possible impairment of renal production of $1,25(OH)_2D_3$ in this disorder. Brewer *et al.* (1977a) studied vitamin D metabolism in vitamin-D-deficient rats with the experimental Fanconi syndrome induced by the intravenous administration of maleic acid. The injection of maleic acid results in typical dysfunctions of the proximal tubule, with increased urinary excretion of phosphate, bicarbonate, and α-amino acids. At 5 hr after the intravenous administration of maleic acid, $[^3H]-25(OH)D_3$ was given intravenously, and labeled $1,25(OH)_2D_3$ was measured in the kidney, intestinal mucosa, and serum. The quantities recovered were one third to one half those found in tissues of control rats that had received either acetazolamide or saline, or were only subjected to the surgical procedure. The $25(OH)D_3$-1-hydroxylase activity found in renal homogenates from vitamin-D-deficient chicks was significantly diminished within 1 hr after the intravenous administration of maleic acid. Furthermore, the addition of maleic acid, *in vitro*, also inhibited the production of $1,25(OH)_2D_3$ from $25(OH)D_3$ by isolated chick renal tubules. Although one cannot exclude a direct toxic effect of maleic acid on renal 1-hydroxylase and renal tubules, these results raise the possibility that the renal production of $1,25(OH)_2D_3$ may be defective in the Fanconi syndrome; such an abnormality could underlie the bone disease characteristic of this syndrome.

Brewer *et al.* (1977b) also reported their observations of vitamin D metabolism in 5 nonazotemic children with the Fanconi syndrome; thus, $[^3H]-1,25(OH)_2D_3$ could *not* be detected in blood after the injection of $[^3H]-25(OH)D_3$. This occurred despite the presence of hypophosphatemia and increased levels of circulating iPTH, both of which should stimulate $1,25(OH)_2D_3$ synthesis by the kidney. However, it is not known whether significant amounts of $[^3H]-1,25(OH)_2D_3$ would be found in the plasma of normal healthy children after a similar injection of $[^3H]-25(OH)D_3$. The lack of data from control subjects makes this study inconclusive; further data may be needed to prove their hypothesis, although ethical considerations may preclude the performance of the appropriate experiments in normal children.

11.3.3. Other Disorders with Uncertain Relationship to Vitamin D

11.3.3.1. Neonatal Hypocalcemia

The pathogenesis of this clinical entity was recently reviewed (Coburn and Hartenbower, 1977). It is a general consensus that more than one factor is usually operative in most instances. Kooh *et al.* (1976) reported the successful treatment of 6 infants with protracted hypocalcemia with intravenous or oral $1,25(OH)_2D_3$, 0.05 μg/kg per day, for 5–12 days. Plasma calcium levels began to rise within 24 hr after treatment with the sterol was started, and reached the normal range within 8 days. Four of the infants remained normocalcemic after treatment was discontinued, but 2 infants required treatment with $1,25(OH)_2D_3$ for a longer period. The oral administration of $1\alpha(OH)D_3$ was also reported to be effective in the treatment of a case of neonatal hypocalcemia (Doxiadis and Lapatsants, 1977).

Turner *et al.* (1977) reported 104 cases with symptomatic infantile hypocalcemia. The patients were randomly allocated to treatment with calcium, phenobarbital, or magnesium sulfate. The experience of these investigators demonstrates that infants treated with magnesium sulfate achieved higher plasma calcium concentrations within 48 hr after treatment and had fewer convulsions during and after the treatment. Although the precise mechanism responsible for an increase in plasma calcium following magnesium treatment in neonatal hypocalcemia is not known, the prevention of convulsions may be due to well-known effects of magnesium as an anticonvulsant. However, the greater rise in plasma calcium in the magnesium-treated group speaks for a possible role of magnesium depletion in contributing to altered calcium homeostasis in this clinical syndrome. Moreover, mean serum magnesium rose from a moderately low value (1.18 ± 0.34 mEq/liter) to normal (1.75 ± 0.41 mEq/liter) in the group treated with magnesium, while serum magnesium levels remained low in the other two treatment groups.

11.3.3.2. Familial Hypophosphatemic Vitamin-D-Resistant Rickets

Familial vitamin-D-resistant hypophosphatemic rickets is an inherited sex-linked disorder characterized by low plasma phosphate, high renal clearance of phosphate, normocalcemia, and normal circulating iPTH. This disorder was reviewed recently by Fraser and Scriver (1976). It has been suggested that the primary defect is an inability of renal tubules to conserve phosphate, while abnormal vitamin D metabolism probably does not exist. Consistent with this hypothesis are the reports showing that vitamin D or one of its metabolites, $25(OH)D_3$ or $1,25(OH)_2D_3$, was ineffective in reversing the phosphate wasting of this disorder. Moreover, serum concentrations of $25(OH)D$ and $1,25(OH)_2D$ have been found to be normal. Thus, there is no evidence of a reduced ability of these patients to synthesize $1,25(OH)_2D_3$. However, a low plasma phosphate level is believed to be a potent stimulus for renal production of $1,25(OH)_2D_3$, and the finding of normal levels of $1,25(OH)_2D$ in the face of hypophosphatemia may indicate renal 1α-hydroxylase enzyme activity that is inappropriately low. The varied clinical expression of this syndrome is pointed out in a recent study: A family of 133 members spanning six generations with vitamin-D-resistant rickets and hypophosphatemic osteomalacia was reported by Frymoyer and Hodgkin (1977). Members of this kindred were atypical in that hypophosphatemic children did not have rickets or evident bone disease, while the hypophosphatemic adolescent and adult patients were progressively disabled by skeletal disease. Whether this family represents a variant of the typical syndrome or is a separate disorder is unknown.

11.3.3.3. "Itai-Itai" Disease

It seems well established that the syndrome "itai-itai" disease is a form of osteomalacia that is endemic in cadmium-polluted areas of Japan. Recently, studies were carried out in experimental animals in an effort to clarify the pathogenesis of this syndrome. In a study of Ando *et al.* (1977), young rats were given cadmium chloride, 10 mg/kg body weight per day for 1, 2, or 3 months. Following pretreatment with cadmium, each rat was given $^{47}CaCl_2$ intravenously for the evaluation of ^{47}Ca turnover. In other studies, ^{47}Ca was administered orally, and body retention of the administered ^{47}Ca was evaluated. The results indicated decreased intestinal absorption of ^{47}Ca in cadmium-treated rats compared to their controls; also, a substantially greater amount of ^{47}Ca was recovered in the feces of cadmium-treated rats given ^{47}Ca intravenously. Moreover, the bone uptake of the intravenous ^{47}Ca was also reduced in cadmium-treated animals. Such observations suggest that chronic cadmium ingestion may produce abnormal intestinal calcium absorption and altered deposition of calcium in bone. In a preliminary study, we also found evidence for decreased intestinal transport of radiocalcium in cadmium-treated rats. Although it is appealing to attribute this abnormality to a defect of the action or bioconversion of vitamin D, such an abnormality has not, as yet, been established.

11.3.3.4. Metabolic Acidosis

Chronic metabolic acidosis is associated with positive acid balance accompanied by hypercalciuria and a negative calcium balance. Bone is the major source of the calcium appearing in the urine; thus, the carbonate content of bone also decreases during chronic metabolic acidosis. Since carbonate-deficient apatite may be formed when the extracellular fluid concentration of bicarbonate is low, chronic metabolic acidosis may lead to a relative reduction in bone formation with the net loss of bone calcium. Coe *et al.* (1975) reported that metabolic acidosis stimulates PTH secretion, resulting in increased bone resorption and negative calcium balance. The hypophosphatemia that may accompany chronic metabolic acidosis could activate renal production of $1,25(OH)_2D_3$, which may add to the increased net bone resorption. To gain insight into the mechanism responsible for the negative calcium balance that develops during chronic metabolic acidosis, Weber *et al.* (1976) evaluated plasma $25(OH)D_3$ turnover, serum iPTH, and acid and calcium balances in 6 normal human subjects during a control period and during stable chronic metabolic acidosis induced by ammonium chloride ingestion. In this well-designed study, they found a positive balance for H^+ ion and a negative balance for calcium secondary to hypercalciuria during the period of metabolic acidosis. There was *no* significant augmentation of net intestinal absorption of calcium, phosphate, or magnesium during acidosis. Also, chronic metabolic acidosis was not accompanied by significant change in either serum iPTH or in the turnover of plasma $25(OH)D$ pool. Serum $25(OH)D$ levels and the plasma $25(OH)D$ pool size were reduced slightly during acidosis (although this was statistically *not* significant); there was an accelerated disappearance of serum radioactivity of ^3H- or ^{14}C-labeled $25(OH)D_3$, which was considered to be due to the smaller plasma pool of $25(OH)D$, and its daily turnover did not change. The absence of any significant change in serum iPTH during chronic acidosis in this report contrasts with previous observations reported by Coe *et al.* (1975), who found an increase in serum iPTH during both an acute and chronic acidosis. The reasons for these discrepant reports are not obvious. However, differences in the sensitivity or specificity of the immunoassays for PTH and/or a larger daily acid load in the study of Weber *et al.* (1976) could be responsible, at least in part, for the discrepant results. Levels of plasma inorganic phosphorus fell significantly during acidosis in the study of Weber and colleagues, but did not change in the study of Coe and colleagues. Although Weber *et al.* (1976) did not detect an accelerated turnover of $25(OH)D$ during acidosis, this does not exclude the possibility of increased plasma levels of $1,25(OH)_2D_3$ in chronic acidosis, since only a minute fraction (i.e., $\approx 1\%$) of total radioactivity may appear as $1,25(OH)_2D_3$ with the method employed; thus, a small but significant change in plasma $1,25(OH)_2D_3$ could not be detected in this study.

Sauveur et al. (1977) studied the effects of metabolic acidosis on vitamin D metabolism in vitamin-D-deficient chicks. The administration of ^{3}H-labeled vitamin D_3 was followed by the appearance of lower levels of $[^3H]-1,25(OH)_2D_3$ in plasma, intestine, and the tibiae of acidotic chicks than in control animals. The production of $1,25(OH)_2D_3$ in vitro from tritiated $25(OH)D$ was also reduced by 40% in kidney homogenates from acidotic birds. Since the acidotic, rachitic chicks had higher plasma phosphorus concentrations (9.5 ± 0.5 mg/dl) than were observed in "control" rachitic chicks (6.4 ± 0.5 mg/dl), these authors suggested that the higher phosphate level may have inhibited renal production of $1,25(OH)_2D_3$. Hyperphosphatemia is not observed in humans with chronic acidosis; thus, such a change in serum phosphorus may have no bearing on observations in other species.

Metabolic acidosis has been reported to occur in patients with vitamin D deficiency. This is characteristically a hyperchloremic acidosis with a normal anion "gap"; it may have certain characteristics of Type II, "proximal" renal tubular acidosis, and it is corrected by the administration of vitamin D. Moreover, the acidosis could lead to bone disease by reducing the bioconversion of $25(OH)D_3$ to $1,25(OH)_2D_3$. Previously, it had been shown that subphysiological pH values reduce the activity of $25(OH)D_3$-1-hydroxylase in isolated tubules (Bickle and Rasmussen, 1975), and a report by Lee et al. (1977) indicates that there is reduced conversion of $25(OH)D$ to $1,25(OH)_2D_3$ in rats given ammonium chloride. To characterize the acid–base status in pure vitamin D deficiency, Booth et al. (1977) compared vitamin-D-deficient chicks with animals receiving the same diet and added vitamin D_3, 100 IU orally 3 times/week. After the chicks had received the vitamin-D-deficient diet for 3, 4, and 5 weeks, heparinized blood was obtained via cardiac puncture. The chicks on the deficient diet exhibited lower plasma bicarbonate and blood pH compared to values in the vitamin-D-repleted group. Also, the P_{CO_2} was significantly higher in the vitamin-D-deficient chicks. At no time were the mean values for P_{CO_2} lower in the D-deficient than in the control birds, suggesting a failure of respiratory compensation. The acidosis present in the vitamin-D-deficient chicks was relatively hyperchloremic and without an increase in the anion "gap." Within 24 hr after initiation of treatment with vitamin D, the degree of acidosis was significantly reduced, plasma bicarbonate increased, and blood P_{CO_2} fell significantly. These data provide the first clear documentation that metabolic acidosis is a predictable phenomenon in experimental vitamin D deficiency and that vitamin D therapy leads to rapid improvement of the acidosis. The hyperchloremic character is similar to that seen in patients with renal tubular acidosis, and it seems likely that impaired renal acidification leads to the metabolic acidosis. The lack of respiratory compensation with hyperventilation and a lower P_{CO_2} could arise due to rachitic deformities of the thoracic cage or as a consequence of muscle weakness, a common feature in vitamin D deficiency. The hyperparathyroidism that arises due to the hypocalcemia could account, in part, for the acidosis; however, these authors feel that PTH alone could not produce the degree of acidosis generated. Hypocalcemia itself can also decrease the renal tubular reabsorption of bicarbonate. Thus, excess PTH, the fall in plasma calcium, hypophosphatemia, and the lack of $1,25(OH)_2D_3$ could each contribute to the development of metabolic acidosis. The authors make an important point that the metabolic consequences of metabolic acidosis must be considered when an experimental model of vitamin D deficiency is employed.

11.3.3.5. Glucocorticoid Treatment

It has long been known that adrenal steroids, given in large quantities, can inhibit the intestinal absorption of calcium and lead to a negative calcium balance. From the results of studies carried out in experimental animals, it has been suggested that adrenal steroids decrease the intestinal calcium transport by antagonizing the end-organ action of vitamin D or by altering vitamin D metabolism. Favus *et al.* (1973a,b) found that glucocorticoids inhibit the active transport of calcium by duodenal gut sacs despite the administration of vitamin D_3, $25(OH)D_3$, or $1,25(OH)_2D_3$. Moreover, they found no effect of steroid treatment on the metabolism of radiolabeled vitamin D. Such data support a view that steroids interfere with calcium transport independent of altered vitamin D metabolism. More recently, Klein *et al.* (1977) found that the hypoabsorption of calcium in patients receiving steroid treatment could be corrected by the administration of $1,25(OH)_2D_3$, 0.4 μg/day. Also, plasma levels of $25(OH)D_3$ were found to be inversely correlated with the daily dose of steroid. These observations of the effects of $1,25(OH)_2D_3$ in overcoming the action of steroids suggest that altered vitamin D metabolism may occur with steroid treatment (Fig. 5).

The effect of steroids on the metabolism of $25(OH)D$ remains somewhat uncertain. Hahn *et al.* (1977) found similar direct relationshps between plasma levels of $25(OH)D$ and the daily vitamin D intake in steroid-treated patients compared to other individuals receiving no steroid treatment. Thus, they concluded that the maintenance of plasma $25(OH)D$ levels is not affected by steroid treatment. They suggest that previous observations that plasma levels of $25(OH)D$ are affected by steroids may be related to differences in the dietary intake of vitamin D.

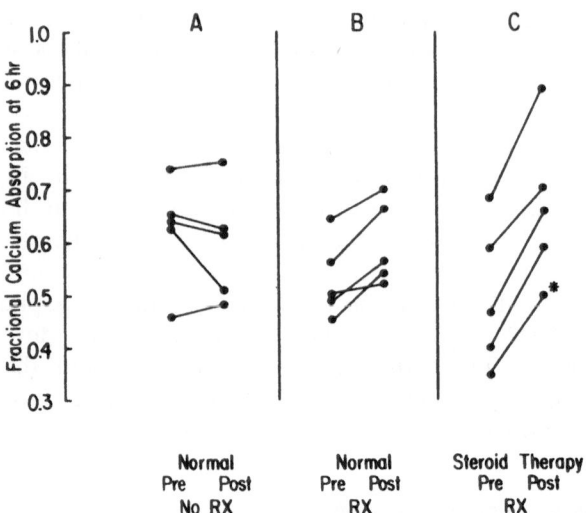

Fig. 5. Fractional intestinal absorption of calcium before and after 7-day course of no therapy (No RX) or oral administration of 1,25(OH)$_2$D$_3$, 0.4 μg/day. (A) No therapy in normal volunteers; (B) 1,25(OH)$_2$D$_3$ daily for 7 days to normal volunteers; (C) 1,25(OH)$_2$D$_3$ to patients receiving high-dose (prednisone 15–100 μg/day) steroid. One patient (*) on high-dose steroid treatment has a clinically active collagen disease. Reproduced from Klein *et al.* (1977) with permission of the publisher.

The implications of some of these observations are of some importance, since it is possible that treatment with an active form of vitamin D might be capable of counteracting certain side effects of steroid treatment, in particular the prevention of steroid-induced osteopenia. Indeed, preliminary studies by Hahn *et al.* (1976) suggest that this may be the case.

11.3.4. Endocrine Disorders with Altered Production of 1,25-Dihydroxy-Vitamin D$_3$

11.3.4.1. Hypoparathyroidism

Since parathyroid hormone (PTH) is considered an important trophic factor that regulates the conversion of 25(OH)D$_3$ to 1,25(OH)$_2$D$_3$, the finding of reduced plasma levels of 1,25 (OH)$_2$D (see Table I) in patients with hypoparathyroidism is not surprising. However, the role of the low levels of 1,25(OH)$_2$D in contributing to the clinical picture remains uncertain. The interaction between vitamin D and PTH may be quite complex. Gerblich *et al.* (1977) reported an elderly female with both idiopathic hypoparathyroidism and dietary deficiency of vitamin D. When the patient was given parathyroid extract (PTE), the urinary excretion of cAMP and phosphate increased; however, the sustained administration of PTE failed to increase serum calcium or augment the urinary excretion of hydroxyproline. When the PTE infusion was repeated after a calcium infusion and after the administration of vitamin D, the hydroxyproline excretion and serum calcium levels both increased. These data substantiate the data obtained in certain animal experiments that suggest that vitamin D is necessary for the skeletal but not the renal actions of PTH. Furthermore, the data suggest that vitamin D deficiency may restrict the skeletal response to PTH by limiting the availability of calcium.

There have been few reports of bone pathology in patients with hypoparathyroidism. Reduced conversion of $25(OH)D_3$ to $1,25(OH)_2D_3$ in patients with long-standing hypoparathyroidism might cause the development of bone disease as a consequence of reduced levels of $1,25(OH)_2D$. Drezner et al. (1977) studied a patient with idiopathic hypoparathyroidism and measured vitamin D levels in the blood. The $25(OH)D$ level was normal and that of $1,25(OH)_2D$ was decreased. The patient was untreated for several years and presented with bone pain, progressive weakness, and bowing of the legs. A bone biopsy showed osteomalacia, which these investigators suggest occurred as a consequence of low levels of $1,25(OH)_2D$. The frequency of this problem is unknown, but it may be rare because such patients may become symptomatic from hypocalcemia and receive treatment with pharmacological doses of vitamin D prior to the development of clinically overt bone symptoms; moreover, such patients have hyperphosphatemia or they lack hypophosphatemia, which may protect them from overt osteomalacia.

Since the plasma levels of $1,25(OH)_2D$ have been found to be low in patients with hypoparathyroidism, it would seem rational to use $1,25(OH)_2D$ or $1\alpha(OH)D_3$ in the long-term treatment of idiopathic hypoparathyroidism. Several studies have appeared reporting the successful use of these active vitamin D compounds in the treatment of idiopathic hypoparathyroidism; Rosen et al. (1977) treated three children with $1,25(OH)_2D_3$. In all three patients, serum calcium rose to the normal range and serum phosphorus was normalized for a period of 6 months to 1 year. Hypercalcemia was infrequent, but it responded readily to discontinuance of treatment with $1,25(OH)_2D_3$. The authors suggest that the use of small quantities of a highly active vitamin D sterol, such as $1,25(OH)_2D_3$, has a significant advantage in such patients; thus, a response occurs quickly, and it is easy to adjust the dosage, making the long-term management easier for the clinician. Davies (1977) noted that serum phosphorus levels fell to normal in association with a rise in serum calcium in 8 patients with hypoparathyroidism treated with $1,25(OH)_2D_3$, 1.0 μg/day by mouth. The fall in serum phosphorus occurred as a consequence of reduction in TmP/GFR, which correlated inversely with the serum calcium level during treatment with $1,25(OH)_2D_3$. The reduction in TmP/GFR could be mediated via changes in the serum or intracellular calcium in a manner previously shown by Eisenberg (1965) in hypoparathyroid patients given a continuous calcium infusion. Hypoparathyroidism has also been effectively treated with $1\alpha(OH)D_3$, a vitamin D analogue currently available for clinical use in the United Kingdom and Europe. The effective dose of $1\alpha(OH)D_3$, 5 μg/day, produced a rapid rise in plasma calcium to normal range in 4 patients with untreated hypoparathyroidism (Brenton et al., 1977). However, as demonstrated by Balsan et al. (1975), $1\alpha(OH)D_3$ was considerably less potent than $1,25(OH)_2D_3$ in hypoparathyroid patients when the two sterols were given at equimolar doses. $1\alpha(OH)D_3$ may still allow a prompt rise in plasma calcium with greater safety compared to vitamin D. We have similar observations; thus, the relative potency of $1\alpha(OH)D$ compared to $1,25(OH)_2D_3$ is lower in patients with hypoparathyroidism compared to uremic patients, an observation suggesting that PTH may possibly augment the 25-hydroxylation of $1\alpha(OH)D_3$ to $1,25(OH)_2D_3$.

The relative safety of vitamin D and related sterols in various hypocalcemic disorders was evaluted by Kanis and Russell (1977). The reversal of hypercalcemia or hypercalciuria following the discontinuation of treatment with vitamin D, dihydrotachysterol, $1\alpha(OH)D_3$, and $1,25(OH)_2D_3$ was evaluated in normal subjects and in patients with osteoporosis, hypoparathyroidism, renal tubular hypophosphatemia, and chronic renal failure. The half-time for reversal of hypercalcemia was less for $1,25(OH)_2D_3$ than for the other compounds; this occurred independently of the dose given or the length of treatment. Also, the reversal of hypercalcemia and hypercalciuria was less rapid in patients with "vitamin-D-resistant" states than in normal subjects.

11.3.4.2. Pseudohypoparathyroidism

Pseudohypoparathyroidism is a not infrequent cause of hypocalcemia. The syndrome has been subdivided into two subtypes: Type I is characterized by biochemical features of hypoparathyroidism, elevated serum iPTH levels with reduced or absent phosphaturia, and a lack of normally augmented excretion or urinary cAMP in response to parathyroid extract (PTE). The Type II variant, which is less common, exhibits a normally augmented renal excretion of cAMP following the administration of PTE; however, there is little or no phosphaturia. The latter response to PTE may be normalized when serum calcium is restored to normal by calcium infusion.

We suggested previously (Coburn and Hartenbower, 1977) that low levels of $1,25(OH)_2D$ may play a role in the pathogenesis of pseudohypoparathyroidism. Our preliminary observations were extended by Sinha *et al.* (1977) when $1,25(OH)_2D_3$ was administered for 12 days to a patient with pseudohypoparathyroidism. Thus, fecal calcium decreased, serum and urinary calcium rose, and iPTH levels fell toward normal. These authors suggested that the diminished intestinal absorption of calcium, the hypocalcemia, and the secondary hyperparathyroidism may arise due to defective formation of $1,25(OH)_2D_3$ in pseudohypoparathyroidism; therefore, $1,25(OH)_2D_3$ may be a useful and specific means of treatment. This point was further emphasized by Metz *et al.* (1977), who evaluated a patient who had hypocalcemia, elevated serum iPTH, and normal phosphaturia, and a rise in urinary cAMP following the administration of PTE; however, there was no increase in serum calcium. The serum level of $1,25(OH)_2D$ was extremely low, and treatment with $1,25(OH)_2D_3$, 1 μg/day, restored the calcemic response to PTE to normal. These authors suggested that this patient with pseudohypoparathyroidism had skeletal resistance but no renal resistance to PTH. They suggested that this may be due to the lack of $1,25(OH)_2D_3$. Treatment with $1,25(OH)_2D_3$ restored the skeletal response to PTH without an increase in base-line serum calcium and while the patient received a diet restricted in calcium to minimize an intestinal action of $1,25(OH)_2D_3$. They proposed a direct and specific effect of $1,25(OH)_2D_3$ on bone. The serum $25(OH)D$ level was normal, excluding a deficiency of the precursor to $1,25(OH)_2D_3$. Since the stimulation of the renal production of $1,25(OH)_2D_3$ by PTH may be mediated via cAMP (Horiuchi *et al.*, 1977), this patient could have a defect in cAMP-activated $25(OH)D_3$-1α-hydroxylase while the cAMP-mediated phosphaturia is intact.

11.4. Phosphorus Metabolism

11.4.1. Regulation of Phosphorus by the Kidney

It is now clear that the kidney plays a central role in the regulation of the concentration of inorganic phosphorus (P) in body fluids and thus indirectly in the maintenance of the intracellular stores of organic high-energy phosphates. The past year has seen further intensive investigation of hormonal and nonhormonal factors controlling the adaptive response of the kidney to variations in phosphate load (from diet or soft tissues or both). This adaptive response can free the urine of phosphorus within 1 day during P restriction or, during high-phosphorus intake, decrease the tubular reabsorption of P to the point where almost 100% of the filtered load is excreted in the urine.

The nephron segments responsible for this striking variation in the tubular reabsorption of P have been delineated by a number of micro-puncture and microperfusion studies, and these studies were analyzed in detail by Knox *et al.* (1977a) in an excellent review. Their findings and those of others are summarized below:

The proximal tubule (convoluted segment and pars recta) is the principal site of phosphate reabsorption in the mammalian kidney, accounting for reabsorption of at least 80% of filtered P. Baumann *et al.* (1975) and Dennis *et al.* (1977), utilizing the stationary microperfusion technique in TPTX rats and the isolated perfused rabbit tubule, respec-tively, demonstrated that the rate of P transport decreases progressively as fluid traverses the proximal tubule from the glomerulus to the pars recta. The reabsorptive rate in the latter is less than half that found in the proximal convoluted tubule. Knox uses the term "*intra*nephron heteroge-neity" to refer to the differences in transport along the proximal segments of the same nephron.

Phosphate reabsorption by nephron segments between the late proxi-mal and early distal tubule has been evaluated in free-flow micropuncture studies in normal animals, during phosphate and/or saline loading, and following acute and chronic TPTX. The results suggest that phosphate is reabsorbed in one or more nephron segments between late proximal and early distal tubule and that this reabsorption is inhibited by PTH. DeRouffignac *et al.* (1973) studied phosphate transport in psammomys and found that fractional delivery of phosphate from the superficial proximal convoluted tubule was 40%, at the tip of Henle's loop 10%, and to the early distal convoluted tubule 24%. These findings suggest that there is either net reabsorption along the descending limb with the subsequent net *addition* of phosphate along the ascending limb or hetero-geneity of phosphate transport between superficial and deep nephrons, since only the latter would be subject to micropuncture at the papillary tip. Internephron heterogeneity was documented more recently by Knox *et al.* (1977b) in free-flow micropuncture studies in the phosphate-loaded Wistar rat. They collected urine from deep nephrons (juxtaglomerular, ascending limb of loop of Henle in the papilla), superficial nephrons (distal tubules in the cortex), and urine (duct of Bellini). The fractional delivery of P to the ascending limb of the loop of Henle in deep nephrons was 78% ± 10% (S.E.), a value significantly greater than the 51% ± 6% delivered to the distal convoluted tubules of superficial nephrons and the 72% ± 10% fractional excretion of phosphate in the urine (Knox *et al.*, 1977b).

In general, free-flow micropuncture data are consistent with phosphate reabsorption occurring in terminal nephron segments (late distal convoluted tubule and collecting duct). These data have shown that phosphate delivery from superficial distal nephrons is consistently higher than that present in ureteral urine, and this "ultimate" reabsorption is influenced in the appropriate manner by the presence or absence of PTH. However, *in vitro* and *in vivo* microperfusion studies generally have not demonstrated phosphate reabsorption in these segments. A possible explanation for the discrepancy comes from the work of Knox *et al.* (1977b), which demonstrated internephron heterogeneity with more avid phosphate reabsorption by deep nephrons.

11.4.1.1. Effect of Restriction of Phosphorus Intake

As mentioned earlier, when phosphorus is removed from the diet, the kidney responds by freeing the urine of P (Shikita *et al.*, 1962). Until recently, it was considered that this striking "adaptation" was due to phosphate depletion and hypophosphatemia. However, it is clear that such a change may occur within the first 24 hr after phosphorus is removed from the diet (Cuisinier-Gleizes *et al.*, 1976a) and while the animal or human is normophosphatemic and not obviously phosphorus-depleted; moreover, it is not dependent on a change in circulating PTH (Cuisinier-Gleizes *et al.*, 1976a,b) or on the presence of vitamin D or its metabolites. The profound hypophosphaturia observed in the first day of dietary P restriction is always accompanied by marked hypercalciuria, evidence of enhanced bone resorption, and, in certain species, a rise in serum calcium (Cuisinier-Gleizes *et al.*, 1976a,b). It is not known how quickly these changes in divalent ion excretion occur after P has been removed from the diet. However, Baylink *et al.* (1977) recently found that the enhanced bone resorption and an increase in serum calcium may occur in the rat as early as 6 hr after P restriction. The rapidity with which these biochemical events take place suggests a true homeostatic adaptation to the absence of P in the diet. This leads to the speculation that the gastrointestinal tract in some way "senses" a deficiency of P in the diet and, possibly by a humoral mechanism, signals both bone and the kidneys to respond as they do. Steele (1976, 1977), Steele and DeLuca (1976), and Goldfarb *et al.* (1977) found that the tubular reabsorption of P continues almost completely in either rats or dogs subjected to chronic P depletion for 2 weeks or longer. Moreover, this occurs despite infusion of phosphate to increase serum P and its filtered load by 4- to 5-fold and despite the administration of PTH.

Lau *et al.* (1977) and Goldfarb *et al.* (1977) studied P-depleted rats and dogs using standard renal clearance techniques and free-flow micro-puncture methods; they concluded that the critical tubular adjustments of calcium and phosphorus reabsorption occurred in the terminal, i.e., late distal and collecting duct, portions of the nephron of the P-depleted animal. These observations must be accepted with a note of caution until it can be shown that the findings cannot be explained by nephron heterogeneity. Goldfarb *et al.* (1977) further observed that P depletion led to a reversible sustained inhibition of proximal tubular reabsorption of sodium and water in the dog.

11.4.1.2. Adaptation to High-Phosphorus Intake

The studies of Tröhler *et al.* (1976a,b) and Steele and DeLuca (1976) clearly demonstrated the renal tubular capacity to adapt to high-P diets. While this adaptation was also observed in the TPTX animal, it was significantly blunted in comparison to results in the normal animal. Bonjour *et al.* (1977) suggested that the impaired capacity of the TPTX animal to increase the fractional excretion of phosphate or lower the TmP/GFR may be due both to the absence of PTH and to a deficiency of $1,25(OH)_2D_3$, which may accompany the hypoparathyroid state. Therefore, they studied the renal handling of phosphate in sham-operated and TPTX rats either supplemented or not with $1,25(OH)_2D_3$, 2×13 pmol/day, an amount believed to be "physiologic" since it normalized but did not overcorrect the impaired intestinal absorption of Ca and P observed in TPTX rats. In rats with intact thyroid and parathyroid glands that were fed a high-P diet and then given an acute infusion of phosphate, $1,25(OH)_2D_3$ had no effect on the fractional excretion of phosphate (FEP). In contrast, the $1,25(OH)_2D_3$ returned FEP to normal in TPTX rats; however, $25(OH)D_3$ in a dose 100 times greater did not increase FEP in such animals. The authors concluded that $1,25(OH)_2D_3$, when administered in "physiologic" amounts to hypoparathyroid rats, restores to normal the capability of the renal tubule to excrete phosphorus and to adapt to large variations in dietary P.

Swenson *et al.* (1975) had previously observed a normal adaptation to changes in dietary P intake in TPTX dogs with various degrees of renal failure created by stepwise ablation of renal mass when serum calcium was maintained normal with high doses of supplemental vitamin D. It is not known whether the high-dose vitamin D may have led to the synthesis of physiological amounts of $1,25(OH)_2D_3$ by the remnant kidney, thus allowing the kidney to adapt in a manner comparable to the TPTX rats of Bonjour *et al.* (1977). The mechanism by which $1,25(OH)_2D_3$ produces the effect is unknown. It could be a direct permissive action on the renal

Table IV. Modification of Tubular Handling of Phosphate following Changes in Dietary Intake: Fractional Reabsorption of Phosphorus (× 100)

	Dietary P	
	0.2%	1.8%
Glomerulus to early proximal tubule	20	−10
Early proximal tubule to late proximal tubule	50	57
Late proximal tubule to distal tubule	48	17
Distal tubule to final urine	0	−64

tubule or it could act elsewhere, e.g., on bone, to influence indirectly the adaptive response of the kidney to varying P loads.

The same group of investigators (Muhlbauer *et al.*, 1977) continued their studies on the renal adaptation of P with free-flow micropuncture techniques in rats fed either a low (0.2%)- or high (1.8%)-phosphorus diet. The investigation was carried out as filtered loads of P were increased to similar levels by the acute infusion of P. Their results of fractional reabsorption of P at a comparable filtered load are shown in Table IV.

The findings suggest that there are adaptations of tubular P reabsorption in the early segment of the proximal tubule, and between the end of the accessible proximal tubule to late distal tubule and in the terminal nephron. The apparent tubular secretion in the terminal nephron segments could also be explained by heterogeneity of nephrons, with the deeper, inaccessible tubules reabsorbing less P throughout and thereby contributing more P to the final urine.

11.4.1.3. Effect of Parathyroid Hormone

Walker (1977) studied the relationship between the phosphaturic response to PTH and the simultaneous rate of cAMP excretion in normal human subjects and in patients with primary hyperparathyroidism studied both before and after surgery. In these subjects, he infused a purified (Medical Research Council) preparation of bovine parathyroid hormone at varying rates for a number of hours. In both normals and patients, the renal handling of P was expressed in terms of maximum tubular reabsorption of phosphate/glomerular filtration rate (TmP/GFR) in a manner recommended by Bijvoet (1969). Before the infusion, the serum concentration of immunoreactive PTH (iPTH) in the normals ranged from undetectable (<0.15 ng/ml) to 0.9 ng/ml, and there was no correlation between serum iPTH, urinary cAMP, and TmP/GFR. The infusion of the

PTH at a rate of 0.25–0.5 U/kg/hr, a very low, questionable physiological rate, caused a marked decrease of TmP/GFR into the range seen in patients with hyperparathyroidism and a fall in serum phosphate, but *no* rise in cAMP excretion or in the concentration of iPTH in the plasma. The results indicate that there was a striking dissociation between the parameters, TmP/GFR and urinary cAMP, in the state of mild hyperparathyroidism.

In the patients with primary hyperparathyroidism, as in the normals, there was no correlation between the preoperative plasma iPTH, the TMP/GFR, or the urinary cAMP. However, there was no overlap between the preoperative TmP/GFR (0.2–0.8 mmol/liter) in the patients and the base-line TmP/GFR of the normal subjects (0.8–1.5 mmol/liter). At 3 weeks after parathyroid surgery, there was a significant rise of the TmP/GFR in each patient.

11.4.1.4. Effects of Estrogen on Phosphate Metabolism

Lindsay *et al.* (1977) have contributed to our understanding of the rise in plasma inorganic P seen in the postmenopausal period and after oophorectomy. The latter change in plasma is due to estrogen deficiency. Also, the TmP/GFR is inversely related to the plasma level of estradiol, and both the increased concentration of plasma phosphate and the increased TmP/GFR can be returned toward normal by exogenous estrogen replacement. This recent study confirms and amplifies the earlier investigations of Nassin *et al.* (1956) and Aitken *et al.* (1971). However, we still do not know whether this estrogen-dependent alteration of tubular phosphate transport is a direct action on the nephron or arises secondary to extrarenal effects of the hormone.

11.4.1.5. Growth Hormone and Renal Phosphate Reabsorption

Some years ago, Corvilain *et al.* (1964) found that chronic administration of growth hormone (GH) caused effects on phosphate handling by the kidney that were opposite those of PTH but occurred in the absence of PTH. These actions could explain the enhanced tubular reabsorption of phosphate, the hyperphosphatemia, and the hypercalciuria present in both experimental and clinical states of growth hormone excess. Recently, Westby *et al.* (1977) also studied the effect of the short-term administration of bovine GH on calcium and phosphorus excretion. They were unable to observe any changes in the renal handling of these ions under these experimental conditions, and they concluded that the results of Corvilain *et al.* (1964) and other similar findings in patients with acromegaly probably represent indirect effects of the GH on the kidney. They suggested that such effects may be mediated through somatomedin.

11.4.1.6. Other Factors That Affect Renal Handling of Phosphorus

Following the relief of unilateral ureteral obstruction, there is characteristically a decrease in the fraction of filtered phosphate appearing in the urine. Moreover, this occurs even though there is an *increase* in the fractional excretion of sodium. The mechanism(s) responsible for this unilateral hypophosphaturia were studied by Chaimovitz *et al.* (1977). Volume expansion with saline and infusion of parathyroid extract in dogs either with intact parathyroid glands or following parathyroidectomy demonstrated that under all conditions the kidney excreted significantly less phosphorus after unilateral ureteral obstruction. This pattern was closely duplicated by hypoperfusion of the left kidney secondary to constriction of the aorta between the origin of the renal arteries. The results strongly suggest that the ipsilateral hypophosphaturia that follows the relief of unilateral ureteral obstruction is due to enhanced proximal tubular reabsorption of phosphorus secondary to reduced GFR/nephron. The dissociation between fractional excretion of sodium and phosphorus probably arises secondary to decreased sodium reabsorption at a site distal to the proximal tubule. The results of this study have physiological significance beyond the hypophosphaturia of unilateral ureteral obstruction. They may indicate that any cause of functional decrease of GFR/nephron could cause hypophosphaturia, a factor that must be considered as a major variable in any study of other renal or extrarenal factor(s) that influence the tubular reabsorption of phosphorus.

11.4.2. Phosphate-Depletion Syndrome

In the prior edition, Coburn *et al.* (1978) reviewed in some detail the background, pathophysiology, and clinical characteristics of phosphate depletion, and we have discussed earlier in this chapter more recent data on certain biochemical and physiological characteristics and the feature of phosphate depletion. Additional clinical and experimental studies have contributed further to our understanding and delineation of this syndrome.

An osteomalacic skeletal disease that is histologically identical to the osteomalacia of vitamin D deficiency is characteristic of chronic phosphate deficiency in animals and humans. There is evidence of a change in bone function soon after the removal of phosphorus from the diet of an experimental animal. Hypercalciuria and hypercalcemia occur within 1 day of dietary P restriction in the rat (Cuisinier-Gleizes *et al.*, 1976a); also, these effects occur in parathyroidectomized animals as well (Cuisinier-Gleizes *et al.*, 1976a,b). Our preliminary observation suggests that such biochemical changes cannot be explained by enhanced absorption of calcium from the gastrointestinal tract, and thus they must result from increased liberation of calcium from the skeleton. In the rat, phosphate depletion increases osteoclastic and periosteocytic bone resorption and decreases appositional bone formation rate (Baylink *et al.*, 1971).

It seems likely that the enhanced bone resorption, hypercalcemia, hypercalciuria, and hypophosphaturia do not arise because of actual depletion of body stores of phosphorus, but represent features of very acute adaptation (?homeostatic) to the single factor of removing phosphorus from the diet. How the latter information is transmitted to kidney and bone to bring about the adaptive changes is unknown.

Previously, Gold *et al.* (1973) demonstrated that chronic depletion of phosphorus in the dog caused a significant impairment in the renal tubular reabsorption of bicarbonate. This impairment was completely reversible when phosphorus was added to the diet. However, despite bicarbonate wasting, acidosis did not occur in these animals. To investigate the effect of phosphate depletion on acid–base balance, Emmett *et al.* (1977) carried out a series of experiments in the chronically P-depleted rats. They confirmed first that P depletion caused a defect in the tubular transport of bicarbonate and bicarbonate wasting, and second that this defect may not cause systemic acidosis because the enhanced bone resorption of P depletion liberated sufficient amount of alkaline to replace bicarbonate lost in the urine.

Additional clinical features of the syndrome of P depletion that have appeared include a report of acute respiratory failure due to ventilatory depression that required tracheostomy and mechanically assisted respiration (Newman *et al.*, 1977) and a report of pseudomyopathy with diffuse and profound involvement of proximal limb girdle musculature with painful tender muscles and inability to raise the arms or to rise from a sitting position or climb stairs (Searles *et al.*, 1977). Other patients have been described with marked impairment or alterations of circulatory function with cardiac failure and peripheral circulatory collapse (O'Connor, L. R., *et al.*, 1978; Ljunghall and Hedstrand, 1977).

ACKNOWLEDGMENTS

Some of the work cited herein has been supported by USPHS Grant AM 14750 and by Veterans Administration Research Funds.

The authors are indebted to Harriet Goldware-Sorkin and Patti Kentor for their assistance in the preparation of this manuscript.

References

Aitken, J. M., Hart, D. M., and Smith, D. A., 1971, The effect of long term mestranol administration on calcium and phosphorus homeostasis in oophorectomized women, *Clin. Sci.* **41**:233–236.

Ando, M., Sayato, Y., Tonomura, M., and Osawa, T., 1977, Studies on excretion and uptake of calcium by rats after continuous oral administration of cadmium, *Toxicol. Appl. Pharmacol.* **39**:321–327.

Arnaud, S. B., Matthusen, M., Gilkinson, J. B., and Goldsmith, R. S., 1977, Components of 25-hydroxy-vitamin D in serum of young children in upper midwestern United States, *Am. J. Clin. Nutr.* **30**:1082–1086.

Aschinberg, L. C., Solomon, L. M., Zeis, P. M., Justice, P., and Rosenthal, I. M., 1977, Vitamin D-resistant rickets associated with epidermal nevus syndrome: Demonstration of a phosphaturic substance in the dermal lesions, *J. Pediatr.* **91**:56–60.

Balsan, S., Garabedian, M., Sogniard, R., Holick, M. F., and DeLuca, H. F., 1975, 1,25-Dihydroxy-vitamin D_3 and 1α-hydroxy-vitamin D_3 in children: Biologic and therapeutic effects in nutritional rickets and different types of vitamin D resistance, *Pediatr. Res.* **9**:586–593.

Barragry, J. M., France, M. W., Carter, N. D., Auton, J. A., Beer, M., Boucher, B. J., and Cohen, R. D., 1977, Vitamin D metabolism in nephrotic syndrome, *Lancet* **2**:629–632.

Baumann, K., de Rouffignac, C., Roinel, N., Rumrich, G., and Ullrich, K. J., 1975, Renal phosphate transport: Inhomogeneity of local–proximal transport rates and sodium dependence, *Pfluegers Arch.* **356**:287–298.

Baylink, D. J., 1977, Effect of phosphate depletion on bone, Proceedings of the 3rd International Phosphate Workshop, Madrid, Spain.

Baylink, D. J., Wergedal, J., and Stauffer, M., 1971, Formation, mineralization and resorption of bone in hypophosphatemic rats, *J. Clin. Invest.* **50**:2519–2530.

Bickle, D. D., and Rasmussen, H., 1975, The ionic control of 1,25-dihydroxy-vitamin D_3 production in isolated chick renal tubules, *J. Clin. Invest.* **55**:292–298.

Bijvoet, O. L. M., 1969, Relation of plasma phosphate concentration to renal tubular reabsorption of phosphate, *Clin. Sci.* **37**:23–36.

Bonjour, J. P., Preston, C., and Fleisch, H., 1977, Effects of 1,25-dihydroxy-vitamin D_3 on the renal handling of P_i in thyroparathyroidectomized rats, *J. Clin. Invest.* **60**:1419–1428.

Booth, B. E., Tsai, H. C., and Morris, R. C., Jr., 1977, Metabolic acidosis in the vitamin D-deficient chick, *Metabolism* **26**:1099–1105.

Bordier, P., Ryckwaert, A., Marie, P., Miravet, L., Norman, A. W., and Rasmussen, H., 1977, Vitamin D metabolites and bone mineralization in man, in: *Vitamin D: Biochemical, Chemical and Clinical Aspects Related to Calcium Metabolism* (A. W. Norman, K. Schaefer, J. W. Coburn, H. F. DeLuca, D. Fraser, H. G. Grigoleit, and D. v. Herrath, eds.), pp. 897–911, Walter de Gruyter, Berlin and New York.

Bouillon, R., van Baelen, H., and de Moor, P., 1977, 25-Hydroxy-vitamin D and its

binding protein in maternal and cord serum, *J. Clin. Endocrinol. Metab.*
45:679–684.

Boyle, I. T., Omdahl, J. L., Gray, R. W., and DeLuca, H. F., 1973, The biological
activity and metabolism of 24,25-dihydroxy-vitamin D$_3$, *J. Biol. Chem.*
248:4174–4180.

Brenton, D. P., Dent, C. E., and Gertner, J. M., 1977, The treatment of hypoparathyroidism with 1α-hydroxycholecalciferol, *Calcif. Tissue Res.*
22(Suppl.):545–552.

Brewer, E. D., Tsai, H. C., Szeto, K. S., and Morris, R. C., Jr., 1977a, Maleic acid–
induced impaired conversion of 25(OH)D$_3$ to 1,25(OH)$_2$D$_3$; Implication for
Fanconi's syndrome, *Kidney Int.* **12**:244–252.

Brewer, E. D., Tsai, H. C., and Morris, R. C., 1977b, Fanconi syndrome and its
relationship to vitamin D, in: *Vitamin D: Biochemical, Chemical and Clinical
Aspects Related to Calcium Metabolism* (A. W. Norman, K. Schaefer, J. W.
Coburn, T. F. DeLuca, D. Fraser, H. G. Grigoleit, and D. v. Herrath, eds.),
pp. 937–949, Walter de Gruyter, Berlin and New York.

Brickman, A. S., Hartenbower, D. L., Norman, A. W., and Coburn, J. W., 1977,
Actions of 1α-hydroxy-vitamin D$_3$ and 1α,25-dihydroxy-vitamin D$_3$ on min-
eral metabolism in man. I. Effects on net absorption of phosphorus, *Am. J.
Clin. Nutr.* **30**:1064–1069.

Brumbaugh, P. F., Hughes, M. R., and Haussler, M. R., 1975, Cytoplasmic and
nuclear binding components for 1α,25-dihydroxy-vitamin D$_3$ in chick parathyroid glands, *Proc. Natl. Acad. Sci. U.S.A.* **72**:4871–4875.

Care, A. D., Bates, R. F. L., Pickard, D. W., Peacock, M., Tomlinson, S., Riordan, J.
L. H., Mawer, E. B., Tailor, C. M., DeLuca, H. F., and Norman, A. W., 1977,
The effects of vitamin D metabolites and their analogues on the secretion of
parathyroid hormone, *Calcif. Tissue Res.* **21**(Suppl.): 142–146.

Chaimovitz, C., Dickmeyer, J., Friedler, R. M., Kurokawa, K., and Massry, S. G.,
1977, Studies on mechanism of hypophosphaturia after relief of unilateral
ureteral obstruction, *Nephron* **19**:333–341.

Chertow, B. S., Baylink, D. J., Wergedal, J. E., Su, M. H. H., and Norman, A. W.,
1975, Decrease in serum immunoreactive parathyroid hormone in rats and in
parathyroid hormone secretion *in vitro* by 1,25-dihydroxycholecalciferol, *J.
Clin. Invest.* **56**:668–678.

Clark, M. B., and Potts, J. T., Jr., 1977, 25-Hydroxy-vitamin D$_3$, *Calcif. Tissue Res.*
22(Suppl.):29 -34.

Cloix, J. G., Ulmann, A., Bachelet, M., and Funck-Bretano, 1976, Cholecalciferol
metabolites binding in porcine parathyroid glands, *Steroids* **28**:743–749.

Coburn, J. W., and Hartenbower, D. L., 1977, Physiology of calcium, phosphorus
and magnesium and disorders affecting their metabolism, in: *Current
Nephrology* (H. C. Gonick, ed.), Vol. I, pp. 99–171, Pinecliff Medical Publishing Co., Pacific Palisades, California.

Coburn, J. W., Brickman, A. S., Sherrard, D. J., Singer, F. R., Baylink, D. J.,
Wong, E. G. C., Massry, S. G., and Norman, A. W., 1977, Clinical efficacy of
1,25-dihydroxy-vitamin D$_3$ in renal osteodystrophy, in: *Vitamin D: Biochemi-
cal, Chemical and Clinical Aspects Related to Calcium Metabolism* (A. W. Norman,
K. Schaefer, J. W. Coburn, H. F. DeLuca, D. Fraser, H. G. Grigoleit, and D. v.
Herrath, eds.), pp. 657–666, Walter de Gruyter, Berlin and New York.

Coburn, J. W., Hartenbower, D. L., and Kleeman, C. R., 1978, Divalent ion metabolism, in: *The Year in Metabolism 1977* (N. Freinkel, ed.), pp. 327–377, Plenum Medical Book Company, New York and London.

Coe, F. L., Firpo, J. J., Hollandsworth, D. L., Segil, L., Canterbury, J. M., and Reiss, E. M., 1975, Effect of acute and chronic metabolic acidosis on serum immunoreactive parathyroid hormone in man, *Kidney Int.* **8**:262–273.

Colston, K. W., Evans, I. M. A., Spelsberg, T. C., and MacIntyre, I., 1977, Feedback regulation of vitamin D metabolism by 1,25-dihydroxycholecalciferol, *Biochem. J.* **164**:83–89.

Compston, J. E., and Thompson, R. P., 1977, Intestinal absorption of 25-hydroxyvitamin D and osteomalacia in primary biliary cirrhosis, *Lancet* **1**:721–726.

Corvilain, J., Abramow, M., and Bergans, A., 1964, Effect of growth hormone on tubular transport of phosphate in normal and parathyroidectomized dogs, *J. Clin. Invest.* **43**:1608–1612.

Cuisinier-Gleizes, P., Thomasset, M., and Mathieu, H., 1976a, Homeostasis of P and Ca in phosphorus deprivation, in: *Phosphate Metabolism, Kidney and Bone* (L. Avioli, Ph. Bordier, H. Fleisch, S. Massry, and E. Slatopolsky, eds.), pp. 381–386, Nouvelle Imprimerie Fournie, Toulouse.

Cuisinier-Gleizes, P., Thomasset, M., Sainteny-Debove, F., and Mathieu, H., 1976b, Phosphorus deficiency, parathyroid hormone, and bone resorption in the growing rat, *Calcif. Tissue Res.* **20**:235–249.

Davies, M., 1977, Effects of 1,25-dihydroxycholecalciferol on calcium and phosphorus metabolism in hypoparathyroidism, *Calcif. Tissue Res.* **22**(Suppl.):68–73.

DeLuca, H. F., 1977, Vitamin D endocrine system, *Adv. Clin. Chem.* **19**:125–174.

Dennis, V. W., Bello-Reuss, E., and Robinson, R. R., 1977, Response of phosphate transport to parathyroid hormone in segments of rabbit nephron, *Am. J. Physiol.* **233**:F29–F38.

DeRouffignac, C., Morel, F., Moss, N., and Roinel, N., 1973, Micropuncture study of water and electrolyte movements along the loop of Henle in psammomys with special reference to magnesium, calcium and phosphorus, *Pfluegers Arch.* **344**:309–326.

Doxiadis, S. A., and Lapatsants, P. D., 1977, 1α-Hydroxy-vitamin D in neonatal hypocalcaemia (letter), *Lancet* **1**:426.

Drezner, M. K., and Feinglos, M. N., 1977, Osteomalacia due to 1α,25-dihydroxycholecalciferol deficiency, *J. Clin. Invest.* **60**:1046–1053.

Drezner, M. K., Neelon, F. A., Jowsey, J., and Lebovitz, H. E., 1977, Hypoparathyroidism: A possible cause of osteomalacia, *J. Clin. Endocrinol. Metab.* **45**:114–122.

Eastwood, J. B., Stamp, T. C. B., De Wardener, H. E., Bordier, P. J., and Arnaud, C. D., 1977, The effect of 25-hydroxy-vitamin D_3 in osteomalacia of chronic renal failure, *Clin. Sci. Mol. Med.* **52**:499–508.

Eisenberg, E., 1965, Effects of serum calcium level in parathyroid extracts on phosphate and calcium excretion in hypoparathyroid patients, *J. Clin. Invest.* **44**:942–946.

Emmett, M., Goldfarb, S., Agus, Z. S., and Narins, R. G., 1977, The pathophysiology of acid–base changes in chronically phosphate-depleted rats, *J. Clin. Invest.* **59**:291–298.

Fairney, A., Naughten, E., and Oppe, T. E., 1977, Vitamin D and human lactation, *Lancet* **2**:739–741.

Favus, M. J., Kimberg, D. V., Millar, G. N., and Gersham, E., 1973a, Effects of cortisone administration on the metabolism and localization of 25-hydroxycholecalciferol in the rat, *J. Clin. Invest.* **52**:1328–1335.

Favus, M. J., Walling, M. W., and Kimberg, D. V., 1973b, Effect of 1,25-dihydroxycholecalciferol on intestinal calcium transport in cortisone-treated rats, *J. Clin. Invest.* **52**:1680–1686.

Fournier, A. E., Bordier, P. J., Gueris, J., Chanard, J., Marie, P., Ferriere, C., Osario, M., Bedrossian, J., and DeLuca, H. F., 1976, 1α-Hydroxycholecalciferol in renal bone disease, *Proc. Eur. Dial. Transplant Assoc.* **12**:227–236.

Fraser, D., and Scriver, C. R., 1976, Familial forms of vitamin D–resistant rickets revisited: X-linked hypophosphatemia and autosomal recessive vitamin D dependency, *Am. J. Clin. Nutr.* **29**:1315–1329.

Frymoyer, J. W., and Hodgkin, W., 1977, Adult-onset vitamin D–resistant hypophosphatemic osteomalacia: A possible variant of vitamin D–resistant rickets, *J. Bone Joint Surg.* **59A**:101–106.

Gerblich, A. A., Genuth, S. M., and Haddad, J. F., 1977, A case of idiopathic hypoparathyroidism and dietary vitamin D deficiency: The requirement for calcium and vitamin D for bone, but not renal responsiveness to PTH, *J. Clin. Endocrinol. Metab.* **44**:507–513.

Gold, L. W., Massry, S. G., Arieff, A. I., and Coburn, J. W., 1973, Renal bicarbonate wasting during phosphate depletion: A possible cause of altered acid–base homeostasis in hyperparathyroidism, *J. Clin. Invest.* **52**:2556–2562.

Goldfarb, S., Westby, G. R., Goldberg, M., and Agus, Z. S., 1977, Renal tubular effects of chronic phosphate depletion, *J. Clin. Invest.* **59**:770–779.

Goldstein, D. A., Oda, Y., Kurokawa, K., and Massry, S. G., 1977, Blood levels of 25-hydroxy-vitamin D in nephrotic syndrome: Studies in 26 patients, *Ann. Intern. Med.* **87**:664–667.

Haddad, J. G., Jr., and Walgate, J., 1976, Radioimmunoassay of the binding protein for vitamin D and its metabolites in human serum, *J. Clin. Invest.* **58**:1217–1222.

Haddad, J. G., Min, C., Mendelsohn, M., Slatopolsky, E., and Hahn, T. J., 1977, Competitive protein-binding radioassay of 24,25-dihydroxy-vitamin D in sera from normal and anephric subjects, *Arch. Biochem. Biophys.* **182**:390–395.

Hahn, T. J., Halstead, L. R., Scharp, C. R., and Halic, B. H., 1976, Mineral metabolism and response to 25-hydroxyvitamin D therapy in patients with steroid induced osteopenia, *Endocrine Soc. Annu. Meeting* **58**:62.

Hahn, T. J., Halstead, L. R., and Haddad, J. G., 1977, Serum 25-hydroxy-vitamin D concentrations in patients receiving chronic corticosteroid therapy, *J. Lab. Clin. Med.* **90**:399–404.

Harrison, H. C., and Harrison, H. E., 1976, Inhibition of vitamin D–stimulated active transport of calcium of rat intestine by diphenylhydantoin–phenobarbital treatment, *Proc. Soc. Exp. Biol. Med.* **153**:220–224.

Haussler, M. R., and McCain, T. A., 1977, Basic and clinical concepts related to vitamin D metabolism and action, *N. Engl. J. Med.* **297**:974–983 and 1041–1050.

Haussler, M. R., Hughes, M. R., McCain, T. A., Zerwekh, Z. E., Brumbaugh, P. F., Jubiz, W., and Wasserman, R. H., 1977, 1,25-Dihydroxy-vitamin D_3: Mode of action in intestine and parathyroid glands, assays in humans and isolation of its glycoside from *Solanum malacoxylon*, *Calcif. Tissue Res.* **22**(Suppl.):1–18.

Henry, H. L., Taylor, A. N., and Norman, A. W., 1977, Response of chick parathyroid glands to the vitamin D metabolites, 1,25-dihydroxycholecalciferol and 24,25-dihydroxycholecalciferol, *J. Nutr.* **107**:1918–1926.

Holick, M. F., Kleiner-Bossaler, A., Schnoes, H. K., Kasten, P. M., Boyle, I. T., and DeLuca, H. F., 1973, 1,24,25-Trihydroxy-vitamin D_3: A metabolite of vitamin D_3 effective on intestine, *J. Biol. Chem.* **248**:6691–6696.

Holick, M. F., Baxter, L. A., Schrautrogel, P. K., Tavela, T. E., and DeLuca, H. F., 1976, Metabolism and biological activity of 24,25-dihydroxy-vitamin D_3 in the chick, *J. Biol. Chem.* **251**:397–402.

Horiuchi, N., Suda, T., Takahashi, H., Shimazawa, E., and Ogata, E., 1977, *In vivo* evidence for the intermediary role of $3',5'$-cyclic AMP in parathyroid hormone–induced stimulation of $1\alpha,25$-dihydroxy-vitamin D_3 synthesis in rats, *Endocrinology* **101**:969–974.

Imawari, M., and Goodman, D. S., 1977, Immunological and immunoassay studies of the binding protein for vitamin D and its metabolites in human serum, *J. Clin. Invest.* **59**:432–442.

Jubiz, W., Haussler, M. R., McCain, T. A., and Tolman, K. G., 1977, Plasma 1,25-dihydroxy-vitamin D levels in patients receiving anticonvulsant drugs, *J. Clin. Endocrinol. Metab.* **44**:617–621.

Kanis, J. A., and Russell, R. G. G., 1977, Rate of reversal of hypercalcaemia and hypercalciuria induced by vitamin D and its 1α-hydroxylated derivatives, *Br. Med. J.* **1**:78–81.

Kanis, J. A., Heynen, G., Russell, R. G. G., Smith, R., Walton, R. J., and Warner, G. T., 1977, Biological effects of 24,25-dihydroxycholecalciferol in man, in: *Vitamin D: Biochemical, Chemical and Clinical Aspects Related to Calcium Metabolism* (A. W. Norman, K. Schaefer, J. W. Coburn, H. F. DeLuca, D. Fraser, H. G. Grigoleit, and D. v. Herrath, eds.), pp. 793–795, Walter de Gruyter, Berlin and New York.

Kleeman, K., and Kleeman, C. R., 1979, Parathyroid hormone, in: *Contemporary Endocrinology*, Vol. 1 (S. Ingbar, ed.), pp. 305–339, Plenum Medical Book Company, New York.

Klein, R. G., Arnaud, S. B., Gallagher, J. C., DeLuca, H. F., and Riggs, B. L., 1977, Intestinal calcium absorption in exogenous hypercorticism, *J. Clin. Invest.* **60**:253–259.

Knox, F. G., Osswald, H., Marchand, G. R., Spielman, W. S., Haas, J. A., Berndt, T., and Youngberg, S. P., 1977a, Phosphate transport along the nephron, *Am. J. Physiol.* **233**:F261–F268.

Knox, F. G., Haas, J. A., Berndt, T., Marchand, G. R., and Youngberg, S. P., 1977b, Phosphate transport in superficial and deep nephrons in phosphate loaded rats, *Am. J. Physiol.* **233**:F150–F153.

Kooh, S. W., Fraser, D., Toon, R., and DeLuca, H. F., 1976, Response of protracted neonatal hypocalcaemia to $1\alpha,25$-hydroxy-vitamin D_3, *Lancet* **2**:1105–1107.

Kumar, R., and DeLuca, H. F., 1976, Side chain oxidation of 25-hydroxy-(26,27-

14C)vitamin D₃ and 1,25-dihydroxy-(26,27-14C)vitamin D₃ *in vivo* by chickens, *Biochem. Biophys. Res. Commun.* **69**:197–200.

Kumar, R., and DeLuca, H. F., 1977, Side chain oxidation of 1,25-dihydroxyvitamin D₃ in the rat: Effect of removal of the intestine, *Biochem. Biophys. Res. Commun.* **76**:253–258.

Kumar, R., Harnden, D., and DeLuca, H. F., 1976, Metabolism of 1,25-dihydroxyvitamin D₃: Evidence for side-chain oxidation, *Biochemistry* **15**:2420–2422.

Larsson, S. E., and Lorentzon, R., 1977, Excretion of active metabolites of vitamin D in urine and bile of the adult rat, *Clin. Sci. Mol. Med.* **53**:373–377.

Lau, K., Agus, Z. S., Goldberg, M., and Goldfarb, S., 1977, Chronic phosphate depletion: Changes in segmental calcium and phosphate reabsorption, *Kidney Int.* **12**:458.

Lee, S. W., Russell, J., and Avioli, L. V., 1977, 25-Hydroxycholecalciferol to 1,25-dihydroxycholecalciferol: Conversion impaired by systemic metabolic acidosis, *Science* **195**:994–996.

Levin, M. E., Boisseau, V. C., and Avioli, L. V., 1976, Effects of diabetes mellitus on bone mass in juvenile and adult-onset diabetes, *N. Engl. J. Med.* **294**:241–245.

Lieberherr, M., Pezant, E., Garabedian, M., and Balson, S., 1977, Phosphatase content of rat calvaria after *in vivo* administration of vitamin D₃ metabolites, *Calcif. Tissue Res.* **23**:235–239.

Lim, P., Jacob, E., Tock, E. P. C., and Pwee, H. S., 1977, Calcium and phosphorus metabolism in nephrotic syndrome, *Q. J. Med.* **46**:327–338.

Lindsay, R., Coutts, J. R. T., and Hart, D. M., 1977, The effect of endogenous estrogen on plasma and urinary calcium and phosphorus in oophorectomized women, *Clin. Endocrinol.* **6**:87–93.

Ljunghall, S., and Hedstrand, H., 1977, Serum phosphate inversely related to blood pressure, *Br. Med. J.* **1**:553–554.

Llach, F., Coburn, J. W., Brickman, A. S., Kurokawa, K., Norman, A. W., Canterbury, J. M., and Reiss, E., 1977, Acute actions of 1,25-dihydroxyvitamin D₃ in normal man: Effect on calcium and parathyroid status, *J. Clin. Endocrinol. Metab.* **44**:1054–1060.

Lumb, G. A., Mawer, E. B., and Stanbury, S., 1971, The apparent vitamin D resistance of chronic renal failure: A study of the physiology of vitamin D in man, *Am. J. Med.* **50**:421–441.

Matthews, C., Heimberg, K. W., Ritz, E., Agostini, B., Fritzsche, J., and Hasselbach, W., 1977, Effect of 1,25-dihydroxycholecalciferol on impaired calcium transport by the sarcoplasmic reticulum in experimental uremia, *Kidney Int.* **11**:227–235.

Mawer, E. B., and Reeve, A., 1977, The use of an isolated perfused liver to study the control of cholecalciferol-25-hydroxylase activity in the rat, *Calcif. Tissue Res.* **22**(Suppl.):24–28.

Mawer, E. B., Lumb, G. A., Schaeffer, K., and Stanbury, S. W., 1971, The metabolism of isotopically labeled vitamin D₃ in man: The influence of the state of vitamin D nutrition, *Clin. Sci.* **40**:39–53.

Meema, H. E., and Meema, S., 1975, Improved roentgenologic diagnosis of osteomalacia by microradioscopy of hand bones, *Am. J. Roentgenol. Radium Ther. Nucl. Med.* **125**:925–935.

Metz, S. A., Baylink, D. J., Hughes, M. R., Haussler, M. R., and Robertson, R. P., 1977, Selective deficiency of 1,25-dihydroxycholecalciferol: A cause of isolated skeletal resistance to parathyroid hormone, *N. Engl. J. Med.* **297**:1084–1090.

Michalska, L., Wrobel, J., and Szczepanska-Konkel, M. S., 1976, The effect of calcium restriction in the diet on calcium transport in rat small intestine, *Acta Biochim. Pol.* **23**:109–114.

Miravet, L., Redel, J., Carre, M., Queille, M. L., and Bordier, P., 1976, The biological activity of synthetic 25,26-dihydroxycholecalciferol and 24,25-dihydroxycholecalciferol in vitamin D–deficient rats, *Calcif. Tissue Res.* **21**:145–152.

Mosekilde, L., Melsen, F., Christensen, M. S., Lund, B., and Sørensen, O. H., 1977, Effect of long-term vitamin D_2 treatment on bone morphometry and biochemical values in anticonvulsant osteomalacia, *Acta Med. Scand.* **201**:303–307.

Mountokalakis, T. H., Virvidakis, C., Singhellakis, P., Alevizaki, C., and Ikkos, D., 1977, Intestinal calcium absorption in the nephrotic syndrome, *Ann. Intern. Med.* **86**:746–747.

Muhlbauer, R. C., Bonjour, J. P., and Fleisch, H., 1977, Tubular localization of adaptation to dietary phosphate in rats, *Am. J. Physiol.* **233**:F342–F348.

Nassin, J. R., Saville, P. D., and Mulligan, L., 1956, The effect of stilbesterol on urinary phosphate excretion, *Clin. Sci.* **15**:367–371.

Newman, J. H., Neff, T. A., and Ziporin, P., 1977, Acute respiratory failure associated with hypophosphatemia, *N. Engl. J. Med.* **296**:1101–1103.

Nishii, Y., Kumaki, K., Fukushima, M., Shimizu, T., Ono, M., Okawa, H., Niki, R., Matsunaga, I., Ochi, K., Tohira, Y., Sasaki, S., and Suda, T., 1977, Metabolism of 25-hydroxy-vitamin D_3 and 1α-hydroxy-vitamin D_3 in experimental rats with chronic renal failure, in: *Vitamin D: Biochemical, Chemical and Clinical Aspects Related to Calcium Metabolism* (A. W. Norman, K. Schaefer, J. W. Coburn, H. F. DeLuca, D. Fraser, H. G. Grigoleit, and D. v. Herrath, eds.), pp. 179–181, Walter de Gruyter, Berlin and New York.

O'Connor, L. R., Wheeler, W. S., and Bethune, J. E., 1978, Effect of hypophosphatemia on myocardial performance in man (letter), *N. Engl. J. Med.* **298**:341.

O'Connor, P., 1977, Vitamin D–deficiency rickets in two breast-fed infants who were not receiving vitamin D supplementation, *Clin. Pediatr.* **16**:361–363.

Omdahl, J. L., and Evan, A. P., 1977, Kidney mitochondria metabolism of 25-hydroxy-vitamin D_3: Evaluation of *in vitro* cation modulation, *Arch. Biochem. Biophys.* **184**:179–188.

Peacock, M. (ed.), 1977, The clinical uses of 1α-hydroxyvitamin D_3, *Clin. Endocrinol.* **7**(Suppl.).

Pento, J. T., Waite, L. C., Tracy, P. J., and Kenney, A. D., 1977, Adaptation to calcium deprivation in the rat: Effects of parathyroidectomy, *Am. J. Physiol.* **232**:E336–E342.

Pierides, A. M., Ward, M. K., Alvarez-Ude, F., Ellis, H. A., Peart, K. M., Simpson, W., Kerr, D. N. S., and Norman, A. W., 1976, Long term therapy with $1,25(OH)_2D_3$ in dialysis bone disease, *Proc. Eur. Dial. Transplant Assoc.* **12**:237–244.

Pierides, A. M., Ellis, H. A., Ward, M. K., Simpson, W., and Kerr, D. N. S., 1977, 1α-Hydroxycholecalciferol in renal osteodystrophy, *Calcif. Tissue Res.* **22**(Suppl.):105–111.

Pike, J. W., Toverud, S., Boass, A., McCain, T., and Haussler, M. R., 1977, Circulating 1α,25-(OH)$_2$D during physiological states of calcium stress, in: *Vitamin D: Biochemical, Chemical and Clinical Aspects Related to Calcium Metabolism* (A. W. Norman, K. Schaefer, J. W. Coburn, H. F. DeLuca, D. Fraser, H. G. Grigoleit, and D. v. Herrath, eds.), pp. 187–189, Walter de Gruyter, Berlin and New York.

Popovtzer, M. M., and Robinette, J. B., 1975, Effect of 25(OH)-vitamin D$_3$ on urinary excretion of cyclic adenosine monophosphate, *Am. J. Physiol.* **229**:907–910.

Popovtzer, M. M., Blum, M. S., and Flis, R. S., 1977, Evidence for interference of 25(OH)-vitamin D$_3$ with phosphaturic action of calcitonin, *Am. J. Physiol.* **232**:E515–E521.

Puschett, J. B., Moranz, J., and Kurnick, W. S., 1972, Evidence for a direct action of cholecalciferol and 25-hydroxycholecalciferol on the renal transport of phosphate, sodium and calcium, *J. Clin. Invest.* **51**:373–388.

Puschett, J. B., Beck, W. S., and Jelonek, A., 1975, Parathyroid hormone and 25-hydroxy-vitamin D$_3$: Synergistic and antagonistic effects on renal phosphate transport, *Science* **190**:473–475.

Rasmussen, H., Wong, M., Bikle, D., and Goodman, D. B. P., 1972, Hormonal control of the renal conversion of 25-hydroxycholecalciferol to 1,25-dihydroxycholecalciferol, *J. Clin. Invest.* **51**:2502–2504.

Rizzoli, R., Fleisch, H., and Bonjour, J. P., 1977, Role of 1,25-dihydroxy-vitamin D$_3$ on intestinal phosphate absorption in rats with a normal vitamin D supply, *J. Clin. Invest.* **60**:639–647.

Roelofs, J. M. M., and Raymakers, J. A., 1976, Calculation of three hour calcium absorption from a double isotope test: A simplified method, *Clin. Chim. Acta* **67**:53–62.

Rosen, J. F., Fleischman, A. R., Finberg, L., Eisman, J., and DeLuca, H. F., 1977, 1,25-Dihydroxycholecalciferol: Its use in the long-term management of idiopathic hypoparathyroidism in children, *J. Clin. Endocrinol. Metab.* **45**:457–468.

Rutherford, W. E., Bordier, P., Marie, P., Hruska, K., Harter, H., Greenwalt, A., Blondin, J., Haddad, J., Bricker, N., and Slatopolsky, E., 1977, Phosphate control and 25-hydroxycholecalciferol administration in preventing experimental renal osteodystrophy in the dog, *J. Clin. Invest.* **60**:332–341.

Sauveur, B., Garabedian, M., Fellot, C., Mongin, P., and Balsan, S., 1977, The effect of induced metabolic acidosis on vitamin D$_3$ metabolism in rachitic chicks, *Calcif. Tissue Res.* **23**:121–124.

Schmidt-Gayk, H., Schmitt, W., Grawunder, L., Ritz, E., Tschöpe, W., Pietsch, V., Andrassy, K., and Bouillon, R., 1977, 25-Hydroxy-vitamin D in nephrotic syndrome, *Lancet* **2**:105–108.

Schneider, L. E., Schedl, H. P., McCain, T., and Haussler, M. R., 1977, Experimental diabetes reduces circulating 1,25-dihydroxy-vitamin D in the rat, *Science* **196**:1452–1454.

Schoenfeld, P., Martin, J. H., Barnes, B., and Teitelbaum, S. L., 1977, Amelioration of myopathy with 25-hydroxy-vitamin D₃ therapy in patients on chronic hemodialysis, *Abstract Book*, p. 160 (Third Workshop on Vitamin D, Asilomar, California).

Searles, R. P., Bankhurst, A. D., Ahlin, T. D., and Messner, R. P., 1977, Antacid induced hypophosphatemia: An unusual case of pseudomyopathy, *J. Rheumatol.* **4**:176–178.

Shikita, M., Tsurufuji, S., and Ito, Y., 1962, Adaptation in renal phosphorus excretion under the influence of parathyroids: A study in unilaterally catheterized rats, *Endocrinol. Jpn.* **9**:171.

Sinha, T. K., DeLuca, H. F., and Bell, N. H., 1977, Evidence for a defect in the formation of 1α,25-dihydroxy-vitamin D in pseudohypoparathyroidism, *Metabolism* **26**:731–738.

Skinner, R. K., Sherlock, S., Long, R. G., and Wills, M. R., 1977, 25-Hydroxylation of vitamin D in primary biliary cirrhosis, *Lancet* **1**:720–721.

Steele, T. H., 1976, Renal resistance to parathyroid hormone during phosphorus deprivation, *J. Clin. Invest.* **58**:1461–1464.

Steele, T. H., 1977, Renal response to phosphorus deprivation: Effect of the parathyroids and bicarbonate, *Kidney Int.* **11**:327–334.

Steele, T. H., and DeLuca, H. F., 1976, Influence of dietary phosphorus on renal phosphate reabsorption in the parathyroidectomized rat, *J. Clin. Invest.* **57**:867–874.

Swenson, R. S., Weisinger, J. R., Ruggeri, J. L., and Reaven, G. M., 1975, Evidence that parathyroid hormone is not required for phosphate homeostasis in renal failure, *Metabolism* **24**:199–204.

Tanaka, Y., Castillo, L., and DeLuca, H. F., 1976, Control of renal vitamin D hydroxylase in birds by sex hormones, *Proc. Natl. Acad. Sci. U.S.A.* **73**:2701–2705.

Taylor, C. M., 1977, The measurement of 24,25-dihydroxycholecalciferol in human serum, in: *Vitamin D: Biochemical, Chemical and Clinical Aspects Related to Calcium Metabolism* (A. W. Norman, K. Schaefer, J. W. Coburn, H. F. DeLuca, D. Fraser, H. G. Grigoleit, and D. v. Herrath, eds.), pp. 541–543, Walter de Gruyter, Berlin and New York.

Taylor, C. M., DeSilva, P., and Hughes, S. E., 1977, Competitive protein-binding assay for 24,25-dihydroxycholecalciferol, *Calcif. Tissue Res.* **22**(Suppl.):40–44.

Tröhler, U., Bonjour, J. P., and Fleisch, H., 1976a, Renal tubular adaptation to dietary phosphorus, *Nature (London)* **261**:145–146.

Tröhler, U., Bonjour, J. P., and Fleisch, H., 1976b, Inorganic phosphate homeostasis, renal adaptation to the dietary intake in intact and thyroparathyroidectomized rats, *J. Clin. Invest.* **57**:264–273.

Turner, T. L., Cockburn, F., and Forfar, J. D., 1977, Magnesium therapy in neonatal tetany, *Lancet* **1**:283–284.

Van Stone, J. C., Frank, D. E., and Bradford, W. R., 1977, The effect of decreased renal function with and without reduction in renal mass on 1,25-dihydroxycholecalciferol production in rats, *J. Lab. Clin. Med.* **89**:1168–1174.

Walker, D. A., 1977, Control of renal tubular phosphate reabsorption by parathyroid hormone in man, *Clin. Sci. Mol. Med.* **53**:431–438.

Walling, M. W., 1977, Intestinal Ca and phosphate transport: Differential responses to vitamin D_3 metabolites, *Am. J. Physiol.* **233**:E488–E494.

Walling, M. W., Hartenbower, D. L., Coburn, J. W., and Norman, A. W., 1977, Effects of $1\alpha,25$-, $24R,25$- and $1\alpha,24R,25$-hydroxylated metabolites of vitamin D_3 on calcium and phosphate absorption by duodenum from intact and nephrectomized rats, *Arch. Biochem. Biophys.* **182**:251–257.

Weber, H. P., Gray, R. W., Dominguez, J. H., and Lemann, J., Jr., 1976, The lack of effect of chronic metabolic acidosis on 25-OH-vitamin D metabolism and serum parathyroid hormone in humans, *J. Clin. Endocrinol. Metab.* **43**:1047–1055.

Westby, G. R., Goldfarb, S., Goldberg, M., and Agus, Z. S., 1977, Acute effects of bovine growth hormone in renal calcium and phosphorus excretion, *Metabolism* **26**:525–530.

Witmer, G., Margolis, A., Fontaine, O., Fritsch, J., Lenoir, G., Broyer, M., and Balsan, S., 1976, Effects of 25-hydroxycholecalciferol on bone lesions of children with terminal renal failure, *Kidney Int.* **10**:395–408.

Wyman, A. L., Paradinas, F. J., and Daly, J. R., 1977, Hypophosphataemic osteomalacia associated with a malignant tumour of the tibia: Report of a case, *J. Clin. Pathol.* **30**:328–335.

Metabolism of Amino Acids and Organic Acids

Kay Tanaka and Leon E. Rosenberg

12.1. Pyruvate Metabolism and Its Disorders

To those interested in mammalian biochemistry and metabolism, it has become axiomatic that pyruvate is a key intermediate in such major pathways as those concerned with anaerobic glycolysis, gluconeogenesis, and alanine formation. Until recently, there was a widespread belief among clinical investigators that inborn errors of pyruvate metabolism would not be found. This skepticism had two foundations: First, it was argued, serious defects in utilization of such a key intermediate would be incompatible with successful embryonic or fetal development, and thus affected humans would not survive the gestational interval. Second, since it has been known for some time that pyruvate metabolism is under major regulation by other events such as the redox state of the cell, it was held that the accumulation of pyruvate observed under diverse circumstances would always be secondary to some major tissue insult, rather than being a reflection of a primary, inborn enzymatic disturbance in pyruvate formation or disposition.

There was ample experimental support for the latter position. The classic studies of Huckabee (1961a,b) and associates demonstrated convincingly that pyruvate and lactate could accumulate to massive proportions in patients with tissue anoxia produced by a variety of stresses

KAY TANAKA and LEON E. ROSENBERG • Department of Human Genetics, Yale University School of Medicine, New Haven, Connecticut 06510.

(hemorrhagic shock, trauma, hypotension). This is probably the most frequent cause of severe, metabolic acidosis in adults. Lactic acidosis also occurs in adults taking biguanide drugs such as phenformin. These obviously acquired courses of pyruvate accumulation, which have been reviewed recently (Alberti and Nattrass, 1977; Relman, 1978), are not the only "secondary" forms of this chemical disturbance. Pyruvate and lactate accumulation are known to occur in a growing number of inherited enzymatic disturbances such as glycogen storage disease (type I), fructose-1,6-diphosphatase deficiency, methylmalonic acidemia, propionic acidemia, and isovaleric acidemia (Tanaka, 1975).

Nonetheless, it has become clear in the past decade that primary, inborn errors of pyruvate metabolism *do* exist in man and must be considered in the differential diagnosis of such diverse symptom complexes as acute metabolic acidosis, chronic neurological impairment, or hemolytic anemia. Such disorders are surely rare. Their importance, however, cannot be judged by their frequency. As has so often been true, tissues from patients with these specific enzymatic defects are beginning to give us an idea about the molecular mechanism and modulatory role of several enzymes in this pathway, while the patients themselves reveal something of the pathophysiological mechanisms of their clinical disturbances.

12.2. Pyruvate Metabolism and Its Regulation

As shown in Fig. 1, several enzymes are directly involved with pyruvate metabolism. These enzymes have been studied intensively for many years, but much new information continues to appear. Thus, it is apparent that activities of these enzymes are coordinately regulated according to the metabolic "state" of the cell. For instance, pyruvate carboxylase activity is high under gluconeogenic circumstances but low in the glycolytic "state." Conversely, the activity of the pyruvate dehydrogenase complex is low in the former situation and high in the latter. Such regulation is achieved mainly by modulating the concentration of effectors such as acetyl-CoA, free CoA, NAD^+, and NADH. New, too, is a large body of information, which will be now discussed, about the molecular structure and function of these catalysts.

12.2.1. Pyruvate Kinase

The major exogenous sources of pyruvate are glucose and several amino acids, including alanine. Glucose is metabolized via the glycolytic pathway (Embden–Meyerhof pathway) through several steps to phosphoenolpyruvate (PEP); PEP is then converted to pyruvate with a transfer of its phosphate to ADP by the action of pyruvate kinase (Fig. 1).

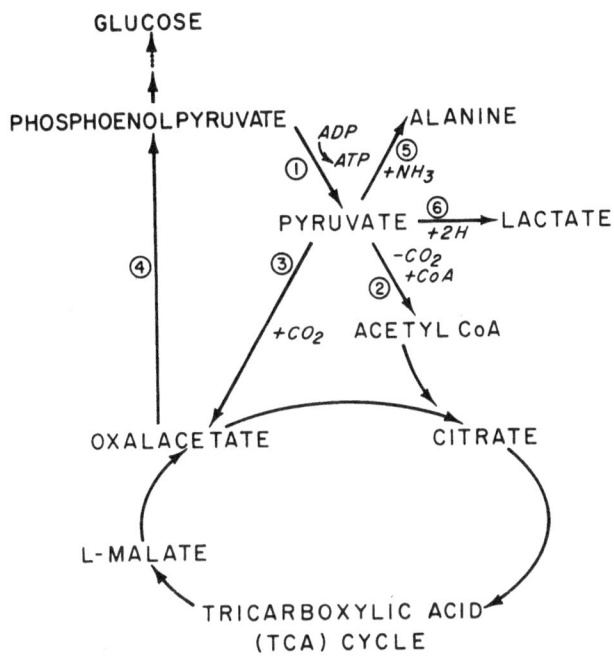

Fig. 1. Schematic representation of key reactions in pyruvate metabolism. The circled numbers denote the following enzymes: ① pyruvate kinase; ② pyruvate dehydrogenase; ③ pyruvate carboxylase; ④ phosphoenolpyruvate carboxykinase; ⑤ pyruvate-alanine transaminase; ⑥ lactate dehydrogenase.

Three pyruvate kinase isozymes designated L(I), K(II), and M(III) have been detected in mammalian tissues (Bigley *et al.*, 1968). These three isozymes are not interconvertible. Type L is the major form found in mammalian liver and erythrocytes; M, the major isozyme present in skeletal muscle, brain, heart, and leukocytes; and K, the predominant form in kidney cortex. L and K isozymes are subject to allosteric regulation by the positive and negative effectors, fructose-1,6-diphosphate and ATP, respectively (Kapoor, 1976). Human erythrocyte pyruvate kinase has been purified and characterized. It has been reported to be a tetramer with a molecular weight variably estimated at 150,000 to 266,000 (Valentine and Tanaka, 1978). The precise subunit composition has not been defined.

12.2.2. The Pyruvate Dehydrogenase Complex

During glycolysis, the major fate of pyruvate is its conversion to acetyl-CoA by oxidative decarboxylation (Fig. 1). This reaction is successively catalyzed by three enzymes that together form a tight multienzyme

Table I.   Enzymes of the Pyruvate Dehydrogenase Complex and
Their Prosthetic Groups and Cofactors

Enzymes	Prosthetic groups (P) and cofactors (C)
Pyruvate decarboxylase (E_1)	Thiamine pyrophosphate (P)
Dihydrolipoyl transacetylase (E_2)	Lipoic acid (P)
	CoA (C)
Dihydrolipoyl dehydrogenase (E_3)	Flavin adenine dinucleoside (P)
	NAD^+ (C)
PDH_a kinase	ATP (substrate)
PDH_b phosphatase	Mg^{2+} (C)
	CA^{2+} (C)

complex called pyruvate dehydrogenase (PDH) (Table I). The PDH complex, located in the inner membrane of mitochondria, is found in all tissues examined. Thiamine pyrophosphate (TPP) and lipoamide are the essential prosthetic groups bound to the first (E_1, pyruvate decarboxylase) and second (E_2, dihydrolipoyl transacetylase) enzymes of the complex, respectively. CoA is also a required cofactor for the transacetylase. The initial step of the reaction is the transfer of the acetaldehyde unit from pyruvate to the TPP bound to pyruvate decarboxylase* (E_1) (Fig. 2). This step removes CO_2 from the carboxyl group of pyruvate. In the second step, the "active acetaldehyde" thus formed is transferred to an SH group of a lipoamide unit that is linked to dihydrolipoyl transacetylase (E_2), thus forming acetyllipoamide. Finally, the acetyl group is transferred to an SH group of CoA, resulting in the formation of acetyl-CoA. This reaction liberates the disulfhydryl form of lipoamide, which is subsequently reoxidized to the disulfide form by dihydrolipoyl dehydrogenase (E_3). Acetyl-CoA is then available for the tricarboxylic acid cycle or fatty acid biosynthesis. The sequence of reactions is summarized in Fig. 2.

In addition to E_1, E_2, and E_3, two other enzymes are known to be components of the PDH complex. These are Mg^{2+}-ATP-dependent pyruvate dehydrogenase kinase (PDH_a kinase) and pyruvate dehydrogenase phosphatase (PDH_b phosphatase) (Reed *et al.*, 1972). These two enzymes catalyze phosphorylation and dephosphorylation, respectively, of E_1, thus comprising a regulatory system for the activity of the PDH complex (Fig. 3).

Mammalian E_1 is an $\alpha_2\beta_2$ tetramer (Barrera *et al.*, 1972). The α subunit (mol. wt. 40,000) catalyzes the first step of pyruvate decarboxylation, the formation of α-hydroxyethylthiamine pyrophosphate, and is the subunit that undergoes an inactivation–activation cycle by the phospho-

*In some papers, pyruvate decarboxylase (E_1) is referred to as pyruvate dehydrogenase.

$$\text{Pyruvate} + \text{TPP-}E_1 \longrightarrow \text{Hydroxyethyl-TPP-}E_1 + CO_2 \tag{1}$$

$$\text{Hydroxyethyl-TPP-}E_1 + \underset{S}{\overset{S}{\rceil}}\text{-Lip-}E_2 \longrightarrow$$
$$\text{Acetyl-S-Lip(SH)-}E_2 + \text{TPP-}E_1 \tag{2}$$

$$\text{Acetyl-S-Lip(SH)-}E_2 + \text{CoA-SH} \longrightarrow$$
$$\text{Acetyl-S-CoA} + \underset{HS}{\overset{HS}{\rceil}}\text{-Lip-}E_2 \tag{3}$$

$$\underset{HS}{\overset{HS}{\rceil}}\text{-Lip-}E_2 + \text{FAD-}E_3 \longrightarrow \underset{S}{\overset{S}{\rceil}}\text{-Lip-}E_2 + H_2\text{-FAD-}E_3 \tag{4}$$

$$H_2\text{-FAD-}E_3 + NAD^+ \longrightarrow \text{FAD-}E_3 + NADH + H^+ \tag{5}$$

$$\text{Pyruvate} + \text{CoA-SH} + NAD^+ \longrightarrow \text{Acetyl-S-CoA} + CO_2 + NADH + H^+$$

Fig. 2. Reactions of the PDH complex. The net result of this sequence is shown below the solid line. (Lip) lipoic acid; (TPP) thiamine pyrophosphate.

rylation–dephosphorylation process mentioned above. The β subunit (mol. wt. 30,000) catalyzes the second step, i.e., the reductive acetylation of the lipoyl moiety of E_2 (Roche and Reed, 1972; Hübner *et al.*, 1978). Mammalian E_2 is a monomer with a molecular weight of about 50,000. Sixty E_2 molecules comprise the core of the PDH complex. The kinase is known to be attached to E_2, but the site of attachment is not known. Although there is disagreement concerning the number of other enzyme components, it has been generally agreed that up to 60 units each of E_1, E_3, and E_1-kinase and -phosphorylase are organized in an ordered fashion with E_2 to form a functional unit. The molecular weight of the whole mammalian PDH complex is estimated to be 7.4–8.0 million (Hayakawa *et al.*, 1969; Barrera *et al.*, 1972), and one bovine kidney mitochondrion is said to contain about 15 molecules of this macromolecular complex.

The activity of the PDH complex is intricately and decisively regulated by tissue concentrations of substrates and products through the

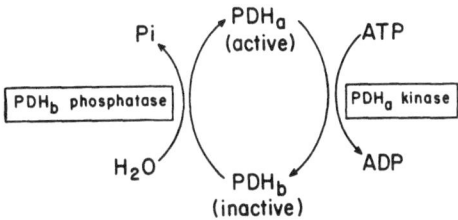

Fig. 3. Phosphorylation (inactivation)–dephosphorylation (activation) cycle of the PDH complex. See the text for details.

kinase–phosphatase cycle. Knowledge of the molecular structure of PDH and of its metabolic regulation is very important for the understanding of mechanisms of several inborn defects of the PDH complex. PDH_a kinase is stimulated by NADH, ATP, and acetyl-CoA, the net result being formation of the inactive form (PDH_b) (Fig. 3). Conversely, ADP, NAD^+, free CoA, and TPP inhibit PDH_a kinase activity. In addition, the response of PDH_a kinase to the aforenamed effectors may be influenced by fluctuations in the levels of free Mg^{2+} and K^+. Thus, the PDH_a kinase activity is modulated by changes in the intramitochondrial ATP/ADP ratio, NADH/NAD^+ ratio, and acetyl-CoA/CoA ratio. Moreover, PDH is under substrate control, pyruvate being stimulatory, fatty acids being inhibitory (Wieland *et al.*, 1973; Cate and Roche, 1978).

12.2.3. Pyruvate Carboxylase

In gluconeogenesis, pyruvate is produced from several amino acids, mainly alanine. To enter the gluconeogenic pathway, pyruvate must first be converted to phosphoenolpyruvate (PEP). Although the pyruvate kinase reaction is reversible, the conversion of pyruvate to PEP by the reversal of this reaction plays a minor role in gluconeogenesis, since the forward reaction has a very high ΔF (Axelrod, 1967). The conversion of pyruvate to PEP is accomplished, therefore, by a means other than reversal of the pyruvate kinase reaction. The phosphorylation of pyruvate is achieved in two steps, first by conversion of pyruvate to oxaloacetate by pyruvate carboxylase and then to PEP by PEP carboxykinase (see Fig. 1).

Vertebrate pyruvate carboxylase is a biotin-containing enzyme present as a tetramer in liver and kidney mitochondria. No significant activity is present in other tissues (Keech and Utter, 1963). There is still some disagreement as regards its molecular weight (280,000 or 600,000 per tetramer), its biotin content (2 or 4 molecules per tetramer), and its molecular organization (Gottschalk *et al.*, 1976; Frey and Utter, 1977). It requires ATP and Mg^{2+}. Its activity is greatly enhanced by acetyl-CoA and K^+, and is inhibited by malonyl-CoA, methylmalonyl-CoA, and glutamate. Interestingly, pyruvate carboxylase is significantly inhibited by phenylpyruvate and p-hydroxyphenylpyruvate, which accumulate in patients with phenylketonuria and tyrosinemia, respectively (Scrutton and White, 1974).

12.2.4. Phosphoenolpyruvate Carboxykinase and the Malate Shuttle

Oxaloacetate synthesized from pyruvate must be converted to PEP by PEP carboxykinase to enter the gluconeogenic pathway. Intracellular distribution of this enzyme differs greatly in different species. In rat liver,

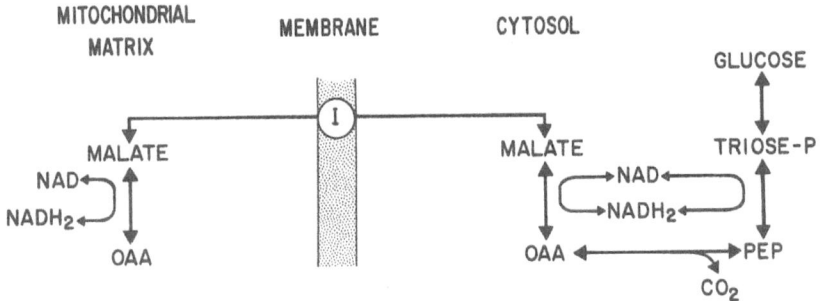

Fig. 4. Schematic representation of transmitochondrial malate transport. (OAA) oxalacetate; (PEP) phosphoenolpyruvate; (P) phosphate.

it is mostly (90%) found in the cytosol, and little if any activity is mitochondrial (Nordlie and Lardy, 1963). Therefore, since oxaloacetate itself cannot be transported, it must be converted to malate and transported from inside the mitochondrion to the cytosol by the malate shuttle system (dicarboxylate transporter). There, malate is again oxidized to oxaloacetate (Fig. 4) (Lardy *et al.*, 1965; Chappel, 1968).

In human and rabbit tissues, however, 80 and 100%, respectively, of PEP carboxykinase activity is located in mitochondria. The PEP produced in mitochondria is transported out to the cytosol in exchange for malate by another transport system, the tricarboxylate transporter. Despite the existence of this second system, malate transport from the inside to the outside of mitochondria by the dicarboxylate transporter is still the rate-limiting step, as shown by experiments using an inhibitor (butylmalonate) of the dicarboxylate transporter (Robinson, 1971; Söling *et al.*, 1973).

The molecular weight of PEP carboxykinase is 70,000–74,500 in most vertebrates. The mitochondrial and cytosolic isozymes in rat are immunologically distinct, although their kinetic and physical properties are similar (Ballard and Hanson, 1969; Utter and Kolenbrander, 1972). PEP carboxykinase requires GTP (or ITP) as the source of high-energy phosphate, and its activity is stimulated by divalent metal ions such as Fe^{2+}, Mn^{2+}, and Ca^{2+} (Bentle and Lardy, 1976). Its activity is also enhanced by fasting, low blood glucose, acute metabolic acidosis, cyclic AMP, and glucocorticoid hormones (Iynedjian *et al.*, 1975; Moreno *et al.*, 1975).

The molecular nature of the dicarboxylate transporter is not well defined, but its regulatory mechanisms have been elucidated. Malate is transported by this system in exchange for inorganic phosphate. It is inhibited by malonate, succinate, and 2-alkyl substituted malonates such as 2-methylmalonate and 2-butylmalonate (Tanaka, 1975). It is also inhibited by glutaryl-CoA but not by free glutarate (Tanaka and Kerley, 1975).

12.2.5. Metabolic Regulation of Pyruvate Metabolism

As discussed above for each of the individual enzymes, pyruvate metabolism is intricately regulated by other metabolic events. For instance, when carbohydrates are available as fuel for energy, pyruvate is oxidized mainly via the PDH complex and tricarboxylic acid cycle because E_1 is kept in the active PDH$_a$ form. When glycolysis wanes, the activity of the PDH complex is inhibited, since increased fatty acid oxidation results in the phosphorylation of E_1. Then, pyruvate metabolism is "switched" from oxidation to the direction of gluconeogenesis. This metabolic switch is triggered by the activation of pyruvate carboxylase resulting from acetyl-CoA produced from fatty acid oxidation. It should also be emphasized that in addition to the metabolic adaptations produced by such normal physiological sequences, pyruvate metabolism can also be greatly influenced by accumulation of abnormal metabolites. For instance, the accumulation of methylmalonic acid in patients with methylmalonic acidemia may cause inhibition of pyruvate carboxylase and the malate shuttle, resulting in inhibition of gluconeogenesis and hypoglycemia.

12.3. Specific Disorders of Pyruvate Metabolism

12.3.1. Erythrocyte Pyruvate Kinase Deficiency

This condition was described much earlier than the other disorders of pyruvate metabolism (Tanaka *et al.*, 1962), and was recently reviewed extensively (Valentine and Tanaka, 1978). Over 250 patients have been reported. Unlike the other errors of pyruvate metabolism, in which the disposal of pyruvate is inhibited, it is the production of pyruvate that is impaired in this condition. Pyruvate kinase deficiency is also unlike the other disorders of pyruvate metabolism in that its clinical manifestations result from chronic hemolytic anemia. This reflects both the tissue distribution of the deficient isozyme, PK I (L form), and the uniqueness of red cell metabolism. Because it lacks a nucleus and mitochondria, the mature erythrocyte is deprived of many metabolic processes that are present in other tissues. Its needs for energy are satisfied only by the glycolytic pathway, which is also peculiar in that in erythrocytes, 1,3-diphosphoglycerate is converted to 3-phosphoglycerate via 2,3-diphosphoglyceate (Rapoport–Luebering shunt), thereby circumventing the phosphoglycerokinase reaction that yields ATP in other tissues (Fig. 5). For this reason, pyruvate kinase activity in erythrocytes is the only mechanism of ATP synthesis, and deficient activity of the enzyme leads to ATP depletion. The low ATP concentration results in a shortened life span of affected

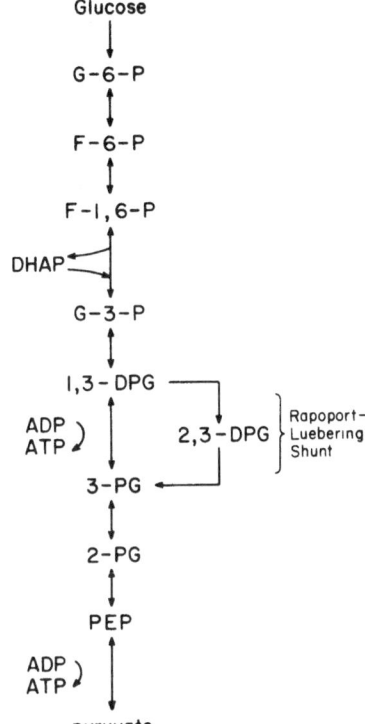

Fig. 5. The glycolytic pathway and Rapoport–Luebering shunt.

erythrocytes, since vital functions such as cationic gradients cannot be maintained.

Clinically, patients with this disease have symptoms of chronic hemolysis such as jaundice, moderate splenomegaly, and an increased incidence of gallstones. The clinical severity ranges from extreme neonatal anemia to a fully compensated hemolytic process in apparently healthy adults. Erythrocytes are normochromic with slight anisocytosis and poikilocytosis (Valentine and Tanaka, 1978).

Pyruvate kinase deficiency is not associated with specific organ dysfunction other than hemolytic anemia due to the presence of the two other isozymes (PK II and PK III) in other organs. Pyruvate kinase activity in leukocytes and muscle is normal in patients with this disease. Activity in liver is reduced, since PK I is the major isozyme found in that organ; unlike the erythrocyte, however, liver contains PK III as well.

Erythrocyte pyruvate kinase deficiency is inherited as an autosomal recessive trait. It is most common in people of Northern European ancestry, but it has also been detected in Mediterranean populations, Orientals, and blacks.

12.3.2. Pyruvate Carboxylase Deficiency

Shortly after the description of lactic acidosis in adults by Huckabee in 1961, a number of newborn babies or children with chronic or recurrent lactic acidosis or pyruvic acidemia were reported. Although the lactic acidosis in these infants appeared to be due to a congenital defect, the nature of the enzyme defect was not then defined (Tanaka, 1975).

In the late 1960's, two patients with an inborn defect of pyruvate carboxylase were reported, their clinical and biochemical features differing widely. The first child, reported by Hommes *et al.* (1968), was an 11-month-old male with neurological manifestations consistent with the diagnosis of Leigh's necrotizing encephalomyelopathy. His neonatal period was uneventful; at age 4 months, he developed vomiting and diarrhea. By the age of 11 months, irritability, lethargy, and mental retardation were observed. Muscles were hypotonic, and deep tendon reflexes were depressed. Biochemical investigation revealed slight hypoglycemia (46 mg/100 ml), generalized aminoaciduria, and modestly elevated blood concentrations of pyruvate (0.3 mM) and lactate (3.4 mM). Normal values are less than 0.2 and 2.0 mM, respectively. The high values of blood pyruvate and lactate, together with the low fasting blood glucose, suggested an impairment of gluconeogenesis. This thesis was supported by the observation that pyruvate carboxylase activity in the patient's liver homogenate was about 1% that of control tissue, whereas PEP carboxykinase activity was similar to that of the controls.

The second child was a 10-year-old girl reported by Yoshida *et al.* (1969) who manifested recurrent vomiting, mental retardation, and severe motor dysfunction. The blood levels of pyruvate and lactate were similar to those found in the patient reported by Hommes *et al.* (1968), again much lower than those observed in adult lactic acidosis. Pyruvate carboxylase activity in liver was approximately 10–25% of that of controls, whereas that of pyruvate decarboxylase was in the normal range.

Since the description of these two children, several additional cases of pyruvate carboxylase deficiency have been reported. Clinical symptoms have ranged from acute fulminant acidosis with death at 4 weeks to chronic psychomotor retardation with hypoglycemia. A progressive subacute course leading to death as in Leigh's necrotizing encephalomyelopathy completes the clinical spectrum.

In vitro findings in these patients with presumed primary pyruvate carboxylase deficiency have been puzzling. In the child reported by Grover *et al.* (1972) with a clinical course typical of subacute necrotizing encephalomyelopathy and death at 38 months of age, hepatic pyruvate carboxylase was assayed on two occasions. At 10 months of age activity, in a biopsy specimen was quite normal (5.6 U/g tissue), whereas that of autopsy material obtained 6 hr after death was markedly reduced (0.18 U/ g tissue). Similar autopsy specimens from five controls had activities ranging from 1.81 to 14.70 U/g tissue. These data suggest that the reduced carboxylase activity observed in the final stage of this child's illness may have been secondary to chronic illness, rather than being a primary disturbance.

Brunette *et al.* (1972) reported a female infant who manifested recurrent metabolic acidosis and seizures of the "jackknife" variety. Her plasma alanine and urinary lactate were greatly increased, but responded dramatically to thiamine administration. These workers claimed to have shown that there were two pyruvate carboxylases in normal human liver mitochondria from the biphasic nature of Lineweaver–Burk plots and that mitochondria from the patient's liver had only one enzyme with high K_m. The enzyme with low K_m was said to be missing. However, the total activity of pyruvate carboxylase(s) was not significantly lower than their control values. Pyruvate decarboxylase activity in leukocytes and fibroblasts was normal. Scrutton and White (1974) pointed out subsequently that biphasic Lineweaver–Burk plots have previously been noted for normal pyruvate carboxylases from other species, and need not imply either molecular or functional heterogeneity of the enzyme. They argued that the absence of the biphasic relationship seen in the patient's liver was more consistent with the low steady-state concentration of acetyl-CoA in the assay system, and emphasized that a major problem in interpretation of the biochemical findings in patients with alleged pyruvate carboxylase deficiency involved unclear definition of the maximal catalytic capacity of pyruvate carboxylase in human tissues. For example, control values in these studies of patients with pyruvate carboxylase deficiency ranged from 0.03 to 14.7 U/g wet weight of liver. Furthermore, modification of the assay procedures originally described for chicken liver mitochondria had been employed. These caveats are particularly important, since it is now known that although catalytic properties of human liver pyruvate carboxylase are similar to those for other vertebrate liver pyruvate carboxylases including that of the chicken liver enzyme, marked differences in effector properties exist between mammalian and avian liver enzymes (Scrutton and White, 1974).

The relationship between pyruvate carboxylase deficiency and Leigh's subacute necrotizing encephalomyelopathy remains a subject of controversy. Leigh's disease was first described in 1951, and was extensively reviewed by Ebels *et al.* (1965). It is an unusual, infantile encephalomyelopathy characterized by bilateral symmetrical lesions in the brainstem that are strikingly similar to those observed in Wernicke's encephalopathy due to thiamine deficiency. It often becomes asymptomatic in the first year of life and usually progresses to a fatal outcome within 12 months.

However, 4 of 28 cases reviewed by Ebels and co-workers died after the age of 10 years. Symptoms vary considerably from case to case, but the ones most frequently observed are: muscle weakness; hypotonia or hypertonia; difficulties in sitting, feeding, and walking; ataxia; and absence of pupillary reaction to light. Worsley *et al.* (1965) observed high serum lactate and pyruvate concentrations in two sibs with this disease. Clayton *et al.* (1967) made similar observations later in three sibs.

Because of the histological similarity to Wernicke's encephalopathy, Pincus *et al.* (1969) investigated thiamine metabolism in patients with Leigh's disease. They showed that the thiamine triphosphate content of the brain of two such patients was very low, but the tissue content of other thiamine derivatives, such as the pyrophosphate (TPP) and monophosphate (TMP), was normal. They further demonstrated the presence of a substance in the blood and the urine that strongly inhibits thiamine triphosphate synthesis (Cooper *et al.*, 1970). This inhibitor was detected, without exception, in urine samples from 10 confirmed cases with subacute necrotizing encephalomyelopathy, in 3 cases with the clinical diagnosis, and in 2 normal sibs of patients, but not in 13 controls. They also noted high serum lactate and pyruvate concentrations, and found that pyruvate dehydrogenase, α-ketoglutarate dehydrogenase, and transketolase activities in the patients' brains were normal.

In a child with the clinical findings of Leigh's disease and enzymatic demonstration of pyruvate carboxylase deficiency (Tang *et al.*, 1972), the urinary inhibitor of thiamine triphosphate synthesis was demonstrated, raising the possibility that all the chemical findings could be reconciled. However, Saudubray *et al.* (1976) found normal hepatic pyruvate carboxylase activity in biopsy specimens from seven children with Leigh's necrotizing encephalomyelopathy diagnosed clinically. These data seem to indicate that some, but not all, children with that clinical constellation called Leigh's disease may have pyruvate carboxylase deficiency.

A variety of treatments including administration of biotin (10 mg/day), thiamine, thiamine propyldisulfide (30 mg/day), and lipoic acid (20 mg/day) have been tried in children with Leigh's disease or pyruvate carboxylase deficiency. Effects have been variable. Brunette *et al.* (1972) reported that thiamine administration resulted in amelioration of acidosis and reduction in urinary lactate. They attributed the effect to an enhancement of PDH complex activity that would have provided a "shunt" mechanism for pyruvate disposal. Tang *et al.* (1972) made the interesting observation that administration of glutamine (150 mg every 3 hr) plus pyridoxine (25 mg four times a day) resulted in marked clinical improvement and reduction of blood lactate and pyruvate concentrations in their patient. The infant (4 months old) became more alert and active and less hypertonic, and began to roll over from a prone position. They believe

that glutamine provided four carbon dicarboxylic acids including oxaloacetate via the tricarboxylic acid cycle. From this discussion, it should be
apparent that little clarity exists about the significance or management of
pyruvate carboxylase deficiency.

12.3.3. Phosphoenolpyruvate Carboxykinase Deficiency

Hommes *et al.* (1976) described two male infants, a 3-day-old and a
19-month-old, who suffered from extreme hypoglycemia and liver
impairment. The newborn exhibited apnea, liver enlargement, and hypotonia. Slight jaundice and metabolic acidosis were found. Blood glucose
was undetectable. Other routine blood chemistries were normal, including
lactate, pyruvate, and β-hydroxybutyrate. Blood glucose was very difficult
to maintain despite continuous, high-dose dextrose infusion, and the
patient died 5 days after admission. The second child was developing
reasonably well until 19 months of age, except for moderate delay in
motor skills. At 19 months, he developed seizures and became comatose
concomitant with a respiratory infection. Severe hypoglycemia (9 mg/100
ml) was noted. As in the first case, blood glucose could not be maintained
despite constant glucose infusion, and the patient died 10 days after
admission.

At autopsy, extensive fat accumulation was observed in liver and
kidney of both patients. Hepatic activities of pyruvate carboxylase, glu-
cose-6-phosphatase, and fructose-1,6-diphosphatase were either normal
or increased in the first infant, but that of PEP carboxykinase was 5–10%
of control values (as expressed in units per gram wet weight). A similarly
severe reduction of PEP carboxykinase activity was also noted in the
second child's liver.

12.3.4. Pyruvate Dehydrogenase Complex Mutants

12.3.4.1. Pyruvate Decarboxylase Deficiency

Since pyruvate decarboxylase (E_1) deficiency was first described by
Blass *et al.* (1970), at least eight confirmed cases of this disease have been
reported. Clinical manifestations range from mild intermittent neurological symptoms such as ataxia and choreoathetosis to an acute fatal lactic
acidosis. The severity of symptoms seems to correlate with the degree of
E_1 deficiency.

The first patient reported by Blass *et al.* (1970) was an 8-year-old boy
who had experienced intermittent episodes of ataxia two to six times a
year since he was 16 months old. These episodes usually occurred after a
febrile illness or other stress and lasted for intervals ranging from a few

hours to over a week. On examination, the patient had cerebellar ataxia, mild choreoathetosis, and minimal dystonic posturing. Irregular "wandering" eye movements were also observed, but true nystagmus was not present. Intelligence was estimated to be high average to superior. Signs of severe acidosis were not observed. The pyruvate concentration in the blood was 0.19–0.31 mM, about three times normal. The concentration of alanine in the plasma was also increased to twice normal, but the blood lactate concentration was not increased. There were excessive fat droplets in skeletal muscle. Pyruvate oxidation to CO_2 by the patient's white blood cells and fibroblasts was 4–10% of control values, and the oxidation of acetate and glutamate was normal. E_1 activity in cell-free preparations of the patient's fibroblasts was only 20% of control. Mixing experiments ruled out the possibility that the defect in E_1 activity was the result of the presence of a soluble inhibitor. Pyruvate oxidation and E_1 activity of cells from the patient's father were intermediate, between those of the patient and of controls. Values in the mother's cells were at the lowest range of normal. Thiamine administration had little effect, although the frequency of attacks seemed to decline after 19 months of treatment. Significantly, two siblings from another family who exhibited similar intermittent ataxia had E_1 activities about 10–25% of normal.

The male infant reported by Farrell et al. (1975) is a typical example of the severe, acute form of E_1 deficiency. He exhibited metabolic acidosis and high plasma pyruvate concentrations (0.65 mM) on the first day of life, and died at 6 months of age after a progressive, deteriorating clinical course. There was no measurable PDH complex activity (<5% of control) or E_1 activity (<1%) in liver and brain homogenates, but E_2 and E_3 activities were within the normal range. Mixing different ratios of liver homogenate from the patient and a control resulted in a threefold increase in the activity of the PDH complex compared with the expected activity (calculated as the simple sum of activities of two homogenates), but E_1 activities in the mixture were only as expected. These experiments indicated that E_1 activity is not rate-limiting in the PDH complex. They also indicate that mammalian E_1 can participate in "intercomplex" exchange, as has been suggested for E_3 (Barrera et al., 1972). Another patient with markedly reduced activity of E_1 (4% of control) and of the PDH complex (8% of normal) suffered from lactic acidosis and died at 3 weeks of age (Stromme et al., 1976).

12.3.4.2. Dihydrolipoyl Transacetylase Deficiency

Cederbaum et al. (1976) described a 9-year-old boy with severe mental and growth retardation and slight elevation of blood pyruvate (0.21 mM) and lactate (2.1 mM) while he was on a normal diet. Neuromuscular changes such as flexion deformities of the hands, dystonia, and choreoathetoid movements were also present. He developed life-threatening lactic acidosis on a high-carbohydrate diet. His two sisters had similar neuromuscular symptoms and died with spontaneous lactic acidosis at 6 and 2½ years of age. PDH complex activity in cultured skin fibroblast homogenates from this patient was less than 20% that of controls. In contrast, E_1 activity and the activity of the α-ketoglutarate dehydrogenase (KGDH) complex, which appears to share E_3 with the PDH complex, were normal. From this evidence, a deficiency of dihydrolipoyl transacetylase (E_2) has been postulated as the cause of this disease, although E_2 activity was not assayed directly. The intermediate value of PDH activity ($\approx 50\%$ of normal) observed in both parents' cells, and the pattern of occurrence in the family, are consistent with autosomal recessive inheritance. Further biochemical investigation is necessary to confirm the E_2 deficiency.

12.3.4.3. Dihydrolipoyl Dehydrogenase Deficiency

Deficiency of dihydrolipoyl dehydrogenase (E_3) was first suggested as a cause of chronic metabolic acidosis in three siblings from an American Indian family (Haworth *et al.*, 1976). Each had mental retardation, seizures, and other neurological abnormalities. Plasma concentrations of alanine and glutamate, which may be produced by transamination of pyruvate and α-ketoglutarate, respectively, were consistently elevated. The activities of the PDH and KGDH complexes in cultured skin fibroblast homogenates from one of the sibs were 13 and 39% of control, respectively, but E_1 (PDH) activity was normal. E_2 and E_3 activities were not measured. The suggestion of primary E_3 deficiency in these cases may not be valid unless a deficiency of E_3 is proved by direct assay, since, as discussed earlier, the activities of these two enzyme complexes are known to be subject to several kinds of metabolic regulation.

The only confirmed case of E_3 deficiency is that recently reported in a newborn male by Robinson *et al.* (1977). The patient developed normally until 6 weeks of age; at 8 weeks, he exhibited intervals of lethargy and hypotonia alternating with irritability and hypertonia. Low blood glucose (35–42 mg/100 ml) was noted occasionally. Chemical examination revealed raised blood lactate (2.6–8.7 mM), pyruvate, α-ketoglutarate (0.103–0.147 mM vs. normal <0.054 mM), and branched-chain amino acids (leucine, isoleucine, and valine: 2–4 times normal) (Taylor *et al.*, 1978). These findings were highly suggestive of a lesion involving some aspect of oxidative decarboxylation common to several substrates. Activities of citrate synthetase and several gluconeogenic enzymes in liver were all in the normal range, despite the hypoglycemia. Activities of the PDH complex, KGDH complex, and α-ketoisocaproate dehydrogenase in several different tissues were 3–28, 1–13, and 5–20% of controls, respectively. The activities of E_1 of PDH and α-ketoisocaproate decarboxylase (the equivalent of E_1) were normal in five tissues, but E_3 activity was deficient, ranging from 5 to 10% of normal activity in all the tissues tested.

The enzyme studies in this patient unequivocally establish a deficiency of E_3 as the cause of this disease. They also offer an interesting insight into the structures of different α-ketoacid dehydrogenase complexes. It has been shown that E_1 and E_2 of the PDH complex are different proteins from those of the KGDH complex and that E_1 of the KGDH complex does not catalyze decarboxylation of pyruvate (Hayakawa *et al.*, 1969; Koike *et al.*, 1974). In contrast, E_3 isolated from the PDH complex and that from the KGDH complex share many physicochemical characteristics such as ultracentrifugal analysis, absorption spectra, flavin content, amino acid analyses, group analyses, peptide mapping, and immunological properties, suggesting the identity of these two enzymes (Sakurai *et al.*, 1970). They are also interchangeable with regard to both their functions and their ability to form a catalytically active complex with other components of the PDH and KGDH systems. The two E_3's were, however, separable by starch gel electrophoresis and showed some difference in optical rotatory dispersion and circular dichroism. It was assumed that these differences were due to conformational differences around the active site.

The results of Robinson *et al.* (1977) lend support to the identity of E_3 from the PDH and KGDH complexes. Moreover, they indicate that the same E_3 component is also shared by the branched chain α-ketoacid dehydrogenase(s). Deficient activity of the branched-chain α-ketoacid dehydrogenase complex has been found in several forms of "maple syrup urine disease," in which the three branched-chain amino acids (leucine, isoleucine, and valine) and their α-keto analogues accumulate. In this respect, the child with E_3 deficiency may be considered to have a new variant of "maple syrup urine disease."

12.3.5. Pyruvate Dehydrogenase Phosphatase Deficiency

Robinson and Sherwood (1975) described a male newborn who was well developed at birth but became acidotic on the first day of life. Blood lactate and pyruvate were elevated but no unusual organic acid was found in his urine, nor was any amino acid except alanine excreted in excess. With infusion of sodium bicarbonate and glucose, blood lactate fell from the previous range of 15–20 mM to 6 mM, but exacerbation of ketoacidosis occurred intermittently. Neurological damage became evident, and the patient died at 6 months of age.

Hypoglycemia was not observed throughout his clinical course. Consistent with that observation, activities of gluconeogenic enzymes in his liver were all in the control range. PDH activities in his tissues were normal when assayed in the ordinary fashion. When tissue preparations were incubated with ATP prior to assay, PDH activity in the patient's tissues and those of controls was reduced by 60–75% because of the inactivation by PDH_a kinase. Addition of Ca^{2+} and Mg^{2+} to the inactivated enzyme caused a prompt restoration of activity to normal in control tissue but not in the tissues from the patient. From these experimental results, the metabolic defect in this patient was attributed to a markedly reduced activity of pyruvate dehydrogenase phosphatase. The fact that the pyruvate dehydrogenase activity in his postmortem tissue was fully activated was explained by some residual activity of the phosphatase. Since postmortem ATP content in all tissues falls rapidly to extremely low levels, it was proposed that inactivation of PDH_a by the kinase does not occur.

12.3.6. Decreased Activity of Pyruvate Oxidation in Patients with Friedreich's Ataxia and Other Neuromuscular Diseases

Ataxia is a major neurological sign in a variety of inborn errors of metabolism including several lipid storage diseases, aminoacidurias, and disorders of pyruvate metabolism. The brain is metabolically unique in that although carbohydrates are the major source of its energy, its PDH complex activity appears to be only about twice that required to catabolize a normal pyruvate load (Cremer and Teal, 1974; Jope and Blass, 1976). Therefore, a moderate reduction in PDH activity may theoretically lead to central nervous system dysfunction.

Kark et al. (1974) studied pyruvate oxidation in muscle slices from 49 patients with various neuromuscular diseases and from 8 normal controls. They found that pyruvate oxidation in 7 of 19 patients with spinocerebellar degeneration (including 4 patients with Friedreich's ataxia) and in 8 of 19 patients with motor neuropathy was reduced to 19–21% of control values. Pyruvate oxidation in these patients was considerably lower than that observed in 11 myopathic controls, who had about 64% of control activity. These changes were independent of several physiological variables such as succinate oxidation and of the ratios of Type I/Type III muscle fibers. The severity of neuropathic changes did not correlate with the rate of pyruvate oxidation.

Blass et al. (1976) further studied pyruvate and α-ketoglutarate oxidation in cultured skin fibroblasts from 5 patients with Friedreich's ataxia. They found that pyruvate and α-ketoglutarate oxidation in cells from these patients was 43 and 50%, respectively, of those in 16 controls, whereas E_1 (PDH) and cytochrome C oxidase activities were maintained at normal levels. Mixing experiments gave no evidence of soluble enzyme inhibitors or activators. The possibility of a K_m mutant was also excluded. From this evidence, they speculated that decreased activity of E_3 in these patients is the underlying mechanism of this disease, and that 40–50% of normal PDH activity, together with 50% of normal KGDH activity, may be associated with an ataxia beginning in puberty and progressing slowly. This interesting hypothesis must be verified by the direct assay of E_3 in more patients with Friedreich's ataxia.

References

Alberti, K. G., and Nattrass, M., 1977, Lactic acidosis, *Lancet* **2**:25–29.

Axelrod, B., 1967, Glycolysis, in: *Metabolic Pathways*, Vol. 1 (D. M. Greenberg, ed.), pp. 112–145, Academic Press, New York.

Ballard, F. J., and Hanson, R. W., 1969, Purification of phosphoenolpyruvate carboxykinase from the cytosol fraction of rat liver and the immunological demonstration of differences between this enzyme and the mitochondrial phosphenolpyruvate carboxykinase, *J. Biol. Chem.* **244**:5625–5630.

Barrera, C. R., Namihira, G., Hamilton, L., Munk, P., Eley, M. H., Linn, T. C., and Reed, L. J., 1972, α-Keto acid dehydrogenase complexes. XVI. Studies on the subunit structure of the pyruvate dehydrogenase complexes from bovine kidney and heart, *Arch. Biochem. Biophys.* **148**:343–358.

Bentle, L. A., and Lardy, H. A., 1976, Interaction of anions and divalent metal ions with phosphoenolpyruvate carboxykinase, *J. Biol. Chem.* **251**:2916–2921.

Bigley, R. H., Stenzel, P., Jones, R. T., Campos, J. O., and Koler, R. D., 1968, Tissue distribution of human pyruvate kinase isozymes, *Enzymol. Biol. Clin.* **9**:10–20.

Blass, J. P., Avigan, J., and Uhlendorf, B. W., 1970, A defect in pyruvate decarboxylase in a child with an intermittent movement disorder, *J. Clin. Invest.* **49**:423–432.

Blass, J. P., Kark, R. A. P., and Menon, N. K., 1976, Low activities of the pyruvate and oxoglutarate dehydrogenase complexes in five patients with Friedreich's ataxia, *N. Engl. J. Med.* **295**:62–67.

Brunette, M. G., Delvin, E., Hazel, B., and Scriver, C. R., 1972, Thiamine-responsive lactic acidosis in a patient with deficient low K_m pyruvate carboxylase activity in liver, *Pediatrics* **50**:702–711.

Cate, R. L., and Roche, T. E., 1978, A unifying mechanism for stimulation of mammalian pyruvate dehydrogenase kinase by reduced nicotinamide adenine dinucleotide, dihydrolipoamide, acetyl coenzyme A, or pyruvate, *J. Biol. Chem.* **253**:496–503.

Cederbaum, S. D., Blass, J. P., Minkoff, N., Brown, W. J., Cotton, M. E., and Harris, S. H., 1976, Sensitivity to carbohydrate in a patient with familial intermittent lactic acidosis and pyruvate dehydrogenase deficiency, *Pediatr. Res.* **10**:713–720.

Chappel, J. B., 1968, Systems used for the transport of substrates into mitochondria, *Br. Med. Bull.* **24**:150–157.

Clayton, B. E., Dobbs, R. H., and Patrick, A. D., 1967, Leigh's subacute necrotizing encephalopathy: Clinical and biochemical study with special reference to therapy with lipoate, *Arch. Dis. Child.* **42**:467–478.

Cooper, J. R., Pincus, J. H., Itokawawa, Y., and Piros, K., 1970, Experience with phosphoryl transferase inhibition in subacute necrotizing encephalomyelopathy, *N. Engl. J. Med.* **283**:793–795.

Cremer, J. E., and Teal, H. M., 1974, The activity of pyruvate dehydrogenase in rat brain during postnatal development, *FEBS Lett.* **39**:17–20.

Ebels, E. J., Blokzii, E. J., and Troelstra, J. A., 1965, A Wernicke-like encephalomyelopathy in children (Leigh), an inborn error of metabolism: Report of five cases with emphasis on its familial incidence, *Helv. Paediatr. Acta* **23**:310–324.

Farrell, D. F., Clark, A. F., Scott, C. R., and Wennberg, R. P., 1975, Absence of pyruvate decarboxylase activity in man: A cause of congenital lactic acidosis, *Science* **187**:1082–1084.

Frey, W. H., and Utter, M. F., 1977, Binding of acetyl-CoA to chicken liver pyruvate carboxylase, *J. Biol. Chem.* **252**:51–56.

Gottschalk, E. M., Mayer, F., Klostermann, A., and Seubert, W., 1976, Determination of molecular weight and molecular structure of rat-liver pyruvate carboxylase, *Eur. J. Biochem.* **64**:411–421.

Grover, W. D., Auerbach, V. H., and Patel, M. S., 1972, Biochemical studies and therapy in subacute necrotizing encephalopathy (Leigh's syndrome), *J. Pediatr.* **81**:39–44.

Hayakawa, T., Kanzaki, T., Kitamura, T., Fukuyoshi, Y., Sakurai, Y., Koike, K., Suematsu, T., and Koike, M., 1969, Mammalian α-keto acid dehydrogenase complexes. V. Resolution and reconstitution studies of the pig heart pyruvate dehydrogenase complex, *J. Biol. Chem.* **244**:3660–3670.

Haworth, J. C., Perry, T. L., Blass, J. P., Hansen, S., and Urquhart, N., 1976, Lactic acidosis in three sibs due to defects in both pyruvate dehydrogenase and α-ketoglutarate dehydrogenase complex, *Pediatrics* **58**:564–572.

Hommes, F. A., Polman, H. A., and Reerink, J. D., 1968, Leigh's encephalomyelopathy: An inborn error of gluconeogenesis, *Arch. Dis. Child.* **43**:423–426.

Hommes, F. A., Bendien, K., Elema, J. D., Bremer, H. J., and Lombeck, I., 1976, Two cases of phosphoenolpyruvate carboxykinase deficiency, *Acta Paediatr. Scand.* **65**:233–240.

Hübner, G., Neef, H., Schellenberger, A., Bernhardt, R., and Khailova, L. S., 1978, Two-center mechanism for the oxidative decarboxylation of pyruvate by the pyruvate decarboxylating component of the pyruvate dehydrogenase complex of pigeon breast muscle, *FEBS Lett.* **86**:6–8.

Huckabee, W. E., 1961a, Abnormal resting blood lactate. I. The significance of hyperlactatemia in hospitalized patients, *Am. J. Med.* **30**:833–839.

Huckabee, W. E., 1961b, Abnormal resting blood lactate. II. Lactic acidosis, *Am. J. Med.* **30**:840–848.

Iynedjian, P. B., Ballard, F. J., and Hanson, R. W., 1975, The regulation of phosphoenolpyruvate carboxykinase (GTP) synthesis in rat kidney cortex, *J. Biol. Chem.* **250**:5596–5603.

Jope, R., and Blass, J. P., 1976, The regulation of pyruvate dehydrogenase in brain *in vivo*, *J. Neurochem.* **26**:709–714.

Kapoor, M., 1976, Pyruvate kinase: A model allosteric enzyme for demonstration of structure–function relationship, *Int. J. Biochem.* **7**:439–443.

Kark, R. A. P., Blass, J. P., and Engel, W. K., 1974, Pyruvate oxidation in neuromuscular diseases, *Neurology* **24**;964–971.

Keech, D. B., and Utter, M. F., 1963, Pyruvate carboxylase. II. Properties, *J. Biol. Chem.* **238**:2609–2614.

Koike, K., Hamada, M., Tanaka, N., Otsuka, K., Ogasahara, K., and Koike, M., 1974, Properties and subunit composition of the pig heart 2-oxoglutarate dehydrogenase, *J. Biol. Chem.* **249**:3836–3842.

Lardy, H. A., Paetkau, V., and Walter, P., 1965, Paths of carbon in gluconeogenesis and lipogenesis: The role of mitochondria in supplying precursors of phosphoenolpyruvate, *Proc. Natl. Acad. Sci. U.S.A.* **53**:1410–1415.

Moreno, F. J., Sanchez-Urruttia, L., Medina, J. M., Sánchez-Medina, F., and Mayer, F., 1975, Stimulation of phosphoenolpyruvate carboxykinase (guanosine triphosphate) activity by low concentrations of circulating glucose in perfused rat liver, *Biochem. J.* **150**:51–58.

Nordlie, R. C., and Lardy, H. A., 1963, Mammalian liver phosphoenolpyruvate carboxykinase activities, *J. Biol. Chem.* **238**:2259–2263.

Pincus, J. H., Itokawa, Y., and Cooper, J. R., 1969, Enzyme-inhibiting factor in subacute necrotizing encephalomyelopathy, *Neurology* **19**:841–845.

Reed, L. J., and Cox, D. J., 1970, Multienzyme complexes, in: *The Enzymes*, Vol 1, 3rd ed. (P. D. Boyer, ed.), pp. 213–240, Academic Press, New York.

Relman, A. S., 1978, Lactic acidosis and a possible new treatment, *N. Engl. J. Med.* **298**:564–565.

Robinson, B. H., 1971, Transport of phosphoenolpyruvate by the tricarboxylate transporting system in mammalian mitochondria, *FEBS Lett.* **14**:309–312.

Robinson, B. H., and Sherwood, W. G., 1975, Pyruvate dehydrogenase phosphatase deficiency: A cause of congenital chronic acidosis in infancy, *Pediatr. Res.* **9**:935–939.

Robinson, B. H., Taylor, J., and Sherwood, W. G., 1977, Deficiency of dihydrolipoyl dehydrogenase (a component of the pyruvate and α-ketoglutarate dehydrogenase complex): A cause of congenital chronic lactic acidosis in infancy, *Pediatr. Res.* **11**:1198–1202.

Roche, T. E., and Reed, L. J., 1972, Function of the nonidentical subunits of mammalian pyruvate dehydrogenase, *Biochem. Biophys. Res. Commun.* **48**:840–846.

Sakurai, Y., Fukuyoshi, Y., Hamada, M., Hayakawa, T., and Koike, M., 1970, Mammalian α-keto acid dehydrogenase complexes. VI. Nature of the multiple forms of pig heart lipoamide dehydrogenase, *J. Biol. Chem.* **245**:4453–4462.

Saudubray, J. M., Marsac, C., Charpentier, C., Cathelineau, C. L., Besson-Leaud, M., and Leroux, J. P., 1976, Neonatal congenital lactic acidosis with pyruvate carboxylase deficiency in two siblings, *Acta Paediatr. Scand.* **65**:717–724.

Scrutton, M. C., and White, M. D., 1974, Purification and properties of human liver pyruvate carboxylase, *Biochem. Med.* **9**:271–292.

Söling, H. D., Kleineke, J., Willms, B., Janson, G., and Kuhn, A., 1973, Relationship between intracellular distribution of phosphoenolpyruvate carboxykinase, regulation of gluconeogenesis and energy cost of glucose formation, *Eur. J. Biochem.* **37**:233–243.

Stromme, J. H., Borud, O., and Moe, P. J., 1976, Fatal lactic acidosis in a newborn attributable to a congenital defect of pyruvate dehydrogenase, *Pediatr. Res.* **10**:62–66.

Tanaka, K., 1975, Disorders of organic acid metabolism, in: *Biology of Brain Dysfunction*, Vol. 3 (G. E. Gaull, ed.), pp. 145–214, Plenum Press, New York.

Tanaka, K., and Kerley, R. C., 1975, Synergistic hypoglycemic effects of lysine and tryptophan with hypoglycin A: Interrelationship between the inhibition of glutaryl CoA dehydrogenase and gluconeogenesis, in: *Hypoglycin* (E. A. Kean, ed.), pp. 163–173, Academic Press, New York.

Tanaka, K. R., Valentine, W. N., and Miwa, S., 1962, Pyruvate kinase (PK) deficiency hereditary nonspherocytic hemolytic anemia, *Blood* **19**:267–295.

Tang, T. T., Good, T. A., Dyken, P. R., Johnsen, S. D., McGreadie, S. R., Sy, S. T., Lardy, H. A., and Rudolph, F. B., 1972, Pathogenesis of Leigh's encephalomyelopathy, *J. Pediatr.* **81**:189–190.

Taylor, J., Robinson, B. H., and Sherwood, W. G., 1978, A defect in branched chain amino acid metabolism in a patient with congenital lactic acidosis due to dihydrolipoyl dehydrogenase deficiency, *Pediatr. Res.* **12**:60–62.

Utter, M. F., and Keech, D. B., 1963, Pyruvate carboxylase. I. Nature of reaction, *J. Biol. Chem.* **238**:2603–2608.

Utter, M. F., and Kolenbrander, H. M., 1972, Formation of oxaloacetate by CO_2 fixation on phosphoenolpyruvate, in: *The Enzymes*, Vol. 6 (P. D. Boyer, ed.), pp. 117–168, Academic Press, New York.

Valentine, W. N., and Tanaka, K. R., 1978, Pyruvate kinase and other enzyme deficiency hereditary hemolytic anemia, in: *The Metabolic Basis of Inherited Disease*, 4th ed. (J. B. Stanbury, J. B. Wyngaarden, and D. S. Fredrickson, eds.), pp. 1410–1429, McGraw-Hill, New York.

Wieland, O. H., Siess, E. A., Weiss, L., Loffler, G., Patzelt, C., Portenhauser, R., Hartmann, U., and Schirmnn, A., 1973, Regulation of the mammalian pyruvate dehydrogenase complex by covalent modification, *Symp. Soc. Exp. Biol.* **27**:371–400.

Worsley, H. E., Brookfield, R. W., Elwood, J. S., Noble, R. L., and Taylor, W. H., 1965, Lactic acidosis with necrotizing encephalopathy in two sibs, *Arch. Dis. Child.* **40**:492–501.

Yoshida, T., Tada, K., Konno, T., and Arakawa, T., 1969, Hyperalaninemia with pyruvicemia due to pyruvate carboxylase deficiency of the liver, *Tohoku J. Exp. Med.* **99**:121–128.

Index